FEMALE REPRODUCTIVE SURGERY

FEMALE REPRODUCTIVE SURGERY

Edited by

John A. Rock, M.D.

Professor of Gynecology/Obstetrics and Pediatrics
The Johns Hopkins University School of Medicine
Chairman
Department of Gynecology and Obstetrics
Union Memorial Hospital
Baltimore, Maryland

Ana Alvarez Murphy, M.D.

Assistant Clinical Professor
Department of Reproductive Medicine
Division of Reproductive Endocrinology
University of California Medical Center
San Diego, California

Howard W. Jones, Jr., M.D.

Professor of Obstetrics and Gynecology
Eastern Virginia Medical School
Norfolk, Virginia

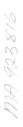

WILLIAMS & WILKINS
BALTIMORE · HONG KONG · LONDON · MUNICH
PHILADELPHIA · SYDNEY · TOKYO

Editor: Charles W. Mitchell
Managing Editor: Victoria M. Vaughn
Copy Editor: Judith F. Minkove
Designer: Wilma E. Rosenberger
Illustration Planner: Ray Lowman
Production Coordinator: Kathleen C. Millet

Copyright © 1992
Williams & Wilkins
428 East Preston Street
Baltimore, Maryland 21202, USA

Accurate indications, adverse reactions, and dosage schedules for drugs are provided in this book, but it is possible that they may change. The reader is urged to review the package information data of the manufacturers of the medications mentioned.

Printed in the United States of America

Library of Congress Cataloging-in-Publication Data

Female reproductive surgery / edited by John A. Rock, Ana Alvarez
  Murphy, Howard W. Jones, Jr.
        p.   cm.
   Includes bibliographical references and index.
   ISBN 0-683-07317-6
   1. Generative organs, Female—Surgery.   I. Rock, John A.   II. Murphy, Ana
Alvarez.   III. Jones, Howard Wilbur, 1910–
   [DNLM: 1. Genitalis, Female—surgery.   2. Infertility, Female—surgery.   WP
468 F329]
RG104.F46   1992
618.1′059—dc20
DNLM/DLC
for Library of Congress   91-30302
                                                                          CIP

                                              92   93   94   95   96
                          1   2   3   4   5   6   7   8   9   10

To our families

PREFACE

In 1983, two of the present authors published *Reparative and Constructive Surgery of the Female Generative Tract*. At that time, the field of reproductive surgery was emerging as a discipline requiring special competence and skill. Today, female reproductive surgery has matured into a specific specialty focus. The specialty has obtained recognition in the American Fertility Society through the formation of the Society of Reproductive Surgeons.

There is little argument that reproductive surgery requires meticulous and troublesome attention to detail, whether endoscopic surgery or surgery through the open abdomen is performed. Reproductive surgery often requires judgment as to what not to do as much as what to do. In contrast to the oncologist, who aspires to remove disease, the reconstructive and reparative surgeon aspires to achieve and restore normalcy.

The widespread availability of advanced reproductive technologies affords a more acceptable alternative to many women with extensive pelvic adhesions due to endometriosis or pelvic inflammatory disease. Nevertheless, some patients do not have the financial resources to consider in-vitro fertilization, and traditional pelvic reconstructive surgical techniques remain their only alternative.

There are specific criteria for the abandonment of an established surgical technique in favor of a new technique. First, it must be established that the new technique is comparable or more effective in the areas of pregnancy success, pain reduction, need for further surgery, and recurrence of symptoms. Second, the new technique must demonstrate specific advantages; that is, reduced morbidity or surgical risks, or reduced costs. Third, complication rates of the new technique must be acceptable. And fourth, the new surgical technique should be easily taught to residents and practitioners in gynecology.

Operative laparoscopy has rapidly advanced over the past decade. New instrumentation and surgical techniques have allowed the use of an endoscopic approach for conditions that have traditionally been treated through the open abdomen. Nevertheless, a precise role for operative laparoscopy is evolving. Clearly, ectopic pregnancy may be effectively treated by laparoscopy. Less clear is the role of operative laparoscopy in ovarian and tubal reconstruction. Carefully designed studies need to be performed to document the efficacy of operative laparoscopic procedures.

The purpose of this text is to bring together specialized procedures that are generally recognized to be efficacious. The ability to successfully perform these techniques is obtained through observation and patient training and through acquisition of delicacy, attention to detail, and judgment that comes with time. Today, training in reproductive surgery may be acquired by fellowships through the Society of Reproductive Surgeons and the Division of Reproductive Endocrinology of the American Board of Obstetrics and Gynecology. Residencies also afford adequate training in some of these specialized surgical techniques. The challenges of the future include the development of specific criteria for training so as to obtain the skills and judgment required to perform specific procedures.

The authors describe, for the most part, surgical techniques adopted in their surgical practice. The authors are aware that many surgeons have made valuable contributions in this field. However, because of the restrictions on the length of this volume, all surgical approaches to a particular entity could not be included.

The authors are grateful to Gere S. diZerega, M.D., David S. Guzick, M.D., Alan H. De-Cherney, M.D., Alan S. Penzias, M.D., and George M. Grunert, M.D. for their excellent contributions to the text. We specifically wish to thank Diane Abeloff for her addition of excellent illustrations for this text. The authors wish to express their sincere appreciation for the cooperation and helpfulness of the staff at Williams & Wilkins in the preparation of this text. We thank Anne D. Terry, Nancy W. Garcia, Pauline M. Clynes, and Esther J. Davison for their assistance in the preparation and editing of this manuscript.

CONTRIBUTORS

Alan H. DeCherney, M.D.
Louis E. Phaneus Professor and Chairman
Department of Obstetrics and Gynecology
Tufts New England Medical Center
Boston, Massachusetts

Gere S. diZerega, M.D.
Professor
Department of Obstetrics and Gynecology
Livingston Reproductive Laboratories
University of Southern California
Los Angeles, California

George M. Grunert, M.D.
Clinical Instructor
Baylor College of Medicine
Director
Assisted Reproductive Technology
Women's Hospital of Texas
Houston, Texas

David S. Guzick, M.D., Ph.D.
Associate Professor
Department of Obstetrics and Gynecology
Director, Reproductive Endocrinology
McGee Women's Hospital
Pittsburgh, Pennsylvania

John Hesla, M.D.
Associate Professor
Department of Gynecology and Obstetrics
Division of Reproductive Endocrinology
The Johns Hopkins University School of
    Medicine
Baltimore, Maryland

Howard W. Jones, Jr., M.D.
Professor of Obstetrics and Gynecology
Eastern Virginia Medical School
Norfolk, Virginia

Ana Alvarez Murphy, M.D.
Assistant Clinical Professor
Department of Reproductive Medicine
Division of Reproductive Endocrinology
University of California Medical Center
San Diego, California

Alan S. Penzias, M.D.
Postdoctoral Associate
Department of Obstetrics and Gynecology
Yale University School of Medicine
New Haven, Connecticut

John A. Rock, M.D.
Professor of Gynecology/Obstetrics and
    Pediatrics
The Johns Hopkins University School of
    Medicine
Chairman
Department of Gynecology and Obstetrics
Union Memorial Hospital
Baltimore, Maryland

CONTENTS

Preface   *vii*
Contributors   *ix*

Section 1. General Considerations

1   THE PERITONEUM: POSTSURGICAL REPAIR AND
    ADHESION FORMATION   2
    Gere S. diZerega

2   DIAGNOSTIC PROCEDURES   19
    Ana Alvarez Murphy

3   INTRODUCTION TO MICROSURGICAL TECHNIQUE
    AND INSTRUMENTATION   31
    Ana Alvarez Murphy

4   LASERS IN GYNECOLOGIC RECONSTRUCTIVE
    SURGERY   61
    George M. Grunert

5   EVALUATION OF SURGICAL RESULTS   77
    David S. Guzick

Section 2. Reparative Surgical Techniques

6   SURGERY OF THE CERVIX   94
    John A. Rock

7   UTERINE RECONSTRUCTIVE SURGERY   113
    John A. Rock

8   RECONSTRUCTIVE SURGERY OF THE OVIDUCT   146
    Ana Alvarez Murphy

9   ECTOPIC PREGNANCY   170
    *Alan H. DeCherney and
    Alan S. Penzias*

10 RECONSTRUCTIVE SURGERY OF THE OVARY   190
    Ana Alvarez Murphy

11 ENDOMETRIOSIS 205
John S. Hesla and
John A. Rock

Section 3. Congenital Anomalies

12 RECONSTRUCTION OF CONGENITAL UTEROVAGINAL
ANOMALIES 246
Howard W. Jones, Jr.

13 SURGICAL PROCEDURES FOR DISORDERS OF SEXUAL
DEVELOPMENT 287
Howard W. Jones, Jr.

14 IN-VITRO ASSISTED AND OTHER REPRODUCTIVE
TECHNOLOGIES 379
Howard W. Jones, Jr.

Index 394

Section I.
General Considerations

1

THE PERITONEUM: POSTSURGICAL REPAIR AND ADHESION FORMATION

Gere S. diZerega

INTRODUCTION

The peritoneum is the most extensive serous membrane in the body. The surface area of the peritoneum is generally equal to that of the skin, ranging from 8,800–12,000 cm² for adults (177 cm²/kg body weight) to 475–1,400 cm² for infants and children (383 cm²/kg body weight), (34). It is composed of mesothelial cells that form a continuous layer resting upon loose mesenchymal connective tissue, a basal lamina, and basement membrane, which is attached to the abdominal wall and viscera by areolar tissue (subserous fascia) (5). The apical surface of the mesothelial cells contains an abundance of long microvilli that increase the functional surface area of the peritoneum for absorption and secretion. The peritoneum is well supplied with blood vessels and lymphatics, which give rise to a rich capillary network. It serves to minimize friction, facilitating free movement between abdominal viscera. It also resists or localizes infection, and stores fat, especially in the greater omentum. (23a).

PERITONEAL FLUID

The peritoneal cavity contains 3–5 ml of serous exudate. The pH of peritoneal fluid ranges between pH 7.5–8.0 and contains significant buffering capacity (53). Peritoneal fluid contains a variety of freely floating cells, including macrophages, desquamated mesothe-lial cells, lymphocytes, eosinophils, mast cells, and in inflammatory exudates, large numbers of polymorphonuclear cells. Excess fluid in the peritoneal cavity is either a transudate (specific gravity <1.010) that accumulates (ascites) from peritoneal obstruction or circulatory differences (failure, portal cardiac hypertension, hypofibriginonemia, etc.) or an exudate (specific gravity >1.020) that arises from inflammation. Peritoneal fluid also contains many plasma proteins including a large amount (50% plasma concentration) of fibrinogen. The amounts of fluid and plasma protein greatly increase in the peritoneal cavity during postsurgical repair or following an inflammatory insult (36).

Fluid is both filtered into and absorbed from the abdominal-pelvic space through the peritoneum. Absorption of colloid and larger particles from the peritoneal cavity occurs through the subdiaphragmatic and mesenteric lymphatics (11). Smaller substances, such as ions, are rapidly equilibrated between capillaries and the lumen of mesothelium-lined spaces (40). Numerous large lymphatic channels lead from the peritoneal surface of the diaphragm. With each diaphragmatic excursion, significant quantities of lymph flow out of the peritoneal cavity into the thoracic duct.

The rate of absorption during equilibration is primarily dependent upon crystalloid osmotic pressure gradients across the peritoneal membrane (39,127). Hypotonic solutions are absorbed more rapidly than isotonic solutions because the osmotic pressure gradient across the peritoneum is greater. Shear et al (126) measured the rate of fluid and electrolyte absorption from the peritoneal cavity in adults. Equilibrium of an albumin dialysate occurred within 2 hr after peritoneal infusion at a rate of 0.5 ml per min. Thereafter, fluid was absorbed at the rate of 30–37 ml per hr. By contrast, when hypertonic saline solutions are instilled into the peritoneal cavity, intraperitoneal fluid volume increases as water moves out of the vascular space.

PERITONEAL REPAIR

In 1919, it was shown that peritoneal healing differs from that of skin (55). When a defect is made in the parietal peritoneum, "the entire surface becomes endothelialized simultaneously and not gradually from the borders as in epidermidalization of skin wounds" (55). While the mesothelial cells surrounding the site of injury contribute to the reparative process after peritoneal injury, the contribution of this process is relatively minor. During the course of repair, the entire surface of the wound becomes epithelialized simultaneously by mesenchymal cells from the underlying connective tissue in such a way that new mesothelium develops in the center of a large peritoneal defect as rapidly as it develops in the center of a smaller one. Peritoneal defects 2 × 2 cm or 0.5 × 0.5 cm are both covered by a continuous sheet of mesothelium 3 days after wounding. The granulation and contraction that occur around the edges of skin wounds do not accompany peritoneal healing (30).

Initially, an inflammatory exudate develops after surgical injury that includes polymorphonuclear leukocytes (PMNs), histocytes, and monocytes in a fibrin exudate. Within 48–72 hr after surgical injury, these cells are replaced by fibroblasts, which then secrete collagen beneath the peritoneal surface (23) (Fig. 1.1). Raftery (102) evaluated postsurgical healing of parietal and visceral peritoneum in rats after excision as well as abrasion of peritoneum. During the first 2 days, wounds were grossly evident, as they were uneven and hemorrhagic. By 5 days, they

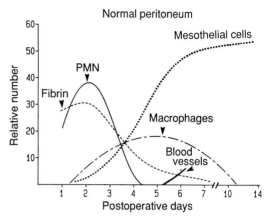

Figure 1.1. Relative change in the number of polymorphonuclear cells (PMN) and macrophages in the abdominal cavity after standardized injury to the parietal peritoneum of rats. The deposition and rate of fibrin removal and rate of mesothelial regeneration as well as the emergence of new blood vessels at the site of injury are also depicted (22).

were smooth and glistening. Wounds of the visceral peritoneum remained through day 10 as shiny, grayish-white, puckered areas. In contrast, wounds of the parietal peritoneum were difficult to identify after 7 days.

Raftery (103) studied the regeneration of parietal and visceral rat peritoneum using electron microscopy. Twelve hours after injury, numerous PMNs were seen entangled in fibrin strands. Very little cellular infiltrate was found in the depths of the wound compared with the wound surface. At 24–36 hr after wounding, the number of cells in the superficial part of the wound was greatly increased due to infiltration by macrophages. Meanwhile, the base of the wound remained relatively acellular. At 2 days, most of the wound surface was covered with a single layer of macrophages supported by a fibrin scaffold. Two additional cell types were also seen on the wound surface: a cell that looked like a primitive mesenchymal cell found in small numbers at the wound base, and mesothelial cells that formed islands within the peritoneal injury. At 3 days, the number of primitive mesenchymal cells on the wound surface increased, although macrophages were still the most prevalent cell type present. The base of the wound contained scattered mesenchymal cells and some proliferating fibroblasts. The cells on the wound surface at 3 days were similar in appearance to the primitive mesenchymal cells located in the deeper layers of the wound. At 4 days, cells resembling primitive mesenchymal cells or proliferating fibroblasts on the wound surface came into contact with one another. In some areas, reepithelialization appeared complete at 5 days because a single layer of mesothelial cells was present on the wound surface, interconnected by desmosomes and tight junctions.

The origin of new mesothelium is unclear because of difficulty in distinguishing between primitive mesenchymal cells and proliferating fibroblasts in the later stages of healing. Some investigators have indicated that metaplasia of fibroblasts within the loose connective tissue beneath the surface of the peritoneum leads to mesothelial regeneration (59,114,152). This work was confirmed by Ellis et al. (30), who found that peritoneal reepithelialization results from the transformation of subperitoneal fibroblasts into an intact mesothelium.

Some discrepancy exists between various studies on the time taken for regeneration of the peritoneum. Ellis et al. (30) and Hubbard et al. (59) reported that reepithelialization of parietal peritoneum occurs in 5–6 days. Glucksman (45) showed that visceral peritoneum reepithelialized in 5 days, while Eskeland (33) found that regeneration of parietal peritoneum is not complete until 8 days. Raftery (102) confirmed the findings of Eskeland (32,33) that the parietal peritoneum of the rat is reepithelialized by 8 days.

FIBRINOLYSIS

The fibrinolytic activity of the peritoneum, which includes the plasminogen activator system, is involved in clearing fibrinous deposits from peritoneal surfaces (86,99). Porter showed that mechanical abrasion reduced the fibrinolytic activity of human peritoneum and speculated that such reductions might play a role in adhesion formation (100). Peritoneal fibrinolysis in the removal of fibrin after surgery and the suppression of fibrinolysis leading to postsurgical adhesion formation were confirmed by Buckman et al. (10). A general correlation was provided between suppression of peritoneal fibrinolytic activity by

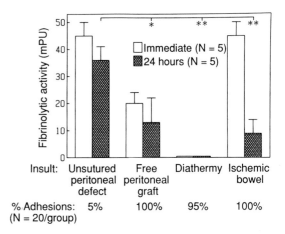

Figure 1.2. Correlation of peritoneal fibrinolytic activity and adhesion formation immediately and 24 hr after various surgical injuries. Persistent fibrolytic activity was seen only when the peritoneal defects were allowed to heal without suturing (adapted from Raftery, 105).

trauma and the extent of subsequent adhesion formation (Fig. 1.2). Raftery (105) determined the changes in peritoneal fibrinolytic activity in rats after various types of trauma. Immediately after each procedure, there was a reduction in fibrinolytic activity. In the case of the unsutured defect, free peritoneal graft, and ischemic bowel, the activity was further reduced over the next 24 hr. Tissue injury induced by electrocautery completely abolished intrinsic fibrinolytic activity, which remained suppressed for 24 hr. The unsutured peritoneal defects showed the smallest reduction in fibrinolytic activity; these defects were associated with the lowest incidence of adhesion formation. Free peritoneal grafting, electrocoagulation, and ischemic bowel resulted in a significant reduction in fibrinolytic activity compared with the unsutured defect, and were associated with a significantly higher incidence of adhesion formation.

Plasminogen activator activity (PAA) of the peritoneal mesothelium may determine whether the fibrin that forms after peritoneal injury is lysed or organized into permanent fibrous adhesions (10,83). The PAA of human peritoneal biopsies was measured using fibrin plate lysis (139). Activity was found in all biopsies from normal parietal and visceral peritoneum (Fig. 1.3). Inflamed peritoneum contained significantly less PAA compared with normal peritoneum; visceral ischemia also

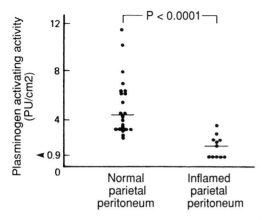

Figure 1.3. Plasminogen activation activity of normal and inflamed human parietal peritoneum (bars show median response) (139).

resulted in a significant decrease of PAA. These reductions in human peritoneal PAA support the view that mesothelial PAA plays a key role in removing fibrin and subsequent adhesion free healing.

ADHESIONS

Incidence

The most common cause of peritoneal adhesions is prior surgery (150). Perry (97) reported that 79% of the 388 patients with abdominal adhesions had a history of surgery. Among those individuals with a history of minor (e.g., appendectomy, exploratory lapa-

roscopy), major (e.g., gastrectomy, aortic bypass), and multiple surgical procedures, adhesions were present in 51%, 72%, and 93%, respectively. Adhesions occurred in 55–100% of fertility-enhancing procedures, as determined by second look laparoscopy performed in a number of large, multicenter studies (1,60) (Table 1.1). Diamond et al. (20) performed second-look laparoscopy to evaluate the location of adhesions in 161 infertility patients after reproductive pelvic surgery. Adhesions developed at 50% of the pelvic sites without adhesions at the time of the initial procedure. In a prospective study of 955 patients undergoing laparoscopic sterilization, Szigetvari et al. (135) confirmed that significant adhesions were more frequent among patients with prior pelvic or abdominal surgery (28% vs. 2% in no prior surgery group). DeCherney and Mezer (18) found that 75% of the 61 infertile females they evaluated after salpingostomy contained adhesions upon follow-up laparoscopy. Appendectomy and gynecologic surgery are the most frequent surgical procedures implicated in clinically significant adhesion formation (101).

The omentum is particularly susceptible to adhesion formation. In Weibel and Majno's studies (150), the omentum was involved in 92% of postoperative adhesions. The omentum was also the predominant organ involved in "spontaneous" adhesions (i.e., those with no prior history of surgery); 100% of the 126 spontaneous adhesions examined by Weibel

Table 1.1. Pelvic Adhesions Noted at Second-Look Laparoscopy[a]

	Time from Initial Procedure	Total No. of Patients	Total No. with Adhesions	% with Adhesions
Diamond (21)	1 wk–12 wk	106	91	86
Decherney and Mezer (18)	4 wk–16 wk	20	15	75
	1 yr–3 yr	41	31	76
Surrey and Friedman (133)	6 wk–8 wk	31	22	71
	≥ 6 mo	6	5	83
Pittaway (153)	4 wk–6 wk	23	23	100
Trimbos-Kemper (141)	8 days	188	104	55
Daniell and Pittaway (17)	4 wk–6 wk	25	24	96

[a]From Diamond MP: In: Sciarra JW, ed. Gynecology and Obstetrics, vol 5. Philadelphia: Harper & Row; 1988;5.

Table 1.2. Incidence of Adhesions at Initial Surgery and Follow-up Laparoscopy[a]

Tissue	Adhesion Rate			
	Initial Surgery[b]		Follow-up Laparoscopy[c]	
	No.	%	No.	%
Ovaries	303/387	78%	207/376	55%
Fimbria	244/384	64%	135/372	36%
Cul-de-sac	87/208	42%	42/208	20%
Omentum	32/208	15%	39/208	19%
Colon	63/208	14%	30/204	15%
Small intestine	30/208	14%	30/208	14%
Pelvic sidewall	124/208	60%	84/208	40%

[a]Adapted from Diamond et al. (20).
[b]Initial surgery performed using CO_2 laser + 35% dextran 70 or non-laser surgical technique with or without dextran. Results are pooled over three initial surgical procedure groups.
[c]Within 12 weeks of initial surgery.

and Majno involved the omentum. These reports raise the question of omentectomy during pelvic surgery, where postoperative adhesion formation is likely to occur. The ovary is the most common site for adhesions to form after reconstructive surgery of the female pelvis (1,20,60) (Table 1.2). Ovarian adhesions were found at second-look laparoscopy on over 90% of cases after ovarian surgery (98).

Laparoscopic Surgery

Although there are obvious advantages to laparoscopy vs. laparotomy with respect to duration of hospitalization and recovery time, no clinical studies have adequately compared the occurrence of adhesions following the two procedures. Luciano et al. (76) found greater postoperative adhesion formation following laparotomy compared with laparoscopy in a rabbit model. In addition, less adhesion formation was noted following salpingoovariolysis by laparoscopy than by laparotomy. In contrast, the mean area of uterine adhesions did not differ significantly between rats after uterine injury by microsurgery involving laparoscopy or laparotomy (37,38). Mecke reported a 52% incidence in pelvic adhesions in 33 patients who previously underwent adhesiolysis during removal of ectopic pregnancy by laparoscopy (82). Although intraoperative bleeding can usually be controlled during laparoscopic surgery, rigorous removal of clot

and complete postoperative hemostasis may be more problematic.

Reperitonealization

Adhesions, delayed healing, and wound breakdown are often attributed to failure of peritoneal suturing or the presence of deperitonealized areas within the abdomen. To reconstruct the pelvis after removal of viscera and peritoneum seems logical for good surgical practice. However, the data indicate that approximation of peritoneum by sutures to cover vascularized areas denuded by the previous dissection may not facilitate peritoneal repair. Clinical reports after cancer surgery demonstrate normal healing of unsutured peritoneum (59,114,152). No instance of bowel obstruction occurred, and at later reoperation, the surgical sites were covered by a smooth, glistening peritoneal surface. Trimpi and Bacon reported 49 cases of abdominoperineal resection of the rectum (143). In 18 patients, the peritoneal floor was closed, and there were four instances of intestinal obstruction. In 28 patients, no reperitonealization was performed, and there were no instances of obstruction. Ulfelder and Quinby found that, after combined abdominoperineal resection, 50% of postoperative intestinal obstructions were due to incarceration of small bowel between sutures of the newly constructed peritoneal floor (148). All experimental evidence indicates that areas denuded of peritoneum will heal satisfactorily (45,59,113,129) and that the suturing of peritoneum actually increases the incidence of adhesions (9,14,30,114,129,138,143,152). This was confirmed by Tulandi in a clinical study using second-look laparoscopy follow-up (146).

CLINICAL SIGNIFICANCE OF ADHESION

Intestinal Obstruction

The most serious complication of intraperitoneal adhesions is intestinal obstruction. In patients presenting with intestinal obstruction due to adhesion formation, the mortality rate is 6–8% (87,97). Menzies and Ellis prospectively evaluated 2,708 laparotomies for an average of 14 months (range 0–19 months); 1% of patients developed intestinal obstruction within 1 yr of surgery (85). In the majority of patients with intestinal obstruction secondary to postoperative adhesion formation, the presenting symptoms occurred long after surgery. Sannella reported that 63% of his 35 patients developed an obstruction of the small bowel longer than 30 days after surgery (122). Raf reported the interval between the initial laparotomy and surgery for obstruction due to adhesion formation was greater than 1 yr in 84% of the 1477 patients evaluated (101). In 17% of the patients in this survey, the interval was greater than 20 years.

Pelvic Pain

Peritoneal adhesions are a major cause of chronic or recurrent pelvic pain. In three surveys, adhesions were identified as the primary cause of chronic pelvic pain in 13–26% of females (48,77,79,108,111). Removal of adhesions in women with pelvic pain often leads to relief of symptoms (79,111). It was suggested that chronic pain arises as a result of the restriction of pelvic organ mobility imposed by adhesions (68).

From a clinical point of view, the relationship between pelvic pain and adhesions is unclear. Rapkin reported that of the 88 infertility patients undergoing laparotomy, 39% had adhesions; however, only 12% of these patients presented with pelvic pain (108). Stovall et al. found that the incidence of adhesions in their patients with chronic pelvic pain (48%) was not significantly different from the overall incidence of adhesion (34%) in their study (132). The only significant predictor of adhesions was prior pelvic surgery, while the only significant physical findings that predicted adhesions were an adnexal mass and decrease in uterine mobility. In this study, approximately one-quarter of all patients with intraperitoneal adhesions had no pelvic pain and a normal physical examination.

Infertility

Adhesion formation is well recognized as a major cause of infertility. Drake and Grunert reported that of 38 infertile females with otherwise normal evaluations, 31% had adhesions upon diagnostic laparoscopy (26). Trimbos-Kemper et al. reported a similar incidence of periadnexal adhesions among 188 infertile women (140). Marked increases in pregnancy rates after adhesiolysis were reported (8,12, 51,58).

PREVENTION OF ADHESION FORMATION

While careful attention to surgical techniques reduces the likelihood of adhesion formation, these efforts alone are unable to prevent adhesion formation (1,20,60). Extensive studies describe various approaches to prevent postoperative adhesion formation. In general, these treatments fall into three categories: prevention of fibrin deposition in the peritoneal exudate, reduction of local tissue inflammation, and removal of fibrin deposits. To date, no single therapeutic approach has proven universally effective in preventing formation of postoperative intraperitoneal adhesions.

Prevention of Fibrin Deposition

Therapeutic attempts to prevent fibrin deposition include peritoneal lavages to dilute or wash away fibrinous exudate, agents affecting coagulation of the fibrinous fluid, surgical techniques to minimize tissue ischemia and barriers to limit apposition of healing serosal surfaces.

Peritoneal Lavage

Prolonged drying of the peritoneum was shown by Ryan et al. to induce significant injury (120). Immediately after drying, intact mesothelial cells were found to be absent in a rat cecal preparation. Four hours later, no mesothelial cells were seen; most of the surface contained only an irregular thin coating of fibrin without cells. Continuous irrigation minimizes tissue desiccation and either dilutes or washes away fibrinous exudates. However, the choice of irrigating solution is important. Kappas et al. demonstrated an increase in adhesion formation in the rat when the temperature of the saline solution exceeded 37°C (65). Although antibiotics are frequently added to intraperitoneal lavage solutions, their efficacy is unproven. Further, it was recently shown that cefazolin and tetracycline irrigation of the abdominal cavity contributes to the formation of adhesion in animal models (109). Serosal damage with swelling of the underlying tissue and cell damage can occur with hypotonic and many nonbuffered irrigating solutions. For this reason, many clinicians perform intraoperative irrigation with Ringer's lactate.

Solutions containing heparin are often used due to their effects on inhibiting coagulation and fibrin formation. Adhesion formation was significantly reduced following the addition of heparinized saline (25 IU/2 ml) prior to peritoneal closure in rats after uterine reanastomosis or surgical trauma (3). However, Fayez and Schneider (35) and Jansen (62) reported no significant reduction in adhesions by the use of heparinized Ringer's lactate (2500–5000 IU/liter) compared with Ringer's lactate alone in patients undergoing infertility surgery. Jansen reported no adverse effects of the heparin solution on blood loss or wound healing. High-dose heparin given intraperitoneally was associated with hemorrhage and delayed wound healing (136).

Procoagulants

Blood together with peritoneal trauma can facilitate adhesion formation (27,46). Lindenberg and Lauritsen reported a reduction in adhesion formation in the rat following the use of a fibrin sealant spray containing thrombin, fibrinogen, and aprotinin (73). This study raised the question of how procoagulants prevent adhesion formation: i.e., did their efficacy represent a barrier effect or an effect on hemostasis. Recently, McGraw et al. reported that a thrombin spray was ineffective in reducing adhesion formation in a rat peritoneal abrasion model (81). Since this spray contained procoagulant activity but provided only a minimal barrier effect, these results support the conclusion that the barrier activity is of primary importance to adhesion prevention. In addition, the results of an experimental study with oxidized cellulose demonstrate that the barrier

effect is directly dependent upon prior hemostasis in the underlying tissue (75). Linsky et al. observed a significant attenuation of the efficacy of oxidized cellulose in preventing adhesion formation in a rabbit model in the presence of autologous blood (75). As Elkins indicated, the use of procoagulants in areas of substantial bleeding seems to promote adhesion formation (27).

Mechanical Barriers

Physical barriers are used in attempts to prevent adhesion formation by limiting tissue apposition during the critical period of peritoneal healing, thereby minimizing the development of fibrin matrix between the tissue surfaces. Barrier agents used for the prevention of postoperative adhesion formation include mechanical barriers as well as viscous solutions.

Gore-Tex surgical membrane is a thin sheet of expanded polytetrafluoroethylene that is used as a pericardial patch. The small pore size ($\leq 1 \mu m$) of the barrier reduces cellular penetration and tissue attachment. The barrier must be sutured in place within the body and is nonabsorbable. Evaluations of its efficacy in reducing adhesion formation after intraperitoneal surgery are limited. Boyers et al. reported significant reductions in the extent, type and tenacity of adhesions with the use of Gore-Tex surgical membrane relative to the control side in a rabbit uterine horn abrasion model (7). Furthermore, no adhesions to the surgical membrane were found 3 weeks after surgery in the 24 animals tested. Conversely, Goldberg et al. found no benefit of the Gore-Tex surgical membrane in rabbit uterine horn abrasion model (47). However, minimal adhesion formation occurred in the control animals, raising the question of the sensitivity of their model to detect treatment-related reductions in adhesion formation.

Ideally, a physical barrier for use in adhesion prevention should be absorbable, nonreactive, and should remain in place without the use of sutures or staples. Barriers made of oxidized regenerated cellulose (ORC) appear to satisfy these criteria. Larsson reported that a knitted fabric made of ORC is effective in preventing adhesions in animal models (71). Raftery found ORC prevented peritoneal adhesion formation in rats (104). Galan confirmed its effect in reducing adhesions using a rabbit uterine horn reanastomosis model (42). ORC was also shown to provide a graded reduction in adhesion formation after uterine trauma and intestinal anastomosis (88,128) in standardized animal models.

However, not all studies demonstrated efficacy of ORC in preventing adhesions. Schroder (124) and Yemini (153) evaluated Surgicel among other modalities and failed to demonstrate a reduction in cecal adhesions in rats. Soules (130) found that Surgicel offered no advantage over no treatment after a standardized cut or scrape of the rabbit uterine horn. Hixson (56) studied the ability of Surgicel to prevent postsurgical adhesions to the fimbria and ovaries; Surgicel did not reduce adnexal adhesions.

Recently, a modification of Surgicel was found to be more effective in preventing adhesion formation in the rabbit (21,74). This new material (Interceed) is also an oxidized regenerated cellulose in a knitted pattern different from that of Surgicel. A prospective, multicenter, randomized clinical evaluation of Interceed was conducted to evaluate clinical efficacy (60,80). Infertility patients (N = 148) in 13 investigational centers underwent lysis of bilateral pelvic sidewall adhesions. Following adhesiolysis, the area of the deperitonealized surface was measured. Interceed was applied in an amount sufficient to completely cover de-peritonealized surfaces on the sidewall; the contralateral sidewall was left uncovered, thereby serving as a control. A second-look laparoscopy was performed between 10 days and 14 weeks after the laparotomy. Interceed barrier was found to significantly reduce the incidence, extent, and severity of postoperative adhesions (Table 1.3). Interceed also significantly reduced adhesion formation between ovaries and peritoneal sidewall. Interceed prevented the reformation of adhesions in over twice as many patients [N=68] as did the control [N=32]. In October 1989, Interceed received approval by the Food and Drug Administration as the first adjuvant to reduce the incidence of postsurgical adhesions.

Larsson suggested that ORC prevents adhesion formation by its transformation into a gelatinous mass that covers the damaged peritoneum and thereby protects it from involvement in adhesion formation (71). Interceed rapidly forms a soft gelatinous mass in the body which persists at the application site longer than Surgicel. This gelatin "cocoon" seems to provide a protective coating over healing tissue during the initial 7–10 days after application (21,74). During this time, reepithelialization of damaged peritoneal surfaces is completed. In preclinical studies, the presence of blood significantly reduced the efficacy of ORC barriers such as Interceed (75). To obtain maximum benefit, it is essential to achieve hemostasis prior to applying the material.

Table 1.3. Clinical Evaluation of Interceed TC7 Following Adhesiolysis Among Infertile Patients[a]

Adhesion Parameter	Treatment Group	
	TC7 (N = 74)	Control (N = 74)
Adhesions @ second-look		
Present	34 (46%)	53 (72%)
Absent	40 (54%)	21 (28%)
Mean area of adhesions (cm³)		
At laparotomy	10.8	8.8
At laparoscopy	1.6	3.1
Adhesion severity @ second-look		
None	72%	53%
Filmy	16%	24%
Severe	13%	24%
Total adhesions @ second-look	116	110

[a]From Malinak (80).

Barrier Solutions

Many years ago, Kajihara reported that chondroitin is useful in adhesion prevention (64). Elkins (28,29) and Fredericks (41) showed that carboxymethyl cellulose prevented formation of adhesions in animal models. Chondroitin sulfate and carboxymethyl cellulose (CMC) both show promise in animal studies as liquid barriers to prevent adhesions. Oelsner et al. (93) compared the two regimens in an animal model and found chondroitin sulfate superior to both carboxymethyl sulfate (CS) or Hyskon in preventing postsurgical adhesion. However, in comparing the regimens in a standardized rat model, Graebe et al. (52) found CMC to be as effective as CS and significantly better than Hyskon, in preventing adhesions. Elkins et al. (28,29) found CMC effective in preventing adhesions in the rat. The clinical utility of these "liquid barriers" awaits the scrutiny of toxicity studies and clinical trials.

Dextran is a water-soluble glucose polymer originally used as a plasma expander. Dextran can be manufactured in a variety of molecular weights; most of the research in adhesion prevention has focused on 32% dextran 70 (Hyskon, Pharmacia; molecular weight, 70,000). Dextran induces an osmotic gradient that draws fluid into the peritoneal cavity. The osmotic gradient from 32% dextran 70 can draw in 2.5–3 times the volume instilled from the vascular space into the peritoneal cavity (69). The basis for dextran's effects on adhesion formation may relate to the mechanical separation of serosal surfaces. Tissues are held apart by the peritoneal fluid, resulting in a "hydroflotation" effect. Dextran also has antithrombotic activity and retards blood clot adherence and deposition of fibrin matrix. Furthermore, dextran tends to modify the fibrin network and makes it more susceptible to lysis. Thirty-two percent dextran 70 was reported to reduce the ability of severe intraperitoneal trauma to depress plasminogen activator activity and to enhance plasminogen activation in vitro (149). Beneficial effects of dextran 70 (either 6% or 32%) on the incidence and/or severity of adhesion formation were widely observed in animal models (see review by Dlugi and DeCherney (24)). Still, failures to observe any beneficial effect with dextran 70 were also reported in animal models (57,137).

Two prospective, controlled clinical studies using infertility surgery reported a significant beneficial effect of 32% dextran 70 on prevention of adhesion formation. In one study, a total of 102 patients undergoing surgery for distal tubal disease, endometriosis, or pelvic adhesions had 250 ml of 32% dextran 70 (N = 55) or saline (N = 47) instilled into the peritoneal cavity prior to closure (1). The extent and severity of adhesions were evaluated at the time of the initial laparotomy and at a second-look laparoscopy performed 8–12 weeks later. Adhesions occurred more frequently at the time of the second-look laparoscopy in control patients than in 32% dextran 70 patients in the gravitationally dependent portions of the pelvis (ovary and cul-de-sac).

In a second prospective study, patients undergoing infertility surgery were randomized to receive 200 ml 32% dextran 70 (N = 23) or 200 ml Ringer's lactate (N = 21) intraperitoneally prior to closure (119). Four–12 weeks after the initial surgery, a second-look laparoscopy was performed. There was a significant difference between the two groups with respect to the net change in patients' adhesion scores at the time of the initial surgery and at laparoscopy. Adhesion scores tended to worsen after receiving Ringer's lactate (mean change = 2.4 units), while they improved after receiving 32% dextran 70 (mean change = − 2.6 units).

Not all clinical evaluations found a therapeutic effect of 32% dextran 70 on adhesion formation. In a prospective, controlled evaluation of 250 ml 32% dextran 70 and saline in 105 patients undergoing salpingoneostomy, fimbrioplasty, or adhesiolysis, Larsson et al. reported no difference between the two treatments in the extent of adhesions at follow-up laparoscopy 4–10 weeks later (72). Jansen also reported no benefit from the addition of 100–200 ml 32% dextran 70 on adhesion scores at follow-up laparoscopy performed 12 days later in patients after infertility surgery (61).

The clinical use of 32% dextran 70 is associated with clinically important side effects.

Ascites is commonly observed after administration of 32% dextran 70. Cleary reported that serum dextran levels gradually increased during a 4-day postoperative period but that clinical ascites was resolved by the 4-week follow-up visit in each of the five patients they evaluated (15). A transient weight gain is commonly observed with 32% dextran 70 (78). Labial edema (1,78,123,145) and accompanying leg edema (145) as well as pleural effusion (2,43,118) and coagulopathy (118) were reported less frequently in patients receiving intraperitoneal 32% dextran 70. Elevations in serum transaminase levels also accompany dextran use (151). Anaphylactic shock or allergic symptoms occur in a small percentage of patients given 32% dextran 70 intraperitoneally (6,142). Stangel reported that two patients treated with intraperitoneal 6% dextran 70 developed disseminated intravascular coagulation and anaphylactic shock (131). Hyskon reduces macrophage phagocytosis in women treated by intraperitoneal administration (110) and was reported to support bacterial growth in vitro (4,67). Recently, King reported a patient who developed a *C. albicans* pelvic infection following intraoperative administration of 32% dextran 70 (67).

Limitations

The complex nature of infertility and pain limits the utility of trials designed to assess the clinical efficacy of adhesion prevention agents. Accordingly, the clinical problems associated with adhesion formation were not evaluated in any of the aforementioned studies. Studies of clinical efficacy can only assess the presence or absence of adhesions and not the clinical benefits of adhesion prevention per se.

Inhibition of Inflammation

Anti-inflammatory drugs were evaluated for their effects on postoperative adhesion formation since they may limit the release of fibrinous exudate in response to inflammation at the surgical site. Two general classes of these drugs were tested: corticosteroids and nonsteriodal anti-inflammatory drugs (NSAIDs). The results of corticosteroid use in animal studies are generally not encouraging; furthermore, clini-

cal use of corticosteroids in a postoperative situation is limited by their other pharmacologic properties. Experimental evaluations of nonsteroidal anti-inflammatory drugs in postoperative adhesion formation show promise; however, clinical evaluation of these drugs for adhesion prevention is needed.

Although Cohen et al. reported significant reductions in adhesions following the use of intraperitoneal solutions containing corticosteroids (16), others did not observe any benefit of these agents on adhesion formation in animal models (49,22,121,125,144). Sanfilippo et al. (121) showed that betamethasone, methylprednisolone, hydrocortisone acetate, and dexamethasone do not prevent adhesions in rats; although in some cases they diminish fibrosis. Clinical use of glucocorticoids in intraperitoneal surgery also yielded mixed results (35,54,58, 112,134). In some of these studies, the antihistamine promethazine was also administered along with the glucocorticoid. Because of the potential for high-dose glucocorticoids to cause immunosuppression and poor wound healing, these agents should be used with caution in patients undergoing surgical procedures. Additionally, Magyar et al. reported that two of 25 patients who received corticosteroids for adhesion prophylaxis (dexamethasone, 20 mg) during peritoneal surgery expressed short-term suppression of the hypothalamic-pituitary-adrenal axis as demonstrated by failure to achieve a normal rise in serum cortisol during insulin-induced hypoglycemia on postoperative day 6 (78). Although corticosteroid use contains the theoretical risk of enhanced sepsis, no reports document this problem.

There are several possible mechanisms by which NSAID could reduce adhesion formation following peritoneal surgery. Adhesions could be reduced through diminished inflammatory events mediated by prostaglandins including a decrease in leukocyte infiltration and coagulation (which follows platelet aggregation). These approaches may decrease the matrix necessary for fibroblast organization (107). NSAIDs also inhibit platelet aggregation. Macrophages secrete plasminogen activator (PA), which activates the fibrinolytic enzyme, plasmin (13,95). The secretion of PA by resident macrophages may be reduced by prostaglandin synthesis. In a series of in-vitro and in-vivo experiments, Rodgers evaluated various effects of the NSAID tolmetin on cells involved in peritoneal repair and adhesion formation (115). Peritoneal macrophage functions were altered by this NSAID, including reductions in plasminogen activator inhibitor and increases in elastase activities. These changes would enhance overall fibrinolytic activity and, hence, decrease the formation and persistence of fibrin matrix.

Studies with NSAIDs in experimental models of postoperative adhesion formation generally demonstrate reduction in the incidence and severity of adhesions by these drugs. Oxyphenbutazone, administered perioperatively in rats and monkeys, reduced postoperative adhesion formation (66,70). In most studies, the NSAIDs were administered prior to surgery and postoperatively 2–7 days, (Table 1.4).

Nishimura reported that administration of the NSAID ibuprofen after the completion of surgery did not affect adhesion formation (92). However, a significant reduction in adhesion formation was noted with the addition of preoperative dosing (89,90). Intraperitoneal administration of ibuprofen as well as tolmetin through a miniosmotic pump, in hydron polymer or in a liposome carrier, reduced adhesion formation in animals (96,116,117). Taken together, these studies suggest that prolonged treatment of the peritoneal injury by NSAIDs may provide a useful approach to adhesion prevention.

Table 1.4.   Animal Studies Performed to Assess the Efficacy of Nonsteroidal Anti-inflammatory Drugs as Adjuvants to Prevent Formation of Postsurgical Adhesions

Author	Animal Model	Ibuprofen Dosage[a]	Results	Reference
Siegler et al.	Rabbit uterine horn transection with unilateral reanastomosis and contralateral cautery	7 mg/kg three times daily × 2 days, IV	5/9 control—dense adhesions 7/7 treated—filmy adhesions	Fertil Steril 34:46, 1980
Bateman et al.	Rabbit uterine horn linear incisions with repair and contralateral abrasion	10 mg/kg three times daily × 4 days, IV or 10 mg/kg, IP	Mean adhesion score in control 0.9; IV, 0.2; IP, 0.5	Surg Forum 32:603, 1981
Holtz	Rabbit uterine horn crush and abrasion with lysis of adhesions 2 weeks later	12.5 mg/kg two times daily × 3 days, IM	No significant reduction in reformation	Fertil Steril 37:582, 1982
Bateman et al.	Rabbit uterine horn crush and abrasion	10 mg/kg three times daily × 4 days, IV	Significant reduction	Fertil Steril 38:107, 1982
O'Brien et al.	Oophorectomy and contralateral salpingo-oophorectomy in ewes	5 mg/kg three times daily × 2 days, IM	No significant reduction	Obstet Gynecol 60:373, 1982
Nishimura et al.	Rabbit uterine horn abrasion, crushing or devascularization	70 mg/kg × 2, IM or 70 mg/kg four times daily	No reduction with 2 doses; significant with 5 doses	J Surg Res 34:219, 1983
Luciano et al.	Rat uterine horn transection with unilateral reanastomosis and contralateral cautery	12.5 mg/kg three times daily × 2 days, IP	No significant reduction	Am J Obstet Gyn 146:88, 1983

[a]IV, intravenous; IP, intraperitoneal; IM, intramuscular.

Removal of Fibrin Deposits

Proteolytic enzymes such as pepsin, trypsin, and papain augment the local fibrinolytic system and theoretically should limit postoperative adhesion formation. Unfortunately, these enzymes are rapidly neutralized by peritoneal exudates, rendering them virtually useless for adhesion prophylaxis. Fibrinolytics, such as fibrinolysin, streptokinase, and urokinase, were also advocated in adhesion prophylaxis (31, 44). One potential complication to the clinical use of these enzymes in postoperative therapy is excessive bleeding resulting from their administration.

Recently, topical application of a recombinant tissue plasminogen activator (rt-PA) was shown to reduce adhesion formation in a variety of animal models (25,84,94). No deleterious effects of rt-PA on wound healing or bleeding were observed in this study. These studies underscore the importance of fibrin deposition in adhesion formation. At the same time, they identify the postoperative window when adhesion prevention by these medications is feasible. Ongoing efforts are focused on delivery systems designed to provide drugs to the surgical site.

SURGICAL ADHESION LYSIS

When the existence of adhesions is thought to play a contributory role in infertility, adhesiolysis can be used to promote fertility. Tulandi et al. reported that the cumulative pregnancy rate was significantly higher among infertile patients who underwent salpingoovariolysis for

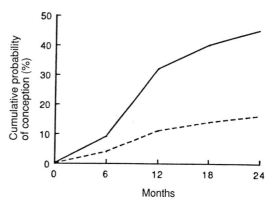

Figure 1.4. Cumulative probability of conception in women with periadnexal adhesions who were treated by salpingoovariolysis (*solid line*) and who were not treated (*broken line*) (147).

periadnexal adhesions (37% at 24 months) compared with patients who received no treatment for their adhesions—15% at 24 months (Fig. 1.4) (147). Gomel (51) and Bronson and Wallach (8) reported an overall pregnancy rate of approximately 60% following adhesiolysis by laparoscopy and laparotomy, respectively. Table 1.5 summarizes the overall pregnancy rate and rate of ectopic pregnancy in four studies employing a second-look laparoscopy during which adhesions were separated and/or lysed.

The interval between the initial surgery and the second-look laparoscopy varied in these studies. In studies in which either a control group that did not undergo second-look laparoscopy was included (147) or the interval between the initial surgery and second-look laparoscopy varied (106,133), the benefits of second-look laparoscopy are thought to be

Table 1.5. Summary of Pregnancy Rates Following Second-Look Laparoscopy (SLL)

Reference	Interval Between Original Surgery and SLL	Number of Patients	Percent of Patients	
			Pregnant	Ectopic Pregnancy
Raj and Hulka[a] (147)	4–8 weeks	51	20%	14%
Surrey and Friedman (148)	6–8 weeks	31	52%	0%
	≥ 6 months	6	17%	17%
Trimbos-Kemper et al. (151)	8 days	188	30%	10%
Tulandi (145)	12 months	19	67%[b]	47%[b]

[a]Originally, 60 patients were evaluated, nine of whom had no postoperative adhesions and were excluded. The majority of the 60 patients (83%) had SLL after 4–8 weeks; three patients had SLL ≤ 2 weeks, and seven patients had SLL > 12 weeks postoperatively.
[b]Cumulative probability at 36 months using life-table analysis.

greater the shorter the postoperative interval prior to the procedure. This clinical impression may be related to the finding that although adhesions per se do not form at the postsurgical site after 7–10 days from the surgical injury (91), adhesion density and organization appear to increase as the postoperative interval increases (19,106,133). Swolin (134), Osada (personal communication), Trimbos-Kemper et al. (141), and Jansen (63) reported success with early second-look laparoscopy.

CONCLUSION

Adhesions are not a prerequisite for peritoneal repair. They are a major cause of postoperative morbidity and failure of surgical therapy and cannot be prevented by surgical technique alone. The development of adjuvants to prevent postsurgical adhesion formation is encumbered by differences between the process of skin and peritoneal healing, access to the peritoneal cavity, interspecies differences in peritoneal physiology, limitations of animal models, and the complexities of transperitoneal transport. Clinical utilization of adhesion prevention regimens is slowed by the ambiguities of efficacy assessment. The clinical benefits of adhesion prevention are only a part of the multifactorial problems of pain, bowel obstruction, and infertility. A direct cause-and-effect relationship between adhesion prevention and amelioration of disease is difficult to establish.

To date, no treatment has proven uniformly effective in preventing postoperative adhesion formation. Surgical techniques that limit tissue ischemia, as well as absorbable, nonreactive mechanical barriers, provide clinical benefits to patients today. Ongoing evaluations of liquid barriers, drugs that modify the local inflammatory response (e.g., nonsteroidal anti-inflammatory drugs), and agents that promote plasminogen activator activity (e.g., recombinant tissue plasminogen activator) show promise for limiting adhesion formation in the future.

References

1. Adhesion Study Group. Reduction of postoperative pelvic adhesions with intraperitoneal 32% dextran 70: a prospective, randomized clinical trial. Fertil Steril 1983;40:612–619.

2. Adoni A, Adatto-Levy R, Mogle P, et al. Postoperative pleural effusion caused by dextran. Int J Gynecol Obstet 1980;18:243–244.

3. Al-Chalabi HA, Otubo JAM. Value of a single intraperitoneal dose of heparin in prevention of adhesion formation: an experimental evaluation in rats. Int J Fertil 1987;32:332–335.

4. Bernstein J, Mattox J, Ulrich J. The potential for bacterial growth with dextran. J Reprod Med 1982; 27:77–79.

5. Bloom W, Fawcett DW. A textbook of histology. 9th edition. Philadelphia: WB Saunders 1975;186–188.

6. Borten M, Seibert CP, Taymor ML. Recurrent anaphylactic reaction to intraperitoneal dextran 75 used for prevention of postsurgical adhesions. Obstet Gynecol 1983;61:755–757.

7. Boyers SP, Diamond MP, DeCherney AH. Reduction of postoperative pelvic adhesions in the rabbit with Gore-Tex surgical membrane. Fertil Steril 1988;49:1066–1070.

8. Bronson RA, Wallach EE. Lysis of periadnexal adhesions for correction of infertility. Fertil Steril 1977;28:613–619.

9. Brunschwig A, Robbins GF. Regeneration of peritoneum: Experimental observations and clinical experience in radical resections of intra-abdominal cancer. In: Bruxelles, Henri de Smedt. XV Congr Soc Internat Chir, Lisbonne 1953. 1954;756–765.

10. Buckman RF, Woods M, Sargent L, et al. A unifying pathogenetic mechanism in the aetiology of intraperitoneal adhesions. J Surg Res 1976;20:1–5.

11. Casley-Smith JR. Endothelial permeability—the passage of particles into and out of diaphragmatic lymphatics. J Exp Physiol 1964;49:365–383.

12. Caspi E, Halpern Y, Bukovsky I. The importance of peritoneal adhesions in tubal reconstructive surgery for infertility. Fertil Steril 1979;31:296–300.

13. Chapman HA, Vavrin Z, Hibbs JB. Macrophage fibrinolytic activity: identification of two pathways of plasmin formation by intact cells and of a plasminogen activator inhibitor. Cell 1982;28:653–662.

14. Chester J. The use of free peritoneal grafts in intestinal anastomosis. Surg Gynec Obstet 1948;89:605–608.

15. Cleary RE, Howard T, diZerega GS. Plasma dextran levels after abdominal instillation of 32% dextran 70: Evidence for prolonged intraperitoneal retention. Am J Obstet Gynecol 1985;152:78–79.

16. Cohen BM, Heyman T, Mast D. Use of intraperitoneal solutions for preventing pelvic adhesions in the rat. J Reprod Med 1983;28:649–653.

17. Daniell JF, Pittaway DE. Short-interval second-look laparoscopy after infertility surgery: a preliminary report. J Reprod Med 1983;28:281–283.

18. DeCherney AH, Mezer HC. The nature of posttuboplasty pelvic adhesions as determined by early and late laparoscopy. Fertil Steril 1984;41:643–646.

19. DeCherney AH, Mezer HC. The nature of posttuboplasty pelvic adhesions as determined by early and late laparoscopy. Fertil Steril 1984;41:643–646.

20. Diamond MP, Daniell JF, Feste J, et al. Adhesion formation and de novo adhesion formation after

reproductive pelvic surgery. Fertil Steril 1987; 47:864–866.

21. Diamond MP, Linsky CB, Cunningham T, et al. A model for sidewall adhesions in the rabbit: reduction by an absorbable barrier. Microsurgery 1987;8:197–200.

22. diZerega GS, Hodgen GD. Prevention of postsurgical tubal adhesions: Comparative study of commonly used agents. Am J Obstet Gynecol 1980;136:173–178.

23. diZerega GS. The peritoneum and its response to surgical injury. In: diZerega GS, Malinak LR, Diamond M, Linsky C, eds. Treatment of postoperative surgical adhesions. New York: Wiley-Liss, 1990;1–11.

23a. diZerega GS, Rodgers KE: The peritoneum. New York: Springer-Verlag, 1992.

24. Dlugi AM, DeCherney AH. Prevention of postoperative adhesion formation. Sem Reprod Endocrin 1984; 2:125–129.

25. Doody KJ, Dunn RC, Buttram VC Jr. Recombinant tissue plasminogen activator reduces adhesion formation in a rabbit uterine horn model. Fertil Steril 1989;51:509–512.

26. Drake TS, Grunert GM. The unsuspected pelvic factor in the infertility investigation. Fertil Steril 1980; 34:27–31.

27. Elkins TE. Can a pro-coagulant substance prevent adhesions? In: diZerega GS, Malinak LR, Diamond MD, Linsky CP, eds. Treatment of postsurgical adhesion. New York: Wiley-Liss, 1990.

28. Elkins TE, Bury RJ, Ritter JL, et al. Adhesion prevention by solutions of sodium carboxymethylcellulose in the rat. I. Fertil Steril 1984;41:926–928.

29. Elkins TE, Ling FW, Ahokas RA, et al. Adhesion prevention by solutions of sodium carboxymethylcellulose in the rat. II. Fertil Steril 1984;41:929–932.

30. Ellis H, Harrison W, Hugh TB. The healing of peritoneum under normal and pathological conditions. Br J Surg 1965;52:471–476.

31. Ellis H. The cause and prevention of postoperative intraperitoneal adhesions. Surg Gynecol Obstet 1971;133:497–511.

32. Eskeland G. Growth of autologous peritoneal cells in intraperitoneal diffusion chambers in rats. I. A light microscopical study. Acta Pathol Microbiol Scandinav 1966;68:481–500.

33. Eskeland G, Kjærheim Å. Regeneration of parietal peritoneum in rats. I. A light microscopical study. Acta Pathol Microbiol Scandinav 1966;68:353–378.

34. Esperanza MJ, Collins DL. Peritoneal dialysis efficiency in relation to body weight. J Ped Surg 1966; 1:162–169.

35. Fayez JA, Schneider PJ. Prevention of pelvic adhesion formation by different modalities of treatment. Am J Obstet Gynecol 1987;157:1184–1188.

36. Felix M, Dalton AJ. A phase contrast microscope study of free cells native to the peritoneal fluid of DBA/a mice. J Natl Cancer Inst 1955;16:415–445.

37. Filmar S, Jetha N, McComb P, et al. A comparative histologic study on the healing process after tissue transection. II. Carbon dioxide laser and surgical

microscissors. Am J Obstet Gynecol 1989;160:1068–1072.

38. Filmar S, Jetha N, McComb P, et al. A comparative histologic study on the healing process after tissue transection. I. Carbon dioxide laser and electromicrosurgery. Am J Obstet Gynecol 1989;160:1062–1067.

39. Flessner MF, Dedrick RL, Schultz JS. A distributed model of peritoneal-plasma transport: theoretical considerations. Am J Physiol 1984;246:R597–R607.

40. Flessner MF, Dedrick RL, Schultz JS. Exchange of macromolecules between peritoneal cavity and plasma. Am J Physiol 1985;248:H15–H25.

41. Fredericks CM, Kotry I, Holtz G, et al. Adhesion prevention in the rabbit with sodium carboxymethylcellulose solutions. Am J Obstet Gynecol 1986; 155:667–670.

42. Galan N, Leader A, Malkinson T, Taylor PJ. Adhesion prophylaxis in rabbits with Surgicel and two absorbable microsurgical sutures. J Reprod Med 1983; 28:662–664.

43. Gauwerky JF, Heinrich D, Kubli F. Complications of intraperitoneal dextran application for prevention of adhesions. Biol Res Pregnancy Perinatol 1986;7: 93–97.

44. Gervin AS, Puckett GL, Silver D. Serosal hypofibrinolysis: A cause of postoperative adhesions. Am J Surg 1973;125:80–88.

45. Glucksman D. Serosal integrity and intestinal adhesions. Surgery 1966;60:1009–1011.

46. Golan A, Winston RML. Blood and intraperitoneal adhesion formation in the rat. J Obstet Gynaecol 1989;9:248–252.

47. Goldberg JM, Toledo AA, Mitchell DE. An evaluation of the Gore-Tex surgical membrane for the prevention of postoperative peritoneal adhesions. Obstet Gynecol 1987;20:846–848.

48. Goldstein DP, deCholnoky C, Emans SJ, Leventhal JM. Laparoscopy in the diagnosis and management of pelvic pain in adolescents. J Reprod Med 1980; 24:251–256.

49. Gomel V. Recent advances in surgical correlation of tubal disease producing infertility. Curr Prob Obstet Gynecol 1978;1:1–60.

50. Gomel V. Salpingo-ovariolysis by laparoscopy in infertility. Fertil Steril 1983;40:607–611.

51. Gomel V. Salpingo-ovariolysis by laparoscopy in infertility. Fertil Steril 1983;40:607–611.

52. Graebe RA, Oelsner G, Cornelison TL, et al. An animal study of different treatments to prevent postoperative pelvic adhesions. Microsurgery 1989; 10:53–55.

53. Greenwald D, Nakamura R, diZerega GS. Determination of pH and pKa in human peritoneal fluid. Curr Surg 1988;45:217–218.

54. Grosfield JL, Berman IR, Schiller M, et al. Excessive morbidity resulting from the prevention of intestinal adhesions with steroids and antihistamines. J Pediatr Surg 1973;8:221–226.

55. Hertzler AA. The peritoneum. Vol. I, C.V. Mosby Co., St. Louis, MO, 1919.

56. Hixson C, Swanson LA, Friedman CI. Oxidized

cellulose for preventing adnexal adhesions. J Reprod Med 1986;31:58–60.

57. Holtz G, Baker E, Tsai C. Effect of thirty-two per cent dextran 70 on peritoneal adhesion formation and re-formation after lysis. Fertil Steril 1980;33:660–662.

58. Horne HW Jr, Clyman M, Debrovner C, et al. The prevention of postoperative pelvic adhesions following conservative operative treatment for human infertility. Int J Fertil 1973;18:109–115.

59. Hubbard TB, Khan MZ, Carag VR, et al. The pathology of peritoneal repair: its relation to the formation of adhesions. Ann Surg 1967;165:908–916.

60. Interceed (TC7) Adhesion Barrier Study Group. Prevention of postsurgical adhesions by Interceed (TC7), an absorbable adhesion barrier: a prospective, randomized multicenter clinical study. Fertil Steril 1989;51:933–938.

61. Jansen RPS. Failure of intraperitoneal adjuncts to improve the outcome of pelvic operations in young women. Am J Obstet Gynecol 1985;153:363–371.

62. Jansen RPS. Early laparoscopy after pelvic operations to prevent adhesions: safety and efficacy. Fertil Steril 1988;49:26–31.

63. Jansen RPS. Failure of peritoneal irrigation with heparin during pelvic operations upon young women to reduce adhesions. Surg Gynecol Obstet 1988;166:154–160.

64. Kajihara Y. The use of chondroitin sulfuric acid for the prevention of peritoneal adhesions. J Kurume Med Assoc 1960;23:4641.

65. Kappas AM, Fatouros M, Papadimitrious K, et al. Effect of intraperitoneal saline irrigation at different temperatures on adhesion formation. Br J Surg 1988;75:854–856.

66. Kapur BML, Talwar JR, Gulati SM. Oxyphenbutazone-anti-inflammatory agent-in prevention of peritoneal adhesions. Arch Surg 1968;98:301–302.

67. King IR. Candida albicans pelvic abscess associated with the use of 32% dextran-70 in conservative pelvic surgery. Fertil Steril 1989;51:1050–1052.

68. Kresch AJ, Seifer DB, Sachs LB, Barrese I. Laparoscopy in 100 women with chronic pelvic pain. Obstet Gynecol 1984;64:672–674.

69. Krinsky AH, Haseltine FP, DeCherney A. Peritoneal fluid accumulation with dextran 70 instilled at time of laparoscopy. Fertil Steril 1984;41:647–649.

70. Larsson B, Svanberg SG, Swolin K. Oxyphenbutazone—an adjuvant to be used in prevention of adhesions for operations for fertility. Fertil Steril 1977;28:807–808.

71. Larsson B, Nisell H, Grunberg I. Surgicel—An absorbable hemostatic material—in prevention of peritoneal adhesions in rats. Acta Chir Scand 1978;144:375–378.

72. Larsson B, Lalos O, Marsk L, et al. Effect of intraperitoneal instillation of 32% dextran 70 on postoperative adhesion formation after tubal surgery. Acta Obstet Gynecol Scand 1985;64:437–441.

73. Lindenberg S, Lauritsen JG. Prevention of peritoneal adhesion formation by fibrin sealant. Ann Chir Gynecol 1984;73:11.

74. Linsky CB, Diamond MP, Cunningham T, Constantine B, DeCherney A, diZerega GS. Adhesion reduction in the rabbit uterine horn model using an absorbable barrier, TC-7. J Reprod Med 1987;32:17–20.

75. Linsky CB, Diamond MP, Cunningham T, et al. Effect of blood on the efficacy of barrier adhesion reduction in the rabbit uterine horn model. Infertility 1988;11:273–280.

76. Luciano AA, Maier DB, Koch EI, et al. A comparative study of postoperative adhesions following laser surgery by laparoscopy versus laparotomy in the rabbit model. Obstet Gynecol 1989;74:220–224.

77. Lundberg WI, Wall JE, Mathers JE. Laparoscopy in evaluation of pelvic pain. Obstet Gynecol 1973;42:872–876.

78. Magyar DM, Hayes MF, Moghissi KS, Subramanian MG. Hypothalamic-pituitary-adrenocortical function after dexamethasone-promethazine adhesion regimen. Obstet Gynecol 1984;63:182–185.

79. Malinak LR. Operative management of pelvic pain. Clin Obstet Gynecol 1980;23:191–200.

80. Malinak LR. Interceed (TC7) as an adjuvant for adhesion reduction: clinical studies. In: diZerega GS, Malinak LR, Diamond M, Linsky C, eds. Treatment of postoperative surgical adhesion. New York: Wiley-Liss, 1990;193.

81. McGraw T, Elkins TE, DeLancey JOL, et al. Assessment of intraperitoneal adhesion formation in a rat model: Can a procoagulant substance prevent adhesions? Obstet Gynecol 1988;71:774–778.

82. Mecke H, Semm K, Freys I, et al. Incidence of adhesions in the true pelvis after pelviscopic operative treatment of tubal pregnancy. Obstet Invest 1989;28:202–204.

83. Menzies D, Ellis H. Intra-abdominal adhesions and their prevention by topical tissue plasminogen activator. J R Soc Med 1989;82:534–535.

84. Menzies D, Ellis H. Intra-abdominal adhesions and their prevention by topical tissue plasminogen activator. Journal of the Royal Society of Medicine 1989;82:534–535.

85. Menzies D, Ellis H. Intestinal obstruction from adhesions—how big is the problem? Ann R Coll Surg 1990;72:60–63.

86. Myhre-Jenson O, Larsen SB, Astrup T. Fibrinolytic activity in serosal and synovial membranes: rats, guinea pigs, and rabbits. Arch Pathol 1969;88:623–630.

87. Nemir P Jr. Intestinal obstruction; ten-year statistical survey at the Hospital of the University of Pennsylvania. Ann Surg 1952;135:367–375.

88. Nishimura K, Bienarz A, Nakamura RM, diZerega GS. Evaluation of oxidized regenerated cellulose for prevention of postoperative intraperitoneal adhesions. Jpn J Surg 1983;13:159–163.

89. Nishimura K, Nakamura RM, diZerega GS. Biochemical evaluation of postsurgical wound repair:

prevention of intraperitoneal adhesion formation with ibuprofen. J Surg Res 1983;34:219–226.

90. Nishimura K, Nakamura RM, diZerega GS. Ibuprofen inhibition of post-surgical adhesion formation: A time-and dose-response biochemical evaluation. J Surg Res 1984;36:115–124.

91. Nishimura K, Nakamura RM, diZerega GS. Ibuprofen inhibition of postsurgical adhesion formation: a time and dose response biochemical evaluation in rabbits. J Surg Res 1984;36:115–124.

92. Nishimura K, Shimanuki T, diZerega GS. Ibuprofen in the prevention of experimentally induced postoperative adhesions. Am J Med 1984;77:102–106.

93. Oelsner G, Graebe RA, Pan SB, et al. Chondroitin sulphate. A new intraperitoneal treatment for postop-erative adhesion prevention in the rabbit. J Reprod Med 1987;32:812–814.

94. Orita H, Girgis W, diZerega GS. Inhibition of post-surgical adhesions in a standardized rabbit model: intraperitoneal administration of tissue plasminogen activator. Int J Fertil (in press).

95. Orita H, Campeau JD, Gale JA, et al. Differential secretion of plasminogen activator activity by postsurgical activated macrophages. J Surg Res 1986;41:569–573.

96. Orita H, Girgis W, diZerega GS. Prevention of postsurgical peritoneal adhesion formation by intraperitoneal administration of ibuprofen. Drug Devel Res 1986;10:97–105.

97. Perry JF Jr, Smith GA, Yonehiro EG. Intestinal obstruction caused by adhesions. A review of 388 cases. Ann Surg 1955;142:810–816.

98. Pittaway DE, Daniell JF, Maxson WS. Ovarian surgery in an infertility patient as an indication for a short-interval second-look laparoscopy: a preliminary study. Fertil Steril 1985;44:611–614.

99. Porter JM, McGregor FH, Mullen DC, Silver D. Fibrinolytic activity of mesothelial surface. Surg Forum 1969;20:80–82.

100. Porter JM, Ball AP, Siver D. Mesothelial fibrinolysis. J Thorac Cardiovasc Surg 1971;62:725–730.

101. Raf LE. Causes of small intestinal obstruction; a study covering the Stockholm area. Acta Chir Scand 1969;135:73–76.

102. Raftery AT. Regeneration of parietal and visceral peritoneum. A light microscopical study. Br J Surg 1973;60:293–299.

103. Raftery AT. Regeneration of parietal and visceral peritoneum: an electron microscopical study. J Anat 1973;115:375–392.

104. Raftery AT. Absorbable haemostatic materials and intraperitoneal adhesions formation. Br J Surg 1980;67:57–58.

105. Raftery AT. Effect of peritoneal trauma on peritoneal fibrinolytic activity and intraperitoneal adhesion formation. An experimental study in the rat. Eur Surg Res 1981;13:397–401.

106. Raj SF, Hulka JF. Second-look laparoscopy in an infertility surgery: Therapeutic and prognostic value. Fertil Steril 1982;38:325–329.

107. Randall RW, Eakins KE, Higgs GA. Inhibition of arachidonic acid cyclooxygenase and lipo-oxygenase activities of leukocytes by indomethacin and compound BW755. Agents Actions 1980;10:553–555.

108. Rapkin A. Adhesion and pelvic pain, UCLA, Obstet Gynecol 1986;68:13–15.

109. Rappaport WD, Holcomb M, Valente J, et al. Antibiotic irrigation and the formation of intraabdominal adhesions. Am J Surg 1989;158:435–437.

110. Rein MS, Hill JA. 32% dextran 70 (hyskon) inhibits lymphocyte and macrophage function in vitro: a potential new mechanism for adhesion prevention. Fertil Steril 1989;52:953–957.

111. Renaer M. Chronic Pelvic Pain in Women. New York, Springer-Verlag 1981;78.

112. Replogle RL, Johnson R, Gross RE. Prevention of postoperative intestinal adhesions with combined promethazine and dexamethasone therapy: Experimental and clinical studies. Ann Surg 1966;163:580–588.

113. Rhoades JE, Schwegman CW. One-stage combined abdominoperineal resection of the rectum (Miles) performed by two surgical teams. Surgery 1965;58:600–606.

114. Robbins GF, Brunschwig A, Foote FW. Deperitonealization: clinical and experimental observations. Ann Surg 1949;130:466–479.

115. Rodgers KE. Nonsteroidal anti-inflammatory drugs (NSAIDs) in the treatment of postsurgical adhesion. In: diZerega GS, Malinak LR, Diamond MD, Linsky CP, eds. Treatment of adhesions. New York: Wiley-Liss, 1990;119–130.

116. Rodgers KE, Girgis W, Johns D, et al. Intraperitoneal tolmetin prevents postsurgical adhesion formation in rabbits. Int J Fertil 1990;35:40–45.

117. Rodgers KE, Bracken K, Richer L, et al. Inhibition of post surgical adhesion by liposomes containing nonsteroidal antiinflammatory drug. Intl J. Ferti 1990;35:315–320.

118. Rose BI. Safety of hyskon for routine gynecologic surgery. A case report. J Reprod Med 1987;32:134–136.

119. Rosenberg SM, Board JA. High-molecular weight dextran in human infertility surgery. Am J Obstet Gynecol 1984;148:380–385.

120. Ryan GB, Grobety J, Majno G. Mesothelial injury and recovery. Am J Pathol 1973;71:93–112.

121. Sanfilippo JS, Cox JG, Nealon NA, et al. Comparison of corticosteroid therapy in the prevention of pelvic tissue reaction and adhesion formation. Int J Fertil 1986;30:57–61.

122. Sannella NA. Early and late obstruction of the small bowel after abdominoperineal resection. Am J Surg 1975;130:270–272.

123. Sauer M, Rodi I, Bustillo M. Unilateral vulvar edema after intraperitoneal Hyskon administration. Fertil Steril 1985;44:546–547.

124. Schroder M, Willumsen H, Hansen JPH, Hansen OH. Peritoneal adhesion formation after the use of oxidized cellulose (Surgicel) and gelatin sponge (Spongostan) in rats. Acta Chir Scand 1982;148:595–596.

125. Seitz HM Jr, Schenker JG, Epstein S, et al. Postoperative intraperitoneal adhesions: a double-blind assessment of their prevention in the monkey. Fertil Steril 1973;24:935–940.

126. Shear L, Swartz C, Shinaberger JA, Barry KG. Kinetics of peritoneal fluid absorption in adult man. New Engl J Med 1965;272:123–127.

127. Shear J, Harvey JD, Barry KG. Peritoneal sodium transport; enhancement by pharmacologic and physical agents. J Lab Clin Med 1966;67:181–188.

128. Shimanuki T, Nishimura K. Localized prevention of postsurgical adhesion formation and reformation with oxidized regenerated cellulose. J Biomed Mat Res 1987;21:173–185.

129. Singleton AO Jr, Rowe EB, Moore RM. Failure of reperitonealization to prevent abdominal adhesions in the dog. Am J Surg 1952;18:789.

130. Soules MR, Dennis L, Bosarge A, Moore DE. The prevention of postoperative pelvic adhesions: An animal study comparing barrier methods with dextran 70. Am J Obstet Gynecol 1982;143:829–834.

131. Stangel JJ, Nisbet JD II, Settles H. Formation and prevention of postoperative abdominal adhesions. J Repro Med 1984;29:143–156.

132. Stovall TG, Elder RF, Ling FW. Predictors of pelvic adhesions. J Reprod Med 34:345–348.

133. Surrey MW, Friedman S. Second-look laparoscopy after reconstructive pelvic surgery for infertility. J Reprod Med 1982;27:658–660.

134. Swolin K. Die Einwirkung van grossen, intraperitonealen Dosen glukokortikoid aud die Bildung von postoperativen Adhaesionen. Acta Obstet Gynec Scand 1967;46:1–15.

135. Szigetvari I, Feinman M, Barad D, et al. Association of previous abdominal surgery and significant adhesions in laparoscopic sterilization patients. J Reprod Med 1989;34:465–466.

136. Tarvady S, Anguli VC, Pichappa CV. Effect of heparin on wound healing. J Biosci 1987;12:33–40.

137. ten Kate-Booij MJ, van Geldorp HJ, Drogendijk AC. Dextran and adhesions in guinea-pigs. J Reprod Fert 1985;75:183–188.

138. Thomas JW, Rhoads JE. Adhesions resulting from removal of serosa from an area of bowel: failure of "oversewing" to lower incidence in the rat and the guinea pig. Arch Surg 1950;61:565–576.

139. Thompson JN, Paterson-Brown S, Harbourne T, et al. Reduced human peritoneal plasminogen activating activity: possible mechanism of adhesion formation. Br J Surg 1989;76:382–384.

140. Trimbos-Kemper TCM, Trimbos JB, van Hall EV. Adhesion formation after tubal surgery: results of the eighth-day laparoscopy in 188 patients. Fertil Steril 1985;43:395–400.

141. Trimbos-Kemper, TCM, Trimbos JB, van Hall EV. Adhesion formation after tubal surgery: results of the eighth-day laparoscopy in 188 patients. Fertil Steril 1985;43:395–400.

142. Trimbos-Kemper TC, Veering BT. Anaphylactic shock form intracavitary 32% Dextran-70 during hysteroscopy. Fertil Steril 1989;51:1053–1054.

143. Trimpi HD, Bacon HE. Clinical and experimental study of denuded surfaces in extensive surgery of the colon and rectum. Amer J Surg 1952;34:596–602.

144. Tschoepe R, Wright KH, Gizang E. The effect of dexamethasone and promethazine administration on adhesion formation, tubal function and ultrastructure following microsurgical anastomosis in rabbit oviducts. Fertil Steril 1980;34:162–171.

145. Tulandi T. Transient edema after intraperitoneal instillation of 32% dextran 70. A report of five cases. J Reprod Med 1987;32:472–474.

146. Tulandi T, Hum HS, Gelfand MM. Closure of laparotomy incisions with or without peritoneal suturing and second-look laparoscopy. Am J Obstet Gynecol 1988;158:536–537.

147. Tulandi T. Treatment-dependent and treatment-independent pregnancy among women with periadnexal adhesions. Am J Obstet Gynecol 1990; 162:354–357.

148. Ulfelder H, Quinby WC Jr. Small bowel obstruction following combined abdominoperineal resection of the rectum. Surgery 1951;30:174–177.

149. Wagaman R, Ingram JM, Rao PS, et al. Intravenous versus intraperitoneal administration of dextran in the rabbit: Effects of fibrinolysis. Am J Obstet Gynecol 1986;155:464–470.

150. Weibel MA, Majno G. Peritoneal adhesions and their relation to abdominal surgery. Am J Surg 1973; 126:345–353.

151. Weinans MJN, Kauer FM, Klompmaker IJ, et al. Transient liver function disturbances after the intraperitoneal use of 32% dextran 70 as adhesion prophylaxis in infertility surgery. Fertil Steril 1990;53:159–161.

152. Williams DC. The peritoneum. A plea for a change in attitude towards this membrane. Br J Surg 1955; 42:401–405.

153. Yemini M, Meshorer A, Katz A, Rozenman D, Lancet M. Prevention of reformation of pelvic adhesions by "barrier" methods. Int J Fertil 1984;29:194–196.

2

DIAGNOSTIC PROCEDURES

Ana Alvarez Murphy

INTRODUCTION

Constant improvements in diagnostic techniques have afforded greater accuracy in the identification of certain factors associated with infertility. Furthermore, diagnostic techniques such as hysterosalpingography, hysteroscopy, and laparoscopy have been found to have therapeutic value. A combination of these techniques usually helps to establish a definitive diagnosis while providing therapy in many cases. These techniques may also be helpful in evaluating the response to treatment. Moreover, at the time of evaluation, further therapy may be provided, as in the case of early second-look laparoscopy. This chapter describes these techniques and provides a summary of their diagnostic and therapeutic advantages.

EXAMINATION OF THE UTERINE CAVITY

Hysterosalpingography (HSG) and hysteroscopy are currently the most practical clinical methods for evaluating the uterine cavity. HSG is a safe and simple nonoperative procedure that can provide information on the contour of the uterine cavity and tubal lumina. It is an integral part of the evaluation of the uterine cavity for the presence of congenital anomalies, myomas, and synechiae in patients with repeated pregnancy wastage. However, it cannot distinguish a septate uterus from a bicornuate uterus. The addition of a pelvic exam and ultrasound to HSG can increase the accuracy of the diagnosis to 90% (21). Obviously, the combination of HSG or hysteroscopy and laparoscopy can make a definitive diagnosis.

HSG is commonly used in the evaluation of infertility not only to assess the uterine cavity but to assess tubal patency as well. Although the HSG is a good nonoperative method of evaluating the uterine cavity, abnormalities reported on HSG may not always be confirmed by hysteroscopy. False-positive uterine HSG findings were confirmed in 21% of patients by Siegler (24), while Valle (25) noted a 57% false-positive rate.

Proximal tubal obstruction may be seen on HSG. Ostry (19) examined 1,830 HSGs and noted 240 (13%) with bilateral proximal obstruction. Of 158 who returned for more testing, 108 had tubal patency. Of the remaining 50, 44 had a tuboplasty. Results of preoperative testing with anesthesia resulted in 26 patent tubes. Of the 18 women who had a laparotomy, five showed normal patency. These findings indicate the need for repeated testing and hysteroscopic or fluoroscopic transcervical fallopian tube catheterization prior to surgery for proximal tubal obstruction. False-positive laparoscopic findings of cornual obstruction may be expected in 3% of patients (22).

In contrast to hysteroscopy, the HSG can provide a crude evaluation of rugal pattern in patients with distal tubal obstruction. However, it is not a substitute for the evaluation of pelvic structures by laparoscopy. As would be expected, in a study of 500 infertile patients, HSG was found to be particularly ineffective when compared with laparoscopy for diagnosis of pelvic adhesions and endometriosis (10). Duff (11) noted similar results when HSG was compared with laparoscopy. HSG could not distinguish peritubular adhesions from tubal obstruction (Table 2.1).

Table 2.1. Accuracy of Hysterosalpingography in Detecting Tubal Disease[a]

	Diagnostic Accuracy (%)
	Overall + SEM
Specificity	20.6 ± 4.2
Sensitivity	67.1 ± 14.1
False-positive rate	20.6 ± 4.2
False-negative rate	44.9 ± 9.6

[a]Adapted from Duff DE et. al. Am J Radiol 1983;141:762.

Hysteroscopy is useful to document suspected uterine pathology on HSG or clinical history. It is a very useful adjunct in the evaluation of patients with abnormal uterine bleeding to delineate the presence of organic pathology such as endometrial polyps or submucous myoma. It may provide confirmation of congenital anomalies and uterine synechiae noted on HSG as well as provide therapy. Lindemann and Mohr reported a 29% rate of uterine abnormalities in 1100 diagnostic hysteroscopies. Siegler and coauthors (23) reported adequate observation of the uterine cavity in 92% of 257 patients with a variety of suspected uterine defects. Intrauterine abnormalities could be demonstrated in approximately 48%.

Which diagnostic method is chosen to evaluate the uterine cavity depends mostly on the suspected diagnosis, physician preference, and familiarity with the techniques. Obviously, a history of iodine allergy is a relative contraindication to HSG. HSG is also contraindicated during bleeding because blood will cause artifacts. With profuse bleeding, only contact hysteroscopy is likely to yield useful information. Panoramic hysteroscopy with high molecular weight dextran (Hyskon) may be selected if the bleeding is not heavy. Mucosal lesions are most accurately evaluated with hysteroscopy. All abnormalities that intrude into the cavity will be more easily identified with hysteroscopy since the characteristics of the lesion will be seen. A filling defect on HSG is less specific. HSG is more accurate when it is important to evaluate the general contour such as when congenital malformations or complex synechiae are suspected. Moreover, the diagnosis of diverticula characteristic of adenomyosis cannot be evaluated by hysteroscopy. These two diagnostic procedures are often complementary. HSG remains an excellent screening method that can be followed up by hysteroscopy when necessary. Although more accurate in many ways and able to provide therapy, hysteroscopy cannot evaluate the lumen of fallopian tubes. HSG should be performed as part of the infertility evaluation unless tuboscopy is to be done. The combination of hysteroscopy and HSG gives maximal information.

Hysterosalpingogram

The HSG is an outpatient radiologic procedure (Table 2.2). It should be performed in the proliferative phase, after menstrual bleeding has stopped and before ovulation. The possibility of reflux fragments of endometrial mucosa obstructing the tubes and irradiation of a possible early pregnancy should be avoided.

We strongly recommend that the requesting reproductive surgeon perform the test with the radiologist in order to obtain maximum information. If it is to be performed in the absence of a gynecologist, it is important to be explicit

Table 2.2. Hysterosalpingography

Technique
  Vacuum cervix adapter
  Foley catheter
  Metal or plastic Rubin's cannula
Contrast media
  Water-soluble contrast medium
  Oil-soluble contrast medium
Time
  Preovulatory
Premedication (if any)
  Demerol or Valium
  Prophylactic antibiotics
Contraindications
  Acute pelvic inflammatory disease
  Bleeding
  Allergy to iodine
  Intrauterine pregnancy
Complications
  Pain
  Perforation
  Hemorrhage
  Granuloma Formation
  Acute flare of pelvic inflammatory disease
  Allergic reactions
  Intravasation
  Endometriosis (theoretic)

about the indication and suspected pathology. As with all procedures, the patient should be given a thorough explanation about the procedure and the possible side effects. Premedication with prostaglandin synthetase inhibitors is useful in minimizing uterine contractions. Although rarely necessary, oral Demerol or Valium may be used in the very apprehensive patient. The efficacy of prophylactic antibiotics for patients with a history of pelvic inflammatory disease undergoing HSG remains to be established. Nevertheless, until this question is resolved, thought should be given to the administration of antibiotics to patients thought to be at risk for possible exacerbation of pelvic inflammatory disease.

A variety of techniques have been described to perform a hysterosalpingogram. A metal or plastic Rubin's cannula, vacuum cervix adapter, or Foley catheter may be used (Fig. 2.1). The vacuum cervix adaptor can provide a more careful study of the endocervical canal. However, the vacuum may be difficult to establish on a small nulliparous cervix. Oil or water contrast media is generally available. It is generally believed that water-soluble media provides the most discriminating images of the cavity and fallopian tubes.

Television fluoroscopy with image intensification is indispensable for selecting the propitious moment for taking the films. Films should be taken during early filling to provide halftone images that outline the details of the mucosa and small filling defects. After complete filling, another film is taken to outline the cavity and determine contour, size, and configuration. This will generally demonstrate congenital malformations, intracavitary myomas, and endometrial polyps as well as diverticuli. When dye has spilled or filled the distal tube, roentgenograms should be obtained of one or both oblique views. These films will help to identify spill and will determine the location of an intracavitary lesion. After removal of the cannula, an overall view of the pelvis allows study of the internal os and endocervix (1). A delayed 15–20 min film has been recommended to confirm whether the tubes are patent with dye freely dispersing in the cavity, trapped in a hydrosalpinx, or loculated in the peritoneal cavity, as is likely with pelvic adhesions. Duff et

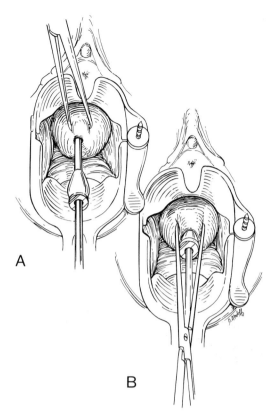

Figure 2.1. A Rubin's cannula is inserted into the cervical os after the position of the uterus has been ascertained. A tenaculum is necessary to manipulate the uterus appropriately when using this type of cannula.

al. (11) have suggested that a preliminary film should not be obtained routinely and a postdrainage film should be obtained only in equivocal cases. They found that the postdrainage film did not aid in the interpretation of the films. Moreover, they confirmed the findings of Horwitz et al. (13), which noted that peritubal involvement was not diagnosed with any accuracy.

False-positive results may be seen if insufficient amounts of contrast media are injected into the uterus (Table 2.3). Air, water, blood, or other foreign material can cause erroneous interpretation of a filling defect. Air shadows in the sacrum may be mistaken for a filling defect. To view the uterine cavity properly, anteversion or retrodisplacement should be corrected with gentle movement of the uterus.

Intravasation may be confused with tubal spill if the roentgenograms are not taken during fluoroscopic examination. Tubal spasm or lo-

Table 2.3. Possible Errors in Hysterosalpingographic Techniques

Air, water, blood, or other foreign material in the syringe and cannula can cause erroneous interpretations of uterine and tubal changes.

Too little contrast fluid may be injected and too few roentgenograms made.

Uterine anteversion or retrodisplacement may prevent adequate study of the fundus.

Too much contrast material has been injected, resulting in obliteration of all the radiographic outlines of the uterus and tubes.

Unfamiliarity with the contrast material to be employed can cause unexpected problems.

Intravasation can be confused with tubal spill.

Air shadows in the sacrum can be mistaken for a polyp or a defect in the fundus.

Pelvic spill from normal salpingograms is identified easily, but mistakes are often made about small collections of spill, significant pelvic adhesions that involve tubes, degrees of tubal occlusion, and even hydrosalpinx.

Tubal spasm can be confused with obstruction.

Localized uterine contraction can occur, resulting in abnormal uterine contour.

Differences in interstitial tubal diameter can occur, resulting in unilateral tubal filling due to the existence of a path of least resistance.

Table 2.4. Complications of Hysteroscopy

Pain
Bleeding
  Cervical laceration
  Uterine perforation
Infection
Endometriosis
Anesthesia risks
Complications related to the medium
  Theoretical cardiovascular overload with intravenous infusion of dextran
  CO_2 acidosis and arrhythmia with possible embolus

bleeding, allergy to iodine, and intrauterine pregnancy. Complications from HSG include pain, perforation, hemorrhage, granuloma formation resulting from water-soluble or oil-soluble contrast media, acute flare of pelvic inflammatory disease, allergic reaction, intravenous and/or lymphatic intravasation, embolism, and possibly endometriosis (Table 2.2).

Hysteroscopy

Hysteroscopy has gained much attention and acceptance as a method of examining the cavity and providing therapy in many cases. The hysteroscopic procedure and its possible side effects should be thoroughly discussed. A decision should be made jointly by the patient and physician about whether the procedure is to be performed in the office or operating room and what type of anesthesia is to be used. Often, dilatation is not necessary if the 4-mm diagnostic hysteroscope is used. In those cases, no anesthesia is usually required. Office procedures may also be performed with paracervical block. Decisions regarding place and form of anesthetic are often influenced by whether a diagnostic procedure and a possible operative procedure are contemplated.

For optimal visualization, hysteroscopy should be performed in the proliferative phase of the cycle. During the secretory phase, the endometrium is lush and can appear somewhat irregular, and normal endometrium can be easily mistaken for small polypi.

The patient is placed in the dorsal lithotomy position, and a posterior weighted speculum is placed as well as a single-tooth tenaculum. The appropriate telescope is selected with attached light cable. The scope is placed in the appropri-

calized uterine contraction may be confused with pathology. In a normal pelvis, tubal spill is usually very easily identified. However, mistakes are often made about small collections of spill, significant pelvic adhesions that involve the tubes, degrees of tubal occlusion, and even hydrosalpinx.

It has been suggested that the HSG may have therapeutic value, probably because mechanical lavage of the tubes may release mucous plugs. A possible stimulatory effect on the cilia of the tubal mucosa has been hypothesized (16). Furthermore, the iodine-containing contrast may have a bacteriostatic effect and may improve cervical mucus. Mackey (16) and DeCherney (9) have reported an increase in conception after HSG with both water- and oil-based contrast media. The reported conception rate with water-soluble contrast media ranges from 13–40%. Wahby (26) showed that HSG increased the pregnancy rate more than tubal insufflation, suggesting that the contrast material itself may be a therapeutic agent.

Absolute contraindications to HSG include acute pelvic inflammatory disease, uterine ate sheath and the medium flushed through the sheath, extruding the air within the sheath (Fig. 2.2).

Distending media may be liquid (Hyskon glycine, saline) or gas (CO_2). Hyskon (dextran 70) is a highly viscous solution of 32% dextran that is optically very clear. It has the obvious advantage of not being miscible with blood. If the sheath is a tight fit with the cervix, distension is easy to maintain, and most diagnostic procedures can be completed with 50 cc. Hyskon can be delivered via a syringe and plastic tubing attached to the intake valve of the hysteroscopic sheath. A pump has also been developed to deliver the medium. Unfortunately, Hyskon is quite messy and sticky. If not cleaned properly, the dried residue can harden and clog the channels or "freeze" movable parts.

Of greatest concern is the "Hyskon reaction," which consists of a bleeding diathesis. Decreased plasma levels of both factor VIII and fibrinogen are seen (17). This is the result of an increase in the rate of fibrin formation. Hyskon can also be absorbed onto the surface of platelets. Platelet adhesion as well as aggregation is decreased (17). Hyskon is predomi-

nantly removed by glomerular filtration (80%) and will remain in the bloodstream for up to 6 weeks. Hypervolemia may also result with noncardiogenic pulmonary edema (14). Rarely, an anaphylactoid reaction is seen. Most commonly, these reactions are seen with the use of large amounts of Hyskon or with procedures damaging the uterine wall with subsequent intravasation.

CO_2 is a safe medium to distend the uterus when instilled with the proper insufflation apparatus. The hysteroinsufflator delivers gas at a rate in cc/min as opposed to the laparoscopic insufflator, which delivers in liters/min. The rate of flow is usually set at less than 100 cc/min, and intrauterine pressure is kept under 150 mm Hg. CO_2 is very clean and ideal for office hysteroscopy. Although it can flatten the mucosa, CO_2 is an excellent diagnostic media. It is not recommended for bloody diagnostic or operative procedures, as CO_2 and blood mix, creating a bubbling reddish foam. CO_2 cannot be used to flush the cavity of debris. Improperly instilled, gas emboli can form, with significant untoward effects.

Normal saline and Ringer's lactate have regained popularity. The medium is delivered

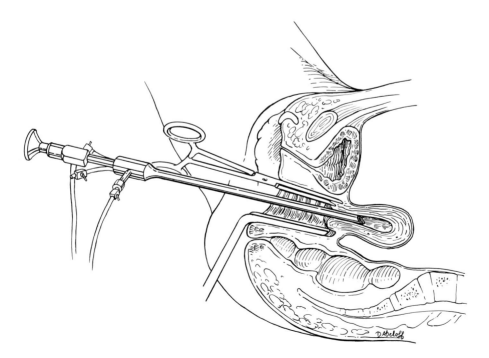

Figure 2.2.   A diagrammatic representation of the instruments necessary for hysteroscopy.

to the hysteroscopic sheath via intravenous tubing that is attached to 3-liter bags mounted on an IV pole and enclosed in a wide blood pressure cuff. The cuff is inflated to 50–100 mm Hg pressure. The cervix can be overdilated to provide a continuous outflow. For diagnostic purposes, a single-channel, and for operating, a double-channel operating sheath are useful to provide outflow through one of the channels. This provides some measure of control since the outflow valve can be regulated to provide the flow necessary to keep the field clear and the cavity properly distended. Unfortunately, to keep the cavity distended, large fluid volumes are necessary. Moreover, these media mix readily with blood, which may obscure the operative field. These media, like 5% glucose in water (D_5W), can result in circulatory overload and pulmonary edema. It is therefore very important that a careful accounting of input and output be kept. Obviously, these electrolyte solutions should not be used with electrical devices, as the media conducts electricity and may result in shock to the patient and endoscopist.

Glycine (1.5%) is commonly used for urologic procedures requiring the resectoscope. Glycine, as a distending media, has the same properties as sterile water with the advantage of being safer than electrolyte solutions for electrosurgery. It has problems with electrolyte and water imbalances, which may lead to pulmonary edema. Glycine is absorbed and metabolized to ammonia and finally to urea. Glycine should therefore not be used in patients with hepatic dysfunction because they are at risk for ammonia intoxication. Patients with renal impairment may achieve toxic levels of urea.

For diagnostic purposes, it is best to avoid cervical dilatation, if possible. Dilators can cause trauma to the endocervix and endometrium. The obturator is carefully inserted to the level of the internal cervical os, the insert removed, and the telescope introduced and fixed in the encasing sheath. If fluid is the distension media, the system should be primed prior to placing the instrument in the cervix to avoid introducing bubbles. Exploration of the uterine cavity is then performed. Depending on the type of endoscope used, straightforward or

foreoblique, the amount of rotation necessary to fully view the entire cavity will differ. A discussion of the different types of available instruments is provided in Chapter 3, Introduction to Microsurgical Technique and Instrumentation.

The endometrium in the proliferative phase appears smooth and pink. The four walls of the uterine cavity must be examined carefully. The cornua can be seen on either side. The tubal ostia are visible at the extremity of the cornua and show great anatomic variation. Once one ostia is found, the other can usually be found in the symmetrical position on the other side. Distortion of the cavity with myomata or synechiae may distort these anatomic landmarks. The isthmus is the narrow portion of the uterine cavity above the internal os. The os appears as a constriction at the top of the endocervical canal. The canal is best viewed at the end of the procedure as the telescope is being withdrawn. The canal has folds that form papillae and clefts.

The examination may be recorded with still photographs or video. At the very least, a standardized report form and/or operative note should contain a description of the normal and abnormal findings (Fig. 2.3). Contraindications to hysteroscopy include recent or existing uterine infection, pregnancy, and profuse uterine bleeding. Complications include pain, bleeding from cervical or uterine perforation, infection, complications related to the distension media, and risk of anesthesia. (Table 2.4) Hysteroscopy is a safe procedure in experienced hands and has achieved a definite place in the evaluation of the uterine cavity.

EXAMINATION OF THE PELVIC CAVITY AND FALLOPIAN TUBE

Salpingoscopy

Hysterosalpingography and laparoscopy are the standard methods of evaluating the fallopian tube prior to tubal microsurgery. Recently, evaluations of the tubal mucosa by microbiopsies (4) or operating microscope (2) have suggested that the HSG and laparoscopy may be inadequate to fully evaluate the fallopian tubes and provide prognostic data. The

THE JOHNS HOPKINS HOSPITAL
REPRODUCTIVE SURGERY
HYSTEROSCOPY REPORT FORM

Patient name:_____
History number:_____
Date: _____
Cycle day:_____ LMP:_____

Surgeon:
Preoperative diagnosis:

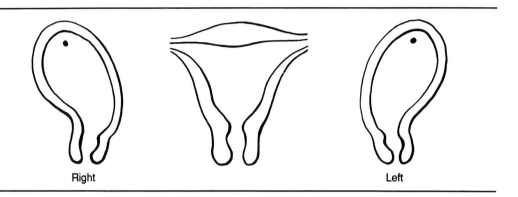

Right   Left

Anesthesia:

Distension medium used: Volume used:

Anatomical findings:

    Cervix:

    Endocervical canal:

    Isthmus:

    Uterine cavity

        Right uterotubal ostium and cornu

        Left uterotubal ostium and cornu:

        Fundus:

        Right lateral uterine wall:

        Left lateral uterine wall:

        Posterior uterine wall:

        Anterior uterine wall:

Photographs: Voltage: Exposure: Film no.:

Biopsy: Site:

Operative procedure performed via hysteroscopy (described):

Postoperative diagnosis:

Surgeon signature _____

Figure 2.3.   The Johns Hopkins standardized form to record hysteroscopic findings.

degree of tubal mucosal damage is probably the major factor in establishing the prognosis for pregnancy after tubal reconstruction. HSG gives some information on the state of the tubal mucosa, particularly if the films are taken when the tubes are incompletely filled.

Endoscopic exploration of the ampullary mucosa has recently become possible. Modified hysteroscopes inserted through an ancillary incision or the operating channel of the laparoscope (3) as well as flexible bronchoscopes (5) have been used. The tubal mucosa can be evaluated at the time of microsurgical laparotomy (12) or at diagnostic/operative laparoscopy (3,8).

The salpingoscope is probably most commonly used through the operating channel of the laparoscope (Fig. 2.4). It is a rigid sheath with an obturator and an endoscope that measures 2.6 mm (Richard Wolf, Knittlingen, FRG). The sheath is connected to a saline drip. The distal fallopian tube must be mobilized prior to tuboscopy even if microsurgical laparotomy is anticipated. If the tube is occluded, a small incision is made in the dimple. The blunt-tipped obturator is then used to enter the fallopian tube. An atraumatic grasper is placed at the distal end of the tube to hold the salpingoscope sheath in place. The endoscope is introduced after removal of the obturator. A slow saline drip is begun to distend the lumen and to allow appropriate visualization. The mucosa is inspected as the endoscope is withdrawn from the ampullary-isthmic junction to the fimbriated end. Adhesions, agglutination, and flattened mucosa have been described. Preliminary evidence suggests that these findings may correlate with subsequent pregnancy

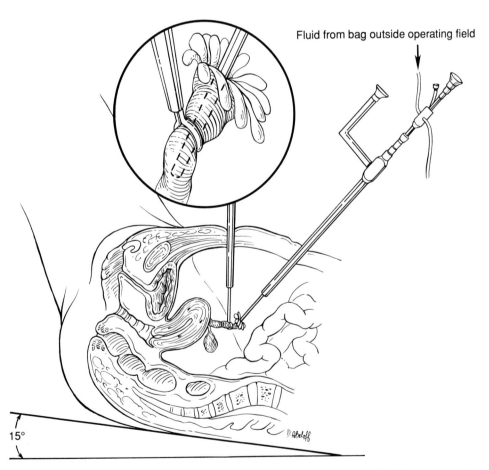

Fluid from bag outside operating field

15°

Figure 2.4. A diagrammatic representation of a salpingoscopy performed using a modified hysteroscope inserted through the operating channel of the laparoscope.

success following salpingoplasty. Puttemans (20) has introduced a classification of the ampullary mucosa. This will allow uniformity of evaluation, thus simplifying the comparison of results in prospective studies.

Laparoscopy

Laparoscopy has been established as an important diagnostic method in the evaluation of the infertile female. It permits evaluation of tubal and peritoneal factors and allows the selection of appropriate treatment (7). Certainly, prior to laparoscopy, an infertility survey should be performed that includes an evaluation of ovulatory status, semen analysis, and uterine and tubal assessment by hysterosalpingography. Other indications for laparoscopy in the infertile patient include a history or clinical findings suggestive of endometriosis, failure to conceive after six ovulatory cycles in the anovulatory patient, failure to conceive after 12 months of well-timed frozen donor insemination, history of puerperal fever, pelvic inflammatory disease, ectopic pregnancy, ovarian wedge resection, or prior tubal surgery. It may also be used to reevaluate the patient after surgery or after an appropriate trial of therapy. The indications for operative laparoscopy will be discussed in separate chapters.

Absolute contraindications to laparoscopy include bowel obstruction, ileus, peritonitis, intraperitoneal hemorrhage with unstable vital signs, diaphragmatic hernia, and severe cardiorespiratory disease. The first three contraindications recognize the very high rate of bowel perforation in patients with distended bowel. Patients with the latter three contraindications may experience exacerbation of cardiac or respiratory symptoms induced by position and pneumoperitoneum. Relative contraindications include inflammatory bowel disease, extreme body weight, and very large abdominal masses. In the latter, visualization may be impossible, and the mass easily punctured. Patients with Crohn's disease or ulcerative colitis may have adhesive bowel disease and fistula formation. These patients have a higher incidence of bowel perforation.

Obviously, informed consent should be obtained, which encompasses the nature of the procedure, risk, complications, and alternatives, if appropriate. The risk of bleeding requiring transfusion and its attendant risk, infection, damage to bowel, bladder, or other pelvic organ requiring further surgery including a laparotomy, and the risk of anesthesia should be discussed.

The procedure is usually performed in the early to midfollicular phase. One should avoid manipulating preovulatory follicles and corpus luteum, as these are very fragile vascular structures and can be traumatized easily. Moreover, the chances of operating on an early pregnant patient are greatly diminished.

General anesthesia is strongly recommended for diagnostic laparoscopy, which requires meticulous inspection of the peritoneal cavity. These patients should be intubated and receive assisted ventilation because the Trendelenburg position and pneumoperitoneum place the patient at increased risk of hypercarbia. Correct placement of the patient in lithotomy position with the patient's buttocks protruding slightly from the edge of the table will facilitate uterine manipulation. Our personal preference is for the use of the Rubin's cannula for manipulation and chromopertubation and a straight laparoscope with an ancillary puncture site (Fig. 2.5). The basic techniques of laparoscopy have been described in detail elsewhere (6,18).

A systematic inspection of the cavity including the upper abdomen should be performed prior to placing the patient in the Trendelenburg position. An ancillary puncture site is usually necessary to perform a thorough evaluation. The sites often poorly examined include the uterovesical fold, the lateral portions of the ovary, the ovarian fossa, and the proximal portions of the fallopian tube. It is important to aspirate the fluid in the posterior cul-de-sac, as it may obscure areas of endometriosis. If adhesions obliterate an adnexa, it may be necessary to lyse adhesions to properly evaluate the area including the fimbriated end. If tuboscopy is to be performed, extensive lysis is sometimes required. It is important that the patient be informed of the possibility of extensive lysis to properly evaluate the pelvis. Since the vast majority of our operative procedures are done laparoscopically, this situation rarely exists. Chromotubation may be performed with methylene blue or indigo carmine. A

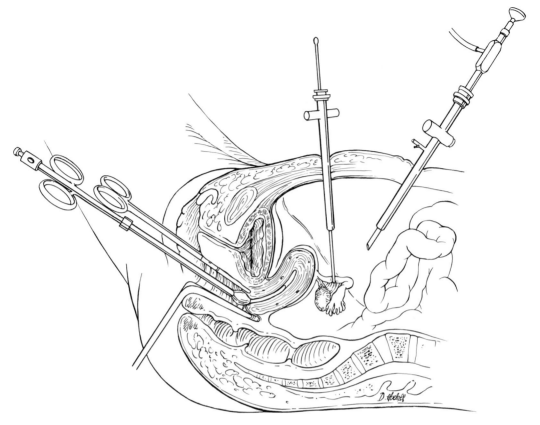

Figure 2.5. A diagnostic or straight laparoscope is inserted through the trumpet valve trocar sleeve. A 5-mm probe has been inserted through a secondary trocar sleeve. A Rubin's cannula is placed into the uterus for manipulation during the procedure.

water-tight seal is essential and may be achieved with a Rubin's or Cohen cannula, intrauterine devices with an intrauterine balloon, or an intrauterine pediatric foley.

The sites and amount of adhesions and endometriosis are carefully documented, as well as any abnormalities of the fallopian tubes, ovaries, or uterus. For routine surgical procedures, the dictated operative note is the form most widely used for documentation. It should record findings as well as the details of the operative procedure. It has been suggested and it is our practice to complement the operative report with a drawing of the general anatomy that can accurately identify abnormalities or lesions (Fig. 2.6). The findings are carefully documented on a standardized report form. Moreover, the American Fertility Society (AFS) publishes forms for the staging of endometriosis, adhesive disease, hysteroscopy,

and congenital uterine anomalies. Still photography or video may be used to document visually the extent of disease present in the pelvis. These recorded findings provide essentially the same view to a secondary observer or to the surgeon at a later time.

Our diagnostic capabilities are expanding. Salpingoscopy is now being explored, and its role in the workup of the infertile couple is being defined. We are also better defining the role and limitations of our established diagnostic tools. Appropriate diagnosis is important not only in deciding on the appropriate procedures but also in deciding if *any* procedure is warranted, given the circumstances. With the advent of the assisted reproductive technologies, the most appropriate treatment for severe tubal disease with poor or absent mucosal folds seen on salpingoscopy may not be tuboplasty and neosalpingostomy.

THE JOHNS HOPKINS HOSPITAL
REPRODUCTIVE SURGERY
ENDOSCOPY REPORT FORM

Surgeon:
Preoperative diagnosis:

Patient name: _____
History number: _____
Date: _____
Cycle day: _____ LMP: _____

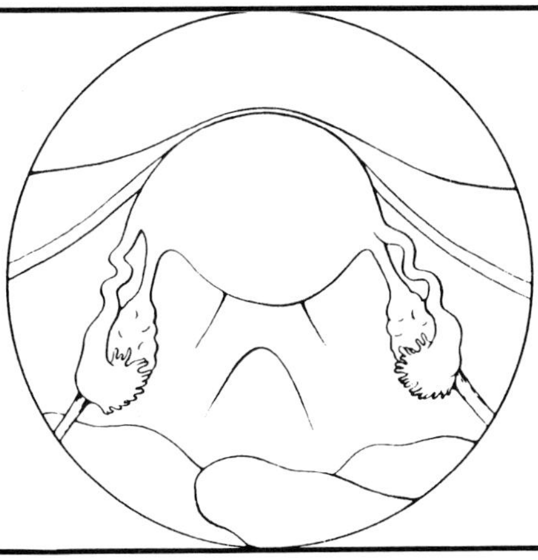

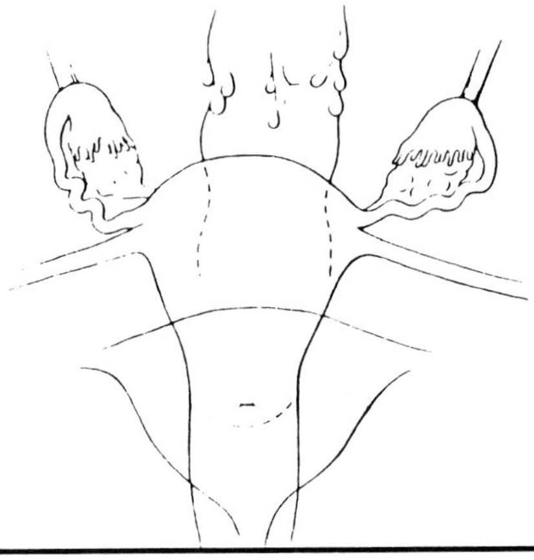

Peritoneum:
  Uterus: Size   Shape   Position
  Uterosacral ligaments:
  Round ligaments:
  Broad ligaments:
  Anterior cul-de-sac:
  Posterior cul-de-sac:

Left ovary: Right ovary:
  Size: Size:
  Shape: Shape:
  Color: Color:
  Surface: Smooth Wrinkled   Surface: Smooth Wrinkled
  Utero-ovarian ligament: Utero-ovarian ligament:
  Infundibulopelvic adhesions: Infundibulopelvic adhesions:

Left tube: Right tube:
  Length: Length:
  Surface: Surface:
  Size: Size:
  Patency: Patency:
  Fimbria: Fimbria:
  Adhesions: Location: Adhesions: Location:
           Consistency: Consistency:
           Extent: Extent:
  Fimbrica ovarica: Fimbria ovarica:

Photographs: Voltage: Exposure: Film no.:
Biopsy: Site:
Operative procedure performed via laparoscopy (described):

Postoperative diagnosis:

                              Surgeon signature _____

Figure 2.6.   The Johns Hopkins standardized report form to record laparoscopic findings.

References

1. Barbot J.: Hysteroscopy and hysterosalpingography. In: Baggish MS, Barbot J, and Valle RF, eds. Diagnostic and operative hysteroscopy: a text and atlas. Chicago: Year Book Publishers, 1989;121.
2. Boer-Meisel ME, TeVelde ER, Habbema JD, et al: Predicting the pregnancy outcome in patients treated for hydrosalpinges: a prospective study. Fertil Steril 1986;45:23.
3. Brosens I, Boeckx W, Delattin P, et al: Salpingoscopy: a new pre-operative diagnostic tool in tubal infertility. Br J Obstet Gynecol 1987;94:768.
4. Brosens IA, Vasquez G: Fimbrial microbiopsy. J Reprod Med 1976;16:171.
5. Cornier E: L'ampulloscopie per-coelioscopique. J Gynecol Obstet Biol Reprod 1985;14:459.
6. Corson SL: Operating room preparation and basic techniques. In: Phillips JM, ed. Laparoscopy. Baltimore: Williams & Wilkins, 1977;88.
7. Corson SL: Use of the laparoscope in the infertile patient. Fertil Steril 1979;32:359.
8. De Bruyne F, Puttemans P, Boeckx W, et al: The clinical value of salpingoscopy in tubal infertility. Fertil Steril 1989;51:339.
9. DeCherney AH, Kort H, Barney JB, et al: Increased pregnancy rate with oil-soluble hysterosalpingography dye. Fertil Steril 1980;33:407.
10. Donnez J, Langerock S, Lecart C, et al: Incidence of pathological factors not revealed by hysterosalpingography but disclosed by laparoscopy in 500 infertile women. Eur J Obstet Gynecol Reprod Biol 1982; 13:369.
11. Duff DE, Fried AM, Wilson EA, et al: Hysterosalpingography and laparoscopy: a comparative study. Am J Radiol 1989;141:761.
12. Henry-Suchet J, Loffredo V, Tesquier L, et al: Endoscopy of the tube (= Tuboscopy): its prognostic value for tuboplasties. Acta Eur Fertil 1985;16:139.
13. Horwitz RC, Morton RCG, Shaff MI, et al: A radiological approach to infertility-hysterosalpingography. Br J Radiol 1979;53:255.
14. Leake J, Murphy AA, Zacur HA: Noncardiogenic pulmonary edema: a complication of operative hysteroscopy. Fertil Steril 1987;48:497.
15. Lindemann HJ and Mohr J: CO_2 hysteroscopy: diagnosis and treatment. Am J Obstet Gynecol 1976; 124:129.
16. Mackey RA, Glass RH, Olsen LE, et al: Pregnancy following hysterosalpingography with oil- water-soluble dye. Fertil Steril 1971;22:504.
17. Mishler JM: Synthetic plasma volume expanders—their pharmacology, safety and clinical efficacy. Clin Haematol 1984;13:75.
18. Murphy AA: Diagnostic and operative laparoscopy. In: Thompson JD, Rock JA, eds. TeLinde's operative gynecology. Philadelphia: JB Lippincott (in press).
19. Ostrey EI: An investigation of tubal implantation for tubal block. Am J Obstet Gynecol 1957;73:409.
20. Puttemans P, Brosens I, Dlattin P, et al: Salpingoscopy vs. hysterosalpingography in hydrosalpinges. Human Reproduction 1987;2:535.
21. Reuter KL, Daly DC, Cohen SM: Septate uterus versus bicornuate uteri: errors in imaging diagnosis. Radiology 1989;172:749.
22. Rock JA, Jones HW Jr: Comparative evaluation of hysterography and laparoscopy for tubal disease. Unpublished manuscript, 1980.
23. Siegler AM, Kemmann E, Gentile GP: Hysteroscopic procedures in 257 patients. Fertil Steril 1976;27: 1267.
24. Siegler AM: Hysterography and hysteroscopy in the infertile patient. J Reprod Med 1977;18:143.
25. Valle RF: Hysteroscopy in the evaluation of female infertility. Am J Obstet Gynecol 1980;137:425.
26. Wahby O, Sabrers AJ, Epstein JA: Hysterosalpingography in relation to pregnancy and its outcome in infertile women. Fertil Steril 1966;22:504.

3

INTRODUCTION TO MICROSURGICAL TECHNIQUE AND INSTRUMENTATION

Ana Alvarez Murphy

INTRODUCTION

The microsurgical approach is a philosophy of gentle technique that applies to laparotomy and laparoscopy. It can be broadly defined as a technique that stresses gentle tissue handling, delicate instruments, precise hemostasis with a minimum of coagulation, fine needles and suture (only when absolutely necessary), and magnification. The weight of clinical and experimental evidence suggests that ischemia of the peritoneum resulting from inflammation, trauma, coagulation, or foreign materials leads to adhesion formation secondary to a local failure of the intrinsic peritoneal fibrinolytic system (7,8). The microsurgical technique, therefore, stresses minimization of tissue trauma, coagulation/vaporization, sutures, with avoidance of reperitonealization, and graft placement. The desired result is the restoration of normal pelvic anatomy and function.

Strictly defined, the microsurgical technique demands the use of the operating microscope. However, Gomel (11) broadened its definition to include surgery performed under magnification provided by a loupe, hood, or microscope. The laparoscope can magnify up to $10\times$ depending on the working distance, so it too may be included in this broadened definition.

Microsurgical techniques have been employed in most surgical specialties only within the past two decades. The initial proponents were the otolaryngologists, who found magnification essential for operating within the restrictive confines of the middle ear. Subsequently, ophthalmologists became dependent on microsurgical techniques for repair and reconstruction of deformities within the anterior chamber of the eye. In the 1950s, Jacobson et al. (17) used microsurgical techniques to repair blood vessels less than 2 mm in diameter.

The use of magnification for tubal surgery in gynecology was introduced by Swolin (33,34), who used both the loupe and the operating microscope for salpingolysis and salpingostomy. Reports by Winston (35,36) and Gomel (11) suggested improved pregnancy success following reversal of sterilization procedures in which an operating microscope was used for magnification.

Microsurgery is an acquired skill whose execution requires a magnification system, delicate microinstruments, meticulous hemostasis, and fine microsutures. A delicate manual task is performed, requiring eye-hand coordination in a restricted operative field. Special care is taken to excise adhesions precisely using gentle, delicate, atraumatic methods. Accurate knowledge of normal and abnormal anatomy, disease states, and their clinical implications provide the basis of good surgical judgment for microsurgery either through a laparotomy or laparoscopy incision. The principals of microsurgery remain the same regardless of the incisional approach. It must be stressed that good surgical judgment remains the cornerstone of all successful surgery.

MICROSURGICAL TECHNIQUES

Laparotomy

Good exposure is essential in microsurgical cases as it is for all laparotomies. A vaginal pack may be placed to elevate the uterus, especially for a tubal reanastomosis. In most instances, the tubes are slightly below the level of the incision. Additionally, the cul-de-sac is packed with pads to support the uterus and adnexa to the level of the abdominal incision after excision of cul-de-sac or adnexal disease. Frequent irrigation, which maintains moist tissues, is an important feature of microsurgery performed through a laparotomy incision.

The correct positioning of the hands allows accurate fingertip movement without fatigue. The hands, wrists, and forearms should rest on an immovable surface. In most instances, this is the patient's upper thigh and lower abdomen. Without proper hand and wrist support, the placement of suture and tying techniques are most difficult, if not impossible.

Instruments should be held in the writing position. This position gives more stability than any other. When placing the needle in the needle holder, the suture should be grasped with the forceps in the left hand, which will stabilize the suture while the needle is positioned in the holder. Minor adjustments of the needle in the needle holder can be made by touching the needle with the left-handed forceps. The needle is in the stable position if it is set at 90° to the axis of the tips of the forceps. The needle should be grasped just behind its midpoint so that the needle tip points horizontally.

When placing the needle through tissue, it should pass perpendicular to the surface of the tissue. At times this is most difficult to achieve, if the tissue edge is not everted a little to provide the necessary distortion. The edge of the tissue may be elevated with left-handed forceps while simultaneously placing the needle through tissue or by simply pressing the tubal lumen with the forceps very gently while passing the needle. Grasping the thickness of the tissue with the jaws of the forceps should be avoided, as this is a

breach of atraumatic technique. The width of the bite of tissue obtained with the needle should be between two to three times the thickness of the needle itself. The bite on the opposite tissue should be equal in width to the original segment. Once the needle has been placed through the opposite side, pulling the suture in one straight movement should be avoided, as this can cause distortion of the tissue and enlargement of the needle hole. Gentle pulls in line with the needle holes are effective. Furthermore, using the tissue forceps to keep the tail of the suture in line with the exit hole avoids damage to tissue caused by angulation of the thread at the entry hole.

Knot placement with delicate instruments in a restricted field may be a principal source of frustration for the surgeon. Knot tying consists of five maneuvers (Fig. 3.1): 1. The suture is first grasped with the right-handed forceps or needle holder approximately 2 cm from the suture site. That length of suture is referred to as the "loop length." The suture should be rotated so that it is brought across as the hand is pronated. 2. A loop is made with the long tail of the suture. A double loop may be made if the knot is to be placed under some tension. The loop should be well onto the tip of the left-handed forceps and loose. If not, the loop will easily fall off the tip of the forceps, and additional movements will be necessary. 3. The short end of the suture is grasped. Usually, this is not difficult, unless the suture is too short. 4. Once the short end of the suture has been grasped, the loop may be pulled off the left-handed forceps. The knot is tightened without bunching the tissue. 5. The sequence of movements is repeated in reverse. Release the short tail from the left-handed pickup and take hold of the long tail next to the right-handed needle holder. Lift the long tail with the pickup and wrap the suture under and over the slightly opened forceps. The short tail is then grasped with the forceps or needle holder and pulled through the loop and tightened. Each knot is square. An additional throw is placed if the suture is absorbable.

Laparoscopy

The atraumatic techniques discussed above for laparotomy should be followed as closely as possible at laparoscopy. The "closed" nature of the procedure keeps the tissue moist, so constant irrigation is not necessary. Suturing is not commonly used in operative laparoscopy; however, the instruments are available when the need arises. The needle holders presently available have serrations; therefore, the needle is secure only at 90° to the instrument. The needle holders are spring-loaded, which means the surgeon does not need to keep tension on the instrument to keep it closed. Rather, the surgeon must actively open the needle holder. The needle holders are available in 3 and 5 mm. The spring on the 5-mm instrument is too difficult to open and causes hand fatigue. If only the 5 mm is available, releasing the spring makes suturing easier, even though one has to "actively" keep the instrument closed. The 3-mm instrument with an adapter can be used through 5-mm ancillary ports. The spring on this instrument is easier to manipulate. Good forceps are not available. However, one of several instruments can be used including the 3-mm needle holder with the spring off, a similar instrument without the serrations and no spring lock, a Vancaille suture forceps, or the ampulla dilator. The latter is not recommended because suture pickup is more difficult with this instrument.

Laparoscopic instruments may be placed in

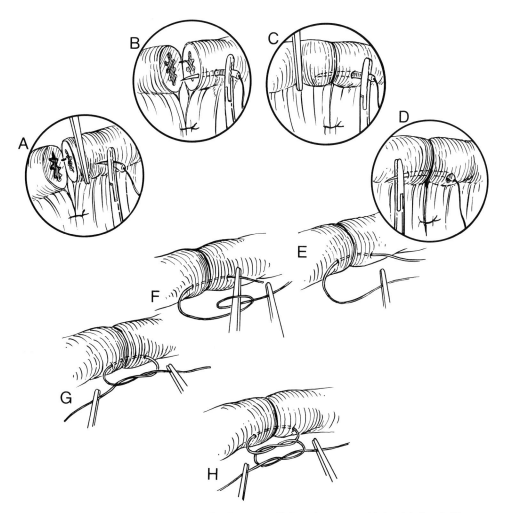

Figure 3.1. Microsurgical knot tying. *A-D*, Needle placement. *E*, Grasping suture with the right-handed forceps, palm up, the suture is brought across while the hand is pronated. *F*, Make the loop about the tip of the left-handed forceps. *G*, Tighten the first throw of the knot. *H*, A second half-knot is placed as the sequence of movements is repeated in reverse.

the palm of the hand. Opening scissor-like instruments such as needle holders and forceps is best accomplished by pushing the bottom handle down with the thumb, using the palm or the first three fingers for counterpressure. Insertion of the fingers in the instrument, especially scissors, may be necessary, but it decreases range of motion and causes awkwardness when the fingers need to be removed for manipulation.

Suturing can be very frustrating through the laparoscope because the field of vision is restricted, and the instruments are not well designed. When placing the needle through tissue, it should pass perpendicular to the surface of the tissue with an open needle holder or Vancaille forceps to provide counterpressure

on the other side of the tissue. This can be most difficult to achieve, if the tissue edge is not everted a little. It is best to elevate the edge of the tissue with left-handed forceps while simultaneously placing the needle through the tissue. One should avoid grasping the thickness of the tissue with the jaws of the forceps, if possible.

The steps outlined above for microsurgical instrument tying can be followed at laparoscopy. A modification of this technique by this author has increased the ease of intraabdominal knot tying at laparoscopy (Fig. 3.2). Knot tying consists of five steps: 1. The right-handed needle holder drives the needle and, if possible, is also used to grasp the needle on the other side of the tissue being sutured. The needle is not dropped. 2. The needle is held at 90° to the

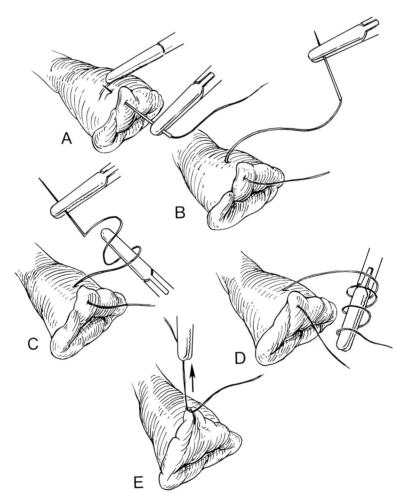

Figure 3.2. Laparoscopic knot tying. *A,* Needle placement. *B,* Grasp needle. *C,* Make the loop about the tip of the other forceps. *D,* Grasp free end. *E,* Tighten the knot.

left-handed needle holder and used to make a single or double loop. Making the loop and keeping the loop on the needle driver while grasping the loose end is the most technically difficult part of the procedure. The 90°-angle made by the needle and suture facilitates making the loop. 3. The left-handed needle holder picks up the other end of the suture. It is important that the suture not be overly long; otherwise, it may fall outside the field of vision. An overly short suture will also be awkward. 4. The knot is drawn tightly, making sure not to bunch the tissue with an overly tight knot. 5. Placing the second half knot repeats the previous movements, but in reverse. The right-hand needle holder is not released. The suture is wrapped over and under the left-handed needle holder in the same manner as described above. The short end is picked up, and the knot is tightened. Note that the needle holders will cross when the suture is tightened to make a square knot. It is less time-consuming not to drop the suture and to regrasp with the opposite needle holder. This is the one exception to the rule of not crossing instruments when working intraabdominally.

Training of the Surgeon and Operating Room Staff

Microsurgical laparotomies require the execution of delicate manual tasks governed by eye-hand coordination and visual acuity. The essential manipulation is a precise, graded pinch-closure between the index finger and thumb, with the instrument supported on the first web space. The size of the operating field is obviously restricted. The skills of knot tying and instrument handling are usually acquired by laboratory training, using animal models. There are courses as well as manuals that outline specific training schedules. Microsurgical technique is routinely taught in reproductive endocrinology fellowships. Many residency programs have also incorporated this technique into gynecologic training. Depending on the surgeon's abilities, the time required to obtain these skills will vary.

Similar skills are required for microsurgery performed through the laparoscope. Unfortunately, laparoscopic instruments are not as well designed and adapted for delicate surgery as those for conventional microsurgery. Moreover, the closed nature of laparoscopic surgery requires that only instruments be used to manipulate tissue. To better achieve the goal of laparoscopic microsurgery, better instruments need to be developed including atraumatic graspers, needle holders, needles, sutures, and microbipolar coagulators. With laparotomy surgery, many surgeons acquire a tactile sense, which can be invaluable. It takes considerable experience to acquire accurate perception of different tissue planes and structures without the "tactile sense" available at open surgery. The experienced laparoscopist develops it through instruments and visualization. Because of the impossibility of handling tissues directly, one needs to have an especially well-developed dexterity with instruments. Moreover, the surgeon must be very familiar with the array of instruments to be used for intricate manipulation and precise repair or removal of tissues. Training in operative laparoscopy can be obtained in various ways. It begins with the skills learned as a gynecologic surgeon and builds on the skills of a surgeon well versed in the use of the laparoscope for diagnostic purposes. More operative laparoscopy courses are being offered, most of which offer didactic lectures and videotapes and a few of which offer hands-on experience with training on models and tissue. Early, hands-on training allows the student to begin acquiring skills that will be useful in the operating room. Ideally, one should observe and operate with an experienced laparoscopic surgeon. Increasingly more complex cases should be attempted as skill improves. Such skills are now being taught in fellowship programs and residency programs to senior residents. Laparoscopic surgery is not for the novice but for the well-trained gynecologic surgeon.

The training of operating room personnel has become much more complex with the advent of new equipment, instruments, lasers, and magnification systems. The nurses who are responsible for the operating room must have additional education to understand the ramifications of new equipment and technology. Preferably, the surgeon, and in some cases, American instrument companies, are providing inservice training on assembling the equipment and the care and cleaning of all the components. It should be scheduled on a regular basis, depending on the turnover of operating room personnel. Ideally, one or two nurses on each shift are directly responsible for the maintenance of the equipment. The staff may also be required to learn the operational characteristics of more than one laser system. Troubleshooting information as well as training on the various laser accessories are paramount.

Preparation of the Operative Field

As with any open abdominal case, the room should be thoroughly prepared for the procedure in advance of the operation. This simply means that all of the appropriate equipment and instruments should be in the room. All instruments and solutions that are necessary to perform the anticipated operation should be on the table and ready to be used. The microscope should be properly adjusted by the surgeons and sterilely draped by the nursing staff prior to beginning the operation. The laser, if to be used, should be tested to make sure it is functional and the appropriate safety measures taken to protect the operating room staff. Once the surgeon is scrubbed and gowned, a final inspection of the equipment should include testing of the working condition of the instruments to be used.

Appropriate lighting can be obtained from the overhead lights with supplementation from a flexible light source or a fiberoptic headlight. Loupes are available that incorporate a fiberoptic headlight (Zeiss Prism Loupe, Carl Zeiss Inc., Thornwood, NY). The movable light source is particularly important with sidewall and cul-de-sac disease. Exposure is key to the proper execution of the manipulations described. Proper exposure may require cutting the rectus abdominus muscles partially or in their entirety. If the muscles are to be transected in their entirety, the inferior epigastric vessels can be easily tied to diminish the possibility of subfascial hematoma. In this case, the muscles should not be dissected from the fascia. Packing the vagina in order to elevate the pelvic organs can be very helpful. After appropriate lysis of adhesions or resection of endometriosis in the cul-de-sac, the area can be packed and a platform made upon which the tubes can be placed. Stabilization of all structures at the same level allows the most efficient use of the operating microscope.

For endoscopy, the procedures are similar; however, due to the greater number of instruments and video apparatus, the setup of the room is more complicated. Additionally, hysteroscopic procedures are usually done under laparoscopic guidance, so laparoscopy equipment also needs to be opened. All equipment must be laid out including the aspirator/irrigator unit and a form of coagulation or suture capable of controlling bleeding from large vessels quickly (preferably a bipolar paddle). It should be remembered that if bleeding occurs during laparoscopy, it occurs in a "closed" space. This space is best approached with laparoscopic instruments that must be immediately available and in working order. It is a wise precaution to keep a sterile laparotomy tray in the room, immediately available for situations that cannot be approached endoscopically.

Magnification System

Magnification may be provided by the microscope, operating hood, binocular lenses, or the laparoscope (Figs. 3.3 and 3.4). Magnification may range from $1\times$ to $20\times$, depending upon the optical system. In the past, the major difficulties with the hood and the binocular lenses have been the excessive weight and short focal length required to obtain an acceptable magnification (4). Modifications involving the use of lighter materials have obviated the weight problem. Lens adjustments have increased the focal lengths, allowing for comfortable working distances and a wider field of vision. In particular, a greater depth of field has been provided. At present, most binocular lenses offer magnifications between $2\times$ and $6\times$. Proper lighting may be provided by using a fiberoptic cable covered by a sterile plastic sheath or a head light.

The operating microscope offers the advantages of a wider range of magnification and a coaxial light system. In general, the range of magnification is dependent on the magnifica-

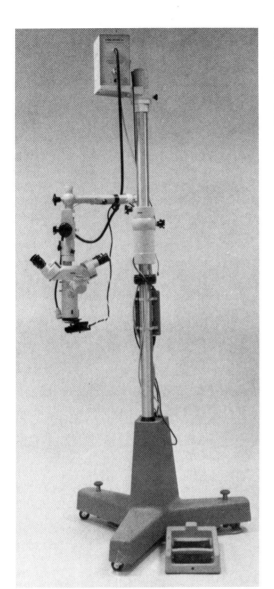

Figure 3.3. Zeiss OpMI-7 operating microscope.

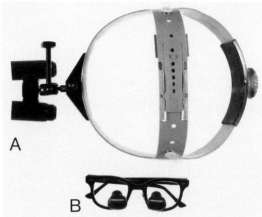

Figure 3.4. Binocular lenses. *A*, Adjustable loupes. *B*, Personalized loupes.

tion coefficient of the eyepiece and the focal length of the objective. Eyepieces of $10\times$ magnification and objective lenses of 250 mm provide a magnification ranging from $3.6\times$ to $16\times$. A manual zoom system for the control of magnification and focusing, photographic attachments, and an assistance binocular observation system are available on many microscopes.

A difference of opinion regarding the advisability of using the various systems appears to focus on the importance of the source and amount of magnification necessary for accurate control of hemostasis and the placement of fine suture. The use of a hood or loupe to provide magnification from $2\times$ to $6\times$ has provided adequate visualization for some ophthalmic and plastic surgery, and its application to the reversal of sterilization in gynecology is very appropriate. Our observations support those of the jewelry repair industry, which have noted that magnification above $6\times$ is associated with increased working time and decreased accuracy. We have determined that magnification greater than $6\times$, in most instances, is unnecessary and not critical in the reversal of sterilization procedures. Pregnancy rates obtained with the microscope are comparable to those obtained with the hood or loupe (27).

Endoscopes are monocular, not binocular, instruments. Depth perception, which is necessary to evaluate the size of an object, is primarily the result of binocular vision. Objects at different distances produce different visual angles at the eye as well as images on different parts of the retina. With binocular vision, the brain learns to interpret these differences in terms of distance from the eye. Magnification, therefore, must be redefined for the endoscope (9). Magnification is usually defined as the ratio of the image size to the object size. The apparent size of an object to an observer is determined by the size of the retinal image, which depends only on the angle subtended at the eye by the object of vision. A close object may subtend a larger angle than an objectively larger object farther away (Fig. 3.5). Magnification for the endoscope therefore must be

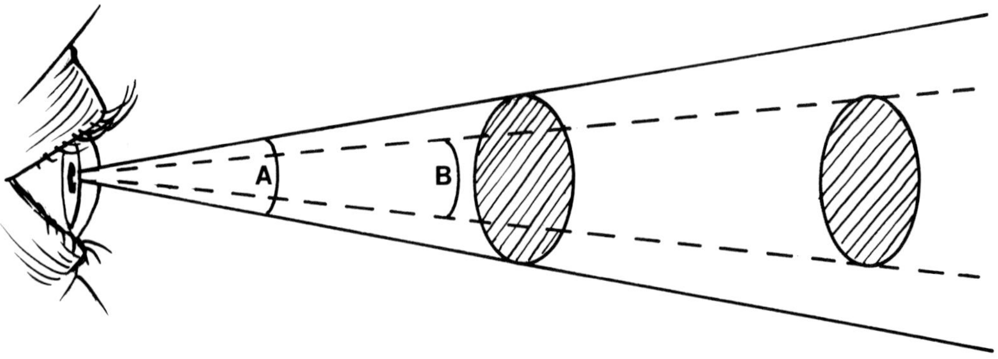

Figure 3.5. Visual angles subtended at the eye by the same size objects at different object distances. (Adapted from Gardner FM: Optical principles of the endoscope. In: Baggish MS, Barbot J, Valle RF, eds. Diagnostic and operative hysteroscopy: a text and atlas. Chicago: Year Book Medical Publishers, 1989;50–57.)

Table 3.1. Range of Magnification Based on Distance

Operating Laparoscope Working Distance	Magnification Rate	
	Wolf[a]	Olympus[b]
3 mm	—	8.2
5 mm	—	5.7
10 mm	3.19	3.2
15 mm	—	2.2
20 mm	1.71	1.7
30 mm	—	1.2
50 mm	0.73	0.7

[a]Personal communication. Richard Wolf Medical Instrument Corporation. Rosemont, Illinois. November 14, 1988.
[b]Personal communication. Olympus Corporation. Lake Success, New York, November 2, 1988.

redefined as the ratio of the angle subtended at the eye by the object to the angle subtended at the eye by the image when the image is at the near point of the eye (250 mm). Consequently, for panoramic endoscopes, the observer sees the near objects at different visual magnifications than those for more distant objects. The visual magnification of the scope is inversely proportional to the object distance. Note the range of magnification depending on the distance to the object (Table 3.1). Naturally, magnification differs with changes in the caliber of the scope.

INSTRUMENTATION

Laparotomy

Specially designed instruments are quite useful in the delicate procedures within the peritoneal cavity designed to enhance or pre-serve fertility. The instruments the authors have chosen are but a few of many forceps, scissors, clamps, and other instruments marketed in the United States and abroad. As a craftsman acquires his set of specialized tools, the reproductive surgeon acquires a set of surgical instruments with which he or she feels most comfortable performing these techniques (5). It must be stressed that what is useful for one surgeon may be awkward for another (37).

ABDOMINAL RETRACTOR

The Kirschner abdominal retractor is useful in gaining maximum visualization through a transverse incision (Fig. 3.6). The retractor arms may be positioned laterally so as to retract only the abdominal wall and not impinge upon the peritoneum or press laterally against the major vessels. The abdominal walls are usually protected with laparotomy packs so that a bloodless field may be obtained. The scalloped edges of the ring and the hooks on the blades interdigitate to allow for adjustment without screws or wing nuts. The lateral blades are much smaller than the bladder blade and the intestinal retractor. A set of deeper blades can also be ordered. In the obese patient, however, this retractor is in most instances unsatisfactory. The traditional Balfour retractor is preferable.

SUCTION/IRRIGATION

Continuous irrigation can be obtained from an intracath tip and a syringe. The intracath tip or an irrigator with manual control on the

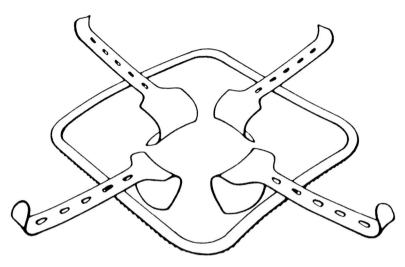

Figure 3.6. Kirschner abdominal retractor (Downs Surgical).

handle can also be connected to a 1000-cc intravenous (IV) bag. This can decrease the manipulations necessary during a long case. A willing assistant is much more useful than the constant drip irrigators that are awkward to position and need to be adjusted when using cautery or laser. Other subspecialties have aspirator-irrigators that can be "borrowed."

UTERINE CLAMPS

There are various clamps manufactured for uterine elevation and transuterine lavage (Fig. 3.7). The Cullen uterine elevator is useful for elevating the uterus in an atraumatic fashion. The blades may be securely placed about the fundus of the uterus with variable pressure, allowing its elevation with minimal trauma.

Depending upon the uterine contour, one of several clamps may be chosen to obstruct the cervical os so dye may pass into the oviducts. In a large parous uterus, the Siegler Hellman clamp is useful in obstructing the lower uterine segment and/or endocervical canal. The Shirodkar clamp may be easily placed to obstruct the endocervical canal in a small nulliparous uterus and is unobtrusive. The swivel jaws feature of the Buxton uterine clamp allows the clamp to be moved laterally so that one may clearly visualize the fallopian tube with the clamp completely out of the field. For tubal perfusion, an intracath may be placed transfundally. The needle is then removed, and chromotubation

with indigo carmine or methylene blue is performed.

While we prefer to use the transfundal approach, others chromotubate from an indwelling device within the uterus. A HUMI or HUI (Unimar, Canooga Park, CA) device may be placed in the uterus with the balloon inflated. Intravenous tubing can be attached to allow the operator to control the device from the operating table. Both methods have some drawbacks. Occasionally, the uterine cavity is hard to find, and several attempts must be made transfundally. The uterus will usually bleed from the transfundal needle; fortunately, it almost always stops spontaneously. The HUMI/HUI devices have been criticized for potentially increasing the risk of infection from the cervix and vagina. Additionally, if uterine manipulation is necessary, those devices are very awkward to use.

FORCEPS

The fallopian tube and ovary forceps are useful for traction puposes. These instruments are designed to hold each structure with a minimum amount of pressure and peritoneal trauma (Fig. 3.8). The brain dressing forceps and microinfertility forceps are useful for gently grasping fine adhesions while excising them. Microforceps should grasp tissue gently and atraumatically. In our experience, the #5 jeweler's forceps is quite useful in both tissue

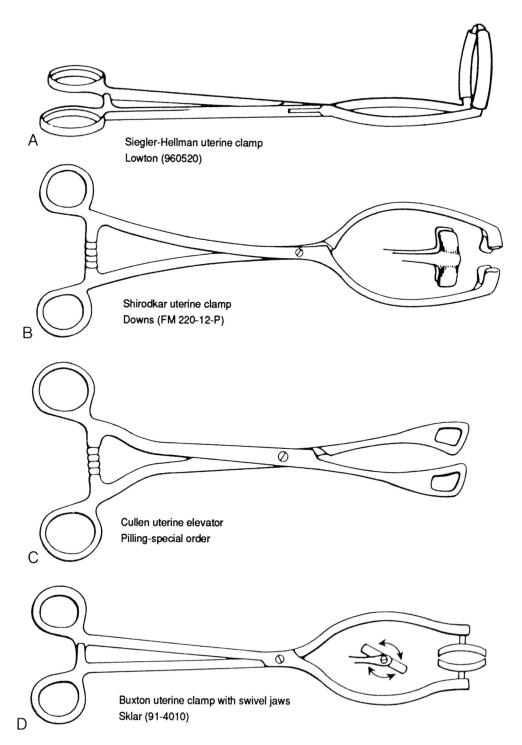

A   Siegler-Hellman uterine clamp
Lowton (960520)

Shirodkar uterine clamp
Downs (FM 220-12-P)
B

Cullen uterine elevator
Pilling-special order
C

Buxton uterine clamp with swivel jaws
Sklar (91-4010)
D

Figure 3.7.   Uterine clamps. *A,* Siegler-Hellman (Lowton) *B,* Shirodkar (Downs) *C,* Cullen (Piling) *D,* Buxton with Swivel jaws (Sklar).

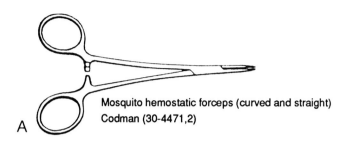

A   Mosquito hemostatic forceps (curved and straight)
Codman (30-4471,2)

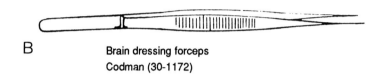

B   Brain dressing forceps
Codman (30-1172)

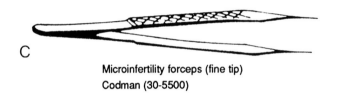

C   Microinfertility forceps (fine tip)
Codman (30-5500)

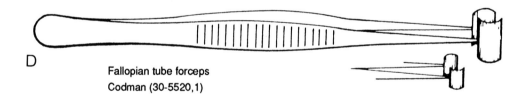

D   Fallopian tube forceps
Codman (30-5520,1)

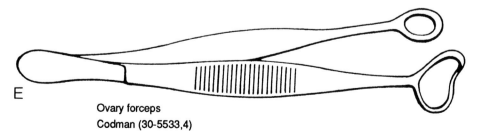

E   Ovary forceps
Codman (30-5533,4)

Figure 3.8. Forceps. *A,* Mosquito hemostatic forceps (curved and straight) (Codman). *B,* Brain dressing forceps (Codman). *C,* Microinfertility forceps (fine-tip) (Codman). *D,* Fallopian tube forceps (Codman). *E,* Ovary forceps (Codman).

handling and suture tying. Longer forceps are necessary for work deep in the pelvis, as jeweler's forceps are quite short. Bayonet microsurgical forceps are also long. The distal curve of this instrument does not obscure the tissue grasped beneath the tips. The Castroviejo forceps with the tying platform and fine 0.3-mm teeth may be useful in grasping tissue when smooth forceps cannot be used. This may be done with minimal trauma, for instance, when placing a fine nylon splint through the oviduct into the uterine cavity. Forceps are also available with small loops on the end which grasp tissue more securely than the smooth microtip forceps. By distributing the force over a wider area, a more secure grasp is achieved without teeth. It is useful to have stops on microinfertility forceps, as this prevents crossing of the tips. Curved and straight mosquito hemostatic forceps are used for clamping small vessels and securing hemostasis along the tube and ovary. Use of forceps with teeth should be avoided when manipulating the tube, ovary, or peritoneal edge.

SCISSORS

Metzenbaum scissors (straight with sharp tips) are useful in releasing adhesions deep in the cul-de-sac, particularly beneath the ovary and adjacent to the uterosacral ligaments (Fig. 3.9). The shorter straight and curved iris scissors may be easily used around structures that may be elevated to the abdominal incision, that is, to release adhesions about the tubes, the uterine fundus, and round ligaments. Full-curved iris scissors are quite useful in releasing adhesions where the curve of the instrument approximates the curve of the viscera. One can release adhesions at the surface of the serosa quite easily with minimal trauma to the serosa itself. The Stevens scissors are useful in releasing rather thick, fibrous adhesions, as one is less likely to damage these scissors on such adhesions, whereas the more delicate instruments described above could be damaged during such use. Delicate microinfertility scissors are useful in cutting or trimming the serosa. These instruments are not to be used in cutting suture but only in trimming delicate tissues. We do not recommend serated scissors because no

improvement in cutting is seen, and they are more difficult to sharpen.

NEEDLE HOLDERS

At times, it is necessary to use very fine needles and suture material. It is therefore important to have a proper needle holder to place these sutures. The classic Castoviejo needle holder is useful in engaging 8–12-mm needles to place sutures near the abdominal incision (Fig. 3.10). However, when sutures must be placed deep in the cul-de-sac, the Crile Wood needle holder with fine tips is in most instances necessary. Finer suture (>6-0) and needles 6 mm or less, should be placed with fine delicate microinfertility needle holders. The microinfertility needle holders with rounded arms are useful in placing suture. With these, all that is required is to rotate the fingers when placing the needle in the tissue. An instrument without a lock enables minimal hand movement when releasing the jaws of the instrument, and this is our preferred needle driver. Some surgeons, however, prefer an instrument lock to secure the needle. Unlocking the needle holder sometimes causes trauma to the tissue.

Most instruments are available in stainless steel, chrome-alloy, or titanium. The steel instruments can become magnetized. Most operating suites, however, have an inexpensive demagnetizer. Steel scissors seem to keep an edge longer and are also easier to sharpen. Titanium instruments are designed for use with a CO_2 laser; however, they are much more expensive than the steel instruments.

PROBES, DIRECTORS, AND REAMERS

Fine metal probes are not only useful to identify the ostium of an incompletely obstructed oviduct, but also to tent adhesions prior to lysis with scissors or electrocautery (Fig. 3.11). A set of lacrimal duct probes of variable diameter is useful for this purpose. A set of plastic, Teflon, titanium, or glass rods assists in retracting the pelvic viscera in an atraumatic fashion. One may have these prepared in different lengths and with blunt or quasipointed tips at varying angles to assist in retraction and manipulation. The Teflon probe can be bent to suit the situation. Quartz or

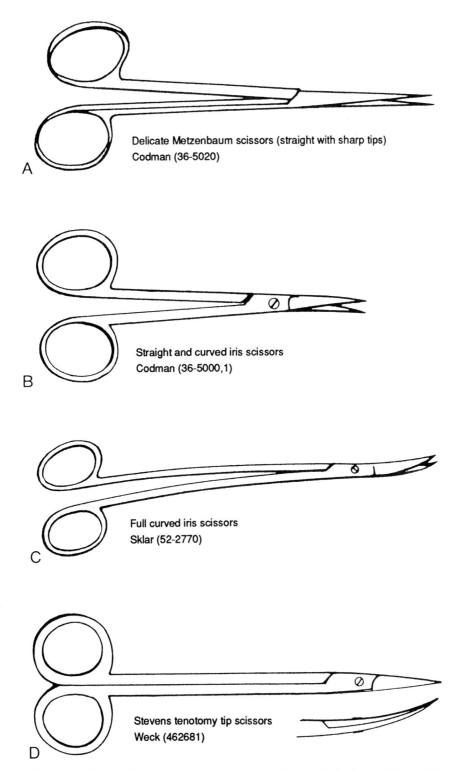

Figure 3.9.   Scissors. *A*, Delicate Metzenbaum scissors (straight with sharp tips). (Codman) *B*, Straight and curved Iris scissors (Codman). *C*, Full curved Iris scissors (Sklar). *D*, Stevens stenotomy scissors (Weck).

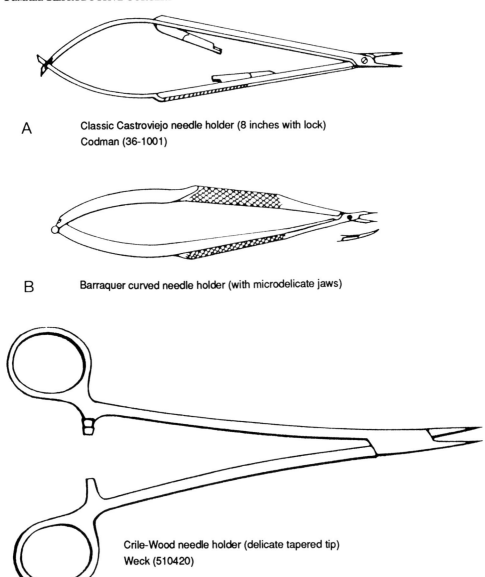

A   Classic Castroviejo needle holder (8 inches with lock)
Codman (36-1001)

B   Barraquer curved needle holder (with microdelicate jaws)

Crile-Wood needle holder (delicate tapered tip)
Weck (510420)

C

Figure 3.10. Needle Holders. *A,* Classic Castroviejo needle holder (8" with lock) (Codman). *B,* Microinfertility or Barraquer curved needle holder. *C,* Crile Wood needle holder (delicate tapered tip) (Weck).

titanium rods are a must if the CO_2 laser is used as Teflon, or glass will be destroyed by the beam. Quartz will only "pit."

ELECTROCAUTERY

Monopolar cautery with a fine delicate needle may be used to remove adhesions as well as to incise a hydrosalpinx (Fig. 3.12). The delicate tip allows precise coagulation of vessels with minimal electrodessiccation temperature. These usually fit into standard electrosurgical units such as Valley Lab (Valley Lab, Boulder, CO).

The microinfertility or neurosurgical bipolar forceps is useful in precise hemostasis where vessels can be identified. The bleeding tissue may be gently grasped with the bipolar forceps and lavaged with warm saline or lactated Ringer's solution to assure complete hemostasis prior to applying current between the tips. Most modern units offer both unipolar and bipolar modes.

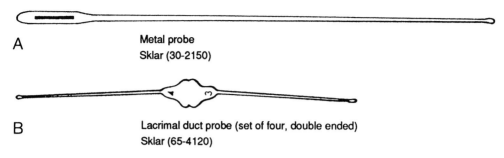

A   Metal probe
     Sklar (30-2150)

B   Lacrimal duct probe (set of four, double ended)
     Sklar (65-4120)

Figure 3.11.   *A,* Metal probe (Sklar). *B,* Lacrimal duct probe (set of four double-ended) (Sklar).

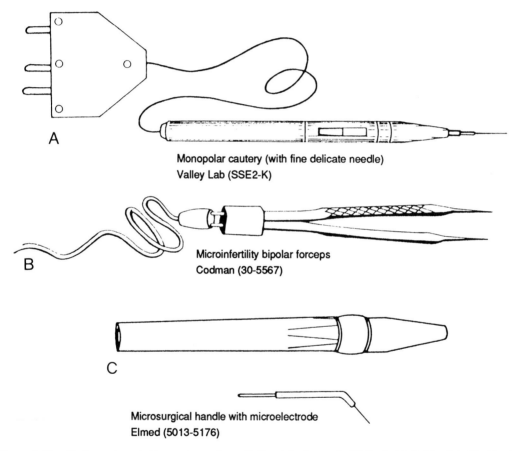

A   Monopolar cautery (with fine delicate needle)
     Valley Lab (SSE2-K)

B   Microinfertility bipolar forceps
     Codman (30-5567)

C

     Microsurgical handle with microelectrode
     Elmed (5013-5176)

Figure 3.12.   Electrocautery. *A,* Monopolar cautery with fine delicate needle (Valley Lab). *B,* Microinfertility bipolar forceps (Codman). *C,* Microsurgical handle with microelectrode (Elmed).

In a unipolar system, the current passes from the generator to the instrument. The current then passes through the path of least resistance to the ground plate and subsequently to the generator. Most units will stop and emit a warning sound if the sensor part of the plate recognizes any change in resistance. Cutting and coagulating current come in "pure" or "blended" form. The cutting current provides a constant high-energy wave form. The coagulating waveform initially has a high voltage component that quickly dissipates and results in desiccation of the outer layer of the tissue and increased tissue resistance (Fig. 3.13). A "blend" literally combines the two and is dispensed, usually through the cutting mode.

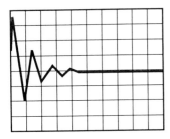

Coagulating wave form

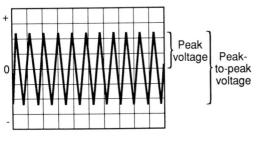

Cutting wave form

Figure 3.13. Cutting and coagulating wave form (Reprinted with permission from Murphy AA: Diagnostic and operative laparoscopy. In: Thompson JD, Rock JA, eds. TeLinde's operative gynecology. Philadelphia: JB Lippincott 1991.)

Cutting currents are best set on "pure" rather than "blend," as the charring effect increases as the current becomes more dampened. It is imperative that the surgeon be familiar with the electrosurgical unit being used. The maximum and minimum power may vary with each unit. The numerical setting needed to achieve a certain power can be determined on a graph frequently found on the top or side of the generator.

Endoscopy

LIGHTING

The amount and quality of light that reaches the telescope is dependent upon the light source as well as the transmitting fiberoptic cable. The simple generators provide 150 W of power, which is sufficient for direct viewing but not adequate for photography or video. These are usually tungsten-type sources that have a red-orange cast. However, they are small and inexpensive. A metal halide source is probably sufficient for photography; however, the light has a noticeable bluish tinge. A

high-intensity light (300 W), ideal for video and still photography, is provided by xenon generators. They also provide variable illumination settings and special filters including flash for still photography.

Regardless of the type and quantity of light generated, what reaches the telescope is dependent on the quality and maintenance of the fiberoptic light cable. Optimal visualization requires that fibers transmitting the light be intact. Broken fibers in the light cable can be identified by looking for dark spots on the lighted end. They can also be identified by looking for illuminated spots along the cladding in a dark room. Liquid light cables provide superior illumination and do not have the above problems. However, the cables are much more heavily clad to prevent explosion and rupture, resulting in less flexibility than glass fiber cables.

VIDEO/PHOTOGRAPHY

Video cameras have become an almost indispensible part of laparoscopy and hysteroscopy. The video cameras have improved immeasurably from the bulky tube cameras used only a few years ago. The new microchip cameras are small, lightweight, and provide great resolution and a wide field. A potent light source is required, preferably the xenon lamp. Besides teaching the dynamic process of diagnostic and operative cases, video cameras allow the operating room staff to assist the surgeon more effectively (Fig. 3.14). Moreover, many endoscopic surgeons are operating from the screen almost exclusively. This technique requires practice since the field is viewed two-dimensionally. Additionally, the nuances of color and texture can be lost on the screen. The great advantage is that the surgeon can stand or sit upright rather than hunched over, thereby reducing operator fatigue.

Beamsplitters supply 80–90% of available light to the video monitor, providing an excellent picture. Operating while viewing the surgical field through the laparoscope may produce eyestrain from the high-intensity xenon light. However, it provides the versatility of operating from the screen, directly, or a combination of both while still allowing the operating room staff to adequately assist.

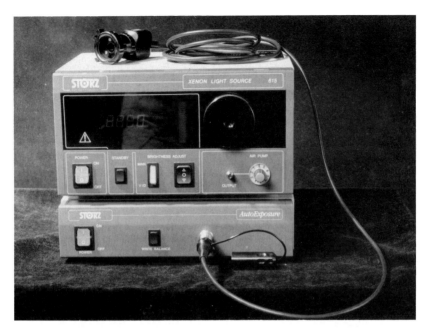

Figure 3.14.   Video camera (Karl Storz, Endoscopy, America).

Still photography is important, especially for documentation. Many cameras are available for this purpose. The pictures are generally brighter and clearer if a flash unit is available, but it is not essential. Generally, daylight ASA 200 film can be used. The easiest way to obtain pictures for documentation is either with a Polaroid system or the "frame grabbing" technology, which allows the production of an instant print from any moment of continuous video recording. The digitally produced hard copy snapshot or slide may soon be the procedure of choice.

TELESCOPES

The standard endoscope consists of an optical component and a lighting mechanism. It can be subdivided into the eyepiece, barrel, and a terminal lens. The inner barrel structures are usually encased in stainless steel. Within this cover is located a group of lenses or rods separated by air spaces. The early endoscopes consisted of a number of lenses separated by long air spaces that allowed the image to be transmitted at unit magnification through a small diameter tube without severely restricting the field of view. The light transmission of the lens relay system was greatly improved by the introduction of the rod-lens system, devised by

H.H. Hopkins (16). The rod-lens system uses long glass rods and short air spaces instead of the long air spaces and thin glass lenses. The optics described allow viewing of objects at different distances from the objective lens. Since the normal eye can create sharp images of objects that lie between optical infinity and 250 mm, the depth of focus can be defined as the range of object distances that fall within the range of the accommodation of the eye. The resolution of the lens-type endoscope is limited by diffraction effects. The image of a point on the object is a diffraction pattern consisting of alternating concentric dark and light bands. The overlap of these patterns causes the viewer to be unable to judge two points as separate (10). A high-quality endoscope has a resolution near the limits set by diffraction theory.

A 4-mm endoscope (outer diameter) is the smallest instrument of choice since smaller scopes do not provide an optimally bright and clear view with a high-intensity light. This is the size most commonly used for hysteroscopy. Diagnostic and operative laparoscopes come in a variety of sizes, from small (5–7 mm) to large (8–11 mm). Although some surgeons prefer to begin using a small laparoscope and then change to the larger bore laparoscope for operative cases, we prefer to begin with a large laparoscope for better visualization. Theoretically, the smaller instruments should be safer since less force is required to enter the abdomen.

Endoscopes are available with different angles of view, either straightforward (0°) or

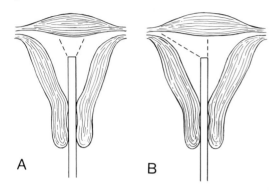

Figure 3.15. Straightforward and fore-oblique endoscope. *A,* Straightforward or 0° angle endoscope. *B,* Fore-oblique or 30–45° angle endoscope.

fore-oblique (30–45°) (Fig. 3.15). The selection of the angle is one of personal preference; the novice will usually prefer a straightforward scope because it requires less adjustment. We prefer the 0° laparoscope and the angled (30°) hysteroscope. The angled hysteroscope allows rapid viewing of the uterine walls and ostia by simply rotating the telescope since the sharpest view is at a 30° angle. A 0° hysteroscope must be severely angled to sharply view the ostia because the sharpest image is straightforward (12).

Laparoscopy

Laparoscopists are divided on the usefulness of operative laparoscopes. Those who prefer to insert all ancillary instruments through separate incision sites claim improved depth perception and a wider field of vision. Proponents of the

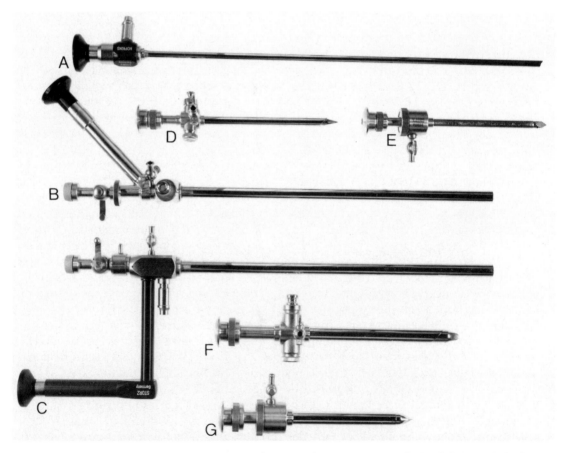

Figure 3.16. Laparoscopes (Storz). *A,* Straight laparoscope. *B,* 45° laparoscope. *C,* Jacob-Palmer. *D,* Ancillary trocars - Trumpet valve. *E,* Ancillary trocars - flapper valve. *F,* Large trocar - Trumpet valve. *G,* Large trocar - flapper valve. (Reprinted with permission from Murphy AA: Diagnostic and operative laparoscopy. In: Thompson JD, Rock JA, eds. TeLinde's operative gynecology. Philadelphia: JB Lippincott 1991.)

operating laparoscope, however, feel that the advantages gained from this unique angle of operation far outweigh its disadvantages.

There are three major types of laparoscopes (Fig. 3.16). The straight laparoscope or photo-laparoscope provides the best (widest) view for any given size. The Jacob-Palmer operating laparoscope has two right angles so that the eyepiece is parallel but offset. The view is identical to the straightforward scope, so it is by far the easiest of the operating laparoscopes to use. Its major disadvantage is the closeness of the instrument to the operator's head, which can easily cause contamination of instruments if care is not taken. The 45° and 90° scopes offer little advantage over the Jacob-Palmer except a slightly wider field of vision and greater distance of instruments from the surgeon's head. The view offered by both of these scopes is confusing, and it takes some time before the operator adjusts to the view (22).

INSUFFLATORS

Laparoscopic surgery is possible only if adequate pneumoperitoneum can be maintained, despite several instrument changes (18). Multiple puncture sites may become sources of gas leaks. Additionally, irrigation and aspiration also deplete intraabdominal gas. It is therefore of utmost importance to use a high-flow insufflator capable of producing at least 5 liters/min or greater at the high-flow setting (Fig. 3.17). There are manual as well as electronic insufflators. The latter can be preset

so that insufflation pressures does not exceed 15 mm Hg. In theory, this pressure should not impede venous return to the heart.

PNEUMOPERITONEAL NEEDLE AND TROCAR

The pneumoperitoneal needle is used to pass carbon dixoide into the abdominal cavity and protect the abdominopelvic contents from accidental puncture by the trocar. There are two needle types. The Touhy needle was commonly used in the past. It was designed for epidural anesthesia and is less expensive than the Verres. The Verres needle was designed to reduce the chances of accidental puncture. It has a spring that allows retraction of the blunt inner point, exposing the sharp outer sheath as it traverses the abdominal wall. The blunt inner part springs out to protect the structures below when it encounters a decrease in pressure (3). A disposable Verres-like instrument is also available.

The trocar pierces the abdominal wall and carries with it the trocar sleeve. The laparoscope or instrument is then placed through the sleeve. There are two basic models: the trumpet valve and the flapper valve. The flapper valve is the more traditional instrument, and it allows the instrument to be inserted and moved easily. Manipulation of instruments is easier with this type of sleeve; however, gas escapes from the sleeve until a finger, another instrument, or trocar is placed. The trumpet valve model must be actively opened to allow instruments to be

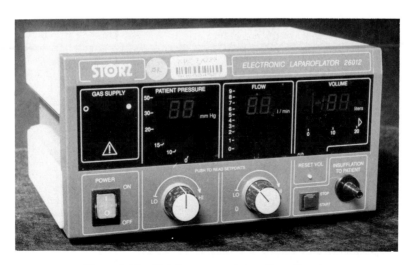

Figure 3.17. High-flow automatic insufflator (Storz).

introduced. Although much less gas escapes when instruments are inserted or withdrawn, the instruments do not glide easily inside the sleeve. Manipulation of the instruments is made easier if the assistant holds the valve open. The trocar tips may be conical or pyramidal. Some argue that the sharp cutting edge of the pyramidal tip is more likely to damage vessels in the abdominal wall and cause a hematoma. The most important issue, however, is sharpness. A dull trocar is more likely to cause damage as more force is necessary for insertion (21). Disposable trocars have a safety shield similar to the Verres needle, which may increase safety. The disposable trocars are always sharp; however, they are very expensive.

PROBES

The prototype of all ancillary instruments is the blunt probe. It is the simplest and probably the most commonly used instrument. It is essential for manipulation of structures that require it for full visualization. Many other instruments can be used as blunt probes as long as the closed instrument is blunt. This reduces the possibility of trauma. The probes are available in a myriad of sizes and lengths to fit

ancillary puncture sites as well as operating channels of laparoscopes. It is helpful to have a probe marked in centimeters because magnification of the laparoscopic lens can make estimation of size difficult (19).

FORCEPS

A range of forceps is essential to any operative set (Fig. 3.18). Their main use is to atraumatically stabilize structures, although traumatic forceps are also used (Fig. 3.19). The atraumatic grasping forceps, also known as tongs or the ampulla dilator, is most frequently used because it is a "gentle" instrument. Traditional atraumatic grasping forceps with springs are too injurious to tissue and should not be used except with tissue that is to be excised. The tongs can be used not only to stabilize a structure but also to gently dilate the distal fallopian tube at fimbrioplasty. Kleppinger or paddle forceps used for bipolar coagulation can also be used as atraumatic forceps. The pressure is distributed over a greater surface area, and they have no spring, so the tissue is not held too tightly or "bunched." Hasson has designed a prototype atraumatic forceps that consists of three prongs on a spring. The tissue

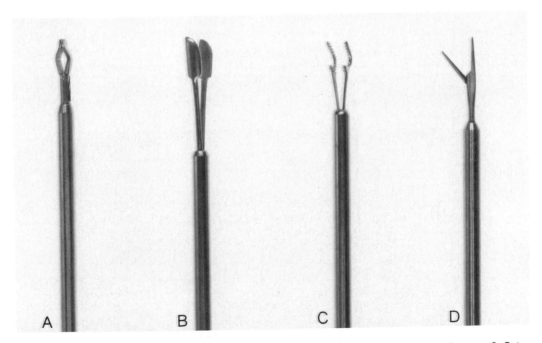

Figure 3.18. Atraumatic grasping forceps (Storz). *A*, Tongs or ampulla dilator. *B*, Dissecting forceps. *C*, Suture forceps. *D*, Grasping forceps.

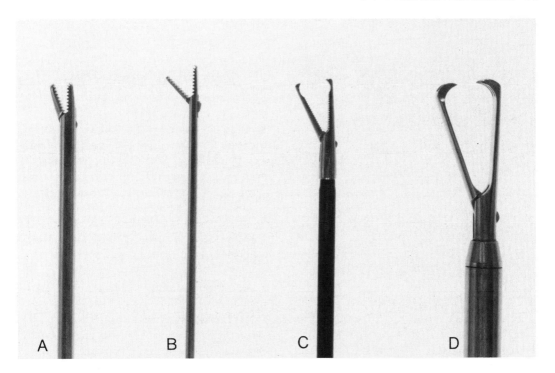

Figure 3.19. Traumatic grasping forceps (Storz). *A*, Needle holder or suture forceps. *B*, Micrograsping forceps. *C*, Claw forceps—5 mm. *D*, Claw forceps—10 mm.

can be grasped more firmly with three prongs, and a screwing mechanism regulates where the spring mechanism stops, thereby causing less trauma to the grasped tissue (13,14). Large-spoon forceps may be used to remove tropho-blastic tissue at salpingostomy as well as other pieces of tissue through the 11-mm trocar sleeve. It has also been used as a grasper.

Traumatic forceps such as the large claw forceps or toothed forceps can be used on tissue that is to be removed such as adnexa or myoma. The hinged jaws of the claw forceps are particularly effective in stabilizing large structures during morcellation as well. This instrument is available in both 5 and 11 mm sizes. The toothed forceps is constructed with a single sharp tooth in one or both jaws to keep the tissue to be biopsied from slipping (Fig. 3.20). The edges should be kept sharp so that biopsied tissue is cut and not avulsed. Microtip biopsy forceps are also available. An incisional biopsy with scissors or knife is more precise and just as easy. Hemostasis, if necessary, should be obtained after the tissue is biopsied so as not to destroy histologic detail.

SCISSORS/SCALPEL

Scissors are an integral part of the instrument set (Fig. 3.21). Many different kinds and sizes are now available. It is essential that they be well maintained and that tissue is cut rather than avulsed when used. The most commonly used scissors are the hook scissors. They tend to maintain their sharpness and can be used for general dissection as well as for cutting suture or tissue. These should always be inserted carefully and under visualization because the tips overlap even when closed and can injure tissue inadvertently. The peritoneal or serrated scissors tend to crush tissue rather than sharply cut it and should be avoided. The microscissors are very delicate and when sharp are perfect for microsurgical work (fine dissection).

Laparoscopic scalpels come in different sizes and shapes. The most useful resembles a number 11 blade (Fig. 3.22). These can be used through the channel of an operating laparoscope or an ancillary site. Frequently, unipolar cautery can be attached to the scalpels and some scissors. This combines cutting and coagula-

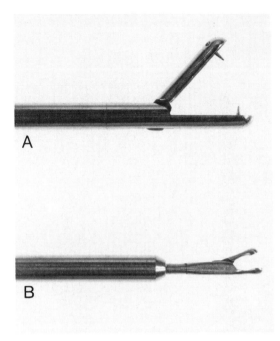

Figure 3.20. Biopsy forceps (Storz). *A,* Toothed biopsy forceps. *B,* Microtip biopsy forceps.

tion, which may be very useful for adhesiolysis or linear salpingostomy.

ASPIRATOR/IRRIGATORS

Laparoscopic needle tip aspirators were once commonly used for oocyte aspiration. Now they are rarely used, except to aspirate simple-appearing ovarian cysts or endometriomas prior to resection. The blunt-tipped cannulas are an integral part of the operating set and are indispensable to effect rapid evacuation of intraabdominal blood. Aspiration can be effected mechanically by suction devices or manually with a large syringe. Combined aspiration/irrigation units are available commercially as well as irrigation units alone. The handle of these units usually has two push-buttons; one each for irrigation and aspiration, and various tips can be substituted (Fig. 3.23). The irrigation portion is frequently used; however, the aspiration unit becomes easily clogged with blood clots. It is easier to connect

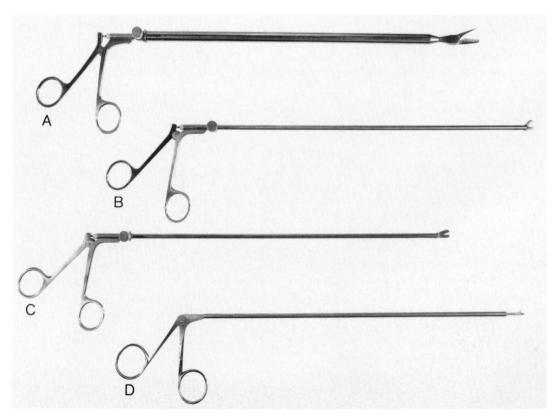

Figure 3.21. Scissors (Storz). *A,* Large 10-mm scissors. *B,* Hook scissors. *C,* Serrated scissors. *D,* Microscissors (Reprinted with permission from Murphy AA: Diagnostic and operative laparoscopy. In: Thompson JD, Rock JA, eds. TeLinde's operative gynecology. Philadelphia: JB Lippincott 1991.)

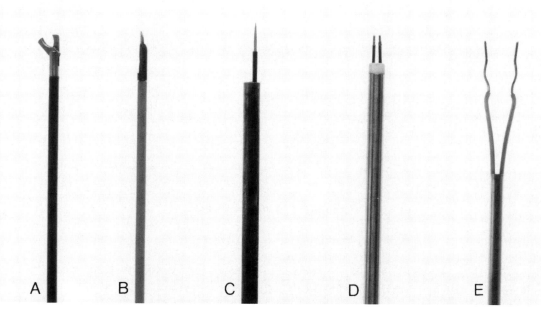

Figure 3.22. Laparoscopic hemostatic instruments. *A*, Scissors with monopolar cautery attachment (Wolf). *B*, Scalpel with monopolar cautery attachment (Wolf). *C*, Microtip monopolar cautery (Cohen cannula or Trident). (Storz) *D*, Microtip bipolar forceps (Storz). *E*, Bipolar paddle forceps or Kleppinger forceps (Storz).

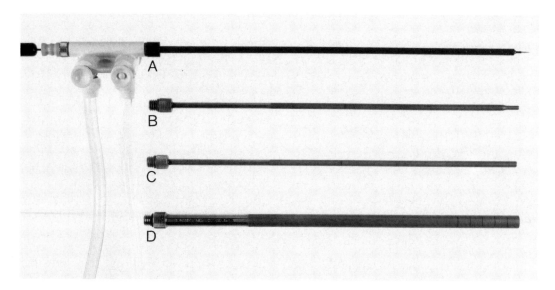

Figure 3.23. Suction/irrigation cannulas (Storz). *A*, Microtip monopolar cautery attachment. *B*, Fine cannula. *C*, Medium cannula. *D*, Large cannula.

the aspiration tubing directly to wall suction. The aspiration portion of the handle can be connected to a bag of intravenous fluid wrapped in a blood pressure cuff to increase the pressure needed for rapid fluid delivery. Marshburn and Hulka (20) recently described an irrigator-aspirator system that may be as-sembled from common operating room supplies.

MORCELLATOR

The morcellator or tissue punch device works by cutting the tissue in small pieces with it's "biting" end and storing the pieces in the

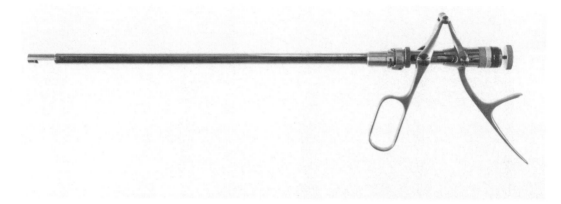

Figure 3.24. Morcellator (Wisap).

sheath (Fig. 3.24). Large pieces of tissue such as myomas and ovaries can be removed in this manner. It is quite cumbersome and very tiring (30,32). It works best when the tissue is held securely with two instruments and the morcellator "bites" are placed in between. Singly held tissue tends to escape as the instrument is closed. Alternatively, the tissue may be cut into smaller pieces and removed through the laparoscopic sleeve. Specimens may also be removed via a small suprapubic incision or a colpotomy incision. Transvaginal or intraabdominal colpotomy is performed in the standard fashion. This will obviously need to be the last step of the procedure because the pneumoperitoneum will be lost.

HEMOSTATIC INSTRUMENTS

The method selected to achieve hemostasis depends on instrument availability, type of proposed surgical procedure, and most commonly on physician preference. This section will be limited to electrosurgical and thermocoagulating instruments. The laser will be discussed separately.

Many instruments can be combined with unipolar cautery, most commonly scissors, scalpels, and point coagulators (Fig. 3.22). The Trident or Cohen Cannula (Karl Storz Endoscopy-America, Inc.) is a combination point coagulator and irrigation instrument. It was designed to facilitate localization and coagulation of bleeding points. However, its fine needle point is very useful for fine dissection when combined with cutting current. It is the laparoscopic version of the needle tip cautery used for many years in microsurgical laparotomies.

The bipolar instruments carry the current from the generator and back. The tissue between the jaws completes the circuit. The bipolar paddles were first used for sterilization. Its use has been generalized and is now widely used to achieve hemostasis during operative cases. Microbipolar forceps can be used for more precise coagulation; however, the only available model cannot be used as a forceps, since the two jaws do not meet. Both cutting and coagulating current can be dispensed through these instruments. As previously seen, the power density achieved is lower with coagulating current than with cutting. It is important to know the difference since the power density in the coagulating mode is insufficient to drive the electrons through an already coagulated tubal muscularis into the endosalpinx. Tubal destruction can be achieved with the bipolar set at the cutting mode (25 W). Not only is it important for sterilization purposes but for partial salpingectomy as well.

It is essential that the cutting current be adjusted by the surgeon and that only the surgeon activate the current. The entire uninsulated tip of the instrument must be kept in view while the current is activated. The lateral spread of current may result in tissue damage. The complications inherent in electrocautery are well known, as are the means for preventing most of these accidents. With knowledge of its limitations, electrocautery can be a valuable, safe, and inexpensive hemostatic method.

Thermocoagulation is an alternative to electrocautery (Fig. 3.25). This system does not use electricity to heat the tissue. Rather, it uses electricity to heat the metal inside the instrument, which in turn delivers the heat. The desired coagulation temperature can be preselected in the range of 20–260°. Generally, 90–120° is necessary to achieve hemostasis. Three instruments may be used with this unit. The crocodile forceps was developed as a means of sterilization and is a jawed, Kleppinger-type instrument. The point coagulator is useful for coagulation of endometriosis and point coagulation; however, the point is fairly large and difficult to use for fine microsurgical work. The myoma enucleator is best suited for resection of intramural myomas. The flat blade-like instrument can be used to dissect and coagulate bleeding points (28,29,31).

Several methods of coagulation for the purpose of tubal sterilization were compared by Riedel et al. (26). The modalities studied included unipolar and bipolar high-frequency current, CO_2 laser, and thermocoagulation. The greatest tissue destruction surrounding the coagulated tissue was found following unipolar coagulation. Decreasing amounts of peripheral destruction were seen with bipolar cautery, thermocoagulation, and CO_2, in that order.

Ridel subsequently demonstrated that the surgeon's experience did not correlate with the extent of coagulation injury, but correlated quite well with the maximum temperature reached in the tissues as well as the coagulation time (25). Murphy et al. (23) subsequently analyzed inflammation and adhesion formation in rat uteri after a standardized incision, with subsequent hemostasis effected by each of the four modalities discussed above. They found significantly less macroscopic adhesive disease following laser treatment, as compared with electrocautery. However, there was no difference between laser and thermocoagulation. Microscopic adhesions, a reflection of periuterine adhesive disease, were not significantly different among groups. Lastly, there was no significant difference in acute or chronic inflammation between the four groups.

Hysteroscopy

INSUFFLATOR

Carbon dioxide is an excellent distention media for hysteroscopy. It is very popular for use in office hysteroscopy. Laparoscopic insufflators should never be used for hysteroscopy, as the maximum flow of CO_2 for hysteroscopy

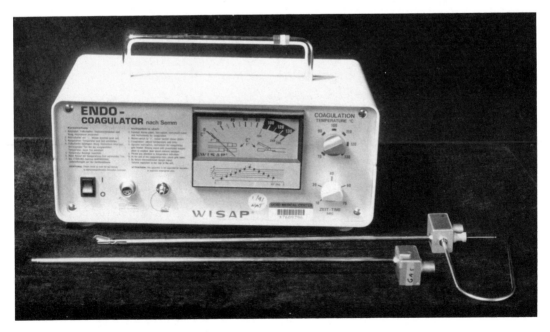

Figure 3.25. Thermocoagulation (Endocoagulator R, Wisap Co.). *A*, Front instrument—point coagulator. *B*, Back—crocodile forceps with hinged upper jaw.

is 100 ml/min (1). Several hysteroscopic insufflators are available, some of which include a vacuum pump for maintaining a cervical suction cannula in place during the procedure. We have not found this to be particularly helpful.

SHEATHS

The telescope must be fitted into a sheath through which the distention media can be infused in order to obtain the necessary distention for panoramic view. The smallest diameter hysteroscope with good optics is 4 mm, and the smallest sheath that fits it is 5 mm. The diagnostic sheaths usually have only one stopcock.

Operative sheaths range from 7–8 mm in outer diameter, while diagnostic hysteroscopes are 4 mm (Fig. 3.26). The most common design consists of an operating channel mounted on the posterior surface, which is fitted with a stopcock and feeds into the common channel. The operating channel needs to be fitted with a rubber gasket to prevent loss of medium. Two stopcocks are placed on either side for the installation of media. Since both stopcocks feed into a common channel, one cannot flush the cavity by opening one. A recently available design provides four isolated channels for the telescope, medium installation, and two operating channels. With this system, the surgeon may flush or aspirate and maintain a telescope and instrument in situ through the other channels. Some sheaths are fitted with a deflector that is manually operated. The deflector is used to angulate flexible instruments or fibers (1).

The urologic resectoscope can be adapted for hysteroscopy (Fig. 3.27). The specialized operating sheath accepts a loop capable of being manipulated forwards and backwards. Unipolar cautery provides coagulating or cutting current. The telescope fits into and locks on the sheath and provides a panoramic view. When manipulated forward, it comes into view but is otherwise retracted. The accessory electrodes include a straightforward loop, a right angle loop, and a loop with a roller ball on the end. The first two accesories are used for resection of uterine septa or myoma. The roller ball is used for endometrial ablation. The recommended media for this instrument is dextran 70 or glycine.

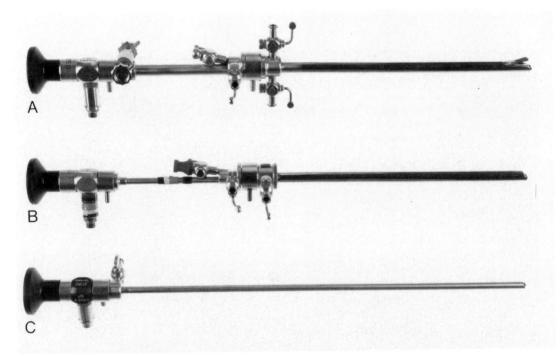

Figure 3.26. Hysteroscopes (Storz). *A*, Operating hysteroscope with deflector. *B*, Operating hysteroscope. *C*, Diagnostic hysteroscope.

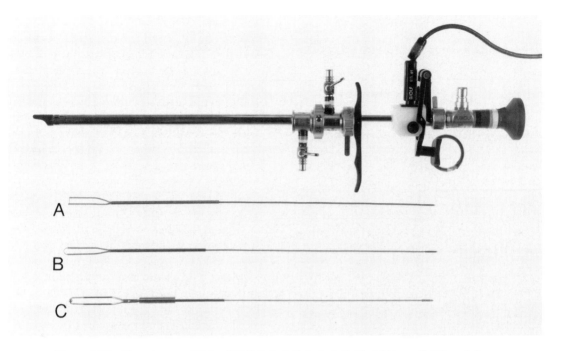

Figure 3.27.   Resectoscope (Richard Wolf Co.). *A*, Rollerball. *B*, Straight loop. *C*, 90° angle loop.

HYSTEROSCOPIC INSTRUMENTS

Various tools for hysteroscopic surgery have been designed and are available in flexible, semirigid, or rigid form (2,38). The flexible and semirigid instruments slide through the operating channel, while the rigid instruments are permanently incorporated into the sheath. The telescope looks through the interior of the rigid operating sheath which is permanently attached to the operating instrument, usually a scissor. Unfortunately, the instrument is at a fixed distance, which is very close to the end of the telescope. The flexible and semirigid instruments have the advantage that they may be pulled out to permit a panoramic view or manipulated for close-up work. The instrument is independent of the telescope.

The flexible instruments are very fragile and difficult to use except with very filmy adhesions and fairly thin septa. The deflectors can be used to try to manipulate the instruments. The semirigid instruments are less delicate and much easier to manipulate (Fig. 3.28). Semirigid scissors are much more suitable for cutting septa, myoma stalk, and dense synechia. Grasping forceps (alligator) and biopsy forceps are also available. Unfortunately, the biopsy forceps are not large enough to obtain a reasonably sized biopsy. Flexible fiber lasers, needles, and aspirators can also be placed through the instrument ports. Lasers are discussed elsewhere. Long needles can be placed to manipulate as well as inject vasoactive solutions. Aspirating cannula are usually 2.0-mm plastic tubing used to flush the cavity and remove blood and debris. It is, however, difficult to find long tubing. Recently, a cannula for hysteroscopic aspiration has been manufactured (Cook Corp., Spencer, IN). The terminal portion of the cannula is marked for measurement and has additional side ports for aspiration. The other end has a Luer-lock fitting that easily attaches to the syringe.

Needle and Suture

Much attention has been given to the effect of adhesion formation between different tissues postoperatively, and to the deleterious effect these adhesions have on fertility. It is generally accepted that the amount of suture material should be kept to a minimum. Riddick (24) has shown that most adhesions in the animal model occur at the site of the surgical knot. The selection of needle and suture type is therefore

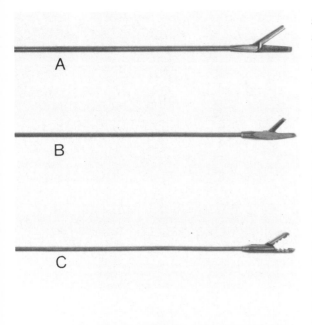

Figure 3.28. Semirigid hysteroscopic instruments (Storz). *A*, Scissors.*B*, Biopsy forceps. *C*, Graspers.

based on "microsurgical" principles with attention to avoidance of tissue trauma and distortion to thereby minimize adhesion formation.

The importance of needle type and suture material has been much debated. Generally, microsurgical needles are curved with a wire diameter of 75 u–14 u and a total length of 4–6 mm, with a chord length of 3–5 mm. This is the smallest size that is useful in gynecologic microsurgery. The most common curve is a 3/8 or 105–135° arc. This provides ease of placement by maintaining the proper axis. Needles may also be obtained in a half-circle or 180°. Taper points are generally held to be less traumatic than cutting and are generally used on the fallopian tube muscularis, but the latter may be more useful for the ovarian capsule.

Microsurgical procedures are generally accomplished using suture sizes between 6-0 and 9-0 gauge. Although some have advised the use of 10-0 for anastomosis, it is questionable whether this smaller diameter offers a discernible advantage. The tensile strength of 10-0 or smaller is such that too much time is spent on replacing broken suture. Interestingly, tensile strength drops off rapidly with decreasing gauge but differs between suture material of the same gauge. 8-0 nylon has twice the break strength of 8-0 polygalactic acid suture. Braided suture such as polygalactic acid, however, is easier to tie because it is more pliable than monofilament suture such as nylon. We usually have a variety of suture gauges available for anastomosis.

The choice of whether to choose a permanent or resorbable suture was quite controversial 15 years ago. The bulk of the evidence presently suggests that pregnancy rates in humans do not differ enough to identify either suture type as superior. Animal data suggest that the absorbable sutures have much less tissue reaction if any at 80 days. Delbeke (6) studied the histologic reaction to nylon, polypropylene, polyglactin, and polydioxanone microsutures in the uterine horn of the rabbit. The first two are permanent, while the other two are absorbable. Only the polyglactin is a braided suture; the other three are monofilament. At 24 days, a marked infiltration of histiocytes was seen around the nylon, polypropylene, and polydioxanone microsutures, whereas the polyglactin was characterized by giant cells. At 80 days, the polydioxanone was almost entirely gone, and the reaction to polyglactin was minimal. Moderate histiocytic infiltration persisted around the nylon and polypropylene. Fibrosis was detected around the latter two but not around polydioxanone or polyglactin.

The variety of suture presently available for use through the laparoscope is meager. Presently, for intraabdominal suturing, only a 4-0 polydioxanone and 4-0 polygalactic is available on a swaged ST-4 straight needle. Other sutures or curved needles can be used if placed through a 10-11-mm puncture site. The technique for intraabdominal suturing was described earlier.

The loop ligature or Endoloop (Ethicon, Somerville, NJ) is a modification of the Roeder loop used for tonsillectomy (Fig. 3.29). This is presently available as 0-chromic or 4-0 plain. The ligature has a preformed "fisherman's knot" that can be tightened using the plastic guide (32). The ligature is loaded onto the applicator by inserting the top end through the bottom of the applicator and by carefully pulling the preformed knot so it does not protrude from the applicator. It is then placed

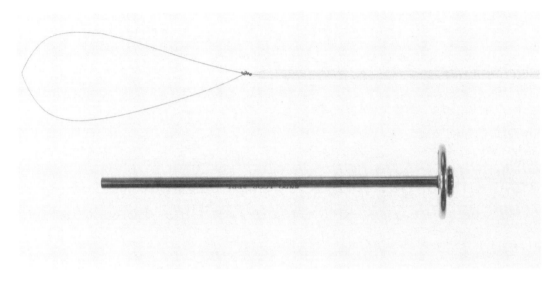

Figure 3.29.   Loop ligature and applicator (Ethicon).

through a 5-mm cannula. The loop is placed around the structure to be excised. The knot guide or forcep can be used to manipulate the loop. The free end of the suture traverses the plastic guide and is embedded into a plastic endpiece. The end is bent so that the plastic guide may be used to push the knot down and close the loop. This sets the knot. Hay (15) suggests that the knot be set in one or, at most, two smooth motions because more manipulation decreases the knot strength significantly. Usually, two to three knots are placed when excising adnexa. Additionally, the suture may be brought outside the abdomen and a "fisherman's slipknot" made. A metal or plastic guide can then be used to close the loop. There have been no clinical studies to assess the uses of different suture material or application technique in the laparoscopy setting. In the final analysis, good surgical judgment and skill are more important than the choice of instrument or method of hemostasis.

References

1. Baggish MS: Instrumentation for hysteroscopy. In: Baggish MS., Barbot J, Valle RF, eds. Diagnostic and operative hysteroscopy. Chicago: Year Book Medical Publishers. 1989;50–57.
2. Baggish MS, Valle RF: Accessory instruments for operative hysteroscopy. In: Baggish MS, Barbot J, Valle RF, eds. Diagnostic and operative hysteroscopy. Chicago: Year Book Medical Publishers, 1989;66–73.
3. Corson SC: Operating room preparation and basic techniques. In: Phillips JM, ed. Laparoscopy. Baltimore: Williams & Wilkins, 1977;86–102.
4. Corson SL: Microsurgical instruments, suture and magnification systems. In: DeCherney AH, Dolan ML, eds. Reproductive surgery. Chicago: Year Book Medical Publishers, 1987;96–114.
5. Corson SL, Smith DC: Principles and instrumentation of microsurgery. Clin Obstet Gynecol 1980;23: 1201.
6. Delbeke LO, Gomel V, McComb PF, et al: Histologic reaction to four synthetic microsutures in the rabbit. Fertil Steril 1983;40:248.
7. Ellis H, Harrison W, Hugh TB: The healing of peritoneum under normal and pathological conditions. Br J Surg 1965;52:471.
8. Ellis H: The cause and prevention of postoperative intraperitoneal adhesions. Surg Obstet Gynecol 1971;133:502.
9. Gardner FM: Optical principles of the endoscope. In: Baggish MS, Barbot J, Valle RF, eds. Diagnostic and operative hysteroscopy. Chicago: Year Book Medical Publishers, 1989;50–57.
10. Gardner FM: Optical physics with emphasis on endoscopes. In: Baggish MS, ed. Clinical obstetrics and gynecology, Vol. 26. Philadelphia: Harper & Row, 1983;p 213.
11. Gomel V: Tubal reanastomosis by microsurgery. Fertil Steril 1977b;28:59.
12. Gomel V, Taylor PJ: The technique of endoscopy. In: Gomel V, Taylor PJ, Yuzpe AA, Rioux JE, eds. Laparoscopy and hysteroscopy in gynecological practice. Chicago: Year Book Medical Publishers, 1986;32.
13. Hasson HM: Ovarian surgery. In: Sanfilippo JS, Levine RL, eds. Operative gynecologic endoscopy. New York: Springer-Verlag 1989;pp 86–106.
14. Hasson HM: Multipronged laparoscopic forceps. J Reprod Med 1976;16:167–170.

15. Hay DL, Levine RL, Von Fraunhofer JA, et al: The effect of the number of pulls on the tensile strength of the chromic gut pelviscopic loop ligature. J Reprod Med, in press.

16. Hopkins HH: Optical principles of the endoscope. In: Berci B, ed. Endoscopy. New York: Appleton-Century-Crofts, 1973.

17. Jacobson JH, Miller DB, Suarez E: Microvascular surgery: a new horizon in coronary artery surgery. Circulation 1960;22:767.

18. Leventhal JM: Techniques. In: Sanfilippo JS, Levine RL, eds. Operative gynecologic endoscopy. New York: Springer-Verlag. 1989;38–56.

19. Levine RL: Instrumentation. In: Sanfilippo JS, Levine RL, eds. Operative gynecologic endoscopy. New York: Springer-Verlag, 1989;19–37.

20. Marshburn PB, Hulka JF: A simple irrigator-aspirator cannula for laparoscopy: the Stewart system. Ob Gyn 1990;75:458.

21. Murphy AA: Operative laparoscopy. Fertil Steril 1987;47:6.

22. Murphy AA: Diagnostic and operative laparoscopy. In: Thompson JD, Rock JA, eds. TeLinde's operative gynecology. Philadelphia: JB Lippincott (in press).

23. Murphy AA, Leake JF, Bobbie DL, et al: A comparison of modalities of hemostasis on inflammation and adhesion formation. Abstract American Fertility Society 44th Annual Meeting Atlanta GA, 1988.

24. Riddick DH, DeGrazia CT, Maenza RM: Comparison of polyglactic and polyglycolic acid sutures in reproductive tissue. Fertil Steril 1977;28: 1220.

25. Riedel HH, Cordts-Kleinwordt G, Semm K: Endocrine findings in rabbits after sterilization. J Reprod Med 1982;27:261.

26. Riedel HH, Semm K: An initial comparison of coagulation techniques in rabbits after sterilization with electrocoagulation. J Reprod Med 1983;28: 665.

27. Rock JA, Bergquist CA, Kimball AW, et al: Comparison of the operating microscope and loope for microsurgical tubal anastomosis: a randomized clinical trial. Fertil Steril 1984;41:229.

28. Roseff SJ, Murphy AA: Pelviscopy. In: Martin DC, Holtz M, Wenoff M, eds. Manual of endoscopy. Santa Fe Springs, New Mexico: American Association of Gynecologic Laparoscopy, 1990;101–102.

29. Semm K: Endoscopic intra-abdominal surgery. Kiel: Kurt Semm, 1983;10–13.

30. Semm K: Friedrich ER, ed. Operative manual for endoscopic abdominal surgery. Chicago: Year Book Medical Publishers, 1987;312.

31. Semm K: Endocoagulation: a new field of endoscopic surgery. J Reprod Med 1976;16:4.

32. Semm K: Tissue puncher and loop ligation: new aids for surgical-therapeutic pelviscopy (laparoscopy)-endoscopic intra-abdominal surgery. Endoscopy 1978;10:110.

33. Swolin K: Die einwirkung grossen intraperitonealen dosen glukokortikoidauf diebildungvon-postoperativen adhasionen. Acta Obstet Gynecol Scand 1967a;46:119.

34. Swolin, K: 50 Fertiltratsoperatronen, Teil I and II. Acta Obstet Gynecol Scand 1967b;46: 204.

35. Winston RML: Microsurgical reanastomosis of the rabbit oviduct in its functional and pathological sequelae. Br J Obstet Gynaecol 1975;2:513.

36. Winston RML: Microsurgical tubocornual anastomosis for reversal of sterilization. Lancet 1977;1:284.

37. Winston RML: Evaluating instrumentation for gynecological microsurgery. Contemp Obstet Gynecol 1980a;15:153.

38. Yuzpe AA, Gomel V, Taylor PJ, et al: Instruments for laparoscopy and hysteroscopy. In: Gomel V, Taylor PJ, Yuzpe AA, Rioux JE, eds. Laparoscopy and hysteroscopy in gynecologic practice. Chicago: Year Book Medical Publishers, 1986;7.

LASERS IN GYNECOLOGIC RECONSTRUCTIVE SURGERY

George M. Grunert

INTRODUCTION

Lasers are the latest new surgical tools of the reproductive surgeon. While the appropriate use of these instruments may reduce time, cost, blood loss, and morbidity, lasers themselves do not determine the results of surgery. The primary determinant of success remains the disease process itself.

In this chapter, I will review the basic principles of lasers, laser-tissue interaction, and the effects of laser light on tissue. I will also outline specific applications of lasers for pelvic reconstructive surgery. By necessity, this is a brief overview and introduction to lasers and laser surgery. Prior to clinical application, the reproductive surgeon must have training and supervised experience in the use of these instruments.

LASER PHYSICS

Bohr, in 1900, described what is now accepted as the basic structure of the atom: a central nucleus composed of protons and neutrons, surrounded by an orbital array of electrons (Fig. 4.1A). He theorized that when an atom absorbs the appropriate quantity of energy (a "quantum"), an electron is shifted from a stable ground state to an excited state at which it is temporarily stable. (Fig. 4.1B) The electron must receive the exact quantum of energy to raise it to its energized state. Some electrons have multiple energy levels, in stair-step fashion. Given sufficient time, the electron will eventually decay back to its ground state, resulting in the release of its stored quantum of energy, a process termed spontaneous emission (Fig. 4.1C).

By using Bohr's law: $V = h (E_2 - E_1)$ (where V = the wavelength of light, h = Planck's constant, and $(E_2 - E_1)$ = the quantity of energy stored), one can determine the wavelength of light that corresponds to a quantum of energy, and vice versa.

In 1917, Einstein proposed the theory of stimulated emission of radiation: if an excited electron is struck by a photon of light whose wavelength corresponds to the quantum of energy stored, the electron can be stimulated to release its energy in the form of a second photon which is identical to and in phase with the first photon (Fig. 4.1D) With reference to the first photon, there has been light amplification by the stimulated emission of radiation (LASER). The first practical operational laser (actually a maser, producing microwave amplification) was designed by Townes in 1953, and constructed in 1954 (54). Maiman built the first ruby laser in 1960 (38). A virtual cascade of lasers followed: the helium-neon (HeNe) in 1961, the carbon dioxide (CO_2) and neodymium:yttrium-aluminum-garnet (Nd:YAG) in 1964, and the argon in 1965.

Lasers transfer energy (electrical, light, chemical, or radio-frequency) from an external power source to the electrons of a target substance (the laser medium). This results in a population of excited electrons (a metastable

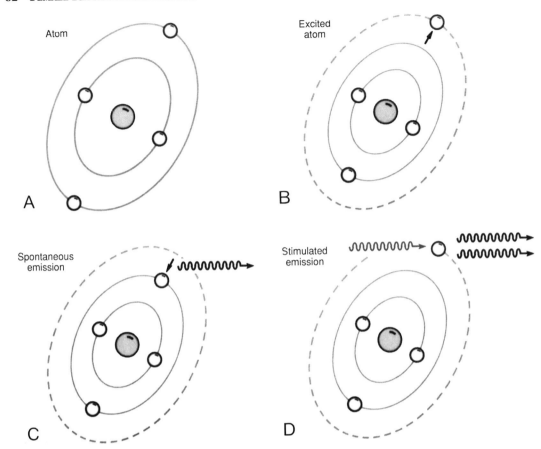

Figure 4.1. *A,* Atoms are composed of a central nucleus surrounded by orbiting electrons. *B,* Energy absorbed by atoms is stored in the electron orbital system. *C,* When an energized electron returns to its ground state, the stored energy is released (spontaneous emission) in the form of a photon. *D,* If a photon of the appropriate energy level strikes the energized electron, the stored energy is released by stimulated emission.

population inversion). Spontaneous emission of radiation from some of the electrons begins a chain reaction of stimulated emission. In lasers using a gas medium (such as the CO_2 or argon lasers), the medium is contained within a sealed chamber. The ends of the chamber are mirrored to promote the propagation of a beam parallel to its long axis. One of the mirrors is partially silvered, allowing some of the beam to be released. The light generated is guided to and focused on the target. The laser light generated is monochromatic (of one frequency) and collimated (in phase and parallel). Monochromatic, collimated light (called coherent light) can be transmitted over long distances without divergence or loss of power.

The electron system used to generate the light determines the energy characteristics and wavelength of the beam. Lasers can be de-

scribed by naming the laser medium, output wavelength, or energy level. As noted above in the discussion of Bohr's law, the terms are interchangeable.

SURGICALLY USEFUL LASERS

Carbon Dioxide

The carbon-dioxide (CO_2) laser emits a beam in the infrared portion of the light spectrum. (Fig. 4.2) The CO_2 laser wavelength is preferentially absorbed by water. (Fig. 4.3) If the energy delivered to the target exceeds the ability of the tissue to absorb and dissipate it, intracellular water is turned into steam, resulting in cellular rupture. The steam, at 100° C, denatures cellular proteins. At lower power levels, the primary effect of this laser is tissue

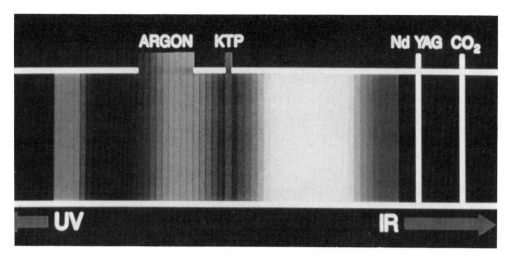

Figure 4.2. Lasers emit light in or near the visible spectrum. The Argon and KTP/532 laser beams are visible, while the Nd:YAG and CO_2 laser are in the invisible, infrared portion of the spectrum.

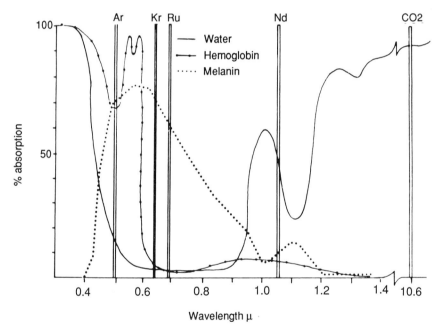

Figure 4.3. The Argon (Ar) laser is preferentially absorbed by hemoglobin and melanin. The KTP/532 laser absorption is similar. The Nd:YAG (Nd) is poorly absorbed by water and pigment, but diffusely absorbed by protein. The CO_2 laser is almost completely absorbed by water. The Krypton (Kr) and Ruby (Ru) lasers are useful for pigmented or melanin-containing lesions.

heating and coagulation. As the power increases, a "blend" of coagulation and vaporization is noted. At high power output, the effect is primarily vaporization with minimal coagulation.

The impact site of a CO_2 laser shows a central area of vaporization surrounded by an area of thermal necrosis 100–200 μm (0.1–0.2 mm) thick, and an outer area of thermal effect 200–400 μm thick (3,6). Cells in the area of thermal necrosis are destroyed, while those in the thermal effect area are edematous but will recover. Small vessels (less than 1–2 mm diameter) are sealed in the area of thermal effect by the swelling of endothelial capillary cells and the external compression of tissue edema. The

microscopic appearance and healing characteristics of this wound are similar to a clean scalpel
incision. The CO_2 laser has been used for all
applications, but is most applicable to adhesolysis, tuboplasty, and procedures requiring fine
incisions or vaporization.

Neodymium:YAG Laser

The Nd:YAG laser uses a synthetic yttrium-
aluminum-garnet crystal doped with neodymium. Although commonly (and technically
incorrectly) referred to as the "YAG" laser, it is
the neodymium that is the laser medium. The
light produced is in the infrared portion of the
spectrum at 1320 and 1064 nm. Commonly,
the 1320 nm beam is filtered and the 1064 nm
beam used. This laser is diffusely absorbed by
tissue proteins and may have wide lateral spread
from the impact site. Unless precisely focused,
the Nd:YAG laser produces diffuse tissue
heating and coagulation.

Examination of the impact site for the
Nd:YAG laser demonstrates central coagulation necrosis without vaporization. The surrounding tissue injury may extend as much as
4–6 mm lateral and deep to the center of the
impact. While focusing the beam may increase
vaporization and decrease local damage, this
laser is primarily used in cases where widespread tissue destruction is desired. As described below, the beam can be focused by
attaching sapphire tips or shaped fibers to the
laser. In this fashion, it is possible to achieve a
mixture of vaporization and coagulation. The
most common use for this laser has been
photocoagulation of the endometrium for
treatment of menorrhagia.

Argon Laser

The Argon laser is a gas-medium laser that
produces multiple wavelengths throughout the
visible spectrum. In the blue-green portion of
the spectrum, the major wavelengths at 488
and 514 nm are utilized because of their
absorption by hemoglobin. This wavelength is
also absorbed by pigmented tissues, but passes
through water and colorless tissues (such as
peritoneum) without significant absorption.

The Argon laser produces a lesion whose
appearance is intermediate between that seen
with the CO_2 and Nd:YAG lasers. There is
central vaporization with surrounding edema
and tissue injury extending to 0.3–1 mm from
the impact. This laser is best utilized for
incision and vaporization of tissues where
surrounding thermal injury is not harmful.
Clinical applications include vaporization and
excision of endometriosis, myomectomy, metroplasty, and salpingotomy for ectopic pregnancy.

KTP/532 Laser

Close in wavelength and similar in effect to
the Argos laser is the KTP/532 laser, which
produces a green beam at 532 nm. The
KTP/532 laser is actually a Nd:YAG laser
whose 1064 nm beam is passed through a
potassium-titanyl-phosphate crystal that halves
its wavelength to 532 nm. The tissue effect and
clinical application of this laser are similar to
that described above for the Argon laser.

Helium-Neon Laser

Because the CO_2 and Nd:YAG lasers are
invisible, they are coupled with a visible laser,
such as the helium-neon (HeNe) laser, which
serves as an "aiming beam." The output of the
HeNe laser is in the red portion of the visible
spectrum. The HeNe laser is employed at an
extremely low power output and exerts no
apparent tissue effect by itself.

Other Lasers

Other lasers, currently under investigation
for surgical use, include minor wavelengths of
the Argon and Nd:YAG lasers, tuneable dye
lasers, free-electron lasers, and the gold-vapor
and copper-vapor lasers. The application of
these lasers depends on their output wavelength and the absorption of this wavelength by
specific tissues.

LASER INSTRUMENTATION

All wavelengths can be transmitted from the
laser to the tissue by reflecting the light along a
series of mirrors. To prevent accidental reflection, the beam and the mirrors are contained in
hollow tubes, forming an articulated arm. After
leaving the arm, lenses focus the light on a

specific area. The CO_2 laser is used almost exclusively in this fashion.

Laser light can also be passed through a quartz fiber that can then be directed to the target. Fibers with diameters of 200, 300, 600, and 800 μm are available for the Argon, Nd:YAG, and KTP/532 lasers. Fibers with shaped tips (tapered for cutting, blunted for coagulation) are available. Sapphire tips can be attached to fibers for the Nd:YAG laser and are available in a variety of shapes and sizes. Although fibers are more compact and maneuverable than an articulated arm system, up to 25% of the output is lost in the fiber. When the beam leaves the tip of the fiber, it diverges so that the area of application increases as the fiber is moved away from the tissue, resulting in a rapid decrease in power density. Fibers for the CO_2 laser have proven to be too cumbersome for practical use. A rigid waveguide that confines the beam in a small straight tube has been developed for the CO_2 laser.

To prevent destruction of fibers, they must be cooled by passing gas or water coaxially or by using the fiber under water. Some fibers are constructed to be used in contact with the tissue while others will burn when touched to tissue. The molded-tip fibers and sapphire tips must be used in contact with tissue. Using the wrong fiber or tip in the wrong way can lead to breakage.

For macrosurgical work, the beam from an articulated arm is passed through a handpiece containing a focusing lens. Handpieces are also available to hold laser fibers. Microsurgery can be performed by using a hand-held laser with the operating microscope. More commonly, the laser is fixed to the microscope and directed to the surgical field by reflecting the beam off of a mirror attached to a joystick. Movement of the joystick moves the beam around the field. The microscope adapter gives the surgeon a stable platform from which to control the laser beam, improving the precision of application.

Laser light can be directed through the operating channel of the laparoscope by attaching the articulated arm to a coupling device. The device aligns the beam so that it passes through the channel without reflecting from the sides. Similarly, the beam can be focused through a hollow second puncture probe. Laser fibers and waveguides can be passed through the laparoscope or through the second puncture site. Because laser vaporization generates smoke, rapid CO_2 insufflation and evacuation systems are employed. When the beam is brought through the laparoscope, gas is passed down the operating channel with the beam. This blows the laser plume out of the way, preventing fogging of the laparoscope lens, and cools the tissue adjacent to the target. Some surgeons have been enthusiastic about the combination of laser laparoscopy and the use of video cameras attached to the laparoscope. This allows the surgeon to operate from a television screen and lets the assistants view the procedure. There is no evidence that this combination improves the results of surgery.

Although the CO_2 laser has been used in hysteroscopy, fiber systems are more commonly employed. The flexible fiber is passed through the operating channel of the hysteroscope and can be moved within the uterine cavity by means of a deflecting albarran. Hyskon or crystalloid solutions are used for uterine distension at laser hysteroscopy. CO_2 should not be used for distension for hysteroscopic laser procedures because of the risk of gas embolism.

To prevent inadvertent injury to tissue deep to the target, it is necessary to stop or attenuate the beam. The tissue itself can be used if depth of penetration is not hazardous. For the CO_2 laser, water stops the beam so that wet tissue or fluid in the cul-de-sac can be used as a backstop. Quartz or burnished metal rods are used in situations where the beam must be stopped rapidly (Fig. 4.4). Because the beam from a quartz fiber diverges rapidly as it leaves the end of the fiber, a backstop is usually not necessary.

A feature unique to laser surgery is the ability to reflect the beam off of a mirror to an inaccessible site, such as the undersurface of the ovary. Front-surfaced mirrors are employed so that the beam does not have to pass through the glass of the mirror. Even with this, mirrors used with high poser-density beams are subject to heating, resulting in pitting or shattering of the glass. To prevent "unintentional mirror surgery," instruments in the operative field should be dulled.

The laser is most commonly triggered by using a foot switch. In the continuous wave mode, the laser emits energy whenever the switch is depressed. Single or repeat pulse

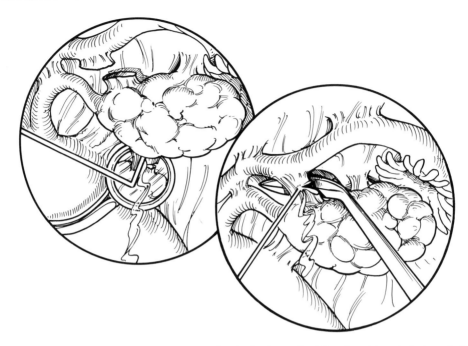

Figure 4.4. To prevent injury from the beam, a nonreflective backstop should be placed deep to the laser incision line (*right*). Laser beams can be transmitted to targets that are not directly accessible by focusing the target in a mirror and reflecting the beam off the mirror (*left*).

modes are available, where a pulse of predetermined duration is emitted either once or in a repeated fashion. The CO_2 laser can also utilize a super-pulse mode whereby short pulses (1000–500 microsecond duration) are released in rapid sequence (200–500 pulses per second). Although the average output is equivalent to the continuous wave mode, the instantaneous peaks may exceed the average 100-fold.

POWER DENSITY

There are three primary determinants of the effect of laser light: the absorption characteristics of the tissue, the wavelength of the laser, and the power output of the laser. The characteristics of the target tissue are fixed and must be known to the surgeon. Unless one is using a laser whose output can be varied, a laser whose output is absorbed by the tissue must be selected for use. Depending on the energy delivered, the tissue can be heated, coagulated, or vaporized. Power density is the power delivered by the laser divided by the area of application, and is expressed as watts per cm.^{2} Every time the laser is used, the power density must be determined to ensure that the desired tissue effect will be achieved.

Because the power density is inversely proportional to the square of the area of application ("spot size"), the power density can be controlled by varying the spot size. This is more efficient than changing the output of the laser.

For the CO_2 laser, power densities below 1000 W/cm^2 cause tissue heating with little vaporization. Increasing the power density results in increased vaporization and decreased coagulation. Because the coagulation of tissue seals small blood vessels, high-power density levels should be used only when hemostasis is not necessary. Colposcopically mounted lasers are used in the range of 500–5000 W/cm,^{2} laparoscopic lasers at 5000–20000 W/cm,^{2} and microscopic lasers above 20000 W/cm^2.

LASER SAFETY

Education, experience, and common sense are necessary for the safe use of lasers. Credentialing for laser surgery is regulated by individual institutions, as is the case for any surgical procedure. Unlike other instruments, however, lasers are regulated by a cascade of federal, state, and local governmental agencies. By federal law, the laser surgeon must be familiar with regulatory guidelines established by the American National Standards Institute (ANSI) (2). Protection of workers exposed to laser energy is also regulated by the Occupational Safety and Health Administration (OSHA). Voluntary institutional guidelines for the credentialing of surgeons for laser use in pelvic reconstructive surgery have been proposed by the Society of Reproductive Surgeons of the American Fertility Society. These guidelines include the satisfactory completion of a didactic course in lasers and laser surgery, laboratory laser exercises, and a preceptorship with an accredited laser surgeon.

The same properties of lasers that make them useful (high-power coherent light, transmission of energy over long distances) also present the potential for inadvertent injury. For the CO_2 laser, the alignment of the aiming beam and laser should be tested each time the laser is used. Because the laser travels in a straight line once it leaves the delivery system, it must have a clear path to the target. The laser must never be fired if the aiming beam cannot be seen. This is especially important in laparoscopy, where the beam is parallel to but separate from the visible path. It is possible to see a lesion while the path from the laser to the lesion is obstructed by another structure. Special care must be taken at laparoscopy to visualize the beam path after it passes through the target and stop or attenuate if necessary.

The eye is an effective light-gathering device that can precisely focus even low levels of laser energy on the retina, causing damage. To prevent injury from an unintentional reflection, protective eyewear should be used by all operating-room (OR) personnel, and should be placed on the patient. For the CO_2 laser, plastic or glass wraparound glasses are sufficient; however, contact lenses are not protective. Laparoscopic or microscopic elements are sufficient protection for the surgeon. Endoscopic cases done under video camera direction where the camera completely covers the eyepiece do not require eye protection.

The shorter wavelength lasers require goggles or glasses whose lenses are specifically designed to block their output. These lenses are wavelength-specific: glasses for the Nd:YAG laser are not protective against Argon laser light. For microscopic or endoscopic applications, protective lenses can be placed over the eyepieces. Some models have shutters that move a filter over the endoscope lens each time the laser is triggered. The operating room windows should be covered, and signs should be placed in and outside the room warning of the danger of invisible laser light. Additional glasses or goggles should be placed outside the OR door so that personnel can put them on before entering the room.

Flammable prep solutions and anesthetic gasses should be avoided. Nonflammable drapes should be used. A fire extinguisher or water-filled prep basin should be kept in the room. The laser should be placed in a stand-by mode (disabling the laser foot switch) to prevent accidental firing. The electronic components of the laser are too complicated for the average person to service, and all covering panels should be left in place. Accidental spills onto the power supply must be avoided.

The plume of steam and debris created by cellular vaporization should be evacuated. This clears material from the beam path, which would otherwise absorb and scatter the light. Removal of the plume also helps cool surrounding tissue, preventing injury adjacent to the target. For plume evacuation, a dedicated stand-alone suction system should be used. If the regular OR wall suction is used, a filter specifically designed to remove laser plume particles should be placed in the suction line to prevent accumulation in the central suction system. Although the impact site itself is sterile, viable tumor cells and viral particles have been recovered from the laser plume (20,24).

Although lasers are generally sturdy, reliable pieces of equipment, they are complex and do break down. They have sophisticated internal monitoring systems designs to prevent use when there is a danger of damage to the instrument. When the laser doesn't operate, a self-diagnostic system alerts the user to the problem. If the problem is corrected and the laser still doesn't operate, a service technician should be called.

SURGICAL APPLICATIONS OF LASERS

Initially, medical lasers were used in ophthalmology, otolaryngology, and dermatology. The first description of laser use at laparotomy in gynecology was by Bellina in 1974 (5). Bruhat, (8) Tadir, (53) and Daniell (14) pioneered the development of CO_2 laser laparoscopy instrumentation in the early 1980s. Goldrath adapted the Nd:YAG laser to hysteroscopy in 1981 (21).

Lasers can be useful in any case where incision, excision, or cautery of tissue is performed. The laser should be employed only in procedures the surgeon is capable of doing with conventional instruments. Competence in difficult multiple-puncture operative laparoscopy, operative hysteroscopy, reconstructive surgery, and microsurgery are prerequisites to using a laser in the same operations. The addition of a laser does not make one a reproductive surgeon any more than magnifying the field with a microscope makes one a microsurgeon.

The aims of reconstructive surgery are the restoration of normal anatomy and function, and the relief of symptoms. Laser technology has evolved in parallel with other advances in surgical techniques. It is possible to separate the specific effects of lasers from other developments in surgery. The addition of the laser to microsurgical procedures has not been proven to decrease postoperative adhesions (18), nor has any significant difference been found in postoperative adhesions when laser and electrosurgical techniques have been compared (55,56). There does appear to be a decrease in adhesion formation at laser laparoscopy compared with laparotomy (36).

Rather than review individual procedures described in detail elsewhere in this text, I will describe how lasers can be used to complement reconstructive surgical techniques. Unless specifically noted, the CO_2 laser can be used for all procedures. If a combination of incision and coagulation is indicated, the Argon, KTP/532, or Nd:YAG (with a tapered tip or sapphire focusing tip) can be used. In cases where coagulation is the primary intent (as in photocoagulation of the endometrium), the Nd:YAG laser with a bare fiber or blunt tip is best.

Adhesolysis

Perhaps the premier application of lasers is the lysis and excision of adhesions. Because of the limited lateral spread of laser energy, adhesions can be vaporized along their lines of attachment to pelvic viscera and excised rather than transected. The CO_2 laser, at power densities in excess of 5,000 W/cm² (power output of 10–25 W with a spot size of 0.2–0.5 mm), can be used within 0.2 mm of the serosa of the tube, ovary, or bowel without injury. Avascular adhesions can be incised with either a continuous or superpulse mode (to increase power density). Vessels that are too large to be sealed with the laser are cauterized with bipolar forceps, and then transected. If a backstop is necessary, it should be held beneath, not in contact with, the adhesions, so that the tissue is not "welded" to the backstop. While thin adhesions can be vaporized in a single pass, it is best to move the laser rapidly back and forth over thick adhesions to allow cooling in one area while another is incised.

Traction and countertraction help structures separate as the adhesions are cut. To minimize trauma, fingers or blunt rods are preferred to pickups and clamps. In this fashion, the laser allows for true "no-touch" surgery. Adhesions that are not directly visible can be vaporized by using mirrors. For proper focus of the laser, the laser should be aimed at the image in the mirror. To allow time to assess results when using mirrors, a pulse or repeat-pulse mode is employed.

Some cases requiring extensive adhesolysis can be done through the laparoscope. The deep cul-de-sac is easier to approach at laparscopy than laparotomy. For laser laparoscopic surgery, the surgeon must be able to identify and separate all structures lateral and deep to the impact site to avoid injury. One must avoid vaporizing adhesions that contain vessels not amenable to laparoscopic hemostasis. The Argon, KTP/532, and Nd:YAG (with tapered tip fiber or attached sapphire tip) have been used for adhesolysis by some surgeons (59), but lack the precise control of the CO_2.

Salpingostomy/Fimbrioplasty

Fimbrial adhesions, constriction rings, and peritubal adhesions are treated as described

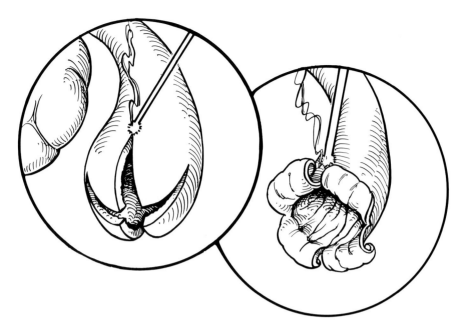

Figure 4.5. The tube is distended with chromotubation fluid, and neosalpingostomy flaps are developed by incision along avascular lines (*left*). Eversion of the flaps is secured by photocoagulating the serosal surface with a defocused (low-power density) beam (*right*). This technique is applicable only for thin-walled hydrosalpinges.

above. In cases of distal tubal occlusion, it is best to operate from the endosalpingeal surface so that fimbrial and salpingeal folds can be identified. A fiberoptic bundle can be attached to the quartz rod backstop to provide transillumination of the tube, helping to identify vessels and cleavage planes.

For salpingostomy, the tube is distended with chromotubation fluid and the distal tube incised along avascular lines. The fluid within the lumen absorbs the CO_2 beam and prevents injury to the endosalpinx. Once the tube is opened, the salpingostomy flaps are developed from the inside of the tube. If the tubal wall is thin, eversion of the flaps is accomplished by using a power density of 100–200 W/cm² (spot size of 5 mm with a poser output of 5–10 W). The beam is rapidly played over the serosal surface of the flaps to produce coagulation and retraction of the serosa. This everts the flaps without the use of sutures (9). In selected cases, where the tubes can be adequately mobilized, this procedure can be done through the laparoscope (Fig. 4.5). Thick-walled tubes are not amenable to this technique and require anchoring sutures.

The prognosis for pregnancy following sur-gery for distal tubal occlusion is related to tubal diameter, wall thickness, endosalpingeal preservation, and associated adhesions, not to the laser (37). Although Kelly reported an improvement in postoperative tubal patency rates with laser salpingostomy, there was no significant change in the chance of pregnancy (28).

The laparoscopic treatment of ectopic pregnancy has been found to be safe and effective (23,27,50,58). Laparoscopy decreases hospital stay, time off work, and expense when compared with laparotomy. Depending on the size and vascularity of the ectopic, it may be helpful to inject the serosa and mesosalpinx with dilute pitressin solution (1 cc in 100 cc diluent). A salpingotomy incision is made with the laser along the antimesosalpingeal border of the tube, over the site of the ectopic. The products of conception are removed from the tube by irrigation or gentle, blunt dissection (Fig. 4.6). Isthmic ectopics can be managed in a similar fashion, or by segmental resection. If bleeding cannot be easily controlled, segmental resection can be performed. All patients with conservative surgery for ectopic pregnancy should be followed with serial postoperative hCG titers.

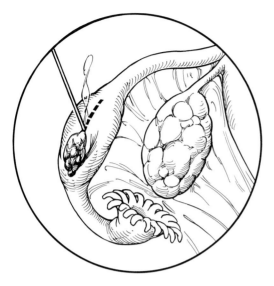

Figure 4.6. Ectopic pregnancies are treated by making a linear salpingotomy incision over the ectopic on the antimesosalpingeal surface of the tube. The products of conception are gently removed by irrigation and counter-pressure on the sides of the tube. Vigorous attempts to remove tissue should be avoided because of the possibility of bleeding.

Tubal Anastomosis

Pathologic occluded tubal segments are excised by transecting the tube with the laser until normal, patent proximal and distal lumens are identified. For reversal of tubal sterilization, preparation of the tubal segments for anastomosis can be done with the CO_2 laser. The hemostatic incision of this beam seals small vessels, decreasing the need for cautery following tubal transection, theoretically decreasing tissue destruction and practically decreasing operative time. If the proximal segment terminates in the isthmus, this section is distended with chromotubation fluid and is rapidly transected, employing a power density above 10,000 W/cm^2 (spot size of 0.2–0.5 mm with a power output of 25–40 W). As with salpingostomy, the fluid in the lumen protects the endosalpinx. For an intramural proximal segment, the laser is used to vaporize myometrium surrounding the tube. Once a normal, patent lumen has been identified, a circumferential ring of myometrium is vaporized to provide a "sewing collar". (Fig. 4.7). If necessary, an obstructed cornual tubal segment can be traced down to the uterine cavity, allowing for a tubouterine anastomosis, a procedure preferable to blind tubal implantation.

If the distal segment begins in the isthmic portion of the tube, the tube is distended by chromotubation through the fimbriated end, and a technique identical to that described for a proximal isthmic segment is used. For anastomosis to a distal ampullary segment, the ampulla is either filled with fluid, or a backstop rod is inserted through the fimbriae to distend the tube and to protect the endosalpinx. A circular incision is made with the laser, matching the size of the incision to the diameter of the proximal lumen. After using fine bipolar cautery to seal any bleeding vessels, anastomosis is performed, as described elsewhere.

Klink (31) reported a technique for tissue welding using the CO_2 laser for tubal anastomosis. Although successful, the laser weld obtained had little tensile strength and required radial sutures for support, negating any advantage over a suture anastomosis.

Ovarian Surgery

Benign ovarian cysts can be excised at laparoscopy (22) or laparotomy by dissecting the cyst lining away from the normal ovarian stroma. The laser can facilitate this dissection (7,46) (Fig. 4.8). Vessels that are not sealed by the laser must be ligated or cauterized before closing the ovarian capsule.

Daniell (15) described a technique for the laparoscopic treatment of polycystic ovaries by puncturing and draining multiple subcapsular cysts with the CO_2 laser. This results in a decrease in intraovarian and circulating androgens and has been associated with the resumption of spontaneous ovulation in the majority of patients treated. Other surgeons have used the shorter wavelength lasers in an additional attempt to coagulate the ovarian stroma surrounding the cysts (25,26,32) (Fig. 4.9).

Endometriosis

Surgery for endometriosis can include any of the techniques described above for adhesolysis, tuboplasty, and ovarian cystectomy. Laser laparoscopic treatment of endometriosis has generated the largest number of studies of any

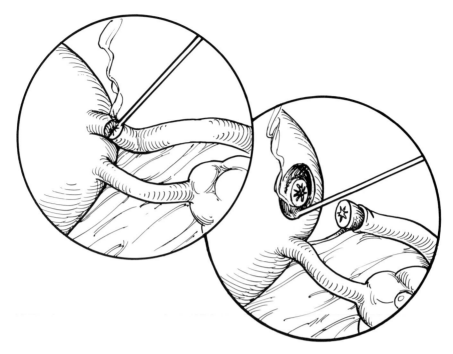

Figure 4.7. Cornual tubal anastomosis can be facilitated by vaporizing a ring of myometrium around the proximal tube.

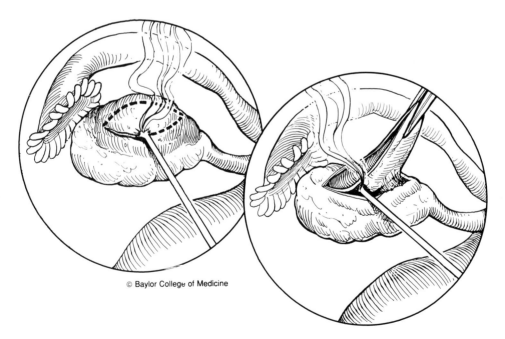

© Baylor College of Medicine

Figure 4.8. Ovarian cysts are excised by incising the ovarian capsule over the cyst (*left*) and dissecting the cyst capsule from the normal ovarian stroma (*right*). If small and hemostatic, the cystectomy site may be left to heal without suture closure.

gynecologic laser procedure (11,16,19,44,47, 48,52). Peritoneal endometriosis can be managed by cautery, vaporization, or excision with any wavelength (Fig. 4.10). Complete vaporization can be assured by the visualization of normal subperitoneal fat at the base of the vaporization site. Implants overlying the lateral

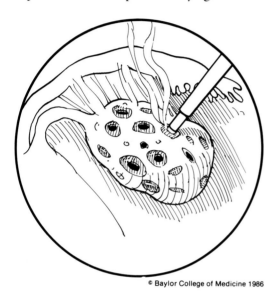

© Baylor College of Medicine 1986

Figure 4.9. The laser is used to treat polycystic ovaries by draining multiple subcapsular cysts. This decreases the intraovarian androgen levels. As illustrated, some surgeons have used fiber lasers in an attempt to coagulate the stroma surrounding the cysts.

Figure 4.10. Depending on the power density used, lesions can be heated to the point of coagulation (A), vaporized (B), or excised by making a circumferential incision and then undercutting the lesion with the laser (C).

pelvis can be elevated away from other structures by injecting saline underneath the peritoneum, providing a protective barrier against the CO_2 laser. (As discussed above in the section on laser safety, water will not attenuate the shorter wavelength lasers.)

A potential problem with vaporization or coagulation of endometriosis is the fact that endometriosis is frequently multifocal and may penetrate deeply into underlying tissues. Excision of implants is preferred by many surgeons (11,16,17,39,45). This allows for a en-bloc removal of multiple implants that may be connected microscopically. It also reduces the chance of leaving deep disease. Most importantly, it allows pathologic confirmation of the disease. As Stripling and Martin have demonstrated, the appearance of endometriosis may vary widely, and lesions that appear "classic" for endometriosis, may occasionally represent other diseases (40,51). The shorter wavelength lasers have also been employed in the surgical treatment of endometriosis (13,29,30,33,41).

Endometriomas create a pseudocapsule by compressing the ovary as they expand and can be excised in a similar manner. The ovary must be examined carefully because endometriomas are frequently irregularly shaped and may be multiple. Leaving active endometriosis behind results in a high risk of recurrence (22). Small

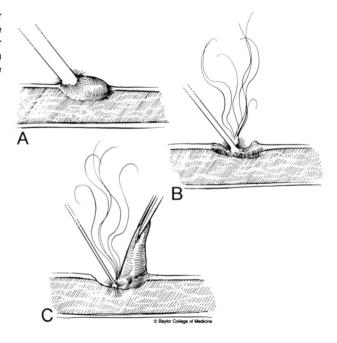

A

B

C

© Baylor College of Medicine

noncomplex endometriomas (under 2 cm diameter) can be managed by completely vaporizing the cyst lining.

Uterine Surgery

Lasers can facilitate myomectomy by making almost bloodless serosal and myometrial incisions. The laser is used to dissect the myoma from its myometrial bed (41). Except for small myomata, the vascular supply to the myoma should be clamped and ligated separately (Fig. 4.11).

Similarly, lasers can be used in place of a scalpel or electrocoagulator to make uterine incisions for metroplasty (Fig. 4.12). Although the majority of patients with uterine septa can be treated at hysteroscopy, laparotomy is indicated for the patient with a broad septum or bicornuate uterus.

Hysteroscopy

Goldrath, in 1981, described photocoagulation of the endometrium with the hysteroscopically directed Nd:YAG laser for the control of menorrhagia (21). This technique is applicable to patients whose bleeding cannot be con-

trolled medically and who have no anatomic basis for bleeding. Neoplasia must be excluded before surgery. The endometrium is reduced in thickness by using a progestin, danocrine, or a GnRH agonist prior to hysteroscopy. The endometrium is coagulated with the Nd:YAG laser fiber in a methodical fashion, beginning in the superior, lateral fundus and moving down to the level of the endocervix (12,34,35). The cervix is not treated so that an egress for blood is retained.

Benign uterine lesions such as adhesions, polyps, myomata, and septa can be cut or excised using a similar hysteroscopic laser procedure. Adhesions (43,49) and septa (10) can be incised avascularly with the laser. If bleeding is encountered, one must be suspicious that the incision has strayed into the uterine fundus or wall. To safeguard against inadvertent injury, simultaneous laparoscopy is advisable. Polyps can be removed by vaporizing their attachment to the uterine wall. Submucous myomata are best approached by serially "shaving" the myoma. Usually, the uterus will contract and push the remaining portion of the myoma into the cavity. If this does not occur, the surgeon must suspect that he/she is seeing

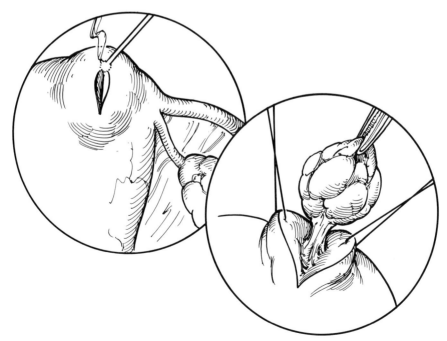

Figure 4.11. Uterine serosal incisions for myomectomy can be made with the laser (*left*). The myoma is dissected from the myometrium with laser assistance. The vascular pedicle of the myoma is clamped and ligated (*right*).

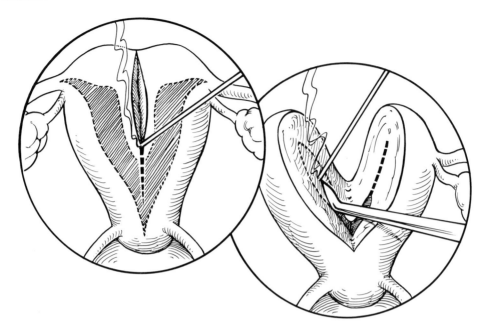

Figure 4.12. Metroplasty for treatment of a septate uterus is accomplished by incising the myometrium over the septum, bivalving the uterus (*left*). Depending on the thickness of the septum, it can be incised (*right*) or excised, and the uterus repaired.

only the intracavitary portion of a larger intramural myoma.

Complications of this technique include those related to hysteroscopy itself plus the possibility of fluid overload from the distending media used. Because endometrial photocoagulation may be recommended for patients medically unable to withstand hysterectomy, the surgeon should keep careful track of the fluid volume used (42,57). Gas should not be used for uterine distension or to cool the laser fiber because of the possibility of vascular injection and gas embolism (4).

CONCLUSION

There are no prospective, blinded studies that show an improvement in surgical results solely due to the addition of the laser. In skilled hands, the laser can reduce the time necessary for a given procedure and reduce the need for tissue handling, thereby decreasing tissue trauma. The ability to simultaneously incise tissue and obtain hemostasis with little injury to adjacent tissues theoretically improves postoperative healing. The laser is a new tool that can be added to procedures the surgeon already knows how to do. Lasers are not a substitute for the observance of basic surgical principles of atraumatic tissue handling and hemostasis. Whatever tools are used for a specific task, success is determined primarily by the materials at hand and the judgment and skill of the surgeon.

References

1. Adamson GD, Lu J, Subak LL: Laparoscopic CO_2 laser vaporization of endometriosis compared with traditional treatments. Fertil Steril 1988;50:704.
2. American National Standards Institute, Ins. American national standard for the safe use of lasers. ANSI 136.1-1986. New York, ANSI, 1986.
3. Baggish MS: High power-density carbon dioxide laser therapy for early cervical neoplasia. Am J Obstet Gynecol 1980;136:117.
4. Baggish MS, Daniell JF: Catastrophic injury secondary to the use of coaxial gas-cooled fibers and artificial sapphire tips for intrauterine surgery: a report of five cases. Lasers Surg Med 1989;9:581.
5. Bellina JH: Gynecology and the laser. Contemp Obstet Gynecol 1974;4:24.
6. Bellina JH: Carbon dioxide microsurgery in gynecology. Int Adv Surg Onc 1978;1:227.
7. Brosens IA, Puttemans PJ: Double-optic laparoscopy. Salpingoscopy, ovarian cycsotcopy and endo-ovarian

surgery with the argon laser. Baillieres Clin Obstet Gynaecol 1989;3:595.

8. Bruhat M, Mage G, Manhes M: Use of the CO_2 laser in laparoscopy. In: Kaplan I, ed. Proceedings of the third international congress for laser surgery. 1979; 274–276.

9. Bruhat MA, Mage G, Pouly JL: The use of the CO_2 laser in neosalpingostomy. In: Kaplan I, ed. Proceedings of the third international congress for laser surgery. 1979;271.

10. Candiani GB, Vercellini P, Fedele L, et al: Argon laser versus microscissors for hysteroscopic incision of uterine septa. Am J Obstet Gynecol 1991:164;87.

11. Chong AP, Keene ME, Thornton NL: Comparison of three modes of treatment for infertility patients with minimal pelvic endometriosis. Fertil Steril 1990;53: 407.

12. Cornier E: Ambulatory hysterofibroscopic treatment of persistent metrorrhagias using the Nd:YAG laser. J Gynecol Obstet Biol Reprod (Paris) 1986;15:661.

13. Corson SL, Woodland M, Frishman G, et al: Treatment of endometriosis with a Nd:YAG tissue-contact laser probe via laparoscopy. Int J Fertil 1989;34: 284.

14. Daniell JF, Brown DH: Carbon dioxide laser laparoscopy: initial experience in experimental animals and humans. Obstet Gynecol 1982;59:761.

15. Daniell JF: Polycystic ovaries treated by laparoscopic CO_2 laser vaporization. Fertil Steril 1989;51:232.

16. Daniell JF: Laparoscopic management of endometriosis with lasers: advantages and disadvantages. Prog Clin Biol Res (US) 1990;323:305.

17. Davis GD, Brooks RA: Excision of pelvic endometriosis with the carbon dioxide laser laparoscope. Obstet Gynecol 1988;72:816.

18. Diamond MP, Daniell JF, Martin DC, Feste J, Vaughn WK, McLaughlin DS. Tubal patency and pelvic adhesions at early second-look laparoscopy following intraabdominal use of the carbon dioxide laser: initial report of the intraabdominal laser study group. Fertil Steril 1984;42:717.

19. Donnez J: CO_2 laser laparoscopy in infertile women with endometriosis and women with adnexal adhesions. Fertil Steril 1987;48:390.

20. Garden JM, O'Banion MK, Sheloitz LS, et al: Papilloma virus in the vapor of carbon dioxide laser treated verrucae. JAMA 1988;259:1199.

21. Goldrath MH, Fuller TA, Segal S: Laser photovaoprization of endometrium for the treatment of menorrhagia. Am J Obstet Gynecol 1981;140:14.

22. Hauuy JP, Madelenat P, Bouquet de la Joliniere J, et al: Laparoscopic surgery of ovarian cysts. Indications and limits as found in a serier of 169 cases. J Gynecol Obstet Biol Reprod (Paris) 1990;19:209.

23. Henderson SR: Ectopic tubal pregnancy treated by operative laparoscopy. Am J Obstet Gynecol 1989; 160:1462.

24. Hoye RC, Ketcham AS, Riggle GC: The airborn dissemination of viable tumor cells by high energy neodymium laser. Life Sci 1967;6:119.

25. Huber J, Hosmann J, Spona J: Endoscopic laser incision of the polycystic ovary. Geburtshilfe Frauenheilkd 1989;49:37.

26. Keckstein J: Laparoscopic treatment of polycystic ovarian syndrome. Ballieres Clin Obstet Gynaecol 1989;3:563.

27. Keckstein G, Wolf A, Wittek S: Status of the fallopian tube following pelviscopic surgery (conventional versus laser) of tubal pregnancy. Arch Gynecol Obstet 1989;245:416.

28. Kelly RW, Robert DK: Experience with the CO_2 laser in gynecologic microsurgery. Am J Obstet Gynecol 1983;146:285.

29. Keye WR, Hansen LW, Astin M, et al: Argon laser therapy for endometriosis: a review of 92 consecutive patients.

30. Keye WR: The present and future application of lasers to the treatment of endometriosis and infertility. Int J Fertil 1986;31:160.

31. Klink F, Grosspietzsch R, vonKlitzing L, et al: Animal in vivo studies and in vitro experiments with human tubes for end-to-end anastomotic operation by a CO_2-laser technique. Fertil Steril 1978;30:100.

32. Kojima E, Yanagibori A, Otaka K, Hirakawa S: Ovarian sedge resection with contact Nd:YAG laser irradiation used laparoscopically. J Reprod Med 1989;34:444.

33. Kojima E, Morita M, Otaka K, et al: Nd:AG laser laparoscopy for ovarian endometriomas. J Reprod Med 1990;35:592.

34. Loffer FD: Hysteroscopic endometrial ablation with the Nd:YAG lasr using a nontouch technique. Obstet Gynecol 1987;69:679.

35. Lomano JM: Photocoagulation of the endometrium with the Nd:YAG laser for the treatment of menorrhagia. A report of ten cases. J Reprod Med 1986;31:148.

36. Luciano AA, Maier DB, Kock EI, et al: A comparative study of postoperative adhesions following laser surgery by laparoscopy versus laparotomy in the rabbit model. Obstet Gynecol 1989;74:220.

37. Mage G, Pouly JL, deJoliniere JB, et al: A preoperative classification to predict the intrauterine and ectopic pregnancy rates after distal tubal microsurgery. Fertil Steril 1986;46:807.

38. Maiman T: Stimulated optical radiation in ruby masers. Nature 1960;187:493.

39. Martin DC, van der Zwagg R: Excisional techniques for endometriosis with the CO_2 laser laparoscope. J Reprod Med 1987;32:753.

40. Martin DC, Hubert GD, van der Zwagg R, et al: Laparascopic appearance of pelvic endometriosis. Fertil Steril 1989;51:63.

41. McLaughlin DS: Micro-laser myomectomy technique to enhance reproductive potential: a preliminary report. Lasers Surg Med 1982;2:107.

42. Morrison LM, Davis J, Sumner D: Absorption of irrigating fluid during laser photocoagulation of the endometrium in the treatment of menorrhagia. Br J Obstet Gynaecol 1989;96:346.

43. Newton JR, MacKenzie WE, Emens MJ, et al: Division of uterine adhesions (Asherman's syndrome)

with the Nd:YAG laser. Br J Obstet Gynaecol 1989; 96:102.

44. Nezhat C, Crowgey SR, Garrison CP: Surgical treatment of endometriosis via laser laparoscopy. Fertil Steril 1986;45:778.

45. Nezhat C, Nezhat FR: Safe laser endoscopic excision or vaporization of peritoneal endometriosis. Fertil Steril 1989;52:149.

46. Nezhat C, Winer WK, Nezhat F: Laparoscopic removal of dermoid cysts. Obstet Gynecol 1989; 73:278.

47. Olive DL, Martin DC: Treatment of endometriosis-associated infertility with CO_2 laser laparoscopy: the use of one- and two-parameter exponential models. Fertil Steril 1987;48:18.

48. Paulson JD, Asmar P: The use of CO_2 laser laparoscopy for treating endometriosis. Int J Fertil 1987;32:237.

49. Siegler AM: Therapeutic hysteroscopy Acta Eur Fertil 1986;17:467.

50. Stangel JJ: Recent techniques for the conservative management of tubal pregnancy. Surgery, laparoscopy, and medicine. J Reprod Med 1986;31:98.

51. Stripling MC, Martin DC, Chatman DL, et al: Subtle appearance of pelvic endometriosis. Fertil Steril 1988;49:427.

52. Sutton C, Hill D: Laser laparoscopy in the treatment of endometriosis. Br J Obstet Gynaecol 1990;97: 181.

53. Tadir Y, Ovadia J, Zuckerman Z: Laparoscopic applications of the CO_2 laser. In: Atsumi K, Nimsakul K, eds. Proceedings of the fourth congress of the international society for laser surgery. 1981;25–26.

54. Townes CH: Production of coherent radiation by atoms and molecules. 1964 Nobel Lecture. IEEE Spectrum (Aug) 1965.

55. Tulandi T: Salpingo-ovariolysis: a comparison between laser surgery and electrosurgery. Fertil Steril 1986;45:489.

56. Tulandi T: Adhesion reformation after reproductive surgery with and without the carbon dioxide laser. Fertil Steril 1987;47:704.

57. Van Boven MJ, Sigelyn F, Connez J, Gribmont BF: Dilutional hyponatremia associated with intrauterine endoscopic laser surgery. Anesthesiology 1989;71: 449.

58. Vermesh M, Silva PD, Rosen GF, Stein AL, Fossom GT, Sauer MV. Management of unruptured ectopic gestation by linear salpingostomy: a prospective, ramdomized clinical trial of laparoscopy versus laparotomy. Obstet Gynecol 1989;74:400.

59. Yanagibori A, Kojima E, Ohtaka K, et al: Nd:YAG laser therapy for intertility with a contact probe. J Reprod Med 1989;34:456.

EVALUATION
OF SURGICAL RESULTS

David S. Guzick

INTRODUCTION

Statistics has been defined as fiction in its most uninteresting form. Although this definition may reflect the attitude of many physicians, an understanding of the basic principles of statistics is a necessary prerequisite to an intelligent interpretation of the medical literature. When a new surgical technique is first suggested, its proponents may have unrealistically high expectations of its benefits. After the technique has been more widely used, the realization that it has some limitations and side effects may result in an overly negative appraisal of its value. Eventually, the surgical technique may reach a level where it is recommended for those who can most benefit and who are least likely to suffer from it. If every new therapy were scientifically scrutinized before being accepted as a standard treatment, the initial extremes might be avoided.

This chapter presents biostatistical concepts and procedures often applied to surgical interventions. The ultimate concern of each surgeon is the health of every patient under his or her care. A clear understanding of basic medical research principles is essential for achieving that goal.

STATISTICAL TESTING

Surgical Trials vs. Jury Trials

Hypothesis development and testing are fundamental to research. To explain hypothesis testing in the context of a surgical study, it may be helpful to illustrate by means of analogy. In a courtroom trial, the defendant is either innocent or guilty. The jury must reach a verdict based on the admissible evidence. The four possible outcomes (Table 5.1) are as follows: (*a*) the defendant may be innocent and the jury may convict; (*b*) the defendant may be guilty and the jury may convict; (*c*) the defendant may be innocent and the jury may release him (finding of innocent or a hung jury); and (*d*) the defendant may be guilty and the jury may release him.

If the jury releases an innocent man or convicts a guilty one, it has made the right decision. But what if it convicts an innocent man or releases a guilty one? One of the difficulties of developing a system of justice is dealing with these two potential mistakes. If the rules are designed to avoid convicting the innocent, the probability of releasing the guilty is increased. If the rules are tightened to ensure that all those who are guilty are convicted, then the number of innocent people convicted for crimes they did not commit will increase. A decision must be made as to which type of error is more serious. In the United States, the judicial system is designed to avoid the error labelled Type I in Table 5.1—finding an innocent person guilty. The basic principle is that a defendant is presumed innocent until proven guilty "beyond a reasonable doubt." To reach a verdict of "guilty," all members of the jury must agree that the state has provided

Table 5.1. Jury Trial Outcomes

	Defendant is	
Jury Decision	Innocent	Guilty
Convict	Type I Error	Correct
Release	Correct	Type II Error

evidence that strongly contradicts the assumption of innocence.

Hypothesis Testing

Statistical hypothesis testing operates on a similar model. The *null hypothesis* (H_o) corresponds to the assumption of innocence until guilt is proven. If two treatments are compared, the null hypothesis is that the two treatments have essentially the same effect. Unless the data provide strong evidence that contradicts this assumption, it cannot be dismissed. One crucial point about hypothesis testing is that the null hypothesis is never "proven"; we state that the available data do not allow us to reject it. The *probability value* or *"p value"* that is associated with statistical testing is a more precise way of expressing "reasonable doubt." If it is true that the two treatments are essentially equal, sample data associated with a p value of 0.05 would occur only five out of 100 times. Researchers have an advantage over juries in that they can place a treatment in double jeopardy; only in very extreme circumstances should a treatment be accepted or rejected on the basis of one trial.

One major difference between jury trials and surgical treatment trials is that in a jury trial, all of the evidence is directed toward making a decision about one defendant, while in a surgical trial, decisions are made about an entire population based on evidence gathered from a sample of individuals. For example, before investing in equipment needed for laser tubal surgery, we may wish to know whether pregnancy rates after tuboplasties performed with the aid of a laser are higher than those performed using cautery. What we really want to know is whether this is true for the entire population of women undergoing tuboplasty. Because there are only limited numbers of patients to study in a given location, however,

we collect information on a sample of patients undergoing one procedure or the other. The method of sampling is critical; ideally, patients sampled from two surgical treatment groups should differ in no important respect, other than the type of procedure performed. Underlying the sampling method is the assumption that the pregnancy rate observed after a specified period of follow-up in the laser-treated sample approximates the pregnancy rate in the entire population of women treated with a laser. We make the same assumption about the pregnancy rate in the microcautery-treated group.

Reformulating these concepts in statistical language, we note that the population is fixed, so the pregnancy rate, although unknown, is a constant; it is called a *population parameter*. The pregnancy rate observed in our sample is a *random variable* because it varies from sample to sample. Such a random variable, calculated from observations in a sample, is a *sample statistic*. The sample pregnancy rate observed in our particular group of patients is an estimate of the population pregnancy rate. As a random variable, it has a certain *probability distribution* associated with it. Given estimates of pregnancy rates in our two treated patient samples (laser and cautery), and given estimates of the associated probability distributions, it is then possible to test the null hypothesis that there is no difference in pregnancy rates between the two groups. This statistical test, which is representative of virtually all statistical tests, is based on estimates of the probability that the difference in the sample pregnancy rates observed between the two groups is reflective of a true difference in the population rather than the particular variability of the samples chosen.

In Table 5.2, we present the possibility outcomes of the test of the hypothesis that the probability of pregnancy associated with laser and cautery treatment is equal. When the null

Table 5.2. Surgery Treatment Trial Outcomes

	Treatments are	
Null Hypothesis	Equal	Not Equal
Rejected	Type I Error	Correct
Not Rejected	Correct	Type II Error

hypothesis is rejected, we claim that one treatment is better than the other. The error labelled Type I is considered the more serious error—claiming that a treatment is a significant improvement, when in reality, it is not. This is also known as an α error. The error labelled Type II occurs when we fail to reject the null hypothesis (i.e., we *cannot* claim that one treatment is significantly better), when in fact one treatment *is* superior. This is a β error, and $1 - \beta$ is defined as the "power" of the test. In the current medical literature, β errors probably occur frequently.

Sample Size Determination

When a study is conducted with a small sample size, it is difficult to obtain a statistically significant result, even if the treatments do in fact differ. For this reason, a sample size determination should precede the initiation of a study. Sample size calculations can help decide whether it is worth attempting a study with the number of patients available. Collaboration with other physicians may be necessary to obtain an adequate number of patients.

In statistical terminology, a small study lacks "power." If one of the two treatments actually *is* superior, this superiority may not be detected with a small sample (6).

To estimate the sample size required for a comparative study of two treatments, the researcher must provide estimates of the following:

1. The level of Type I error (α) allowable. The traditional value of α is 0.05.
2. The allowable level of Type II error (β), or, alternatively, the required "power," which equals $1-\beta$. Note that power does not imply that the observed difference between the proportions pregnant will *equal* the population difference, but only that a statistically significant result in the right direction will be obtained. Suggested levels for power are 0.80 and 0.90.
3. An estimate of the proportion pregnant in the control group (p_1).
4. A realistic guess at what the proportion pregnant might be in the treatment group (p_2). If the value of p_2 is set unrealistically

high, then a nonsignificant result will not contribute new knowledge.

Once these preliminary decisions are made, the researcher can consult tables such as those in Fleiss (5), which give sample sizes for a range of values of p_1, p_2, α, and β. (Note that these tables incorporate a continuity correction.) The required sample sizes are often larger than might be expected. For example, α might be set at 0.05, power at 0.90, and p_1 (the proportion pregnant with the standard treatment) at 0.25. If we think that the new treatment may have a pregnancy rate of 0.35, then the required sample size in *each* group (from the tables in Fleiss) would be 478 patients. If the new treatment is expected to have a success rate of only 0.30, then 1753 patients would be required for each treatment group! This example is meant to emphasize that it is difficult to detect small, but perhaps clinically important differences between treatments.

Sample size calculations are estimates; they should not be used to decide the exact number of patients to be included. Rather, the tables should be entered with several possible values to determine what sort of a difference can be detected with the number of patients available. Consulting sample size tables before beginning studies may have the positive effect of encouraging more collaborative trials. Not only are the size of the study and the chance of reaching a statistically significant conclusion increased, but the results of a collaborative trial can more justifiably be generalized to other geographic areas and other types of hospitals.

THE RANDOMIZED CLINICAL TRIAL

As noted above, our ability to make statistical judgments about whether one treatment group has a better outcome than another hinges on the assumption that there are no differences between the two groups, other than treatment. The best way to protect against a violation of this assumption is to assign individual subjects to treatments prospectively on a random basis. Randomization ensures that the distributions of age, severity of disease, parity, and other potentially confounding factors are essentially the same for the two groups. Often, in the infertility literature, treatments are compared by examining the outcome of patients who received one or another treatment in the course of clinical practice. The very process of clinical decision making that results in a patient being treated one way or another may lead to selection of more favorable patients for a particular therapy. If this treatment is found to be associated with a higher pregnancy rate, it cannot be known whether this is due to better treatment or to a group of patients selected for better prognosis. Moreover, there are several difficulties in comparing prospective data with historical control data because of the possible biases from many different sources (4). Thus, good research design is an absolute prerequisite for sound hypothesis testing. Data obtained from a poor design cannot be used to make reliable inferences no matter how sophisticated the statistical method. Conversely, rigorous research design leads to definitive conclusions with the simplest of statistical tests.

The reluctance of patients and investigators to participate in randomized clinical trials arises in part from a federal regulation (Title 45, Code of Federal Regulations, Part 46) for informed consent, which requires that patients give informed consent before being entered into the study by clinical investigators. This procedure requires the physician to inform the patient about all risks and benefits associated with the trial, alternate therapies available, and the patient's right to withdraw from the study at any time. Furthermore, if treatments are randomly assigned, the patient must be informed. A physician should only participate in such studies if he or she believes that the treatments have potentially equal therapeutic benefits.

The randomized clinical trial remains the strongest and one of the most reliable methods of evaluating surgical therapies. Its application to reproductive surgery is limited by the relatively small patient groups and the amount of time that would be necessary to accumulate the necessary number of patients to answer a particular question. However, with collaboration between institutions, it may be possible to apply this strong method of investigation more frequently in the future.

SPECIAL FEATURES OF INFERTILITY DATA

Measurements of Outcome

The obvious measurement of outcome in an infertility investigation is pregnancy—yes or no. There are, however, variations on this theme. First, one must decide whether the outcome of interest is conception, clinical pregnancy, or term delivery. In the case of tubal surgery, we must pay close attention to the distribution of outcomes among pregnancies that are achieved, especially the proportion that is ectopic.

Another important issue is the duration of follow-up against which the outcome measure is defined. Suppose the outcomes of infertile women undergoing surgery over a number of years were reviewed as of September 1990. Should a patient operated on in June 1990 who is not pregnant at the time of review be classified as "not pregnant" just the same as a woman operated on 2 years earlier? Clearly, such a policy would introduce bias into the analysis, because the patient who is not pregnant after 3 months of follow-up may become pregnant after 6 or 12 months. This problem can be handled by performing a life-table analysis, as discussed later in the chapter, or by requiring that all patients have a specified duration of follow-up (such as 2 years) to be included in the analysis.

Finally, some measurements of outcome other than pregnancy are pertinent to certain types of infertility investigations. Tubal patency and adhesion formation are examples of other important outcome measures.

Dependent Vs. Independent Variables

In statistical terms, outcome is the *dependent* variable. It is variation in this dependent variable that we are trying to explain with one or more *independent* or *explanatory* variables. In a study of pregnancy success after tubal reanastomosis, for example, we might wish to explain the probability of pregnancy (dependent or outcome variable) on the basis of length of tube, type of tubal ligation, luminal discrepancy, and age (independent or explanatory variables). Although it may seem obvious, the distinction between dependent and independent variables is a critical one, and establishing explicit definitions in advance of the planned comparison provides a logical framework for the analysis.

Dichotomous Vs. Continuous Variables

In general, the dependent variables in infertility investigations tend to be *dichotomous,* or *binary* (conception/no conception, fertilization/no fertilization, ovulation/no ovulation). Unfortunately, many of the statistical methods available were developed for continuous dependent variables. Blood pressure, serum cholesterol concentration, temperature, tensile strength of suture material, birth weight, and blood loss at surgery are all continuous variables that commonly serve as measurements of outcome in medical investigations. Standard statistical techniques, such as analysis of variance and multiple linear regression, can be used appropriately when the dependent variable is continuous. When the dependent variable is dichotomous, however, as in most infertility investigations, other techniques should be used.

Impact of Nonuniform Follow-up After Treatment

A fundamental problem in evaluating the outcome of infertility therapy is incomplete or variable follow-up. It is often difficult, for reasons unrelated to the study, to maintain contact with patients over a prolonged period. Furthermore, because patients receive therapy at different times, the duration of follow-up varies among those who are successfully followed until completion of the study.

For these reasons, the pregnancy rate commonly reported in infertility research—defined as the number of patients who conceive divided by the number of patients treated—is a poor measurement of treatment success. It may underestimate the true success of therapy, because an unknown fraction of nonpregnant patients who are lost to follow-up early in the study, or who enter the study at a point close to its completion, become pregnant at a later date. Moreover, as some infertility centers have more successful patient follow-up than others, pregnancy rates after a particular treatment modality reported by different centers cannot be compared reliably. Similarly, if there is variability in the follow-up of patients who differ in severity of disease or other characteristics, a comparison of pregnancy rates according to these patient characteristics is also unreliable.

STATISTICAL TECHNIQUES

Analysis When Follow-Up Is Not Uniform

Over the years, many infertility researchers have recognized the importance of adjusting pregnancy rates for incomplete and variable follow-up. Consensus has grown for uniformity in reporting the results of infertility therapy using a life-table method to adjust for variability in follow-up.

Data appropriate for the life-table method are presented graphically in Figure 5.1. Figure 5.1*A* shows that patients were treated at various times and that those who became pregnant (P) did so after varying periods of observation. Of the nonpregnant group, some patients were lost to follow-up (L). The remaining patients were followed nonpregnant to the time that the study was completed (O). Those who were either L or O are described as "censored." Figure 5.1*B* displays the same data after recording the time of entry into the study (that is, the time of treatment) as time zero. This is the starting point for the pregnancy life-table calculation.

The following life-table calculations are based on the original description by Berkson and Gage (1). Table 5.3 is a life-table constructed from 214 patients with endometriosis who were treated with conservative surgical management at The Johns Hopkins Hospital. Each row represents data for a given interval of time after therapy. During the first 12 months after therapy, 68 patients conceived (column 2). None were censored (column 3), so all 214 patients who entered the study (column 4) were exposed to the possibility of pregnancy (column 5). The probability of pregnancy during this interval was equal to the number of pregnancies (68) divided by the number of women exposed (214), or 31.8% (column 6).

Because 68 patients became pregnant during

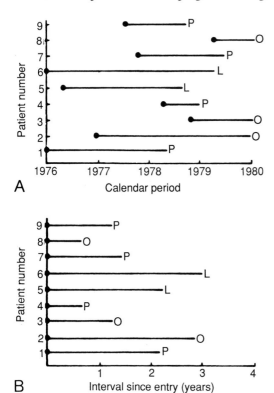

Figure 5.1. Graphic representation of data needed for life-table analysis of nine hypothetical patients treated for infertility. Solid circles = time of treatment; P = pregnancy; L = loss to follow-up; O = nonpregnant at termination of study. A, Patients are treated at various times, and those who become pregnant do so after varying periods of observation. B, Patients are displayed after recording the time of entry into the study (i.e., the time of treatment) as time zero.

the first 12 months, 146 (214 minus 68) entered the second interval (column 4). Of these, 21 conceived (column 2). During this period, however, 39 patients were censored (column 3). We assume uniform dropout of these patients over the 12-month interval; that is, half of them, or 19.5, were exposed. Thus, a total of 146 − 19.5 = 126.5 patients were exposed (column 5), giving a probability of pregnancy for this interval of 21 ÷ 126.5 = 16.6% (column 6).

The cumulative probability of pregnancy is obtained by successively applying the probabilities of pregnancy in each interval to a starting figure of 0% pregnant. Thus, the probability of pregnancy during the first interval is 31.8%. Because none of the patients conceived prior to therapy, the cumulative pregnancy rate is also 31.8% (column 7). In the second interval, we note that 16.6% of the remaining 68.2% of nonpregnant patients conceived, adding an estimated 11.3% patients (0.166 × 0.682) to the pregnancy rate. Thus, in the second interval, the cumulative pregnancy rate is 31.8% + 11.3% = 43.1%. This process continues successively for the remaining intervals.

The cumulative pregnancy curve can be plotted graphically (closed circles in Fig. 5.2). Certain features of the curve can be inferred by examining the plot; that is, the curve seems to level off at a cumulative pregnancy rate of 60–65%, as compared with a crude pregnancy rate of 54% for these same data. To describe the curve more precisely, or to compare two or more such curves for different patient groups, however, a mathematical model is needed.

One model that has been advanced involves the assumption that the pregnancy rate per month (that is, the hazard rate) for all patients

Table 5.3. Calculation of Cumulative Pregnancy Rates by the Life-Table Method

Interval After Treatment (mos)	Last Report		Number Not Pregnant at Beginning of Interval	Number Exposed to Pregnancy	Probability of Pregnancy in Interval	Cumulative Pregnancy Rate (%)
	Pregnant	Not Pregnant				
0–12	68	0	214	214.0	0.318	0.318
13–24	21	39	146	126.5	0.166	0.431
25–36	15	14	86	79.0	0.190	0.539
37–48	7	10	57	52.0	0.135	0.601
49–60	2	10	40	35.0	0.057	0.624
61–72	1	4	28	26.0	0.038	0.639

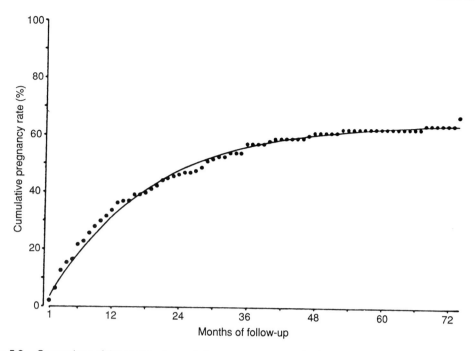

Figure 5.2. Comparison of the observed cumulative pregnancy curve (*solid circles*) age conservative surgery for endometriosis with that predicted by the model of Guzick and Rock (*solid line*).

is constant over time (3). Given a constant monthly pregnancy rate, the predicted cumulative pregnancy rate (CPR) can easily be calculated. Assuming a 20% monthly pregnancy rate, CPR = 20% the first month. During the second month, 20% of the remaining 80% of patients conceive, or an additional 16%. Thus, CPR = 36% after 2 months; similarly, it is 49% after 3 months, 59% after 4 months, and so on.

Applying such a model is straightforward. One simply calculates the average monthly pregnancy rate (or fecundability) by dividing the number of pregnancies by the total months of follow-up, and then predicts CPR as above. Indeed, estimates of fecundability after treatment are now commonly reported in the infertility literature. Interpretation of such estimates is difficult, however, because the underlying assumption of a constant hazard rate is often incorrect. From the endometriosis data in Table 5.3, for example, it can be seen that the hazard rate declines rather markedly over time, as shown in Figure 5.3. It is not surprising, therefore, that the predicted cumulative pregnancy curve based on this model fits the observed data poorly (Fig. 5.4). The CPR

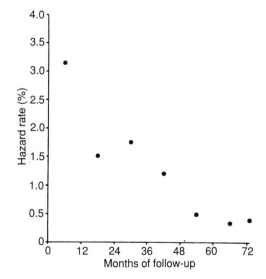

Figure 5.3. Hazard rate (i.e., probability of pregnancy) after conservative surgery for endometriosis as a function of months of follow-up.

predicted by the model initially underestimates and then overestimates the observed CPR.

To develop a model of CPR that better approximates the observed data in a wide variety of infertility investigations (7), let us assume that the observed cumulative pregnancy

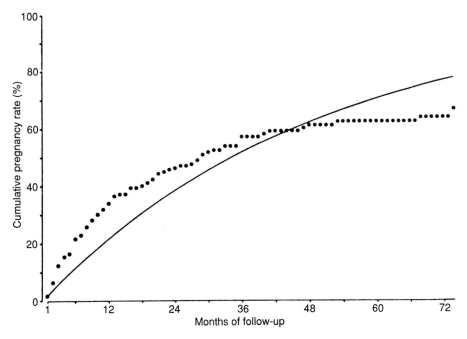

Figure 5.4. Comparison of the observed cumulative pregnancy curve (*solid circles*) after conservative surgery for endometriosis with that predicted by the model of Cramer et al. (*solid line*).

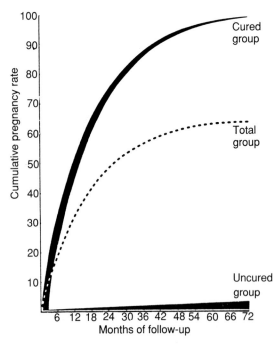

Figure 5.5. Schematic description of cumulative pregnancy model. Relative proportions of patients in the cured and uncured groups over time are represented by the caliber of the line.

curve is a weighted average of two curves; one for patients who will ultimately conceive (the "cured" group), and the other for those who will never conceive (the "uncured" group). The curve for the uncured patients is a horizontal line at 0%. The proportion of patients in the uncured group increases as follow-up advances and pregnant patients in the cured group are progressively deleted from the sample, thus providing greater weight to the overall curve. This concept is shown graphically in Figure 5.5.

More formally, consider a group of women treated for a given, well-documented infertility problem at time zero. The proportion of patients who are cured by treatment can be denoted by c. By "cure" we mean that a patient has the potential, after treatment, to conceive. Depending on the type of infertility problem, this potential may remain lower than that of a nontreated woman without a history of infertility, but the comparison is not relevant to this analysis. The cumulative probability of pregnancy to time t, denoted by $P(t)$, is equal to a weighted average of the cumulative probabilities of pregnancy in the cured $P_c(t)$ and uncured $P_{\bar{c}}(t)$ groups:

$$P(t) = (1-c)P_{\bar{c}}(t) + cP_c(t). \qquad (1)$$

It has been observed that couples with long-standing infertility problems occasionally become pregnant without treatment. In the context of our model, such couples would be included in the cured group, because they obviously had the potential, both before and after treatment, to conceive. The probability of pregnancy in the uncured group, however, is 0, that is, $P_{\bar{c}}(t) = 0$. This causes the term $(1-c)P_{\bar{c}}(t)$ in equation 1 to drop out. We are now left with

$$P(t) = cP_c(t) \qquad (2)$$

If we make the assumption that the probability of pregnancy from month to month in the cured group is the same (that is, if a couple does not conceive 1 month after therapy, this does not change their probability of pregnancy the next month), the second term $P_c(t)$ can be expressed as (7):

$$P_c(t) = 1 - \exp(-\lambda t),^a \qquad (3)$$

where λ = the hazard rate or monthly probability of pregnancy.

Substituting equation (3) into equation (2), we arrive at a simple expression for the cumulative pregnancy rate of the entire population:

$$P(t) = c[1 - \exp(-\lambda t)]. \qquad (4)$$

Thus, the cumulative pregnancy curve derived from life-table analysis for a cohort of treated infertility patients can be expressed in terms of two parameters: the cure rate (c) and the hazard rate (or monthly probability of pregnancy) among those cured (λ). This model can be estimated using nonlinear least squares, or by a maximum-likelihood technique (8). Recently, a program for maximum likelihood

---

$^a\exp(-\lambda t) = e^{-\lambda t}$

estimation of the model has been written for the personal computer (9).

Estimation of the model (equation 4) for the endometriosis data set is as follows:

$$P(t) = 0.645[1 - \exp(-0.056t)].$$

Thus, it is estimated that 64.5% of patients were "cured" of their infertility problem, and among those the monthly probability of pregnancy was 5.6%. The estimated model fits the observed data quite well (see Fig. 5.2). In Figure 5.5, the predicted cumulative pregnancy curve for the sample is the weighted average of two curves, one for the patients who ultimately conceive and one for those who will never conceive. As follow-up advances and pregnant patients in the cured group are deleted from the sample, the relative proportion of patients in the uncured group increases, thus contributing more weight to the probability of pregnancy in the total group.

We have described the life-table method as a procedure to adjust for nonuniformity in the follow-up of patients, and have presented a method for estimating the cure rate and monthly probability of pregnancy represented by a given pregnancy curve. It is often of interest to compare two or more groups of patients with respect to pregnancy after infertility therapy. Is there a difference between a newly proposed form of treatment and the conventionally accepted one? Is there a difference among women of different ages, or among women who differ in severity of disease?

Whenever follow-up is nonuniform, patient dropout or censoring may be different for the different groups. For this reason, the appropriate method of comparing pregnancy success between patient groups is to compare their entire cumulative pregnancy curves or the parameters that describe these curves, rather than their crude pregnancy rates. This can be accomplished by estimating the cumulative pregnancy curve for each patient group using the model described above, and then performing a statistical comparison of the estimated curves. A likelihood-ratio procedure written for a personal computer is available for making such comparisons (9). Unfortunately, the sample size required for this type of estimation (a minimum of 30–40 subjects in each group) is often not available. Nonparametric methods of comparing life-tables (2,11) are available in such instances.

ANALYSIS WHEN FOLLOW-UP IS UNIFORM

If follow-up of patients is uniform, complete, and of sufficiently long duration, the crude pregnancy rate closely approximates the asymptomatic pregnancy rate of the life-table or the cure rate of the model. Under this circumstance, some simple and powerful statistical methods can be applied.

Suppose, for example, that it was of interest to study factors associated with pregnancy success after tubal surgery, and that 200 patients with at least 2 years of follow-up were available. Potential factors that may be associated with pregnancy can be identified on the basis of a theoretical model or previous research findings. From these considerations, suppose that the particular factors hypothesized to be associated with pregnancy success were: surgical technique (microsurgery vs. conventional surgery), severity of disease (mild, moderate, severe), and patient age.

How can we assess the association between pregnancy success and each of these potentially prognostic variables? There are two broad categories of such independent or explanatory variables: categorical (surgical technique, severity of disease) and continuous (age). In our example, the dependent or outcome variable (pregnancy/no pregnancy) is, of course, categorical.

In general, to determine whether a relationship exists between one categorical variable and another, it is appropriate to perform a chi-square test. To determine whether a relationship exists between a dichotomous and a continuous variable, the appropriate test is a t test. Each of these tests allows us to make a decision about whether the observed relationship is greater than would have been expected by some predetermined chance level. That is, we can infer a "statistically" significant association between the variables.

Chi-Square Test

The data for a chi-square test of the relation between pregnancy outcome (pregnant/ nonpregnant) after 2 years of follow-up and surgical technique are shown in Table 5.4. Each cell represents a frequency count of the number of patients who fall into a particular category (for example, 35 patients who had microsurgery conceived). Shown in parentheses below these observed frequencies are the expected frequencies that would occur if the null hypothesis (no difference in pregnancy rate between surgical techniques) were true. These expected frequencies can be calculated from the row and column totals. For example, 29% of the patients conceived (58/200). Thus, if the null hypothesis were true and there were no differences in pregnancy rates, the proportion pregnant for each surgical technique would also be 20%. For example, since 102 patients had microsurgery, it would be expected that 29% of these patients would have conceived, or 29.58 patients.

After the observed (o) and expected (e) frequency counts in each cell have been tabulated, the chi-square statistic can be calculated as follows:

$$\chi_c^2 = \sum_{i=1}^{4} \frac{(|o_i - e_i| - 1/2)^2}{e_i} \qquad (5)$$

Table 5.4. χ^2 Analysis to Test the Difference Between Microsurgery and Conventional Surgery[a]

	Pregnant	Not Pregnant	Total
Microsurgery	35	67	102
	(29.58)	(72.42)	
Conventional Surgery	23	75	98
	(28.42)	(69.58)	
Total	58	142	200

[a]Each cell contains the actual frequency observed and the expected frequency below it in parentheses.

Table 5.5. χ^2 **Analysis with Continuity Correction**

	Pregnant	Not Pregnant	
Microsurgery	a	b	a+b
Conventional	c	d	c+d
	a+c	b+d	N

$$\chi^2_c = \frac{(|ad - bc| - \frac{1}{2}N)^2 \cdot N}{(a+b)\cdot(a+c)\cdot(b+d)\cdot(c+d)}$$

To determine whether this χ^2 value is statistically significant at the 5% level, we consult a χ^2 table and determine the value of χ^2 that represents a 5% probability of falsely rejecting the null hypothesis. In this initial analysis, because our calculated χ^2 value of 2.35 does not exceed this critical value of 2.7, we fail to reject the null hypothesis of no association between microsurgery and conventional surgery.

Equation 5 incorporates a continuity correction (i.e., ½ is substrated from *o-e* before the difference is squared), to adjust for the fact that we are using a continuous distribution to approximate a discrete distribution. A short cut formula for χ^2 that incorporates the continuity correction is shown in Table 5.5. In our example,

$$\chi^2_c = \frac{(|35 \cdot 75 - 23 \cdot 67| - \frac{1}{2} \cdot 200)^2 \cdot 200}{102 \cdot 98 \cdot 58 \cdot 142} = 2.35$$

The short formula for χ^2 can only be used for 2×2 tables. For larger tables, equation 5 (without the continuity correction) is used. For example, Table 5.6 provides the number of pregnant and nonpregnant patients stratified by severity of disease. This is a 3×2 table, with each cell showing the actual number of patients in that category as well as the expected number in parentheses. For Table 5.6, χ^2 equals $(11 - 8.365)^2/8.365 + (18 - 20.635)^2/20.635 + (3 - 2.885)^2/2.885 + (7 - 7.115)^2/7.115 + (1 - 3.75)^2/3.75 + (12 - 9.725)^2/9.725$. Thus, $\chi^2 = 4.02$.

The number of degrees of freedom (df) associated with a χ^2 statistic is calculated by multiplying the number of rows minus one by the number of columns minus one '(rows − 1) · (columns − 1)—. For example, Table 5.6 contains three rows and two columns; thus, the number of degrees of freedom is $(3 - 1) \cdot (2 - 1) = 2 \cdot 1 = 2$. A χ^2 with 2 *df* must exceed 5.99

Table 5.6. χ^2 **Analysis of a 2 × 3 Table[a]**

Initial Severity of Disease	Pregnant	Not Pregnant	Total
Mild	11	18	29
	(8.365)	(20.635)	
Moderate	3	7	10
	(2.885)	(7.115)	
Severe	1	12	13
	(3.750)	(9.725)	
Total	15	17	52

[a]Each cell contains the actual frequency observed and the expected frequency below it in parentheses.

to be significant at the 0.05 level, so the relationship in Table 5.7, with a χ^2 of 4.02, is not statistically significant.

If the data of the previous example are examined more closely, they suggest a direct relationship between extent of disease and pregnancy. As the severity of disease increases, the proportion pregnant decreases. If the ordering of the proportions actually does exist in the population from which the sample was taken, then Bartholomew's test (5) is a more powerful test than the usual χ^2, which ignores ordering. In this case, Bartholomew's χ^2 statistic = 4.0. (See (5) for details).

Student's *t* Test

One use for a *t* test is to examine the relationship between a dichotomous and a continuous variable. Suppose we were interested in the relationship between age (continuous variable, in years) and pregnancy success (dichotomous variable, yes/no).

The formula for the Student's *t* statistic is as follows:

$$t = \frac{\text{difference between means}}{\text{standard error of difference between means}}$$

Conceptually, the *t* statistic is the ratio of the difference between two samples and the vari-

Table 5.7.   Microsurgery Data Stratified by Age Groups

Surgery	n	Age: <25 Proportion Pregnant	n	Age: 25–35 Proportion Pregnant	n	Age: 35 + Proportion Pregnant
Microsurgery	21	0.48 (10/21)	51	0.35 (18/51)	30	0.23 (7/30)
Conventional	49	0.24 (12/49)	39	0.28 (11.39)	10	0.00 (0.10)

ability between them. If the difference between the means of the two samples were high and variability low, the t statistic would be high, and it would be reasonable to conclude that the observed difference between the means reflects a true difference in tube length between the populations of women who do and do not conceive. If the difference between the observed sample means were small and the standard error of the difference large, the t statistic would be low, and we would not reject the null hypothesis that there was no difference between the means—that is, the difference observed would probably be due to sampling variation.

In our example, the observed sample mean age in the pregnant group was 28.3 years, the sample mean age in the nonpregnant group was 33.6 years, and the standard error of difference between the means was 2.1 years. The t statistic is thus (5.3/2.1 = 2.52). This value exceeds the critical value of 1.97 associated with a 0.05 level of significance (as determined from a table of critical points for Student's t). Thus, we conclude that patient age at the time of operation was significantly lower in the pregnant group than in the nonpregnant group.

Adjustment for Confounding Variables

Often, the relationship between two variables (e.g., surgical technique and pregnancy) is confounded by a third variable (e.g., age). Table 5.7 shows pregnancy rates for microsurgery vs. conventional surgery stratified by age. Patients who had conventional surgery were more likely to be in the younger age group. Since we have seen that younger patients have higher pregnancy rates, this predominance of younger patients in the conventional surgery group may have caused an upward bias in the overall pregnancy rate attributed to conventional surgery. Possibly, if we adjusted for this

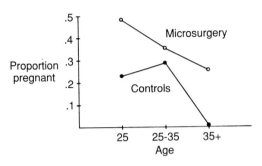

Figure 5.6.   Proportion pregnant within each age group for microsurgery and controls.

age effect, the higher pregnancy rate for microsurgery patients suggested by Figure 5.6, but not reaching statistical significance in the absence of age adjustment, would then reach statistical significance. Such an age adjustment can be accomplished by the Mantel-Haenszel (10) method, which is a way of combining stratified 2 × 2 tables, resulting in a summary χ^2 statistic. In our example, using the data in Table 5.6, the Mantel-Haenszel χ^2 statistic is 4.2, which exceeds the critical value of 2.7. Thus, after adjusting for the effect of age, it can be concluded that the proportion pregnant in the microsurgery group is significantly greater than the proportion pregnant in the control group, with a p value of less than 0.05.

Multivariate Analysis—Logistic Regression

We have seen that our ability to assess a relationship between two variables may be confounded by a third variable. In the above example, there was initially no apparent relationship between surgical technique and the likelihood of pregnancy. However, patients in the conventional surgery group were predominantly younger women who had a higher pregnancy rate. When we adjusted for the effect of age on pregnancy, women who underwent microsurgery were seen to have a higher pregnancy rate than those who underwent conventional surgery.

Suppose it was believed that additional variables, such as severity of disease, further confounded the relationship between other variables in the analysis. For example, disease severity may be greater in older women. How can we simultaneously adjust for the effects of several explanatory variables such that the independent effect of each variable on pregnancy rate could be estimated? The answer lies within the realm of multivariate analysis.

The general purpose of multivariate analysis is to obtain estimates of the effect of a particular explanatory variable on outcome while statistically adjusting for other explanatory variables in an efficient way. Let Y represent the outcome or dependent variable, and let X_1, X_2, X_3, and X_4 represent four explanatory or independent variables. The most commonly used multivariate model in medical research is that of *multiple linear regression:*

$$Y = b_0 = b_1X_1 + b_2X_2 + b_3X_3 + b_4X_4, \quad (5)$$

where b_0 is the intercept when all Xs equal 0, and b_1, b_2, b_3, and b_4 are the regression coefficients of the independent variables. A particular regression coefficient (for example, b_2) represents an estimate of the slope of the relation between Y and X_2 when "all other things" $(X_1, X_3,$ and $X_4)$ are equal.

The difficulty with using this linear model in infertility research is that it is based on the assumption that the dependent variable is continuous and normally distributed rather than dichotomous. Use of dichotomous dependent variables such as pregnancy (yes/no) in this model has been shown to lead to inaccurate estimates of the b's when the probability of outcome deviates much from 50%.

Multiple logistic regression(12) is a technique that was developed in the early 1960s to handle multivariate analysis with a dichotomous dependent variable. As applied to our example where the dependent variable is pregnancy (yes = 1/no = 0), the logistic model specifies that the probability of pregnancy $P = Prob(Y = 1)$ depends on the four explanatory variables $X_1, X_2, X_3,$ and X_4 in the following way:

$$P = Prob(Y = 1) = 1/[1 + \exp - (b_0 + b_1X_1 + b_2X_2 + b_3X_3 + b_4X_4)]. \quad (6)$$

Figure 5.6 shows the general shape of the logistic function, which may be viewed as a basic model for dose-response relationships. The higher the X (dose), the greater the probability of Y (pregnancy, or response).

Two transformations of equation 6 are helpful. First, let Q represent the probability of no pregnancy. From equation 6, a little algebraic manipulation leads to:

$$\frac{P}{Q} = \frac{Prob(Y=1)}{Prob(Y=0)} = \exp(b_0 + b_1X_1 + b_2X_2 + b_3X_3 + b_4X_4). \quad (7)$$

The term P/Q represents the likelihood or odds of a pregnancy occurring with a particular combination of X's.

Taking natural logarithms of both sides of equation 7 so as to linearize the right side of the expression, we have:

$$In(P/Q) = b_0 + b_1X_1 + b_2X_2 + b_3X_3 + b_4X_4. \quad (8)$$

The term $In(P/Q)$ is the log odds, or logit, of pregnancy. The parameters b_i $(b_0, b_1, b_2\ b_3,$ and $b_4)$ are called *logistic regression coefficients*. It can be shown that for a dichotomous independent variable X_i, the antilog of b_i is equivalent to the

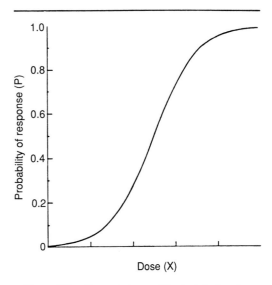

Figure 5.7.   General shape of the logistic function.

odds ratio of pregnancy attributable to X_i, controlling for all other X's. The odds ratio for a given X_i is the odds of pregnancy if X_i were present ($X_i = 1$) divided by the odds of pregnancy if X were absent ($X_i = 0$).

The term *logistic model* is used to refer to either equation 6 or 8, which are algebraically equivalent. Equation 8 is also called a *logit model*. Expressed in terms of logit, a unit change in the variable X_i changes the logit of pregnancy (ln P/Q) by the amount of b_i.

The set of explanatory variables X_i can be dichotomous, continuous, or both. When a categorical variable contains more than two levels, such as severity of disease, we can create dichotomous variable. Thus, we might create the variable "moderate" (yes = 1/no = 0) and the variable "severe" (yes = 1/no = 0). These variables would be entered into the logit model, and their coefficients would be interpreted in relation to the remaining unentered variable, "mild." A logistic coefficient of -0.40 for "severe" means that women who had severe disease had a logit of pregnancy after surgery that was 0.40 units lower than that for women with mild disease. Since the antilog of -0.40 is 0.67, we would conclude that the odds of pregnancy in the severe group is about 2/3 of that in the mild group.

Using our illustrative data set, estimation of the logistic model (using a method of estimation called maximum likelihood that is beyond our present scope) yields results as follows:

ln(P/Q) = 3.9 + 0.52 (microsurgery)
(.21)
$\quad - 0.0135$ (age) $- 0.13$ (moderate)
(.0061) (.10)
$\quad - 0.04$ (severe)
(.19)

Surgical technique (microsurgery) is estimated to have a positive, statistically significant independent impact on the likelihood of pregnancy, while age and severe disease are estimated to have a statistically significant, negative impact where standard errors of the logistic estimates are indicated in parentheses. The logistic estimates indicate the estimated effect of each variable on pregnancy, while adjusting for the other variables in the model.

Besides providing estimates of the independent effects of several variables on pregnancy, an additional benefit of logistic analysis is that it provides a method for estimating the probability of pregnancy given particular combinations of prognostic factors. Using our example as an illustration, we can calculate from equation 9 that a woman who was 30 years old, underwent microsurgery, and had moderate disease would have a logit score (S) of 3.9 + 0.52 − 0.0135(30) − 0.13 = 3.885. The probability of pregnancy in this situation is estimated to be exp(S)/[1 + exp(S)] = 48.67/1.4867 = 32.7%. Similar calculations can be made for patients with other combinations of characteristics.

Computer Software

Fortunately, once the conceptual framework for the statistical techniques is understood, calculations by hand are unnecessary. One needs only the raw data organized in a format that is acceptable as input into preprogrammed computer software. Three major statistical packages for mainframe computers—SAS, SPSS, and BMDP—are widely available at most universities. These packages have been adapted for use with personal computers. Consultation with a statistician is advisable prior to implementing a research design so that suitable statistical methods can be chosen and so that the data can be collected in a manner appropriate for the software available at a particular sight.

SUMMARY

The standard for reaching a verdict in civil trials, such as medical malpractice suits, is "the preponderance of the evidence." This is a valid standard to apply to evaluating the medical literature as well. Every published report should be given weight based on your judgment of its reliability. Larger studies should be weighed more heavily than smaller, randomized trials more heavily than observation studies, rigorously designed trials more heavily than studies that may be biased. If there appears to be a relationship between a factor and an outcome, this does not necessarily imply that the factor causes the outcome. The association could be a result of chance variation between individuals. Statistical testing allows you to rule out chance as a likely cause of the relationship, but this is the *only* explanation ruled out by a significance test. It could be a result of bias—bias in the selection of individuals for the study, bias in measurement of the factor or the outcome, bias in differential loss to follow-up. A thorough analysis of the data is necessary to identify and rule out other possible explanations for the association.

A government agency dealing with environmental regulations experimented with replacing administrative law judges with scientists. It was felt that scientists were better qualified to make the necessary technical evaluations. The experiment was not considered successful because, as one observer remarked: "Judges are used to having to reach a verdict within a short period of time based on whatever evidence is presented—scientists just can't seem to make decisions." This illustrates a similar difference between the role of the researcher and the role of the physician. The physician must decide the best treatment for each patient based only on whatever evidence is available. There is little question, however, what the patient would decide if allowed to choose between receiving the standard therapy and waiting 10 years until conclusive scientific evidence has been obtained. Few patients would choose to wait for an ideal treatment for which they would be too old. Yet, the decisions a physician makes today will be criticized in 10 years, especially by those who have never had to make similar decisions themselves. Some decisions will turn out to be wrong when additional data are available, but physicians must make choices based on the best data currently available. The choice of medicine as a profession implies the acceptance of a life sentence to jury duty: the evidence will never stop accumulating, and the verdict must be continually reevaluated.

References

1. Berkson J, Gage RP: Calculation of survival rates for cancer. Mayo Clin Proc 1950;25:270.
2. Breslow N: A generalized Kreuskil-Willis test for comparing K samples subject to unequal patterns of censorship. Biometrick 1974;57:479.
3. Cramer DW, Walker AM, Schiff I: Statistical methods in evaluating the outcome of infertility therapy. Fertil Steril 1979;32:80.
4. Feinstein AR: Clincial Epidemiology. Philadelphia: WB Saunders, 1985.
5. Fleiss JL: Statistical methods for rates and proportions. New York: John Wiley & Sons, 1973;
6. Freiman JA, Chaimers TC, Smith H, Jr., et al: The importance of Beta, the Type II error and sample size in the design and interpretation of the randomized control trial: a survey of 71 "negative trials." N Engl J Med 1979;299:690.
7. Guzick DS, Rock JA: Estimation of a model of cumulative pregnancy following infertility therapy. Am J Obstet Gynecol 1981;140:573.
8. Guzick DS, Bross DS, Rock JA: A parametric method for comparing cumulative pregnancy curves following infertility therapy. Fertil Steril 1982;37:503.
9. Guzick DS, Bross D: Convenient numerical procedures for estimating cumulative pregnancy curves. Fertil Steril, 1992;57:85.
10. Mantel N, Haenszel W: Statistical aspects of the analysis of data from retrospective studies of disease. J Natl Cancer Inst 1959;22:719.
11. Mantel N: Evaluation of survival data and two new rank order statistics arising in its consideration. Cancer Chemother Rep 1966;50:163.
12. Schlesselman JJ: *Case Control Studies*. Oxford: Oxford University Press, 1982.

Section 2.
Reparative Surgical Techniques

SURGERY OF THE CERVIX

John A. Rock

THE INCOMPETENT UTERINE CERVIX

Since the first description of the repair of an incompetent internal cervical os by Palmer and Lacomme (47), numerous operations for the surgical correction of this condition have been described. The incompetent cervical os is a condition in which there is an abnormally enlarged canal at the corporal cervical junction due to a defect in the ring of the isthmus. The variations in success of these surgical corrections are due primarily to differences in the accuracy of the diagnosis and the adequacy of the surgery. In the past decade, careful attention to the reduction of these errors has brought some consistency in results. The following discussion of the selection of patients and surgical techniques is based on the most recent of these prospective nonconcurrent studies.

INCIDENCE

The incidence of incompetent cervical os has been reported as 3/1000 deliveries (2,49). There has been a noticeable increase to 5/1000 at the Johns Hopkins Hospital. This appears unrelated to our rising numbers of therapeutic terminations of pregnancy. Our observations were similar to those reported from Pennsylvania Hospital (44), where a rising incidence of cervical incompetence was found over a 7-year interval (1966–1973) in the face of a declining number of births. Only three of the 42 patients studied gave a history of previous voluntary interruption of pregnancy. The rise could not be explained on the basis of increasing incidence of therapeutic abortions with dilatation and evacuation.

Etiology

The etiology of cervical incompetence of the internal cervical os remains unclear. Three major etiologies have been suggested.

TRAUMATIC

Overzealous therapeutic or diagnostic dilatation and curettage, laceration from a previous delivery, cervical surgery such as a deep cervical biopsy or Dührssen's incisions, cervical amputation, and poor wound healing after hysterotomy or cesarean section have been considered as contributing to incompetent cervical os.

Miyamoto (39) reported a direct correlation between incompetent cervical os and the incidence of abortions. Other authors (32,61) have found an increased incidence of second-trimester miscarriage in patients who have had a previous first-trimester termination of pregnancy when compared with a control group on the basis of their own data. Thus, it has been suggested that injury to the cervix during a therapeutic termination of pregnancy may be one of the most frequent etiologic factors.

Nwosu et al. (44) noted a rise in incompetent cervical os in the face of a falling delivery rate related to increasing numbers of therapeutic abortions. This rise in incompetent cervical os could not be explained on the basis of traumatic dilatation and curettage at the time of the first-trimester termination. Therefore, at this time, it is unclear whether traumatic dilatation plays a major role in the etiology of the incompetent internal cervical os.

CONGENITAL

Roddick and coauthors (50) suggested that abundant muscle tissue with abnormal sparse connective tissue was responsible for an incompetent os. Eaton and McCusker (15), however, noted a wide variation in fibrous and muscular tissue content. Trythall and Jeremias (58) have suggested that an inadequate lower uterine segment may be responsible. Thirty-two percent of their patients were noted to have an incompetent os of congenital origin.

Kaufman and coworkers (28) described a T-shaped abnormality of the uterine cavity with widening of the isthmus in female offspring of women exposed to diethylstilbestrol (DES) during pregnancy. In 1978, Singer and Hockman (57) reported an incompetent cervical os in a woman exposed to a hormone, presumably DES. Subsequently, Goldstein (16) reported that of 284 DES-exposed women, nine conceived and five developed an incompetent cervical os. More recently, Nunly and Kitchin (43) successfully treated the incompetent cervix in a primigravida exposed to DES in utero.

Clinical evidence suggests that the incompetent cervical os may be present in some patients whose mothers received DES during early pregnancy. It follows that until a clear association has been established in the literature, frequent examinations in these patients should be done during pregnancy as that the incompetent cervical os may be diagnosed and treated appropriately.

PHYSIOLOGIC OR DYSFUNCTIONAL

Some authors (6,41) have suggested that the corporal cervical junction may act as a functional sphincter. Asplund (1) reported combined hysterographic and arteriographic evidence of variations in the isthmic tone, which he considered to be based on hormonal variations in the isthmic tone. Mann and coauthors (37), using a two-stage intrauterine balloon technique capable of causing sequential expansion within the corpus, isthmus, and cervix, were able to demonstrate a hypotonic isthmus in patients with an incompetent cervical os.

There was a close correlation between the isthmic hypotonia in the nonpregnant state and the development of cervical incompetence during pregnancy. The authors concluded that isthmic tone is essential if pregnancy is to reach the state of fetal viability. Furthermore, Hunter and coauthors (23) demonstrated the relaxing influence of papain and bromelin on the cervix. The authors felt that this was an important means of demonstrating the existence of a physiologically incompetent cervical os.

DIAGNOSIS

One may commonly elicit a history of painless effacement and dilatation of the cervix prior to bleeding or labor in the midtrimester from patients with an incompetent internal cervical os. The degree of enlargement of the canal at the corporal cervical junction associated with repeated pregnancy loss is not known. As a consequence, treatment in some cases is based on obstetrical history alone.

The normal isthmus may be hypertonic and atonic, depending upon the phase of the menstrual cycle. During menstruation, the isthmic segment is short and relatively atonic; however, during the early proliferative phase of the cycle, there is a gradual increase in isthmic tone. Isthmic tone is greatest following ovulation. The isthmus progressively lengthens and assumes a hypertonic tubular appearance as the secretory phase progresses. Isthmic relaxation occurs just prior to menstruation (37). The menstrual cycle therefore must be taken into consideration when any diagnostic test is performed.

A variety of methods for diagnosis have been suggested (Table 6.1). The traction test of Bergman and Svenerund (7) consists of pulling a Foley catheter containing 1 ml of water through the internal os of the nonpregnant patient. If this can be performed with less than 600 g of pull, a diagnosis of incompetent cervical os is probable. In the nonpregnant state, the incompetent cervical os will easily admit an 8-mm Hegar dilator. Hysterosalpingogram may demonstrate the widening of the internal os at the isthmus. Mann and coauthors (37), using a two-stage uterine balloon, detected lowered pressure gradients with incompetent cervical os.

Table 6.1. The Incompetent Internal Cervical Os: Methods of Diagnosis

Physical criteria of painless effacement and dilatation of cervix during the second trimester	Danforth (11), Lash and Lash (29)
Previous second-trimester pregnancy loss with typical history of incompetent os	Durfee (14), Lash and Lash (29), Palmer and Lacomme (47), Shirodkar (55)
Passage of #8 Hegar dilator with ease through the internal os of the nonpregnant cervix	Duckman (13), Green-Armytage (18), Lash and Lash (29)
Traction test with Foley catheter and 1 ml of water. A pull of less than 600 g suggests the possibility of an incompetent cervical os	Bergman and Svenerund (7)
The loss of angle (abnormally wide cervical canal at the isthmus funnel) by hysterogram	Jeffcoate and Wilson (24), Lash and Lash (29), Picot et al. (49)
Demonstration of defective cervix or hourglass configuration by radiographic balloon test	Mann (36), Rubovits et al. (51)
Bromelin cervicohysterosalpingogram at ovulation to demonstrate change in cervical lumen caliber	Hunter et al. (23)
Use of olive-tip uterine sound with palpation of vaginal examining finger to detect cervical defect	Durfee (14)
Palpation of cervical defect postdelivery	Johnston (27a)
Two-stage uterine balloon to detect pressure gradients	Mann et al. (37)

The cervical os is most relaxed under the estrogenic influence of the proliferative phase. Results may be misleading with these diagnostic tests unless they are performed toward the end of the cycle. In the usual case, the diagnosis of incompetent cervical os is made on the basis of a history of repeated midtrimester pregnancy loss, in the absence of other identifiable etiologies. Unfortunately, the diagnosis is most frequently suggested during pregnancy. When a patient presents with a convincing clinical picture with or without past history, corrective surgery may be indicated unless ruptured membranes, nearly completely dilated cervix, hydrocephalus, hydramnios, or intrauterine death are present.

The importance of excluding other etiologies for repeated pregnancy loss should be considered before an interval trachelorrhaphy. Other causes of repeated pregnancy loss may be excluded as far as possible through the assessment of history, general health, hysterogram (to detect double uterus or myoma), and endometrial biopsy (to determine adequacy of the postovulatory endometrium). The determination of pregnanediol excretion or serum progesterone during the first and early second trimester will in some instances help to identify patients with progesterone deficiency due to placental inadequacy, who will require progesterone replacement.

It is apparent that there is no truly diagnostic test for cervical insufficiency. Difficulties in establishing a diagnosis are reflected in a wide variation in the use of cervical cerclage. The Medical Research Council of the Royal College of Obstetricians and Gynecologists organized a randomized clinical trial of cervical cerclage to address this issue. Nine-hundred and five women whose obstetricians were uncertain whether to recommend cerclage were randomly allocated to cerclage or no surgery (40). The results for those women allocated cerclage were more favorable in terms of fewer deliveries before 33 weeks. The results suggested that cerclage had an important beneficial effect in one in 20–25 women in the trial.

Blickstein and coauthor compared the outcome of pregnancies complicated by preterm rupture of the membranes after cerclage with cases in which preterm rupture occurred without cerclage (7a). All pregnancies were complicated with preterm (<36 weeks) rupture of membranes. Clinical management was similar in both groups. Under similar conditions and treatment, no significant difference between the outcomes was noted in either group. The authors concluded that the added risks of preterm ruptured membranes to cerclage is low, and the fear of fetal, maternal complications due to cerclage-associated infection should not deter the obstetrician from using a cervical suture when indicated.

THERAPY

Conservative

Except for cases revealing gross defects from trauma or surgery, it is usually difficult to know whether the internal os is giving way because of weakness of the internal os or because of unusually increased pressure (hyperirritability of the uterine muscle or multiple pregnancy). Sherman (54) obtained remarkably good results without surgery by treating patients with repeated midtrimester pregnancy loss with doses approximating 1000 mg of Delalutin for the prevention of premature labor at the time of cerclage procedure and thereafter. Rosenwaks and coauthors (personal communication, unpublished) reviewed 65 patients with cervical incompetence treated by surgical means and Delalutin therapy. A follow-up of the offspring of these patients revealed no intrauterine growth retardation or congenital anomalies other than two newborns with pedunculated postminimi, which have a strong genetic component. They concluded that the incidence of congenital anomalies was not increased over that expected. Therefore, in patients where one cannot clearly demonstrate an incompetent cervical os, conservative management with 500 mg of Delalutin twice weekly may be worthwhile. The use of this regimen is appealing as an adjunct to surgery when uterine irritability is detectable, and may be useful when the diagnosis is uncertain.

The Smith-Hodge pessary appears to have some benefit in patients by changing the location of the cervix so as to bear the weight of the uterine contents through the lower uterine segment, rather than through the weakened os. Some suggest that bed rest will similarly reduce pressure and may be a useful adjunct. These treatments, however, are not practical or sufficient by themselves.

Yosowitz and associates (62) have described an inflatable silicone cuff for the treatment of the incompetent cervical os. This device consists of a plastic ring with two fluid-inflatable balloons attached to its inner and outer surfaces. This may be applied to the internal cervical os during an office visit, obviating the need for anesthesia and surgery. The cuff is placed on the cervix and the cervix pulled through the center of the cuff with the ring forceps. The balloon adjacent to the cervix is inflated with 6 ml of saline. Once the filling tube is ligated with nonabsorbable suture, the outer balloon is inflated with saline and ligated. The excess tubing is cut from the balloons distal to the ligating sutures, and the cuff may be removed at the time of labor by simply cutting the filling tubes, or, as noted in most cases, it slips off the dilating and effacing cervix.

The silicone-plastic cuff is an experimental device that has been applied to the incompetent cervix in a limited number of patients. The pregnancies of a number of these patients have reached viability in gratifying proportions. Its efficacy, however, remains to be established until adequate numbers have used this method in clinical trial.

Surgical

CERCLAGE DURING PREGNANCY

In performing cerclage during pregnancy, the surgeon must anticipate the best gestational age at which to perform the cerclage. Waiting for effacement and even dilatation to occur to confirm the necessity of the procedure is unwise. Attempting surgical correction after dilatation is 3–4 cm is usually unsuccessful. If cerclage is performed prior to effacement and dilatation, one can anticipate a beneficial result. If the procedure is to be performed during pregnancy, as is the general preference, it is best to perform surgery around the 12th week of pregnancy and therefore past the time for most genetically and environmentally predetermined spontaneous abortions. Most surgeons prefer surgery after the 12th week and before the 15th week. The patient should be instructed on the need for close follow-up during this critical interval of time.

Various techniques using various assortments of materials and instruments have been suggested for trachelorrhaphy during pregnancy (Table 6.2). Modifications of the basic techniques described by McDonald (34), Shirodkar (55), and Barter et al. (4), as applied by surgeons at the Johns Hopkins Hospital, will be described in the text that follows. Alternatively, the Wurm technique (20) and the transabdominal cervicouterine cerclage (5), which have also been found useful for certain indications, are described.

McDonald Cerclage

The McDonald encircling cerclage is performed by encircling the cervix with a suture in and out of the cervical mucosa and underlying

Table 6.2.   Various Techniques for the Surgical Repair of the Incompetent Cervix During Pregnancy

Shirodkar (55)	Submucosal cervical cerclage using fascia lata
Baden and Baden (2)	Strip of exocervix denuded for approximately 1 cm and area closed with #0 catgut.
Green-Armytage (18)	Nylon cerclage around cervix after puncture of anterior portio at level of internal os.
McDonald (34)	Endocervix purse-string with 4–6 bites of #4 silk on a Mayo needle.
Barter et al. (4)	Aneurysm needle threaded with fascia lata or merselene.
Page	Cervical cerclage wrapping internal os in cellophane strips coated with dicetyl phosphate. Later, ribbon catgut and strips of oxycel gauze dipped in benzoin and saturated with talc were substituted.
Salles et al. (51a)	Two lateral and one medial "V" sutures placed parallel to axis of cervix with horsehair.
Hefner et al. (20)	Two mattress sutures (#3 braided silk) at level of internal os.
Ritter and Ritter	Merselene band placed beneath uterosacral ligaments and sutured anteriorally.
Benson and Durfee (5)	Transabdominal cervicouterine cerclage.

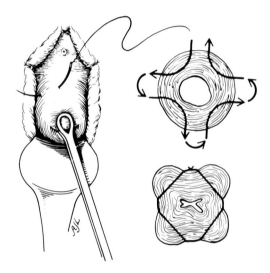

Figure 6.1.   McDonald cerclage: Suture of merselene or braided silk is placed while the cervix is held securely with a suitable atraumatic forceps. Four needle placements are usually necessary at 10, 7, 5, and 2 o'clock.

tissues (34). The procedure's advantages include a simple installation and removal prior to delivery, thereby permitting vaginal delivery. McDonald used #4 braided merselene sewn into the cervical mucous membrane and tissue in four quadrants, encircling the cervix as high as possible (Fig. 6.1). Hofmeister and coauthors (21) modified the technique by using two merselene bands swedged on a large needle and placed 1 cm apart.

Cushner (10) reported the first series of patients with an incompetent cervical os treated by McDonald cerclage at the Johns Hopkins Hospital. Our current approach differs only in the type of suture material employed. Whereas

Cushner used #4-0 white braided silk placed with a Mayo needle, #4 braided merselene suture is now placed with a large half-circle atraumatic needle. The suture is placed at the level of the junction between the smooth mucosa of the portio and the mucosa of the vagina. The needle is directed into stroma, avoiding the endocervical canal. Usually, four "bites" are needed in the following sequence: right anterolateral (10 o'clock), right posterolateral (7 o'clock), left posterolateral (5 o'clock), and left anterolateral (2 o'clock) (Fig. 6.1). The cervix must be held securely with a suitable atraumatic forceps or clamp when each suture is placed. The purse-string suture is tied on the anterior cervix in the midline. The suture is tightened until the cervical os barely admits the assistant's index fingertip.

Equivalent success and morbidity rates between the McDonald and Shirodkar techniques have been demonstrated by Harger (19), who suggests the McDonald approach as the procedure of choice. Unfortunately, the companion groups were not homogeneous indications for the procedure performed. Nevertheless, the authors suggest that the ease of the McDonald cerclage should favor its routine application to cervical incompetence.

The risk of perforation of the membranes is increased when the cervix is dilated, especially if the membranes have hourglassed through the external cervical os. Interestingly, the pregnancy success rate after cerclage is reduced from 92% to 40% if the cervix is dilated and to 23% if there is rupture of the membranes (48). Holman (22a) recommended the use of a Foley catheter to reduce the hourglass membranes when placing the McDonald suture. This practice was further modified by Didolkar (12), who recommended a larger Foley catheter (30 cc) rather than a 5-cc one. Goodlin (17) suggested decompression of the bulging amniotic membranes with installation of antibiotics to lessen the risks of infection. Interestingly, prior to treatment, 10 of 11 women had premature rupture of the membranes. The author placed a 30-cc Foley catheter inside the cervix while placing both a Wurm and a McDonald suture. Ten of 11 patients treated had viable births.

Since 1955, three-quarters of patients with the McDonald technique successfully delivered an infant who survived (10,26). Since Cushner's initial report (1963) of a 52% success rate, Cardwell (9) has reported a pregnancy success rate of 88%, a significant improvement. This is definitely related to improved perinatal care, a more careful selection of patients, and earlier operation. One can generally expect a 70–80% pregnancy success rate using this technique in carefully selected patients.

Shirodkar-Barter Procedure

As originally described by Shirodkar (55), this technique utilizes a 5-mm strip of fascia lata, which is buried beneath the mucosa. Prior to the placement of a band (fascia or merselene), the bladder must be gently advanced. This is done through an incision in the anterior vaginal mucous membrane near the junction with the cervix (Fig. 6.2A and B). This permits the band to be easily placed as high as possible toward the level of the internal cervical os. An incision is made posteriorly in a transverse manner at 6 o'clock at the cervical vaginal junction (Fig. 6.2C). The importance of a high posterior direction in placing the band was emphasized by Shirodkar. He felt that this was of utmost importance in preventing the band from slipping off the cervix. Once both incisions are adequate and the bladder is advanced, an aneurysm needle (3) is brought through both sides (Fig. 6.2D) of the cervix, through which the band is then brought beneath the lateral cervical mucous membrane. A merselene band swedged on a needle may also be used, easing the fixation of the encircling band through the cardinal and uterosacral ligaments.

Care must be taken not to buttonhole the cervical mucous membrane in that a fistula and possible infection may result in these areas. Fistulae are more likely to occur if the mucous membrane has been penetrated at sites other than the incisions. One may avoid a bulky knot by setting only one layer of the knot with an extra loop and securing the arm knots with a transfixing suture of #2-0 silk (Fig. 6.2F and G). Two additional fixation sutures may be placed at 6 o'clock to secure the band (Fig. 6.2H). The anterior and posterior vaginal mucosal incisions may then be closed with several interrupted sutures of #2-0 polyglycolic or chromic catgut suture (Fig. 6.2I).

Occasionally, a fascia lata strip may be preferable to merselene, as some patients may react to this synthetic band. On occasion, multiple fistulae may form, and the band may be rejected. When appropriate, a fascia lata strip can easily be removed from the patient's thigh with a Masson fascial stripper (Fig. 6.3). The fascia lata is exposed, and incisions are made parallel to the direction of the fibers (Fig. 6.3A and B). The width of the strip is usually 102 cm. The inferior end of the band is detached near its insertion to the lateral condyle of the femur. The inferior end of the fascia lata can then be threaded through the eye in the tip of the Masson fascial stripper. The tip of the fascia is held firmly with a straight Kocher forceps (Fig. 6.3C), and the instrument is then pushed in a superior direction along the parallel fibers of the fascia lata (Fig. 6.3D and E). When the full depth has been obtained, the outer sleeve of the instrument is then loosened and stripped over the eye in the tip of the inner tube to cut the fascial strip at its superior end. This produces an adequate fascial cervical band that is placed in a manner similar to that described above with the merselene band.

A temporary Shirodkar procedure has been described by Jennings (25). He buried the cerclage, leaving the ends deliberately exposed for later removal prior to delivery. The installation of the merselene band is simplified by bringing the needle out at 9 and 3 o'clock and sewing back through the same hole. Fistula formation is minimized in this procedure since the band is removed. Jennings reported no infection in 43 cases.

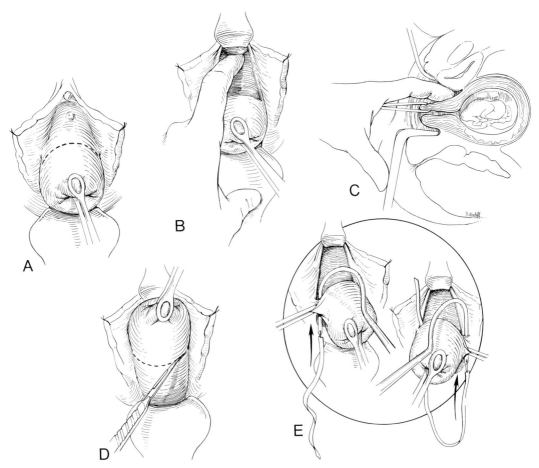

Figure 6.2. Shirodkar-Barter technique for cervical cerclage during pregnancy. *A,* An incision is made through the anterior vaginal mucosa near the junction with the cervix. This may be extended laterally if necessary. *B,* The lower portion of the bladder is gently advanced as high as possible toward the level of the internal os. A small retractor is then gently placed to elevate the bladder in an anterosuperior direction. *C,* The vaginal mucosa is similarly incised at its junction with the posterior cervix. Care must be taken not to enter the posterior cul-de-sac of Douglas. *D,* An aneurysm needle is then passed through the anterior incision submucosally around the right lateral cervix; the merselene band or fascia lata is attached to the needle. The band is then brought around the right lateral cervix. *E,* The other end of the band is then attached to an aneurysm needle inserted through the anterior incision submucosally around the left lateral cervix. This arm of the band is then brought through the left lateral cervix. The cervix must be grasped with a suitable atraumatic stabilizing aneurysm needle. *F and G,* After the operator gently inserts the index finger at the internal os, a single knot is placed anteriorly and tightened so as to allow the fingertip to approach the internal os. The bulky knot may be avoided by setting the knot with one additional throw to square and by securing the arms of the knot with transfixing sutures of #2-0 silk. *H,* Additional #2-0 sutures are placed posteriorly to secure the band. *I,* The anterior and posterior incisions are then closed with interrupted sutures of #2-0 polyglycolic or chromic catgut suture.

Results

Shirodkar (56) reviewed his experience with 305 patients with an incompetent cervical os. Prior to cervical cerclage, the fetal salvage rate was 10%, while the postprocedure salvage rate was 81%. Laurensen and Fuchs (31) reported a success rate of 82% in 143 patients. Similar results have been reported in papers by O'Brien and Murphy (45), Hohlweg-Majert (22), and Cardwell (9). Our own experience with our modified Shirodkar technique has not been dissimilar (26).

There is, however, some difficulty in comparing results of pregnancy success following cervical cerclage in different series. Authors occasionally do not carefully state the criteria for

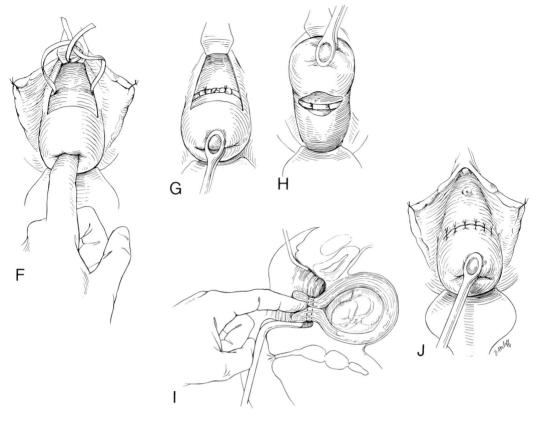

Figure 6.2. *Continued.*

selection of patients, so it is not clear in their results whether those cases that promise to be technical failures have been removed from consideration. Seppälä and Vara (53) suggested the use of an index, the fetal salvage ratio, for reporting results of operations. This ratio is defined as the postcerclage success rate divided by the precerclage success rate. The authors reported a fetal salvage ratio of 2.7 in their operative cases. Block and Rahhal (8) suggested a diagnostic and prognostic scoring system based on clinical and historical criteria. A value of 1 was given to each cerclage indication that the patient met, so that each case was scored from 1–5 (Table 6.3). The pregnancy success rates were significantly different before and after cerclage in those who scored 3 or more but not in those who scored 2 or less. This scoring system, along with a standard method of reporting results such as the fetal salvage ratio, may allow pregnancy success rates in different series to be more closely compared.

Wurm Cerclage

Wurm described a procedure in patients who were found to have considerable dilatation and effacement with bulging membranes in the late second trimester. Hefner and coauthors (20a) described Wurm's technique, whereby two thick mattress sutures were placed across the cervix, one from front to back, the other side to side (Fig. 6.4). They reported that six of nine patients so treated delivered infants who survived. This procedure appeared to be useful in supporting the bulging membranes. Although the technique is appealing in its simplicity, it has not been widely employed nor has its efficacy been established.

Benson-Durfee Transabdominal Isthmic Cerclage

Transabdominal cervical isthmic cerclage, as described by Benson and Durfee (5), presents a method of placing a band quite high to sur-

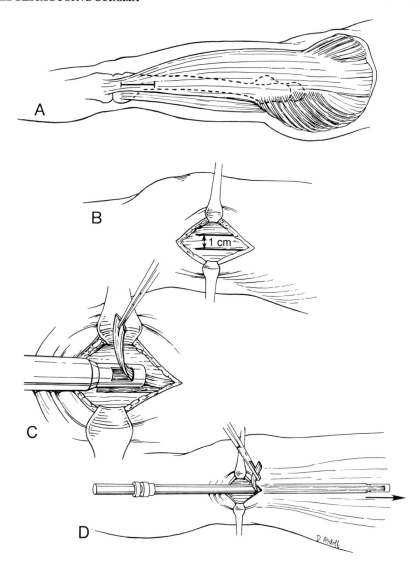

Figure 6.3. Harvesting fiber band cerclage. *A,* The patient is placed in the supine position with exposure of either thigh. After the skin is prepped with a suitable antiseptic agent, an incision is made longitudinally at the lower lateral thigh. *B,* Two incisions are made parallel to the fiber of the fascia 102 cm apart. The strap is then transected above its attachment to the lateral condyle of the femur. *C,* The mobilized 4 cm of fascial strap are threaded through the Masson fascial stripper and held firmly with a Kocher forceps. *D* and *E,* The fascial stripper is then moved firmly superiorly, paralleling the fibers of the fascia for approximately 15 cm. The outer tube of the stripper is slipped toward its tip and over the inner tube, transecting the band of fascia at its superior end. The visible defect in the iliotibial band may be approximated with two or three #2-0 chromic catgut sutures and the skin closed in the usual manner.

round the internal os in selected patients where the cervix has been diminished or amputated by surgery, or when there is a deep uncorrectable laceration. The transabdominal route may assure careful application of the band at the proper level, where it cannot drift downward. The tape should be fixed to the isthmus anteriorally and in the midline just below the attachment of the uterovesical peritoneum to the uterine wall.

Although Benson and Durfee (5) advised dissection of the uterine vessels through a free space that is usually present at the level of the internal os, Mahran (35) modified the technique with a lateral position, avoiding the bleeding complications reported by Benson and Durfee in their original paper. The tape should transverse the isthmus anteriorally, the cardinal ligament laterally, and the uterosacral ligaments posteriorly.

The tape can be drawn gently forward and tied securely in a posterior knot. This knot can easily be inspected by colpotemy, if necessary. Care should be taken in the placement of the tape ligature so that no vessels are caught inside the tape, as uterine ischemia may result.

Table 6.3.   Indications for Cerclage[a]

1. Previous premature delivery or midtrimester abortion without obvious cause.
2. Visual evidence of previous surgical or obstetric trauma to cervix.
3. History of painless premature labor and rapid delivery.
4. Progressive dilatation or dilatation greater than 2 cm on initial examination during midtrimester.
5. Previous diagnosis of cervical incompetence with previous cerclage.

[a]From Block MF, Rahhal DK: Cervical Incompetence: A diagnostic and prognostic scoring system. Obstet Gynecol 1976;47:279.

SURGICAL TECHNIQUES

The peritoneal cavity is entered by a transverse or a midline abdominal incision. The anterior peritoneal reflection is divided transversely, and the bladder is advanced. The space between the ascending and descending branches of the uterine arteries is verified lateral to the uterine isthmus at the cervical uterine junction (Figs. 6.5 and 6.6). This space is carefully delineated with sharp and blunt dissection lateral to the connective tissue of the uterine isthmus; a right-angle forceps is useful for this step (Fig. 6.7). In the process of developing this space, firm upward traction of the uterine fundus is necessary to expose the region of the internal os and to place the vessels on tension. Once the avascular space has been developed to the depth of 1–2 cm, the posterior leaf is opened with a right-angle forceps. A 15-cm segment of mersilin ribbon (0.5 cm

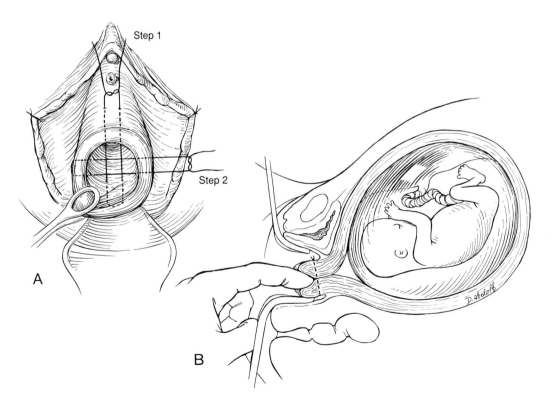

Figure 6.4.   Suturing of the partially effaced and dilated uterine cervix using the Wurm technique (Reprinted with permission from Hefner and coauthors, 1961). A mattress suture of #3 heavy braided silk suture is placed in the cervix at the level of the internal os from 12 to 6 o'clock and back to 12 o'clock (Step 1). A mattress suture is again placed from 3 to 9 o'clock and back to 3 o'clock (Step II). The sutures are tied and the cervical os tested with a finger.

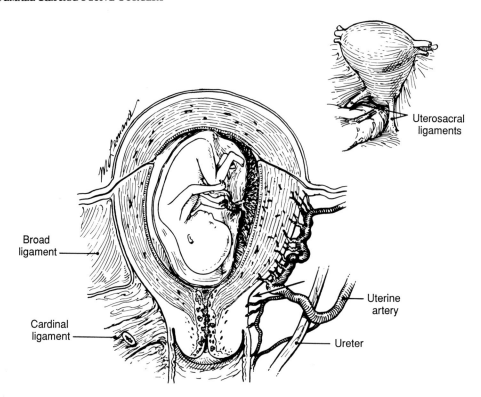

Figure 6.5. Transabdominal Cerclage. Intrauterine gestation at 14 weeks. The arrow marks the free space between the ascending and descending branches of the uterine artery. The uterosacrals are usually attenuated. The band will be placed superior to the posterior uterine insertion.

wide; merselene #5, RS-21, Fcon Inc.) is passed under direct vision (Fig. 6.8). The identical procedure is accomplished on the contralateral side, and the mersilin band is then passed around the zone of the isthmus and over the posterior peritoneum at the level of the insertions of the uterosacral ligaments. The band should lie flat and fit snugly. Once secured anteriorly with a single square knot, the cut ends are fixed to the band with 5-0 proline suture material. (Fig 6.9)

After the procedure, the patient is carefully monitored for uterine irritability, which, in most instances, is uncommon unless there is marked effacement or dilatation of the cervix. The procedure should be performed between 13–16 weeks gestation.

Results

Benson and Durfee (5) reported nine living children in 13 pregnancies in 11 patients so treated. Novy (42) has achieved similar success. Mahran (35), using a modified technique, reported a fetal salvage rate of 70% (Table 6.4). More recently, excellent results have been attained by Wallenburg and Lotgering (59).

CERVICAL REPAIR IN THE NONPREGNANT STATE

When an anatomic defect is clearly demonstrated in the nonpregnant state, prophylactic repair may be preferable. If one is dealing with a congenitally or physiologically incompetent cervix, it is best to make a positive diagnosis during pregnancy. When a cervical defect is apparent, interval trachelorrhaphy may be appropriate. Lash (30) has often stated that repair prior to pregnancy is desirable for severe specific lacerations of the cervix or when previous cerclage has failed. The method as described by Lash has as its goal to restore the normal caliber of the isthmus by excising the scarred tissue in the area of the defect. Defects in the cervix may range from 2–4 cm in length (Fig. 6.10). With a Hegar dilator in the endocervical canal, palpation of the corporal

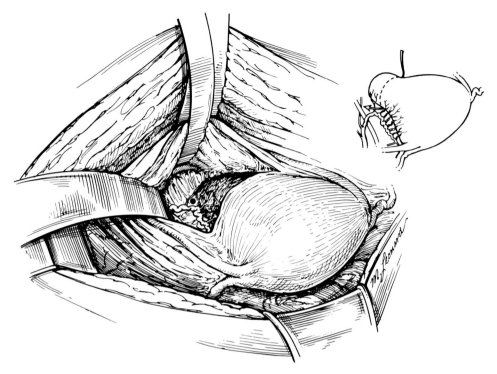

Figure 6.6. Transabdominal Cerclage. The anterior peritoneal reflection is divided transversely, and the bladder is carefully advanced. The space between the ascending and descending branches of the uterine artery is identified.

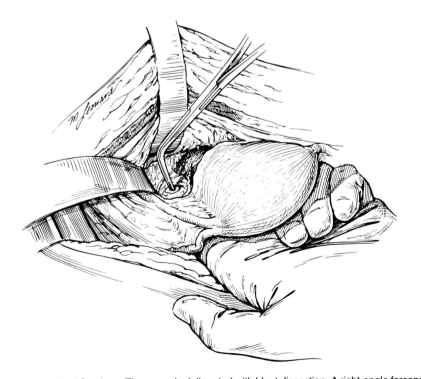

Figure 6.7. Transabdominal Cerclage. The space is delineated with blunt dissection. A right-angle forceps is useful for this dissection.

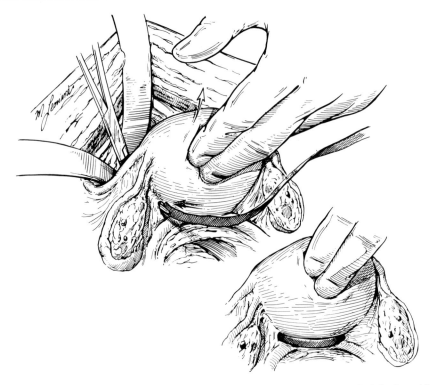

Figure 6.8. Transabdominal Cerclage. Once the space is developed, the posterior leaf of the broad ligament is opened with a right-angle forceps and a 15-cm segment of mersilin ribbon (0.5 cm wide) is passed under direct vision. The identical procedure is accomplished on the contralateral side. The band is passed around the isthmus and over the peritoneum at the level of the insertion of the uterosacral ligaments.

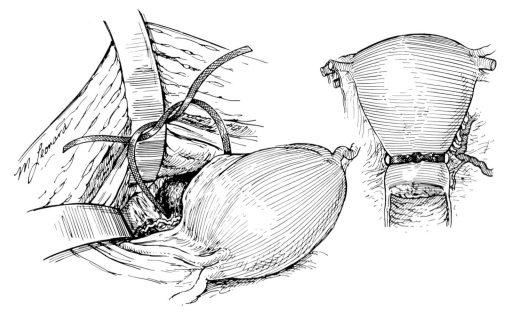

Figure 6.9. Transabdominal Cerclage. Once the band is fitted snugly, it is secured anteriorly with a single square knot. The cut ends are fixed to the band with a #5-0 proline suture.

Table 6.4. Fetal Salvage Before and After Transabdominal Cervical Cerclage (TCC)

Authors	Patients (n)	Before TCC			After TCC		
		Total Pregnancies (n)	Living Infants (n)	Fetal Salvage Rate (%)	Total Pregnancies (n)	Living Infants (n)	Fetal Salvage Rate (%)
Benson and Durfee (5)	10	47	5	11	13	9	69
Watkins (60)	2	9	5	56	2	2	100
Mahran (35)	10	67	7	10[a]	10	7	78
Novy (42)	16	65	13	24	23	21	95
Olsen and Tobiassen (46)	29	101	12	18	35	32	97
Wallenburg and Lotgering (59)	14	50	8	16	16	16[b]	94
Total	81	339	50	17	99	87	91

[a]Number of first trimester abortions not known.
[b]One twin.

junction permits palpation of the defect in the ring, which is usually found anteriorly but may be found obliquely or laterally. At times, longer cervical defects may extend through the external os.

In patients with previously unsuccessful cerclages during pregnancy, one must pay particular attention to the reflection of the bladder, which may be adherent into the cervical defect. The bladder must be gently mobilized and pushed anteriorly so as to avoid perforation. The Lash procedure as modified at the Johns Hopkins Hospital is presented in Figure 6.10. Defects of the internal os that extend to the external cervical os are repaired in a similar fashion. In some instances, the repair may be completed without mobilizing the bladder (Fig. 6.11). If the tissues are poorly vascularized, a merselene or fascia lata strip may be placed across the defect after its closure to lend additional support. The method for obtaining the fascia lata band has been previously described under the discussion of the Shirodkar-Barter technique.

CERVICAL STENOSIS

Conization of the cervix in our experience has been the most common etiology of cervical stenosis. Congenital stenosis is quite rare. The diagnosis may be considered when firm resistance is encountered with an attempt to pass a fine probe into the endocervical canal. Hysterosalpingography may also suggest the diagnosis (Fig. 6.12). Moncrieff and Steel (38) reported cervical stenosis in two postnatal patients. Cervical conization was performed after childbirth when the patients were amenorrheic. Both patients presented with a hematometra. The external os was incised and a Foley catheter left in the uterus for 24 hours. Both patients have resumed menses. Estrogen therapy to improve cervical mucus in patients has been for the most part unsuccessful (52). Usually, attempts to dialate or recanalize a stenotic canal are temporary with a high failure rate. Recently, however, Luesley and coauthors (33) have successfully treated 18 women with cervical stenosis after conization with laser vaporization of the stenotic segment. Once the stenotic tract was identified, a 1-cm diameter cylinder was removed around the probe using a Cavitron carbon dioxide laser with fixed spot (0.4 mm) size on a power density setting of 20 w/cm^2. Vaporization was continued along the length of the probe and 0.5 cm radially until the stenosis was relieved (Fig. 6.13). Relief of the stenosis was accomplished in all but two patients. Twelve patients had relief from dysmenorrhea. Laser dilatation provides a new

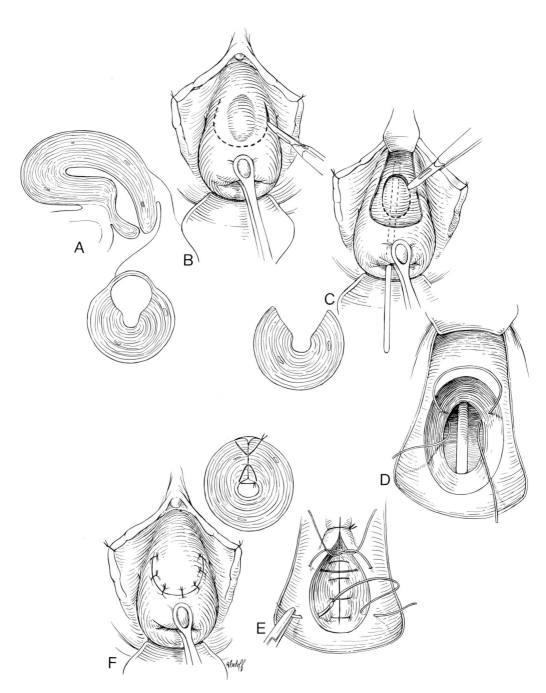

Figure 6.10. Modified Lash procedure for the repair of the incompetent os in the nonpregnant state (defect of cervix). *A,* Incompetent internal os. *B,* A semicircular incision in the vaginal mucosa is made around the defect whereby the mucosal flap is freed and held superiorly with a retractor. If the defect is extensive, the bladder may be pushed superiorly. *C,* The defect in the endocervix is then excised with a suitable dilator in the internal os to mark its position clearly. *D,* The first layer of #0 chromic catgut suture is placed so that the knots are tied within the endocervical canal. *E,* A second layer of #0 chromic catgut suture approximates additional cervical stroma. *F,* The cervical mucosa may then be approximated with #2-0 chromic catgut suture.

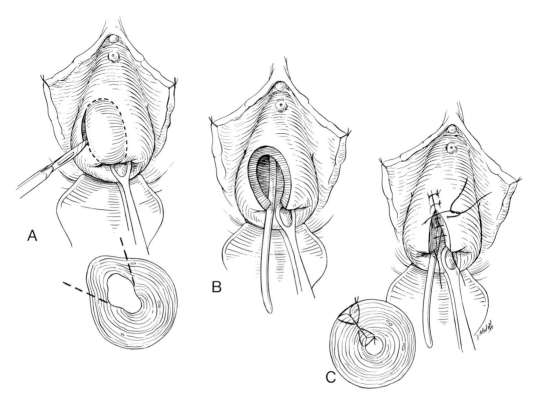

Figure 6.11. *A,* Cervical defect extends to the external cervical os. *B,* The defect is excised, exposing the Hegar dilator. In most instances, the bladder need not be mobilized. *C,* The defect is closed in layers. The first layer of sutures is placed such that the knot is tied within the endocervical canal.

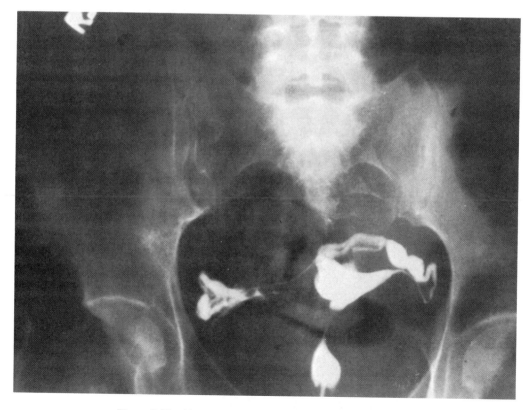

Figure 6.12. Hysterosalpingogram showing cervical stenosis.

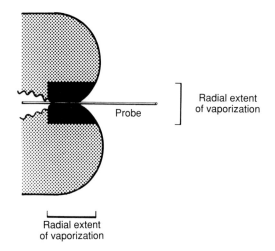

Radial extent
of vaporization

Probe

Radial extent
of vaporization

Figure 6.13. Diagrammatic representation of the technique of laser dilatation. From Luesley and coauthors (33) with permission.

surgical approach to the resolution of postconization cervical stenosis. Further experience with these techniques will better define the rate of subsequent relief of symptoms and resolution of cervical stenosis.

SUMMARY

The diagnosis of the incompetent cervical os may be clearly established by the physician when progressive changes of silent effacement and dilatation of the cervix and intact bulging membranes through the dilated cervical os are observed. A history of repeated pregnancy loss alone is not a sufficient indication for surgical repair. Every effort should be made to identify additional factors that might explain the pregnancy loss. Diagnostic tests such as hysterosalpingography may be of value in delineating the incompetent os in the nonpregnant state. Cervical repair in the nonpregnant state should be done in cases where a definite anatomic defect can be demonstrated. Too often, the diagnosis had previously been considered in a patient who has conceived. In this instance, there are a multitude of trachelorrhaphies beginning with those originally described by McDonald and Shirodkar. If patients are carefully selected, the pregnancy salvage rate should approach 70–80%, regardless of the technique employed. A scoring system such as that described by Seppälä and Vara (53), along with a diagnostic and prognostic scoring system

suggested by Block and Rahhal (8) may provide a method whereby results of different series may be meaningfully compared.

References

1. Asplund J: The uterine cervix and isthmus under normal and pathological conditions. Acta Radiol Suppl 1952;91:3.
2. Baden WF, Baden EE: Cervical incompetence: Current therapy. An J Obstet Gynecol 1960;79:545.
3. Barter RH, Parks J: Myoma uteri associated with pregnancy. Clin Obstet Gynecol 1958;1:519.
4. Barter RH, Dusabech JA, Aiva HL, et al: Closure of the incompetent cervix during pregnancy. Am J Obstet Gynecol 1958;75:511.
5. Benson RC, Durfee RB: Transabdominal cervico-uterine cerclage during pregnancy for the treatment of cervical incompetency. Obstet Gynecol 1965;25:145.
6. Bergman P, Genell S: Incompetence of the internal os of the cervix and habitual abortion. Int J Infertil 1957;2:217.
7. Bergman P, Svenerund A: Traction test for demonstrating incompetence of internal os of the cervix. Int J Fertil 1957;2:163.
7a. Blickstein I, Katz Z, Lancet M, et al: The outcome of pregnancies complicated by preterm rupture of the membranes with and without cerclage. Int J Gynaecol Obstet 1989;28:237–242.
8. Block MF, Rahhal DK: Cervical incompetence: A diagnostic and prognostic scoring system. Obstet Gynecol 1976;47:279.
9. Cardwell MS: Cervical cerclage: a ten year review in a large hospital. South Med J 1988;81:15.
10. Cushner IM: The management of cervical incompetence by purse-string suture. Am J Obstet Gynecol 1963;87:882.
11. Danforth DN: The fibrous nature of the human cervix and its relation to the isthmic segment in gravid and nongravid uteri. Am J Obstet Gynecol 1947;53:541.
12. Didolkar S: Foley catheter and cervical cerclage. Maryland Med J 1986;35:847.
13. Duckman S: Communication in collected letters of international correspondence of society of obstetrics and gynecology, series I. 1960, p. 14.
14. Durfee RB: Surgical treatment of the incompetent cervix during pregnancy. Obstet Gynecol 1958;12:91.
15. Eaton CJ, McCusker JJ: Histopathological study of so-called incompetency in pregnancy. Obstet Gynecol 1961;17:562.
16. Goldstein DP: Incompetent cervix in offspring exposed to diethylstilbestrol *in utero*. Obstet Gynecol 1978;52:735.
17. Goodlin RC: Surgical treatment of patients with hourglass shaped or ruptured membranes prior to the twenty-fifth week of gestation. Surg Gynecol Obstet 1987;165:410.
18. Green-Armytage VB: Habitual abortion due to insufficiency of the internal cervical os. Br Med J 1957; 8:128.

19. Harger JH: Comparison of success and morbidity in cervical cerclage procedures. Obstet Gynecol 1980; 56:543.

20. Hefner JD, Patow WE, Ludwig JM: A new surgical procedure for the correction of the incompetent cervix during pregnancy: the Wurm procedure. Obstet Gynecol 1961;18:616.

20a. Hefner JD, Patow WE, Ludwic JM Jr: A new surgical procedure for the correction of the incompetent cervix during pregnancy. The Wurm procedure. Obstet Gynecol 1961;18:616–20.

21. Hofmeister FJ, Schwartz WR, Vondrak BF, et al: Suture reinforcement of the incompetent cervix. Am J Obstet Gynecol 1968;101:58.

22. Hohlweg-Majert P: Prophylactic and therapeutic operations performed in the clinic for obstetrics and gynecology by Mannheim, between the years 1965 and 1973. Geburtsh U Frauenheik 1974;34:1070.

22a. Holman WR: An aid for cervical cerclage. Obstet Gynecol 1973;42:933.

23. Hunter RG, Henry GW, Civin WH: The action of papain and bromelain on the uterus. III. The physiologically incompetent internal cervical os. Am J Obstet Gynecol 1957;73:875.

24. Jeffcoate TNA, Wilson JK: Uterine causes of abortion and premature labor. NY J Med 1956;56:680.

25. Jennings SL: Temporary submucosal cerclage for cervical incompetence. Am J Obstet Gynecol 1963; 113:1097.

26. Johns Hopkins Hospital Statistics, 1988.

27. Johnston JW: Cervical incompetence and habitual abortion. J Obstet Gynaecol Br Emp 1958;65:208.

27a. Johnston JW, Kernodle JR, Saunders CL Jr: Malignant mesonephroma of the left broad ligament: a case report. Am J Obstet Gynecol 1957;74:1272–1274.

28. Kaufman RH, Binder GL, Gray PM Jr, et al: Upper genital tract changes associated with exposure in utero to diethylstilbestrol. Am J Obstet Gynecol 1977; 128:51.

29. Lash AF, Lash SR: Habitual abortions: The incompetent internal os of the cervix. Am J Obstet Gynecol 1950;59:68.

30. Lash AF: Incompetent internal os of the cervix: diagnosis and treatment. Am J Obstet Gynecol 1960; 79:552.

31. Laurensen NH, Fuchs F: Treatment of the incompetent cervix. Acta Obstet Gynaecol Scand 1973;52: 17.

32. Liu TDY, Melville HAH, Martin T: Subsequent gestational morbidity after various types of abortion. Lancet 1972;2:431.

33. Luesley DM, Williams DR, Gee H, et al: Management of postconization cervical stenosis by laser vaporization. Obstet Gynecol 1986;67:126–128.

34. McDonald JA: Suture of the cervix for inevitable abortion. J Obstet Gynaecol Br Emp 1957;64:346.

35. Mahran M: Transabdominal cervical cerclage during pregnancy. Obstet Gynecol 1979;52:502.

36. Mann EC: Habitual abortion. A report in two parts of 160 patients. Am J Obstet Gynecol 1959;77:706.

37. Mann EC, McLarn DD, Hayt DB: The physiology and clinical significance of the uterine isthmus. Am J Obstet Gyencol 1961;81:212.

38. Moncrieff D, Steel SA: Cervical stenosis after cone biopsy during postpregnancy amenorrhea. Case Reports. Br J Obstet Gynaecol 1988;95:628.

39. Miyamoto J: Background considerations on induced abortion. Int J Fertil 1973;18:5.

40. MRC/RCOG Working Party on Cervical Cerclage. Interim report of the Medical Research Council: Royal College of Obstetricians and Gynaecologists multicenter randomized trial of cervical cerclage. Brit J Obstet Gynaecol 1988;95:437.

41. Nixon CW: Uterine action, normal and abnormal. Am J Obstet Gynecol 1951;62:964.

42. Novy MJ: Managing reproductive failure by transabdominal isthmic cerclage. Contemp Obstet Gynceol 1977;10:17.

43. Nunly WC, Kitchin JD: Successful management of the incompetent cervix in a primigravida exposed to diethylstilbestrol in utero. Fertil Steril 1979;31:217.

44. Nwosu UC, Soffonoff EC, Bolton GC: A new look at the etiology of cervical incompetence. Int Gynecol Obstet 1975;13:201.

45. O'Brien DP, Murphy JF: The value of cervical cerclage in the treatment of cervical incompetence. Irish J Med Sci 1978;147:197.

46. Olson S, Tobiassen T: Transabdominal isthmic cerclage for the treatment of incompetent cervix. Acta Obstet Gynecol Scand 1982;61:473.

47. Palmer R, Lacomme M: La béance de lorifice interne, cause d'avortements á le petition? Une observation de déchirure cervical isthmique reparée chirugicalment, avec gestation á larme consécutive. Gynecol Obstet 1948;47:905.

48. Peters WA, Thigarajah S, Harbert GM: Cervical cerclage: twenty years experience. South Med J 1979;72:933.

49. Picot H, Thompson HG, Murphy CS: Surgical treatment of the incompetent cervix in pregnancy. Obstet Gynecol 1958;12:269.

49a. Ritter HA, Ritter PJ: Surgical repair of the incompetent cervix. Preliminary report of an anatomic modification of the Shirodkar technique. Obstet Gynecol 1961;17:342–345.

50. Roddick JW, Buckingham JC, Danforth DN: Muscular cervix: cause of incompetency in pregnancy. Obstet Gynecol 1961;17:562.

51. Rubovits FE, Cooperman NR, Lash AF: Habitual abortion: a radiographic technique to demonstrate incompetent internal os of the cervix. Am J Obstet Gynecol 1953;66:269.

51a. Salles A de A, Amaral LB, Pinho AL: Diagnosis and treatment of incompetence of the uterine isthmus and cervix during pregnancy. Rev Gynec Obstet 1960; 106:389–98.

52. Scott JZ, Nakamura RM, Davajan V: The cervical factor in infertility diagnosis and treatment. Fertil Steril 1977;28:1289.

53. Seppälä M, Vara P: Cervical cerclage in the treatment of incompetent cervix. Acta Obstet Gynecol (Scand) 1970;49:343.

54. Sherman AJ: Hormonal therapy for control of the incompetent cervical os. Obstet Gynecol 1966;28:198.
55. Shirodkar VN: A new method of operative treatment for habitual abortions in the second trimester of pregnancy. Antiseptic 1955;52:299.
56. Shirodkar VN: Progress in gynecology. Orlando: Grune & Stratton, 1963:260.
57. Singer MS, Hockman M: Incompetent cervix in a hormone exposed offspring. Obstet Gynecol 1978; 51:625.
58. Trythall SW, Jeremias RC: Congenital inadequacy of lower uterine segment as cause of habitual abortion. Int J Fertil 1961;6:67.
59. Wallenburg HCS, Lotgering FK: Transabdominal cerclage for closure of the incompetent cervix. Eur J Obstet Gynecol Reprod Biol 1987;25:121.
60. Watkins RA: Transabdominal cervico-uterine cerclage for the treatment of incompetent cervix. Aust NZ J Obstet Gynaecol 1972;12:62.
61. Wright CSW, Campbell S, Beazley J: Second trimester abortion after vaginal termination of pregnancy. Lancet 1972;1:1278.
62. Yosowitz EE, Haufrect F, Kaufman RH, et al: Silicone-plastic cuff for the treatment of the incompetent cervix in pregnancy. Am J Obstet Gynecol 1972;113:233.

7

UTERINE RECONSTRUCTIVE SURGERY

John A. Rock

INTRODUCTION

Uterine reconstructive surgery requires a thorough understanding of the anatomy and physiology of the uterus, as well as the principles of healing of the smooth muscle of the uterine wall. With current diagnostic techniques, an accurate diagnosis of the extent of uterine disease is often possible. Using the principles of microsurgical technique, the uterus may usually be restored to a near normal configuration. Often, when considering a uterine reconstructive procedure, a decision as to the length and depth of the incision(s) is necessary. Moveover, the surgeon, in some instances, must determine if a less than complete resection (i.e., partial myomectomy) is in order. For if an extensive procedure was performed, infertility or perhaps hysterectomy might be necessary. This judgment may be acquired only through study and experience.

ANATOMY OF THE UTERUS

The uterus is a muscular organ in the true pelvis. It lies between the rectum and bladder, measuring 7–7.5 cm in length, 4.5–5 cm in width, and 2.5–3 cm in thickness. The uterine cavity has an average depth of 6–7 cm and a capacity of 3–8 cc. The uterus is composed of three layers: the perimetrium (serosa), the myometrium, and the endometrium. The perimetrium is continuous with the broad ligament laterally and the bladder and rectal reflections anteriorly and posteriorly, respectively. The myometrium is composed of three layers of smooth muscle fibers: (1) the outer layer (stratum supra vasculare), which is chiefly longitudinal; (2) the middle layer (stratum vasculare) where the fibers are in a circular arrangement and contain many blood vessels; and (3) the inner layer (exaggerated muscularis mucosae) where thin muscle strands are arranged in an oblique and longitudinal fashion. Finally, the endometrium is a mucous membrane composed of tubular glands, stroma, fine connective tissue, and a fine delicate vasculature.

The uterus has a dual blood supply; that is, it receives branches from both the uterine and ovarian arteries. A series of radial arteries branch from the uterine artery as it courses through the uterine body. The radial artery branches into straight arteries, which extend only to the basal layer of the endometrium and into spiral arteries, which are usually coiled and extend through the endometrium. In the superficial layer of the endometrium, "lakes" are formed by capillaries. Venous return is primarily through small veins that drain these capillary plexuses. The vascular picture is quite dynamic, with proliferation and regression associated with cyclic menstruation.

HEALING OF THE SMOOTH MUSCLE IN THE NONPREGNANT UTERUS

Few publications are available concerning the healing of the nonpregnant uterus. This is, in part, due to the lack of surgical specimens immediately following uterine reconstruction for histological study. In particular, one study by Kerr (73) noted that studies of sections from healing uterine incisions revealed a mass of connective tissue from scattered areas of muscle bundles. Furthermore, work by Hartwell (63) summarized the healing process as follows: (*a*) healing of outgrowth of fibroblasts from preexisting structures does not occur; (*b*) a healing cicatrix is formed by exudate cells or macrophages; (*c*) fat is of great importance in the futherance of healing; and (*d*) determination of healing fibrosis is directly related to physical forces; that is, the healing of the uterus may be disturbed by hematoma formation, infection, improper suturing, and constitutional disease.

Siegel (123) emphasized the importance of carefully approximating the layers of the uterus to avoid incorporation of the decidua or endometrium. Inaccurate approximation of the uterine layers may result in adenyomyosis, which may subsequently interfere with healing of the uterine musculature. Additionally, studies of healing in the uterus have revealed that connective tissue formation following incision into the pregnant uterus is abundant and larger in amount than in the nonpregnant uterus.

DIAGNOSTIC TECHNIQUES

Major improvements in diagnostic techniques have afforded a greater accuracy in the identification of uterine factors. Hysterosalpingography and, more recently, hysteroscopy are the current clinical methods for evaluating the uterine cavity. The status of these techniques has been summarized in recent reviews (119,122, 133). The diagnostic applications of hysteroscopy and hysterosalpingography include the evaluations of women with abnormal uterine bleeding or uterine irregularity to delineate the presence of organic pathology, such as endometrial polyps, submucous myoma, or suspected uterine synechiae. Additionally, hysteroscopy may be used to evaluate the patient with repeated abortion, in particular, to determine the extent of congenital uterine anomalies. Operative hysteroscopy requires additional skill in the manipulation of certain instruments, i.e., uterine biopsy forceps and scissors. Repeated hystero-

scopic observation may be performed after lysis of the uterine synechiae to determine if there has been a resolution of uterine scarring. At the same setting, further lysis may be performed, if necessary. Abnormalities with hysterosalpingography may not always be confirmed by hysteroscopy. False-positive hysterographic findings were confirmed in 21% of patients by Siegler in 1977. Therefore, hysterosalpingography should be a complementary procedure usually performed prior to hysteroscopy. Often, organic pathology can be readily identified at the time of hysterosalpingogram, alerting an experienced hysteroscopist as to the location and size of lesions. Furthermore, when multiple lesions are present, as with uterine synechiae or endometrial polyps, the relationship between particular lesions can be more readily studied with a combination of these techniques.

ACQUIRED DEFECTS

Leiomyomata Uteri

The clinical management of leiomyomata uteri has been modified by technologic advances in endoscopy and the introduction of GnRH analogs. The new risks (acquired immunodeficiency syndrome) associated with transfusion also have modified surgical practice. Alternative treatments (e.g., autologous transfusion) have been preferred by patients. Surgeons have taken special care to minimize volume depletion with the use of the cell saver (Haemonetics, Braintree, MA) and more traditional technical methods to minimize blood loss. This section will discuss the medical and surgical management of leiomyomata uteri, with special emphasis on surgical technique.

INCIDENCE

Myomectomy may be indicated for patients with myomas who are being treated for infertility and for those not presently attempting to become pregnant but who wish to maintain their reproductive capacity. Ranney and Frederick (107) reported that 5% of 1022 gynecological operative patients with myomas required myomectomy. Therefore, it is the occasional patient who requires myomectomy to enhance or preserve her fertility.

While many women with myomata have no reproductive difficulty, there are probably others who have reproductive failure consisting of primary infertility, repeated abortion, or premature labor. It is difficult to estimate the magnitude of the problem. Roughly, 40% of women with multiple uterine fibroids have a history of infertility (115). Furthermore, it has been estimated that 5% of infertility patients have a myomatous uterus, which may be partly responsible for their inability to conceive (9). More recently, Ranney and Frederick (107) reported that nine of 51 patients (18%) with infertility thought due to myomas underwent abdominal myomectomy to enhance their ability to conceive. Unfortunately, there are no studies that have documented the numbers of patients with significant fibromyomata who have had term deliveries. These data would serve as a reference to evaluate success following myomectomy.

ETIOLOGY

Enlargement of leiomyomata uteri is usually due to estrogen stimulation. A higher concentration of estrogen receptors has been identified in uterine myomas than in adjacent myometrium in normal uterine tissue (138). Furthermore, uterine myomas bind 20% more estradiol per mg of cytoplasmic protein than does normal myometrium from the same uterus. Maximal growth occurs during the reproductive years when ovarian secretions of estrogen result in significant serum levels. Leiomyoma usually regresses in volume with the onset of menopause; hence the rationale for the use of GnRH analogs to create hypogonadotropic hypogonadism. The enlargement of myomas after menopause raises concern that a malignancy may be present. Nevertheless, the incidence of malignancy arising in a uterine myoma is extremely rare (1 per 200, or 0.5%) (100).

It has been suggested that growth of myomas may also occur as a result of estrogen-progesterone medications including oral contraceptives (70). However, Ross and coauthors (114) have noted that the risk of fibroids was reduced by 30% in women who used oral contraceptive pills (OCP) for 10 years. Furthermore, there are no controlled studies linking OCP to fibroid growth. Currently, the evidence strongly suggests that the underlying risk factor is "unopposed estrogen." Alternatively, androgens and progesterone alone exert an antimitotic effect (57,58).

Leiomyoma are found in approximately 2% of pregnant women. Myomas may increase in size during pregnancy. During pregnancy, the uterine myoma may rapidly enlarge, outgrowing its blood supply. The reduced circulation may result in thrombosis, leading to necrosis of tissue. Dark hemorrhagic colors appear, characteristic of red degeneration. One in 10 women with myoma will have complications related to myomas during pregnancy (71). Patients with complications most commonly experience second or early third trimester pain and, occasionally, bleeding. Other less frequent complications include preterm rupture of membranes, malpresentation, increased cesarean delivery rate, and postpartum endomyometritis. Patients with retroplacental leiomyoma are at increased risk for abruptio placenta (108).

SYMPTOMS

Most patients with leiomyoma are asymptomatic. However, when leiomyoma are large, patients may develop symptoms related to the size and position of the tumors.

More commonly encountered than pain, pressure and increased abdominal girth develop insidiously, are often less apparent, and are usually vaguely described by the patient. As myomas grow, pressure is frequently exerted on adjacent viscera. Pressure on the urinary bladder usually provokes urinary frequency, especially when the myomas are located in the subvesical region, or when a large myomatous uterus fills the entire pelvis. When the myoma is located adjacent to the urethra and bladder neck, acute urinary retention may occur. An enlarging myoma anatomically located just over the cervix may also cause protrusion of the base of the bladder and distension of the anterior vaginal wall, suggesting pelvic relaxation. Stress urinary incontinence may also reflect myomas situated in the vicinity of the bladder neck. Ureteral obstruction is a serious consequence of chronic pressure on the urinary collecting system. Usually silent, this complication results from pressure of the myomatous uterus upon the pelvic brim, obstructing the ureter. This anatomical change is reversible once the pressure is alleviated unless the kidney has suffered parenchymal damage. Chronic obstruction at the level of the bladder neck can also lead to hydroureter and hydronephrosis. Rectal pressure may occur from a solitary large posterior wall myoma extending into the cul-de-sac of Douglas. Constipation may also result from the pressure of a posterior myoma.

DIAGNOSIS

A complete evaluation should be performed on a patient with myomatous uterus and infertility. A hysterogram is indicated to evaluate the relationship of the tumors to the endometrial cavity and to document patency or distortion of the tubes. Hysterosalpingography will identify an intramural myoma, as well as marked distortion of the cavity (Fig. 7.1).

Hysteroscopy is an important diagnostic measure for the detection of submucous myomas. Magnetic Resonance Imaging (MRI) is useful to determine the exact location of the fibroids in relation to the uterine cavity, cervix, and fallopian tubes. The ovulatory, cervical, and male factors should be thoroughly investigated prior to surgery. In patients with repeated pregnancy loss, a karyotype is indicated when normal pregnancies are interspersed with spontaneous abortions, suggestive of a chromosomal abberation. A preoperative intravenous pyelogram may be useful in observing any possible displacement or distortion of the ureters when the fibroids are large and fill the pelvic cavity. Only when a thorough evaluation to identify other factors that might be responsible for infertility or repeated pregnancy wastage (Table 7.1) has been performed should abdominal or endoscopic myomectomy be considered.

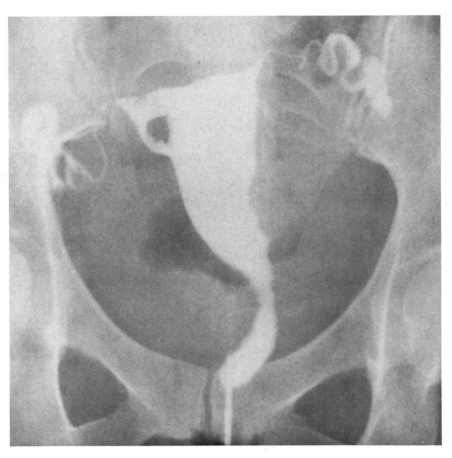

Figure 7.1. Hysterographic representation of fibromyomata distorting the uterine cavity.

Table 7.1.   Preconception Evaluation for Patients with Repeated Pregnancy Loss[a]

Medical history
  Clear description and sequence of all pregnancy loss
  Histologic confirmation
  Chronic illness
  Uterine instrumentation
  Infection
  DES exposure in utero
  Exposure to drugs, radiation, and environmental
    pollutants
Physical examination
  General, with emphasis on signs of metabolic disease;
  Pelvic examination:
    Cervix
      Anatomic changes associated with DES
        exposure in utero
      Laceration
      Infection
    Uterus
      Enlargement or irregularity
      Midline fundal depression
Laboratory testing
  Principle investigations:
    Complete blood count, blood chemistry profile
Uterine reconstructive surgery
  Endometrial biopsy
  Hysterosalpingography and/or hysteroscopy
  Karyotypic analysis
  Antiphospholipid antibodies
Investigations suggested by history and examination
findings:
  Antinuclear factor
  Herpesvirus, cytomegalovirus, toxoplasmosis
  Thyroid profile
Additional investigations recommended for cases of
unexplained habitual abortion:
  Blood group antibody studies
  Cultures for viral infectious agents (e.g., *Mycoplasma*)
  Immunologic testing (e.g., major HLA studies and
    antisperm antibody studies

[a]Adapted from Rock JA, Zacur HA: The clinical management of repeated early pregnancy wastage. Fertil Steril 39:136, 1983. Reproduced with permission of the publisher, American Fertility Society.

PATHOPHYSIOLOGY

The exact mechanisms by which a fibroid uterus interferes with conception are unknown. Possible factors include the mechanical action and local pressure of myomas, distortion and elongation of the endometrial cavity, and myometrial irritation due to the degeneration of intramural and submucous myoma or torsion of a pedunculated myoma (81). Accordingly, anatomic alteration of the uterine cavity may interfere with implantation. Furthermore, a marked distortion of the cavity may result in a cornual occlusion.

A variety of endometrial abnormalities ranging from atrophy to hyperplasia have been reported to be associated with myomas (37,66). Endometrial changes may be seen in up to 80% of patients (15). Abnormal myometrial and endometrial veins have been identified in association with large myomas, and it has been postulated that the obstructive elements produced by myomas cause proximal congestion of myometrium and endometrium due to the absence of valves in these uterine veins. The interference of myomas with normal physiologic myometrial contractility and hormonal factors associated with myomas may also play a role in causing infertility (125). Most authors feel that a combination of the above postulates may explain the infertility observed in a few patients with leiomyomata uteri. The observation that 40–50% of patients conceive after abdominal myomectomy suggests that myomas do interfere with conception. Furthermore, there is a significant improvement in the rate of fetal wastage (Table 7.2).

MEDICAL MANAGEMENT

Reduction in volume of leiomyomata uteri has been documented with the use of several medications. Goodman (58) first noted a reduction of fibroid size following therapy with progesterone. Goldzieher (57) subsequently noted degenerative changes in myomas removed prior to hysterectomy in women treated with large doses of progestogens (medrogestone, 25 mg daily) 14–21 days prior to surgery.

Continho and Goncalves (28) noted reduction in myoma volume following vaginal and oral administration of gestrinone, a 19-norsteroid with antiestrogenic and antiprogesterogenic properties. In 89% of patients, uterine fibroid volume remained below pretreatment values if discontinued at 6 months.

Several studies have demonstrated that treatment with GnRH agonist can cause a reduction in uterine myoma (Fig. 7.2). The GnRH agonist causes pituitary desensitization by down regulation of GnRH receptors. The subsequent hypogonadotropic hypogonadal

Table 7.2.   Spontaneous Abortion Rates in Women with Leiomyomata[a]

		Preoperative		Postoperative	
Author	Total no. Patients	Fetal Salvage	Fetal Wastage	Fetal Salvage	Fetal Wastage
Davids (1957)	1335	498	324	210	30
Ingersoll (1963)	139	10	7	34	8
Stevenson (1964)	107	27	21	39	7
Malone and Ingersoll (1975)	75	13	13	44	13
Loeffler and Nobel (1970)	180	58	48	41	28
Babaknia, et al. (1978)	46	5	16	19	3
Buttram and Reiter (1981)	59	11	12	18	8
Total	1941	622 (59%)	441 (41%)	405 (81%)	97 (19%)

[a]From Buttram V, Reiter R: 1985. Uterine leiomyomata in surgical treatment of the infertile female. Baltimore: Williams & Wilkins, 1985;206.

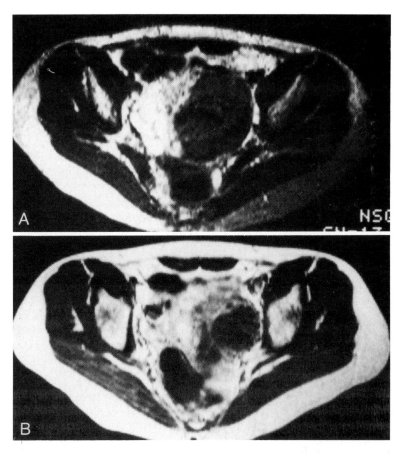

Figure 7.2. Magnetic Resonance Imaging of Pelvis: Transverse section of the pelvis demonstrating uterine myomata. *A,* Before, and *B,* After 24 weeks of depot leuprolide therapy. Normal myometrium emits a much greater (brighter) signal than the more structured myomata. Total myoma volume in this patient was reduced 67% with treatment. (From Schlaff et al., 1989.)

state results in hypoestrogenism. Reduction in myoma size is usually assessed by ultrasound and MRI. Reduction in myoma size has been reported in the range of 30–100% (Table 7.3). Maximal reduction in myoma size occurs within 4 months of treatment.

There are no data to support a specific indication for GnRH agonist in the treatment of uterine myoma. Some surgeons have reported anecdotal experiences, suggesting that a reduction in myoma size allows easier myomectomy. Friedman and coauthors (49) designed a stratified double-blind placebo-controlled study evaluating the efficacy of leuprolide acetate depot before myomectomy. The authors reported that GnRH agonist treatment prior to myomectomy may decrease intraoperative blood loss in women with large leiomyomata uteri.

Another potential use of GnRH agonists has been recommended to create ammenorrhea in women with anemia and hypermenorrhea. This would allow improvement of hematologic status prior to myomectomy. Few argue the role of GnRH agonists prior to resection of a submucous fibroid. A reduction in the size of the submucous myoma facilitates removal with the hysteroscope or resectoscope through the cervical os.

SURGICAL MANAGEMENT
Abdominal Myomectomy

The operative technique of myomectomy is based upon the observation that myomas are tumors that do not invade the uterine myometrium, but rather place pressure on the tissues as they enlarge. This results in distortion and displacement of the myometrium, rather than infiltration. The thinned-out myometrium that encapsulates the myoma, or "pseudocapsule," provides a well-defined place of cleavage between the fibroid and the capsule.

Open Abdomen

Hemostasis is a major consideration at the time of uterine surgery. Myomectomy can often result in considerable blood loss. Vasopressin (Pitressin) may minimize blood loss due to arteriolar vasoconstriction. (Fig. 7.3A).

Dillon (38) suggests vasopressin injection at

Table 7.3. Treatment of Uterine Fibroids with GnRH Agonists

Author	Agonist	Patients	Reduction (%)	Method
Filicori et al. (1983)	D-Tryp⁶	3	78	Ultrasound
Healy et al. (1984)	Buserelin	1	80	Ultrasound
Maheux et al. (1985)	Buserelin	10	80	Ultrasound
Coddington et al. (1986)	Histerlin	6	35–65	Ultrasound
West et al. (1987)	Goserelin	13	55	Ultrasound
Andreyko et al. (1987)	Nafaelin	11	50	MRI
Friedman et al. (1987)	Leuprolide	7	53	Ultrasound
Perl et al. (1987)	D-Tryp⁶	10	10–100	Ultrasound
Friedman et al. (1989)	Leuprolide	38	40	Ultrasound
Schlaff et al. (1989)	Leuprolide	11	30–40	MRI
Letterie et al. (1989)	Histerlin	19	50	Ultrasound
Donnez et al. (1989)	Buserelin	20	35	Cavity size by HSG

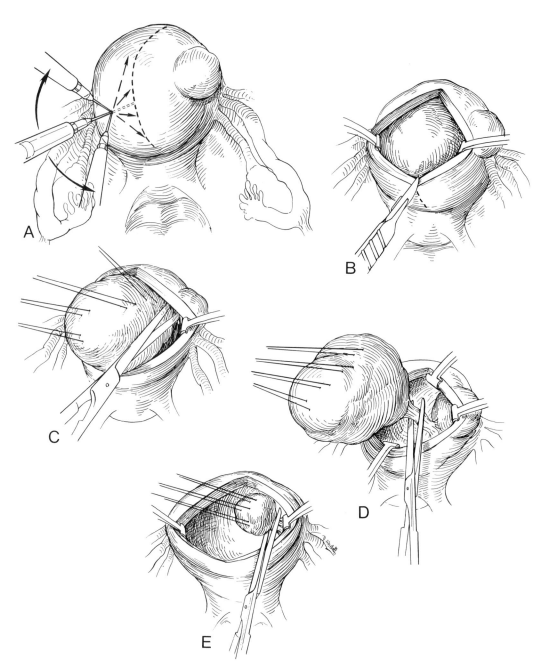

Figure 7.3. Abdominal myomectomy. *A,* After the location of the uterine incision is selected, a dilute solution of vasopressin is injected into the myometrium. *B,* A single vertical incision is most useful in exposing the maximum number of fibroid tumors. *C,* The fibroid may be held under traction with sutures placed into the myoma so as to expose the attachments at the base of the tumor. A fine Metzenbaum scissors may be used to develop the cleavage plane. *D,* A Kelly clamp is applied to the base of the fibroid to free the tumor and to allow suture ligation of the pedicle. *E,* Additional fibroids may be removed through this incision. *F,* Meticulous ligation of bleeders results in minimal blood loss. A purse-string suture is, in some instances, useful to obliterate the dead space at the base of the uterine defect. *G,* The first layer of interrupted 2-0 chromic catgut suture is placed so as to close the defect in the uterine wall and establish hemostasis. A second layer of 3-0 – 4-0 suture material may be placed to approximate subserosal tissues. *H,* The serosa may be closed with a subserosal continuous 4-0 nonreactive suture material.

the junction of the uterus with the myoma or its pedicle. With a dose of 2 units per 10 ml of solution, the effect lasted approximately 30 minutes, at which time additional injections were needed. He noted that arterial bleeding was not masked. With the use of vasopressin, 72% of patients requiring myomectomy did not need blood replacement as compared with 43% of controls. Ingersoll and Malone (65) also found vasopressin injection satisfactory for minimizing blood loss. Our experience has been quite similar. Nevertheless, careful dissection and prompt suturing with the exertion of direct pressure to bleeding vessels by the operative assistant are also necessary to aid in minimizing blood loss. Allis-Adiar or large T-clamps may be used on the incised myometrial walls to minimize bleeding. These clamps should not be applied to the uterine serosa. Gentle traction between the fibroid and its pseudocapsule will allow careful dissection in the plane of cleavage. In this manner, under direct vision, fibers between the fibroid and its pseudocapsule may be carefully lysed. Twisting, pulling, and the use of blunt finger dissection to shell out the tumor should be avoided, as they usually result in excessive bleeding and perhaps the unnecessary invasion

of the endometrial cavity. Furthermore, if dissection is taken laterally, uncontrolled bleeding may occur in the broad ligaments and, occasionally, damage to the ureters may result. Particular care must be taken if myomas are adjacent to the interstitial portion of the oviducts. Inadvertent occlusion of the interstitial portion of the oviduct may occur if wide sutures are placed carelessly so as to encircle the intramural portion of the fallopian tube.

The Myometrial Incision

The location of the uterine incision should be placed so that as many fibroids may be removed through the incision as possible. Traction sutures may be placed at the junction of the round ligaments to elevate the uterus. A single verticle incision is most useful in exposing the maximum number of fibroid tumors (Fig. 7.3A). The location of the uterine incision will vary, but consideration should be given to the fact that the uterine vessels supply the uterus by horizontal concentric loops. As the incision is extended, the myometrium usually retracts over the surface of the tumor (Fig. 7.3B). Often, a tenaculum may be applied to the uterus to elevate the tumor. The myo-

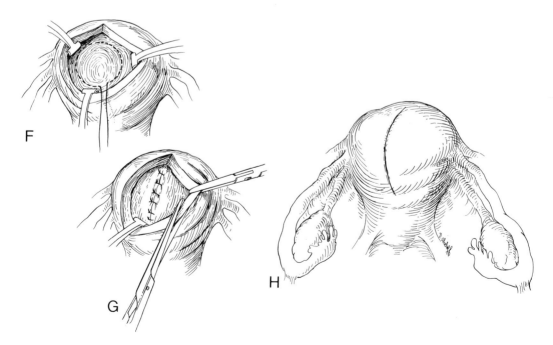

Figure 7.3. *F–H*

metrial incision may be determined by the size and location of the fibroid. Fundal fibroids may have a broad or thin base. A longitudinal elliptical incision easily exposes the pseudocapsule. Multiple subserous fibroids may pose a more difficult decision. Generally, 4–5 fibroids may be removed through a midline incision. With the best technique, 2–3 incisions may be required for complete removal of multiple myomas.

Development of a Cleavage Plane

Vessels along the incised myometrial edge should be suture-ligated. Small bleeders along the incision may be controlled with the placement of Allis-Adair or T-clamps. Furthermore, the proper placement of the T-clamp may be useful for traction, allowing easy dissection with the Metzenbaum scissors along the pseudocapsule (Fig. 7.3C). If additional visualization is needed, the T-clamp may be advanced and readjusted for proper visualization. The fibroid may be held under traction with sutures placed into the myoma so as to expose the attachments at the base of the tumor (Fig. 7.3D,E). A Kelly clamp applied to the base of the fibroid will free the tumor and allow suture ligation of the pedicle. This technique is particularly useful to avoid the risk of tissue retraction where hemostasis could be achieved only with the blind placement of deep sutures.

Repairing the Myometrial Defect

Meticulous ligation of bleeders will result in minimal blood loss. However, a warm, moist pad may be useful in limiting blood loss from small unidentified vessels while the uterine musculature is being repaired. If the uterine cavity is entered, the endometrium should be carefully approximated with interrupted sutures of #3-0 chromic catgut placed in such a manner so as the knots are positioned within the uterine cavity. The uterine defect may be closed in two layers. The endometrium must be carefully approximated to prevent the development of adenomyosis, which may ultimately weaken the uterine scar. A purse-string suture is sometimes useful to obliterate the dead space at the base of the uterine defect (Fig. 7.3F). The first layer of interrupted #2-0 nonreactive

sutures is placed so as to close the defect in the uterine wall and to establish hemostasis (Fig. 7.3G). Care should be taken to ensure that each suture extends down the base of the uterine defect, thus preventing hematoma formation. Depending on the size of the uterine defect, an additional layer of suture may be necessary to approximate the myometrium. Redundant myometrium should be excised to achieve a better approximation of the serosa. The serosa may be closed with a subserosal continuous 4-0 nonreactive suture material or interrupted sutures of fine absorbable suture (Fig. 7.3H).

Prevention of Adhesions

A single vertical incision is less likely to result in adhesions than are multiple incisions. Although all myomas cannot be removed through one incision, often, other fibroids can be removed by pushing them toward the primary incision (20). With posterior uterine incisions, a uterine suspension may be preferable to prevent retrofixation of the uterus. Mobilizing the round ligaments to bring the broad ligament over the incision, or free omental or peritoneal grafts over a posterior incision, may prevent adherence of the small bowel or sigmoid colon. Minimizing postoperative adnexal adhesions should be a primary concern when selecting the uterine incision site. It may be necessary to leave myomas, recognizing that tuboovarian adhesions would surely result if myomectomy was attempted. Attention to the surgical principles limiting blood loss and avoiding adhesion formation will result in minimal operative morbidity and an excellent anatomic result (Table 7.4).

RESULTS

Berkely an coauthors (14) reported only seven of 21 patients over the age of 30 who achieved a pregnancy after myomectomy, whereas 18 of 29 patients under the age of 30 conceived. Babaknia and coauthors (6) noted no pregnancies in women over 35 years of age. Smith and Uhlir (124) noted that half of the patients who achieved pregnancy were over the age of 35, and 32% (5 of 16) were 40 years of age or older. Similarly, Rosenfeld (113) noted that five of eight patients over the age of 35 and two of four patients over the age of 40 became pregnant.

Interestingly, Smith and Uhlir (124) found no significant difference in the weight of myomas removed and the pregnancy success. Berkeley and coauthors (14), however, found an average total weight of fibroid tumors in patients who ultimately conceived to be 194 g as compared with 384 g in those women who did not conceive.

Malone and Ingersoll (83) reported that 40% of 75 patients with uteri greater than twice the normal size conceived following myomectomy. Forty percent of these patients delivered term infants. Roughly two-thirds of these patients had primary infertility. The average duration of infertility was 4 years. The

majority of the pregnancies occurred within the first 2 years postmyomectomy.

Babaknia recorded a similar experience in 67 patients treated with myomectomy at the Johns Hopkins Hospital between 1930–1975 (6). Thirty-six of 67 patients, or 54%, conceived following myomectomy for infertility. Twenty-eight, or 42% of patients had a term delivery that resulted in a living child. Eighty-two percent of the patients who conceived did so within the first 2 years postmyomectomy. Of the 46 patients in the Johns Hopkins study, 42 had a preoperative hysterogram. Nine patients were noted preoperatively to have a distorted endometrial cavity. Of these, five had secondary infertility and three had primary infertility. The remaining 33 patients had endometrial cavities that were normal by hysterosalpingogram. A correlation between the distortion of the endometrial cavity and pregnancy success could not be demonstrated. A current update of our patient series has revealed a term delivery rate of 55% after myomectomy. These results are similar to previous reports, as summarized by Buttram and Reiter (19) (Table 7.2).

Relief of menorrhagia may also be an important goal of abdominal myomectomy. A large distorted uterine cavity may be responsible for excessive blood loss during menses. Following abdominal myomectomy, 81% of women experience relief of symptoms (19) (Table 7.5).

A review of the literature has determined that the risk of occurrence of myomas after myomectomy is 15%, while only 11% of women will require subsequent surgery for symptoms (19). Certain variables may alter the

---

Table 7.4. Surgical Principles of Uterine Myomectomy

1. Limit blood loss by
   a. Using vasopressin myometrial injection
   b. Placing atraumatic hemostasis clamps on the incised myometrial wall
   c. Using moist pads to compress small bleeders
   d. Avoiding digital blunt dissection of fibroids
   e. Using cell saver
2. Avoid adhesion formation by
   a. Atraumatic technique and using nonreactive suture to close the serosa
   b. Selecting fibroids that may be removed without increasing the risk of adnexal adhesions
   c. Choosing a single vertical incision through which several fibroids may be removed
   d. Performing a uterine suspension and/or omental-peritoneal graft when appropriate
   e. Using barriers in conjunction with second-look laparoscopy

---

Table 7.5. Postoperative Reduction or Resolution of Menorrhagia[a]

Author (Year)	No. Patients with Menorrhagia	No. of Patients with Reduction or Resolution of Postoperative Menorrhagia
		(%)
Miller and Tyrone (1933)	57	52 (91)
Counseller and Bedard (1938)	137	113 (82)
Munnell and Martin (1951)	41	38 (93)
Loeffler and Noble (1970)	35	14 (40)
Buttram and Reiter (1981)	15	13 (87)
Total	285	230 (81)

[a]From Buttram V, Reiter R: Uterine leiomyomata in the surgical treatment of the infertile female. Baltimore: Williams & Wilkins, 1985;220.

risk, i.e., completeness of removal of myomas, age of initial myomectomy, and associated pelvic pathology (Table 7.6).

As a rule, the healing of a properly repaired uterine incision in the nonpregnant state is far better than in a gravid uterus. Although some surgeons feel that myomectomy is an absolute indication for delivery be cesarean section, we have been less stringent. Vaginal delivery may be anticipated, unless the uterine scars are known to have been weakened by postoperative infection or if multiple incisions of the uterus were required for a rather extensive myomectomy. Of the 28 term pregnancies in our series, 16 patients delivered vaginally without complications, while 12 were delivered by cesarean section (6).

Laparoscopic Resection

Removal of a myoma through the laparoscope is rarely indicated for resolution in infertility. The uterine defect that results from the removal of a large intramural myoma is difficult to close, as is the serosa. Postoperative adhesion formation may be substantial. Thus, most fibroids are best removed through an abdominal incision. The limitations of the laparoscopic myomectomy are primarily due to the lack of appropriate suture material and instrumentation to accomplish a proper approximation of the muscle and serosa. Nevertheless, there are small fibroids that may result in pain. These may be easily and safely removed through the laparoscope.

Surgical Technique

The pedunculated myoma is grasped with an instrument through a second incision and vasopressin (Pitressin) injected at the base of the myoma through the laparoscope with a needle (Pitressin diluted in 20 ml of saline). The base of the stalk is coagulated with bipolar current, and the myoma freed by incising the stalk. After morcellation, the myoma may be removed through the large trocar, or alternatively, an incision can be made in the poste-

Table 7.6.   Recurrence and Treatment of Leiomyomata Subsequent to Myomectomy[a,b]

Author	Total no. Patients	No. Recurrences of Leiomyomata	No. Patients with Subsequent Treatment
		(%)	(%)
Weiss (1926)	232	17 (7)	9 (4)
Bonney (1931)	210	8 (4)	6 (3)
Miller and Tyrone (1933)	94	8 (9)	8 (9)
Counseller and Bedard (1938)	523	111 (21)	26 (5)
Mussey et al. (1945)	250	75 (30)	50 (20)
Finn and Muller (1950)	274	48 (18)	24 (9)
Munnel and Martin (1951)	236	49 (21)	29 (2)
Brown, A. et al. (1956)	234	66 (28)	35 (15)
Davids (1957)	310		24 (8)
Rubin (1957)	222	37 (17)	12 (5)
McCormick (1958)	66		4 (6)
Ingersoll (1963)	139		14 (10)
Brown, J. et al. (1967)	95		30 (32)
Malone and Ingersoll[c] (1968)	75	22 (29)	12 (16)
Loeffler and Noble (1970)	116	33 (28)	31 (27)
Babaknia, et al. (1978)	46	13 (28)	6 (13)
Ranney and Frederick (1979)	51		14 (27)
Buttram and Reiter (1981)	42	6 (14)	4 (10)
Smith and Uhlir	62	6 (10)	3 (5)
Total	3206	493 (15)	338 (11)

[a]From Buttram V, Reiter R: Uterine leiomyomata in surgical treatment of the infertile female. Baltimore: Williams & Wilkins, 1985;223.
[b]Treatment includes hysterectomy, second myomectomy, or radiation therapy.
[c]Excludes patients in series in whom recurrence of leiomyomata not recorded.

rior cul-de-sac to allow removal through the vagina.

The small subserous or intramural fibroid may also be safely removed, provided the myoma is in a position that does not complicate the procedure. Myomas should not be adjacent to the fallopian tube or lateral in the proximity to the uterine artery.

A dilute portion of a solution of Pitressin (20 units of vasopressin diluted in 20 ml of saline) may be injected at the base of the myoma. A longitudinal incision should expose the myoma, which then may be grasped with an instrument through the second or third incision (Fig. 7.4A). Vessels on the surface of the myoma should be coagulated with bipolar current. With myoma held under traction, a fine scissors may be inserted through the operating channel of the laparoscope and a cleavage plane developed to the base of the myoma (Fig. 7.4B). The bipolar cautery forceps may then be applied to the vascular attachments at the base of the tumor (Fig. 7.4C). This technique should avoid the risk of bleeding from a vascular pedicle, which may retract after it is excised.

The myometrial incision should be closed after hemostasis is established. This usually requires only one layer of interrupted 4-0 PDS (Ethicon). Sutures are placed through the muscularis and serosa and tied securely (Fig. 7.4D,E). The myoma may then be morcellated and removed through a large trocar or an incision in the posterior cul-de-sac.

At present, there are no reports of large series of patients treated by laparoscopic myomectomy. There are no data concerning relief of pain, subsequent fertility, or postprocedure adhesion formation. Until more experience has been obtained, procedures should be performed with the following guidelines in mind:

1. Prophylactic removal of fibroids is rarely indicated;
2. Infertility is rarely an indication for myomectomy;
3. Myomectomy should be performed on centrally located myomas that are not adjacent to the fallopian tube or parametrium;
4. Surgical principles of atraumatic dissection, hemostasis, and myometrial closure should be observed.

With the future development of new laparoscopic instrumentation and special suture material, large fibroids may be safely removed. However, at the writing of this text, laparoscopic myomectomy should be limited to small myomas in accordance with hemostatis, atraumatic removal, myometrial closure, and techniques to limit or prevent subsequent adhesion formation.

Transcervical Myomectomy

Submucous myomas constitute 5% of all uterine myomas (99). Unless there is prolapse of the fibroid, diagnosis may be difficult. The uterus may be minimally enlarged. The most common symptom observed in women with a submucous myoma is profuse vaginal bleeding often associated with significant anemia. GnRH agonist therapy represents a useful adjunct to preoperative reduction in myoma size, which may permit surgical treatment of submucous myoma by hysteroscopy. Furthermore, relief of symptoms, i.e., hypermenorrhea, may allow restoration of normal hemotologic status (40).

Vaginal Myomectomy

Vaginal myomectomy is the treatment of choice for prolapsed submucous myoma. The pedunculated tumor may become necrotic due to impairment of blood supply. Once the tumor has prolapsed through the cervix, the myoma may become infected. Broad-spectrum antibiotics are indicated to prevent endomyometritis.

Vaginal myomectomy is usually a short procedure. The myoma is grasped and twisted free. Rarely, bleeding may occur at the pedicle, requiring a suture ligature. Ben-Baruch and coauthors (10) reported successful vaginal myomectomy in 43 of 46 women. Thirty-four patients, or 8.8%, with a median follow-up of 5.5 years, required a repeat vaginal myomectomy, and 5.9% required hysterectomy. Interestingly, the three failed attempts were patients with large myomas.

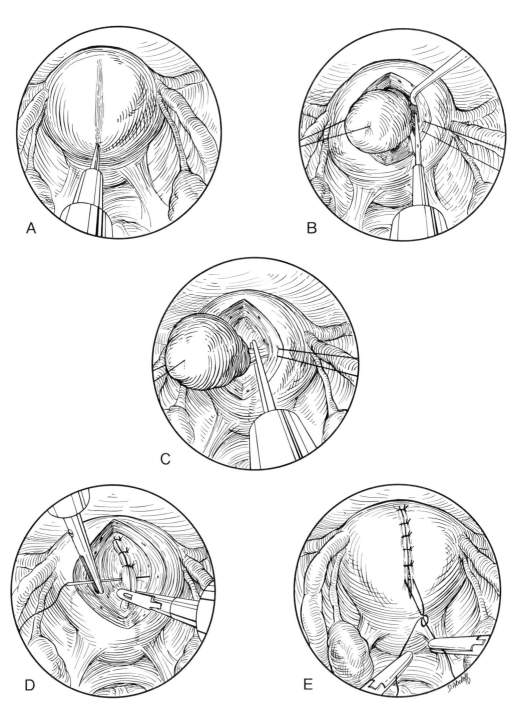

Figure 7.4. Laparoscopic myomectomy. *A,* After a dilute solution of vasopressin has been injected at the site of the incision, a longitudinal incision should expose the myoma. This may be grasped with a suture and held under traction. *B,* The cleavage plane is developed with fine scissors. *C,* After the fibroid is fully mobilized, the pedicle may be clamped and the suture ligated using extracorporal knot-tying technique. *D,* The myometrium is approximated with 4-0 PDS on a straight needle. *E,* The serosa is approximated with 4-0 PDS interrupted sutures.

Hysteroscopic Resection of Submucous Myomas

Hysteroscopy is often useful for the assessment and resection of submucous leiomyomata.

Abnormal uterine bleeding is the usual indication for the endoscopic removal of a submucous myoma through the uterine cervix. Contraindications to this approach include: (*a*) unexplained adnexal mass; (*b*) suspicion of malignancy; (*c*) uterine cavity of greater than 10 cm; and (*d*) when the patient refuses to accept the possibility of hysterectomy. The advantages of hysteroscopic myomectomy include the avoidance of laparotomy, uterine incision, and the need for cesarean section should a subsequent pregnancy occur. Hospitalization is usually limited to same-day surgery or an overnight stay.

The development of the panoramic operating hysteroscope has allowed resection of submucous fibroids with a cautery loop, Nd:YAG laser, and scissors, with excellent anatomic results. The resecting hysteroscope is essentially a modification of the urologic resectoscope (98). Suppression of the menstrual cycle with a GnRH analog, Progestin or danazol, has been recommended to decrease the endometrial lining. GnRH analogs may also result in devascularization and reduction in size of a submucous fibroid. Hyskon (Pharmacia), 32% dextran-70, and 10% dextrose in water solution is often used as a distending medium. Cautery current best suited for a submucous myoma resection is 60–120 W in a small 2-mm depth of burn. The semirigid scissors (131) and the Nd:YAG laser (7) have been used to incise the submucous myoma. The double-channel operating hysteroscope (Weck, Princeton, NJ) permits simultaneous delivery of the Nd:YAG quartz fiber and either an aspirating cannula, long flexible needle, scissors, or forceps. Concurrent laparoscopy is recommended during hysteroscopic resection to avoid perforation of the uterus and to keep the bowel away from the cautery site.

Surgical Technique

The location of the fibroid should be noted. A preoperative hysterogram should be available to view the relationship of the fibroid to the uterotubal os and lower uterine segment. The myoma may be injected with a dilute solution of vasopressin (1 unit to 20 cc of saline) transhysteroscopically with a flexible needle. Large vessels on the surface of the myoma may be coagulated. The needle may also be used to position the myoma (Fig. 7.5). Although semirigid and rigid scissors are adequate for surgical management of pedunculated myomas, a resectoscope or Nd:YAG laser usually is needed if the myoma is partially embedded in the uterine wall or is larger than 4 cm in diameter. It is important to have additional instruments available to grasp the myoma so as to provide traction. Traction may be placed on the edge of the incision in the myoma with forceps, allowing slices of the fibroid to be removed without pushing the myoma against the endometrium. The tumor is shaved down to the base with a cutting current or laser.

If a resectoscope is used, the 90° cutting loop should be used. Resection begins with 60 W of cutting current. The electric loop is placed behind the section to be resected and drawn into the insulated sleeve toward the objective lenses of the hysteroscope. This maneuver is repeated so as to shave away the myoma. The resected fragments may obscure the surgeon's vision. At this point, the scope should be removed, allowing the tissue to flow out with the medium. The resectoscope is then again inserted and the procedure continued. In some instances, tissue may be removed from the uterine cavity with Pollack forceps. Additional dilatation of the cervix may be required to remove large fragments. In cases of postoperative bleeding, a silastic balloon or inflated Foley catheter of large diameter may be inserted into the uterine cavity temporarily for a tamponade effect. The use of prophylatic antibiotics is recommended. The use of an intrauterine device and estrogen-progesterone cyclic therapy are usually unnecessary.

Hysteroscopic resection makes possible the complete removal of pedunculated submucous myomas and partial removal, to the endometrial lining, of sessile tumors. The need for transabdominal myomectomy may be limited to submucous fibroids adjacent to the uterotubal os, where tubal damage may result from cautery. Operative risks include uterine perforation, postoperative infection, and cautery injury.

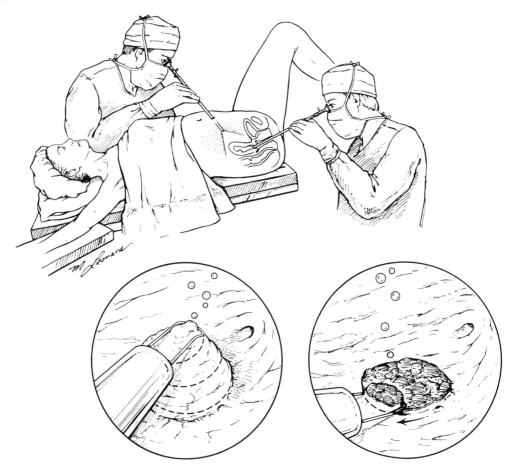

Figure 7.5. Transcervical (hysteroscopic) myomectomy. The submucous fibroid may be shaved with the cutting loop of the resecting hysteroscope. If the fibroid is in a position adjacent to the lateral uterine wall, laparoscopy may be performed at the same setting to limit the risks of perforation of the uterus. The fibroid is carefully shaved down under direct visualization through the hysteroscope. Vasopressin may be injected directly into the submucous fibroid using the injector needle described by Baggish.

Results

The cure rate after hysteroscopic submucous myomectomy for abnormal uterine bleeding has been reported in the range of 60–100% (Table 7.7). The results vary depending on the size and location of the myoma, the type of myoma (pedunculated vs. sessile), and the experience and skill of the surgeon. Recurrence rates reflecting the return of abnormal uterine bleeding requiring further surgery are usually less than 10%.

INTRAUTERINE SYNECHIAE

The phenomenon of intrauterine synechiae was identified by Heindrich Fritsch, who published the first observation of total atresia of the uterine cavity resulting from curettage for postpartum bleeding (52). The full recognition of this syndrome resulted from several publications by Asherman describing its clinical presentation (3–5). Although there are several synonyms for this syndrome, the name intrauterine synechiae has gained wide use and acceptance (53).

The definition of intrauterine synechiae requires the presence of an adherence to the anterior and posterior uterine wall, which results in complete or partial obliteration of the cavity. Depending on the extent of the synechiae, specific clinical symptoms may result. There have been numerous articles describing the etiology, symptoms, and therapy (13,74,127,129). Use of the hysteroscope,

Table 7.7.   Hysteroscopic Myomectomy for Uterine Abnormal Bleeding[a]

Author	No. patients	Type of Myomas Pedunculated	Sessile	Method	IUD[b]	E/P[c]	Antibiotics	Cure (%)	Recurrence (%)
Haning et al. (1980)	1	–	+	Resectoscope	–	+	+	1	–
DeCherney, Polan (1983)	8	+	+	Resectoscope	Foley	+	+	8	–
Neuwirth (1983)	28	+	+	Resectoscope	Intra-uterine	+	+	17 (60.7)	8 (28.5)
Valle, Sciarra (1987)	34	+	–	Semirigid sissors	–	–	+	34	–
Hallez et al. (1988)	300	–	+	Resectoscope	–	–	+	299[d]	–
Baggish et al. (1989)	23	–	+	Nd: YAG laser	–	–	–	100	0
Lin et al.	13	+	–	Resectoscope rigid scissors	–	–	–	9	4
Goldrath (1987)	92[e]	+	–	Lamenaria	–	–	–	80	12[f]
Totals	499							471/499	24/499

[a]Adapted from Seigler AM, Valle RF: Therapeutic hysteroscopic procedures. Fertil Steril 1988;50:685.
[b]IUD, intrauterine device.
[c]E/P, estrogens/progesterones.
[d]1 patient required laparotomy.
[e]3 patients required laparotomy.
[f]Diagnosis by hysteroscopy.

along with several classification systems for uterine synechiae, has provided some consistency in diagnosis and in reporting results. This discussion will present a current overview in the light of these new developments.

Incidence

The incidence of intrauterine synechiae is not known. Nevertheless, it is possible to determine its rate of occurrence in certain patient groups. Eriksen and Koestet (42) noted a 20–25% incidence of intrauterine synechiae in all patients treated with D&C within 2 months postpartum. Dmowski and Greenblatt (39) reported that all patients subjected to hysterograms have a 1.5% incidence of synechiae. When patients were selected for appropriate history and physical examination, in addition to hysterosalpingographic findings, the incidence of 39%. Roughly 5% of all hysterograms done for repeated abortion revealed intrauterine adhesions (106). Thirty-nine percent of patients with a history of previous puerperal curettage will have intrauterine adhesions noted on hysterosalpingogram.

Surgeons in certain countries have reported a high incidence of uterine synechiae thought due to an increased rate of postabortion infection (26,101). Furthermore, this may be related to tuberculosis of the genital organs, which is not uncommon in these areas.

Sugimoto (127) observed intrauterine synechiae by hysteroscopy in 192 of 7000 patients evaluated for abnormal bleeding, infertility, and/or uterine manipulation, while 63 reported a history of postcurettage infection. It is not possible to determine the overall incidence of reproductive difficulty due to uterine synechiae until a reference population is established of patients who have uterine synechiae and who have delivered uneventfully.

Etiology

The etiology of uterine synechiae may be considered from three viewpoints. Although a congenital abnormality has been considered as an etiologic factor, there has been no documentation in this regard nor have cases been reported (55). Trauma is the most frequent antecedent event in patients who develop uterine synechiae. The puerperal D&C results in the highest incidence of uterine synechiae (11). Less frequently, synechiae may result from diagnostic curettage, myomectomy, cesarean section, caustic abortifacients, uterine packing, metroplasty, and hysterotomy. Erikson and Koestet (42) reported that D&C between the 2nd and 4th weeks postpartum resulted in a high incidence of uterine synechiae. This appeared to be the vulnerable phase, as curettage during the first week resulted in a low incidence of uterine synechiae.

Although Asherman (5) originally reported that adhesions resulted from mechanical forces, Rabau and David (106) maintained that infection was the primary etiological factor. The authors noted that cornual adhesions were located where the curette was unable to reach but perhaps where infection could easily spread. An endometrium refractory to estrogen was viewed as a possible explanation for this observation.

Polishuk and coauthors (105) reported that pelvic angiography on patients with significant intrauterine synechiae revealed widespread vascular occlusion of myometrial arteries in seven of 12 patients. The authors suggest that such findings could explain the poor obstetric history in some patients, as well as their greatly reduced menstrual flow. Furthermore, the authors suggest that hypomenorrhea could be a reflection of atrophy or fibrosis of the uterine cavity due to infection or extensive vascular damage.

Tuberculous endometritis may produce uterine synechiae with all the characteristic signs and symptoms. Furthermore, in countries where schistosomiasis is endemic, patients with this parasite may also develop intrauterine synechiae.

Pathophysiology

Asherman hypothesized that sustained myometrial contractions could cause narrowing of the isthmus, resulting in adhesions between opposing endometrial surfaces (4,5). A more reasonable explanation states that trauma to the basal layer of the uterine mucosa and myometrium results in granulation tissue, which persists for several days. If granulation tissue from opposing walls is joined, forming a

bridge of tissue, this may become infiltrated by myometrium and covered by endometrium (42). The resulting synechiae or scarring may involve a large portion of the uterine cavity or may be scattered throughout the fundus. When the endometrial cavity is significantly reduced in size, hypomenorrhea may result.

Symptoms

Traumatic damage to and infection of the endometrium may cause corporal and/or cervical synechiae, which may result in hypomenorrhea-amenorrhea, a symptom of Asherman's syndrome. Originally, menstrual insufficiency was thought to be a frequent symptom of uterine synechiae (93,95). However, contemporary reports reveal that menstrual irregularity may occur in only 20% of women with synechiae (13,128,130). Toaff and Ballas (129) have demonstrated a close correlation between the severity of menstrual insufficiency and the extent of corporal adhesions.

Secondary amenorrhea may be due to complete obliteration of the uterine cavity and/or stenosis or atresia of the internal os. Under these circumstances, the ovarian cycle may continue, but the endometrium becomes refractory to hormonal stimuli. Seldom does hematometra occur. Simple cervical dilatation may restore menstruation in 4–5 weeks. This menstrual insufficiency may be explained by two pathophysiologic mechanisms: (a) reduction of endometrial bleeding area and possible atrophic changes; and (b) unresponsiveness of the endometrium, possibly related to a visceral reflex originating in the area of the internal os (129). Furthermore, the occurrence of severe dysmenorrhea with hypomenorrhea when adhesions are located in the isthmic area may be related to the mechanical obstacle to free flow of menstrual blood. As demonstrated by Carmichael (22), adenomyosis may account for pain in approximately 25% of patients with intrauterine synechiae.

Additional symptoms of uterine synechiae that are commonly recognized are infertility and repeated abortion (Table 7.8). Over 80% of patients who were diagnosed with uterine synechiae in our series complained of repeated pregnancy loss (13). There have been various

Table 7.8. Surgery of the Body of the Uterus

Signs and Symptoms of Intrauterine Synechiae

Infertility
  Primary
  Secondary
Menstrual irregularity
  Amenorrhea
  Hypomenorrhea
  Intramenstrual spotting
Pregnancy abnormalities
  Repeated spontaneous abortion
  Missed second trimester abortion
  Intrauterine fetal demise
  Premature labor
  Ectopic pregnancy
  Obstetrics complication
    Placenta accreta
    Placenta previa

theories for the association of infertility and intrauterine synechiae. Adhesions may impede sperm migration or create an unsuitable endometrial environment for the blastocysts. In some instances, the synechiae may actually obliterate the internal tubal os. In addition, adhesions may cause occult or missed abortion, or, on occasion, intrauterine fetal demise. Forssman (47) recorded a 33% abortion rate, a 33% premature labor rate, and a 33% incidence of ectopic pregnancies, placenta accreta, and placenta previa. Jewelewicz and coauthors (68) noted that of 18 pregnancies in 17 patients treated for Asherman's syndrome, only six had an uncomplicated term delivery. Four patients had premature delivery and neonatal death; three patients, placenta accreta and postpartum hemorrhage; and one patient had a cervical pregnancy. Two patients had incomplete or missed abortion. These studies, along with those by others (12,54,139) indicate a high incidence of fetal wastage in patients who have been treated for intrauterine synechiae.

Diagnosis

A careful history will provide clues to the possible diagnosis of uterine synechiae. A history of a puerperal curettage followed by amenorrhea or hypomenorrhea is significant. Patients with intrauterine adhesions usually have normal ovulatory function, as demonstrated by basal body temperature chart.

The diagnosis of uterine synechiae may be visually confirmed by hysteroscopy. However, hysterosalpingography remains an important adjunct. Synechiae are recognizable by their lacunar pattern with sharply angled edges (Fig. 7.6). When performing hysterosalpingography, it is important to inject only 2 cc of dye to avoid obscuring the view with excess dye (11).

Other methods, such as sounding of the uterine cavity, progesterone withdrawal, and a careful history, may aid in establishing the diagnosis. Sounding with a uterine probe may allow exploration of the uterine cavity with detection of synechiae as irregularities. Failure to bleed with progesterone after proper estrogen priming is suggestive of endometrial sclerosis; however, the differential diagnosis must also include other disease entities such as hypogonadotropic hypogonadism, which must be excluded. The biphasic basal body temperature chart in the presence of amenorrhea is highly suggestive of an unresponsive target organ due to endometrial sclerosis (5). Also, signs of ovulation such as premenstrual molimina and an elevated serum progesterone are presumptive criteria for the diagnosis of intrauterine synechiae in amenorrheic patients. A history of postpartum endometrial infection and subsequent curettage is frequently associated with the presence of intrauterine adhesions.

Occasionally, it is possible to retrieve synechiae with the endometrial curette when exploring the cavity. Grossly, the uterine synechiae are bands identified between the anterior and posterior uterine walls. Histologic examination of the band or scar reveals a core of endometrial stroma with fibrosis of a variable degree surrounded by superficial epithelial cells. Synechiae may contain inflammatory cells. Examination of areas of endometrium away from the synechiae may reveal inactive endometrial glands with fibrosis; however, some areas may have glands that retain their cyclic activity.

Sonography may also be useful in identifying uterine synechiae. Intrauterine adhesions are echogenic rather than sonolucent and are usually asymmetric in their location. Confino et al. (27) localized intrauterine adhesions by sonography in three women. Their echogenic appearance disappeared after lysis.

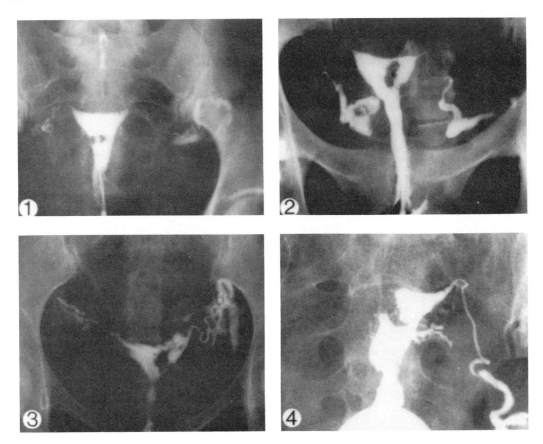

Figure 7.6. Intrauterine synechiae classified by hysterogram according to Toaff and Ballas (1978). *1,* Grade I, small defect well inside the uterus. *2,* Grade II, medium-sized defect occupying one-fifth of the uterine cavity. *3,* Grade III, several defects involving one-third of the cavity, which is asymmetrical due to vaginal adhesion. *4,* Grade IV, large filling defect that occupies most of the uterine cavity and has resulted in tubal obstruction. (From Bergquist and coauthors, 1981.)

Therapy

The therapy for uterine synechiae has as its goals the restoration of normal menstrual function and/or the restoration of fertility. Although almost all authors agree that lysis of synechiae is beneficial in the treatment of this condition, there is little agreement as to the choice of adjunctive therapy such as the use of prostheses and/or hormonal therapy. Because of the lack of carefully controlled randomized treatment groups, it has not been possible to establish the efficacy of any particular treatment regimen. However, it is useful to establish a uniform approach in the treatment of patients with this condition. Our treatment protocol (Table 7.8) has been useful in reestablishing menstrual function and in restoring fertility (13).

HYSTEROSCOPIC LYSIS

Hysteroscopy, as well as lysis under direct visualization, are useful for establishing a visual diagnosis (Fig. 7.7). Curettage is useful in actually removing these fragments of tissue, once lysed. After the hysteroscope is introduced into the endocervix, the adhesions, once identified, should be separated at their midpoint. In our experience, the extensive adhesions should be removed by several separate procedures. As synechiae are lysed with a conventional hysteroscope, blood may obscure vision, and orientation within the cavity may be lost. This problem may in part be alleviated with an operating resectoscope with a flushing system or with a suction cannula through the dual-channel hysteroscope. Simultaneous laparoscopy is advised when there is an increased risk

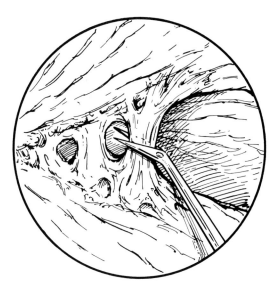

Figure 7.7. Hysteroscopic lysis of intrauterine synechiae. The scissors are introduced through the hysteroscope and the uterine scars lysed under direct visualization.

of perforation. High risk factors include: (*a*) complete obliteration of the uterine cavity as noted on HSG or failed attempts to place a fine probe into the uterine fundus; (*b*) intravasation or tubal occlusion noted on HSG, (*c*) no landmarks noted with attempts to identify the plane of adherence.

Complete obliteration of the uterine cavity or lower portion of the uterine cavity may challenge the hysteroscopist. The endocervix appears as a blind canal. A cleavage plane may not be obvious. An additional procedure may help identify the cleavage plane and facilitate lysis. First, a needle may be placed through the laparoscope and into the uterine fundus. Indigo carmine may then be injected into the uterine cavity. Often, a small opening is demonstrated as the dye is inserted or the plane of dissection may become apparent. In some instances, the cavity still may not be identified. Often, if the surgeon persists in attempting to find the cavity, uterine perforation is accomplished.

Experience dictates that the procedure should be stopped and one of two approaches considered. An interuterine device or Foley catheter may be placed in the endocervix and left in place for 2 weeks. In some instances, constant pressure will open the plane of adherence. Alternatively, a laminaria may be

placed in the endocervix and allowed to expand. These procedures may greatly facilitate the next surgical attempt to open the cavity. In rare instances, hysterotomy and synechiotomy may be required.

ADJUNCTIVE THERAPY

Certain types of prostheses have been recommended to aid in separating the anterior and posterior uterine walls while endometrial proliferation occurs. In particular, polyethylene tubing (90), catheters, drains, and/or balloons (22), and intrauterine devices (79,87,137) have been reported to be of value. Our preference has been a 3-cc #8 pediatric catheter, which once inflated, is left in the uterine cavity for 10 days (Table 7.9). A broad-spectrum antibiotic coverage lessens the likelihood of the seeding of new infection on the traumatized tissue.

Estrogen therapy for endometrial proliferation has been recommended (55,139). Although such therapy is theoretically justifiable, there are no controlled studies supporting its efficacy. Our preference has been for the administration of 2.5 mg of conjugated estrogen daily for 21 days with the initiation of Provera, 10 mg daily, starting on day 16. This is continued for one cycle.

Results

It is difficult to compare pregnancy success rates in different patient series due to the large number of treatment regimens and the use of different adjunctive therapies. Furthermore, there is a lack of strict definition of criteria used for diagnosis. On reviewing the world literature, Klein and Garcia (74) noted that pregnancy rates varied from 0–100% in small

---

Table 7.9. Treatment of Patients with Uterine Synechiae

1. Lysis of adhesions (transhysteroscopic if possible).
2. Placement of 3-cc #8 pediatric catheter for 10 days with broad-spectrum antibiotic coverage.
3. Conjugated estrogen 2.5 mg daily for 21 days with medroxyprogesterone acetate (Provera) 10 mg daily starting on day 16 for 6 days.
4. Repeat hysterogram and/or hysteroscopy in 2 months.

patient groups. In these studies, lysis was performed blindly with scissors or curettage. Various types of adjunctive therapy were administered, including estrogen and cortisone therapy and various types of intrauterine devices. The use of these different types of regimens makes comparison difficult, if not impossible.

Observations based on reports of hysteroscopic lysis of uterine adhesions during the past two decades reflect pregnancy success in the range of 40–90%. Using blind uterine lysis with curved scissors, Caspi and Perpinial (23) noted a 65.5% live birth rate following lysis and Lippes Loop placement. Sequential estrogen therapy was instituted for 3 months,

concluding with the removal of the loop. On the other hand, Oelsner and coauthors (101) reported a 39% pregnancy rate, 30% of which did not result in living children. Patients were treated by uterine lysis and intrauterine device placements of 6 weeks' duration. Estrogen was used in some instances (Table 7.10).

Several classifications have been suggested based on the degree of occlusion of the uterine cavity, especially in the osteal and fimbrial areas. Toaff and Ballas (129) recently reported a classification system based on a semiquantitative evaluation of defects revealed by hysterographic examination (Table 7.11). A correlation of the extent of corporal adhesions and menstrual loss was established in a series of 64

Table 7.10. Hysteroscopic Lysis of Intrauterine Adhesions[a]

Author	No. Cases	Medium Used[b]	Technique	Menses No.	Menses %	Pregnancy No.	Pregnancy %	Term No.	Term %
Levine/Neuwirth (1973)	10	Hyskon	Flexible sissors	5	50	2	20		
Edström (1974)	9	Hyskon	Target abrasion/ biopsy forceps	2	22	1	11		
Siegler/ Kontopoulos (1981)[c]	25	CO_2	Target abrasion/ curettage/ scissors	13	52	11	44	12	44.4
March/Israel (1978)	38	Hyskon	Flexible sissors	38	100	38	100	34	79.1
Neuwirth et al. (1982)	27	Hyskon	Sissors along side of hysteroscope	20	74	14	51.8	13	48.1
Sanfilippo et al. (1982)	26	CO_2	Curettage	26	100	6	100	3	50
Hamou et al. (1983)	69	CO_2	Target abrasion	59	85.5	20	51.3	15	38.4
Sugimoto et al. (1984)	258	Hyskon/ NS	Target abrasion/ forceps	180	69.9	143	76.4	114	79.7
Wamsteker (1984)	36	Hyskon	Scissors/biopsy forceps	34	94.4	17	62.9	12	44.4
Friedman et al. (1986)	30	Hyskon	Resectoscope/ scissors	27	90	24	80	23	76.6
Zuanchong/ Yulian (1986)	70	D_5W	Biopsy forceps/ scissors	64	84.3	30	85.7	17	48.5
Valle/Sciarra (1988)	187	Hyskon/ D_5W	Semirigid scissors	167	89.3	143	76.4	114	79.7
Lancet/Kessler (1988)	98	Unknown	Scissors	98	100	86	87.8	77	89.5
Total	883[d]			773	83.0	535	60.5	435	81.3[d]

[a]Adapted from Siegler AM, Valle RF, Lindemann RJ, et al. (eds): Intrauterine adhesions. In: Therapeutic hysteroscopy: indications and techniques. St. Louis: CV Mosby, 1990;103.
[b]All authors used estrogens, progestogens, and IUDs postoperatively.
[c]Prophylactic antibiotics were used in 50% of the patients.
[d]Based on the number of pregnant patients; based on the number of patients treated the percentage of term pregnancies is 49% (435/883).

Table 7.11. Grading of Corporal Traumatic Adhesions According to Defects Revealed by Hysterogram[a]

I. A single, small, filling defect, frequently well inside the uterine cavity, occupying up to about ⅓ of the uterine area.

II. A. A single, medium-sized filling defect occupying up to ⅕ of the uterine area.
  B. Smaller defects adding up to the same degree of involvement located inside the uterine cavity, whose outline may show minor indentations but no gross deformation.

III. A single, large, or several smaller filling defects involving up to about ⅓ of the uterine cavity, which is deformed or asymmetrical because of marginal adhesions.

IV. Large-sized filling defects occupying most of a severely deformed uterine cavity.

---

[a]Adapted from Toaff R, Ballas S: Traumatic hypomenorrhea-amenorrhea (asherman's syndrome). Fertil Steril 1978;30:79.

---

patients. Caspi and Perpinial (23) using Toaff and Ballas' classification system, could not demonstrate a direct correlation between the extent of adhesions and pregnancy success posttherapy; however, pregnancy results were poorest when large-sized filling defects occupied a major part of the uterine cavity. Buttram and Turati (21) using a similar classification system, experienced difficulty in establishing a correlation between extent of synechiae and pregnancy success. Our own experience has been not dissimilar (13). We found that no correlation could be established between pregnancy success and the extent of synechiae.

Hamou and coauthors (60) described three types of intrauterine adhesions (IUA) at × 20 magnification:

1. Endometrial adhesions appeared white with some glandular and vascular patterns similar to those of the surrounding endometrium. They were easily dissected.
2. Synechiae composed of either fibrous or connective tissue appeared transparent, thin, bridgelike, were poorly vascularized, formed stumps after lysis, and usually their position was central or isthmic.
3. Myometrial adhesions limited uterine distension; general anesthesia was required for lysis. The fibrous adhesions were more common in moderate adhesions. The loca-

tion of adhesions of the endometrial type was usually central, and they had been there less than 1 year. Often, myometrial adhesions were more extensive and had been there longer. Thus, Hamou et al. suggest the following classification:

Mild: Endometrial adhesions are filmy, avascular, and easily disrupted.
Moderate: Fibromuscular adhesions are characteristically thick but may be covered by endometrium and can bleed when divided.
Severe: Connective or fibrous tissue adhesions lack any endometrial lining and do not bleed when divided.

Results of large patient groups verifying the correlation of these findings have not been published as of this writing.

March and coauthors (86) have presented a useful system for categorization based on the amount, character, and site of adhesions. The authors reported a poor correlation between the hysterogram and hysteroscopic findings. However, a direct correlation between menstrual patterns and degree of endometrial scarring was demonstrated.

Valle and Sciarra (133) wrote that removal of mild, filmy adhesions in 43 patients was followed by 35 (81%) term pregnancies; 97 moderate cases of fibromuscular adhesions showed 64 (66%) term pregnancies; and 47 cases with severe connective tissue adhesions resulted in 15 (32%) term pregnancies. Overall restoration of menses occurred in 90%, and the term pregnancy rate was 61%. Of 175 patients reported by March, 69 wanted to become pregnant and had no other infertility factors. Fifty-two (75%) had 62 pregnancies, 54 (87%) going to term. Of 104 patients who complained of amenorrhea, 100 developed normal menses postoperatively, four others had hypomenorrhea, and only one of these four had persistent amenorrhea.

Recently, a classification system has been suggested based on the extent of the cavity involved, type of adhesions, and menstrual pattern (Fig. 7.8). There have been no studies using this system that have confirmed the correlation between relief of symptoms and extent of disease.

THE AMERICAN FERTILITY SOCIETY CLASSIFICATION OF INTRAUTERINE ADHESIONS

Patient's Name _____ Date _____ Chart # _____

Age _____ G _____ P _____ Sp Ab _____ VTP _____ Ectopic _____ Infertile Yes _____ No _____

Other Significant History (i.e. surgery, infection, etc.) _____

HSG _____ Sonography _____ Photography _____ Laparoscopy _____ Laparotomy _____

Extent of Cavity Involved	<1/3	1/3 - 2/3	>2/3
	1	2	4
Type of Adhesions	Filmy	Filmy & Dense	Dense
	1	2	4
Menstrual Pattern	Normal	Hypomenorrhea	Amenorrhea
	0	2	4

Prognostic Classification

	HSG* Score	Hysteroscopy Score
Stage I (Mild) 1-4	_____	_____
Stage II (Moderate) 5-8	_____	_____
Stage III (Severe) 9-12	_____	_____

*All adhesions should be considered dense

Treatment (Surgical Procedures): _____

_____
_____
_____
_____

Prognosis for Conception & Subsequent Viable Infant*

_____ Excellent (> 75%)

_____ Good (50-75%)

_____ Fair (25%-50%)

_____ Poor (< 25%)

*Physician's judgment based upon tubal patency.

Recommended Followup Treatment: _____

_____
_____

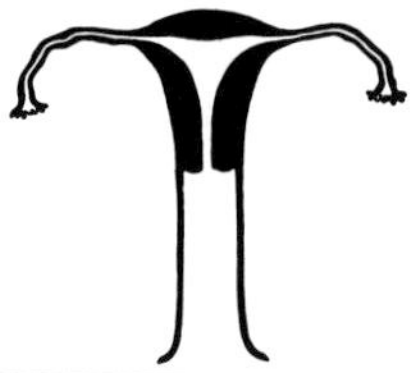

Property of
The American Fertility Society

Additional Findings: _____
_____
_____
_____
_____

DRAWING

HSG Findings

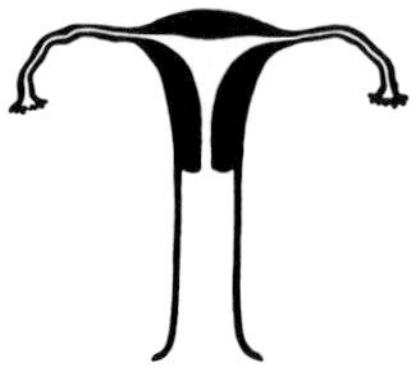

Hysteroscopy Findings

For additional supply write to:
The American Fertility Society
2140 11th Avenue, South
Suite 200
Birmingham, Alabama 35205

Figure 7.8. American Fertility Society classification of intrauterine adhesions.

Congenital Uterine Defects

A classification of uterine anomalies has been suggested to categorize specific uterine type. This classification is useful to discuss the surgical treatment of specific uterine anomalies. (Fig. 7.9). The surgical treatment of Müllerian anomalies is presented in depth elsewhere (Chapter 12). Nevertheless, the hysteroscopic management of the double uterus (nonob-structive failure of the lateral fusion) also will be considered in this section.

NONOBSTRUCTIVE FAILURE OF LATERAL FUSION

Patients with nonobstructed uterine anomalies are the result of the failure or lack of absorption of a uterine septum. In some in-

THE AMERICAN FERTILITY SOCIETY CLASSIFICATION OF MULLERIAN ANOMALIES

Patient's Name _____ Date _____ Chart # _____

Age _____ G _____ P _____ Sp Ab _____ VTP _____ Ectopic _____ Infertile Yes _____ No _____

Other Significant History (i.e. surgery, infection, etc.) _____

HSG _____ Sonography _____ Photography _____ Laparoscopy _____ Laparotomy _____

EXAMPLES

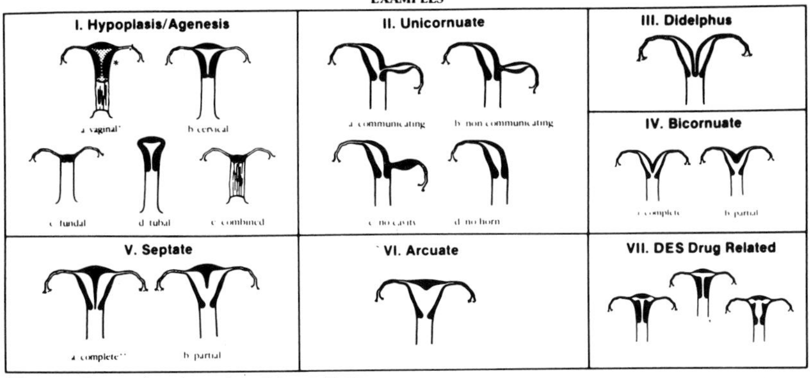

I. Hypoplasia/Agenesis	II. Unicornuate	III. Didelphus
a. vaginal* b. cervical	a. communicating b. non communicating	IV. Bicornuate
c. fundal d. tubal e. combined	c. no cavity d. no horn	a. complete b. partial
V. Septate	VI. Arcuate	VII. DES Drug Related
a. complete** b. partial		

* Uterus may be normal or take a variety of abnormal forms.
** May have two distinct cervices

Type of Anomaly

Class I _____ Class V _____
Class II _____ Class VI _____
Class III _____ Class VII _____
Class IV _____

Treatment (Surgical Procedures): _____
_____
_____

Prognosis for Conception & Subsequent Viable Infant*

_____ Excellent (> 75%)

_____ Good (50-75%)

_____ Fair (25%-50%)

_____ Poor (< 25%)

*Based upon physician's judgment.

Recommended Followup Treatment: _____
_____
_____

Property of
The American Fertility Society

Additional Findings: _____
_____
_____

Vagina: _____
Cervix: _____

Tubes: Right _____ Left _____
Kidneys: Right _____ Left _____

DRAWING

L.   R

For additional supply write to:
The American Fertility Society
2140 11th Avenue, South
Suite 200
Birmingham, Alabama 35205

Figure 7.9. American Fertility Society classification of double uteri.

stances, there is failure of descent of a Müllerian duct, which results in a unicornuate uterus.

The Didelphic and Unicornuate Uterus

In nonobstructed failure of lateral fusion involving both the uterus and vagina (uterus didelphys), there are no symptoms related to menstruation. However, due to narrowness of the vagina, dyspareunia may be a problem. If so, removal of the septum may be required and is not particularly difficult, although sometimes it is very thick and contains a large number of blood vessels that must be secured. At times, there is asymmetry of the two vaginal cavities so that the vaginal function is normal and satisfactory on one side but most difficult with the other.

Overall reproduction seems to be modestly compromised in patients with didelphic uteri. Information is anecdotal and consists of case reports or small series recording examples of primary infertility, pregnancy wastage, and premature labor. A number of examples of simultaneous pregnancies in each have been reported. In some patients, a satisfactory outcome for both pregnancies was reported. The older literature contains examples of vaginal deliveries with sequential labor with significant intervals between the birth of each child. An interval of 24 hr is not unusual, and intervals of several days have been reported. Cesarean section would doubtless be used almost routinely at present.

There is no indication for surgical intervention in a didelphic condition, except for the removal of a longitudinal vaginal septum, which might cause dyspareunia.

The reproductive history of a patient with a unicornuate uterus is not different from that of the didelphic situation. This is not surprising as a didelphic uterus is but a symmetrically inversed duplication of a unicornuate uterus.

As judged by the report of small series, reproduction is somewhat compromised by infertility, pregnancy wastage, and premature labor. However, most pregnancies seem to result in a viable child. Cerclage also has been favorably reported in cases of repeated miscarriage and premature labor.

The Bicornuate and Septate Uterus

A symmetrical nonobstructed double uterus (e.g., septate or bicornuate) may cause a problem in reproduction. Generally, there is no problem in becoming pregnant, but the difficulty arises from abortion, which is often repeated, or from premature labor. In the event pregnancies are carried to term, obstetrical malpresentation and difficulties in delivery are not unusual. Primary infertility in a patient with a symmetrical double uterus is sometimes observed, but the etiological relationship between infertility and the anomaly is unknown.

The type of symmetrical double uterus without obstruction is of great importance. It is necessary to distinguish between the bicornuate uterus and the septate uterus. The bicornuate uterus is usually associated with minimal reproductive problems, whereas the septate uterus is almost always the type that is involved with reproductive failure. The distinction between these two types of uteri cannot be made by hysterogram. Two distinct horns may be felt when palpating a bicornuate uterus. The exterior configuration of the septate uterus may be essentially normal, and many of these uteri cannot be recognized at laparotomy. In some patients, there may be the slightest midfundal indentation. On pelvic examination, one can suspect a septate uterus because of the broadness of the uterus. Ultrasonography may be helpful but cannot be expected to make the critical distinction between a bicornuate and a septate uterus. As may be inferred from the above comments, a bicornuate uterus seldom needs surgical correction.

A special situation pertains to the anomalies associated and probably caused by exposure in utero to diethylstilbestrol (DES). Kaufman et al. (72) called attention to a uterus shaped like a T with some variation in many DES-exposed patients. Haney and coauthors (61) have described the lesion in detail. While the reproductive performance of these uteri has not been specifically determined, Barnes et al. (8) and others have pointed out the unfavorable outcome of pregnancies in DES-exposed women. Nevertheless, repeated pregnancy wastage does not appear to be associated with DES-exposed women. Thus, there is no indication for surgical intervention.

The diagnosis of reproductive wastage due to a double uterus is essentially by exclusion. Considering that reproduction in a double uterus, particularly of the bicornuate type, may be essentially normal, it is necessary to determine whether a particular uterus is responsible for the reproductive problem. It is essential in making the diagnosis of pregnancy wastage due to the double uterus that all other causes of repeated miscarriage be excluded. This investigation should include male factors and such female factors as cervical incompetence, chronic illness, luteal defects, and other endocrine disorders of the adrenal and thyroid, which sometimes result in pregnancy wastage. In addition, the evaluation should require the exclusion of fetal factors, particularly karyoptypic anomalies in one or the other potential parents, which may result in a genetically defective zygote (110).

The characteristic history is an early midtrimester loss associated with a minilabor starting with cramps, followed by bleeding. In a primigravida, the labor may last up to 6 hr or even more, resulting in the delivery of a well-formed, but not viable, fetus. When miscarriages occur in the first trimester or when there is a history of lack of recognition of the embryo, it is necessary to suspect a genetic etiology. On the other hand, histories that differ from the typical one described above are sometimes encountered. In the absence of other causes of miscarriage, such patients may deserve uterine unification.

Hysteroscopy Metroplasty

The septate uterus may be corrected with the operating hysteroscope or resectoscope. The endometrium is suppressed with Danazol or GnRH analog 2 months prior to surgery. A simple uterine septum Class V-B uterus may be incised with scissors or the loop with cutting current under direct vision (Fig. 7.10). The Nd:YAG laser may be used. The procedure is performed under simultaneous laparoscope visualization of the uterine fundus to limit the risks of perforation.

The septum is incised with scissors under direct visualization. Usually, minimal bleeding

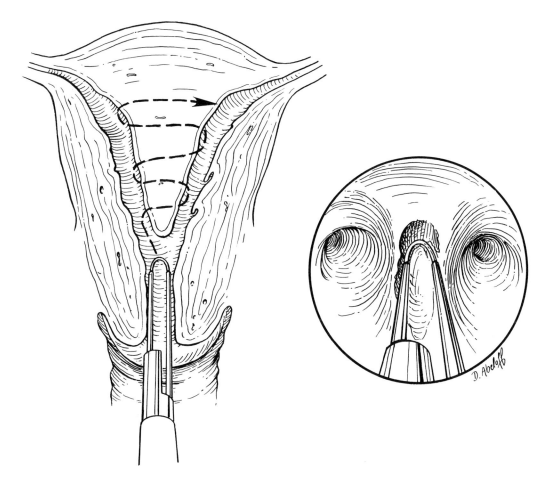

Figure 7.10. Hysteroscopic incision of a septum of a septate uterus. A resectoscope is introduced through the cervix, and the midportion of the uterine septum is incised. The myometrium slowly retracts. The incision should be taken to the point where both intrauterine tubal ostia are visualized. The procedure may be performed under the visualization of the laparoscope to minimize the risks of perforation.

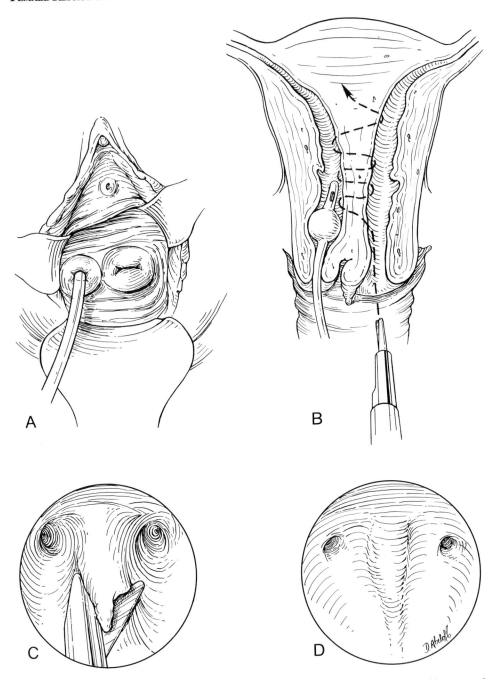

Figure 7.11. The hysteroscopic incision of a septum of a Class V uterus. *A,* Foley catheter is placed in one cervix and the bulb inflated. *B,* Scissors are inserted into the opposite cavity, the septum is incised, and the Foley catheter on the opposite side is visualized. *C,* The septum is then incised. *D,* The septum should be incised until both uterotubal oses may be identified and there is no separation of the uterine cavities.

results from the incision, as the walls of the septum separate and retract. A 3-cc balloon may be inserted if substantial bleeding is encountered, to provide for hemostasis. A 2-month delay prior to attempting pregnancy is suggested to allow complete resorption of the septum.

The Class V-A uterus is a special challenge. This uterus consists of a single fundus, two cervices, and two cavities. The septum should be removed above the internal cervical os. This is accomplished by placing a pediatric Foley catheter in one uterine cavity and the hysteroscope in the other. The septum is incised and the Foley identified in the opposite cavity. The septum may then be incised cephalad (Fig. 7.11).

Fedele and coauthors (44) studied endometrial reconstruction after hysteroscopic metroplasty of a septate uterus by light microscopy and scanning electron microscopy when a uterus was removed 13 days after hysteroscopic incision of a uterine septum. A retraction of the margins of the incised septum was noted. Reepithelialization of the cut surfaces seemed to proceed both centripedally and by proliferation of surrounding endometrium and centripedally from the bottom of the glands present at the base of the septum. Their findings provided the explanation for the low incidence of uterine synechiae after metroplasty and thus no need for an intrauterine device. The authors suggested estrogen supplementation to promote the epithelization process.

A review of reports of patient series reveals pregnancy success rates that are comparable to abdominal metroplasty (Table 7.12). Thus, exploratory laparotomy may be required only for the repair of bicornuate uterus using the Strassman technique.

Table 7.12. Hysteroscopic Metroplasty[a]

Author	No. Patients	Medium	Technique	IUD[b]	E/P[c]	Anti-biotics	Term	Pregnancy Premature	Pregnancy Abortion	Pregnancy In Progress
Edstrom (1974)	2	Dextran 70, 32%	Rigid biopsy forceps	+	—	—	19 wks	—	—	—
Chervenak/ Neuwirth (1981)	2	Dextran 70, 32%	Scissors adjacent to hysteroscope	+	2 mo	+	1	—	—	—
Rosenberg et al. (1981)	1	Dextran 70, 32%	Flexible scissors	N/A[d]	N/A	N/A	N/A	—	—	—
DeCherney et al. (1986)	72	Dextran 70, 32%	Resectoscope	—	—	—	58	—	4	4
Corson/ Batzer (1986)	18	Dextran 70, 32% CO$_2$	Resectoscope and rigid scissors	—	—	—	10	1	2	2
Fayez (1986)	19	Dextran 70, 32%	Rigid scissors	Foley catheter	—	+	14	—	—	—
March/Israel (1987)	91	Dextran 70, 32%	Flexible scissors	+	1 mo	—	44	4	7	7
Valle (1987)	59	D5W/ Dextran 70	Flexible, semirigid rigid scissors	—	1–2 mo	+	44	2	5	—
Daley et al. (1989)	51	Dextran 70, 32%	Scissors	—	2 mo	—	55	5	14	4
Perino et al. (1985)	24	CO$_2$	Flexible, semirigid scissors	+	—	—	10	—	1	5
Totals	331						236/ 331 (71.3%)	13	33	22

[a]Adapted from Siegler AM, Valle RF, Lindemann HJ, et al. (eds): Hysteroscopic metroplasty. In: Therapeutic hysteroscopy: indications and techniques. St. Louis: CV Mosby, 1990;79.
[b]IUD, intrauterine device.
[c]E/P, estrogens/progesterones.
[d]N/A, Not applicable.

References

1. American Fertility Society. The AFS classification of Müllerian anomalies and uterine adhesions. Fertil Steril 1988;49:950.
2. Andreyko JL, Blumenfeld Z, Marshall LA, et al: Use of an agonistic analog of gonadotropin-releasing hormone (nafarelin) to treat leiomyomas: Assessment by magnetic resonance imaging. Am J Obstet Gynecol 1988;158:903.
3. Asherman J: Traumatic intrauterine adhesions and their effects on fertility. Int J Fertil 1957;2:49.
4. Asherman J: Traumatic intrauterine adhesions. J Obstet Gynaecol Br Commonw 1950;57:892.
5. Asherman J: Amenorrhea traumatica (atretica). J Obstet Gynaecol Br Emp 1948;55:23.
6. Babaknia A, Rock JA, Jones HW Jr: Pregnancy success following abdominal myomectomy for infertility. Fertil Steril 1978;30:644.
7. Baggish MS, Sze EHM, Morgan G: Hysteroscopic treatment of symptomatic submucous myomata uteri with the Nd:YAG laser. J Gynecol Surg 1989;5:17.
8. Barnes AB, Colton T, Gundersen J, et al: Fertility and outcome of pregnancy in women exposed *in utero* to diethylstilbestrol. N Engl J Med 1980;302:609.
9. Barter RH, Park J: Myoma uteri associated with pregnancy. Clin Obstet Gynecol 1958;1:519.
10. Ben-Baruch G, Schiff E, Menashe Y, et al: Immediate and late outcome of vaginal myomectomy for prolapsed pedunculated submucous myoma. Obstet Gynecol 1988;72:859.
11. Bergman P: Traumatic intrauterine lesions. Acta Obstet Gynceol Scand 40 (Suppl. 4):1, 1961.
12. Bergman P: Treatment of sterility of intrauterine origin. Clin Obstet Gynecol 1959;2:852.
13. Bergquist CA, Rock JA, Jones HW Jr: Pregnancy outcome following treatment of intrauterine adhesions. Int J Fertil 1981;26:107.
14. Berkeley AS, Polan ML: Abdominal myomectomy and subsequent fertility. Surg Obstet Gynecol 1983;156:319.
15. Bolck F: Die Pathologie der Uterusmyome. Arch Gynaekol 1961;195:166.
16. Bonney V: The technique and results of myomectomy. Am J Obstet Gynecol 1926;11:343.
17. Brown AB, Chamberlain R, TeLinde RW: Myomectomy. Am J Obstet Gynecol 1956;71:759.
18. Brown JM, Malkasian GD, Symmonds RE: Abdominal myomectomy. Am J Obstet Gynecol 1967;90:126.
19. Buttram VC Jr, Reiter RC: Uterine leiomyomata. In: Surgical treatment of the infertile female. Baltimore: Williams & Wilkins, 1985;201.
20. Buttram VC Jr, Reiter RC: Uterine leiomyomata: etiology, symptomatology, and mangement. Fertil Steril 1981;36:433.
21. Buttram VC Jr, Turati G: Uterine synechiae: variations in severity and some conditions which may be conducive to severe adhesions. Int J Fertil 1977;22:98.
22. Carmichael DE: Asherman's syndrome. Obstet Gynecol 1970;36:922.
23. Caspi E, Perpinial S: Reproductive performance after treatment of intrauterine adhesions. Int J Fertil 1975;20:249.
24. Chervenak FA, Neuwirth RS: Hysteroscopic resection of the uterine septum. Am J Obstet Gynecol 1981;141:351.
25. Coddington CC, Collins RL, Shawker TH, et al: Long-acting gonadotropin hormone-releasing hormone analog used to treat uteri. Fertil Steril 1986;45:624.
26. Comninos A, Zourlas P: Treatment of uterine adhesions (Asherman's syndrome). Am J Obstet Gynecol 1969;105:862.
27. Confino E, Friberg J, Giglia RV, et al: Sonographic imagery of intrauterine adhesions. Obstet Gynecol 1985;66:596.
28. Continho EM, Goncalves MT: Long-term treatment of leiomyomas with Gestrinone. Fertil Steril 1989;51:939.
29. Corson S, Batzer FR: CO_2 uterine distension for hysteroscopic septate incision. J Reprod Med 1986;31:713.
30. Counseller VS, Bedard RE: Uterine myomectomy. JAMA 1938;111:675.
31. Daly DC, Maier D, Soto-Albors CE: Hysteroscopic metroplasty: Six years' experience. Obstet Gynecol 1989;73:201.
32. Daly DC, Walters CA, Soto-Albors CE, et al: Hysteroscopic metroplasty: Surgical technique and obstetrical outcome. Fertil Steril 1983;39:623.
33. Davids AM: Myomectomy in the relief of infertility and sterility and in pregnancy. Surg Clin North Am 1957;37:563.
34. DeCherney AH, Maheux R, Polan ML: A medical treatment for myomata uteri. Fertil Steril 1983;39:429.
35. DeCherney AH, Polan ML: Hysteroscopic management of intrauterine leisons and intractable uterine bleeding. Obstet Gynecol 1983;61:392.
36. DeCherney AH, Russell JB, Graebe RA, et al: Resectoscopic management of Müllerian fusion defects. Fertil Steril 1986;45:726.
37. Deligdish L, Loewenthal M: Endometrial changes associated with myomata uterus. J Clin Pathol 1970;23:676.
38. Dillon TF: Control of blood loss during gynecologic surgery. Obstet Gynecol 1962;19:428.
39. Dmowski WP, Greenblatt R: Asherman's syndrome and risk of placenta accreta. Obstet Gynecol 1969;34:288.
40. Donnez J, Schrurs B, Gillerot S, et al: Treatment of uterine fibroids with implants of gonadotropin-releasing hormone agonist. Assessment by hysterography. Fertil Steril 1989;51:947.
41. Edström K: Intrauterine surgical procedures during hysteroscopy. Endoscopy 1974;6:175.
42. Eriksen J, Koestet C: The incidence of uterine atresia after postpartum curettage. Dan Med Bull 1960;7:50.
43. Fayez JA: Comparison between abdominal and hysteroscopic metroplasty. Obstet Gynecol 1986;68:399.
44. Fedele L, Marchini M, Baglioni A, et al: Endometrial

reconstruction after hysteroscopic incisional metroplasty. Obstet Gynecol 1989;73:492.

45. Filicori N, Hall DA, Loughlin JS, et al: A conservative approach to the management of uterine leiomyomata: Pituitary desensitization by a GnRH analog. Am J Obstet Gynecol 1983;147:726.

46. Finn WF, Muller PF: Abdominal myomectomy. Am J Obstet Gynecol 1950;60:109.

47. Forssman L: Posttraumatic intrauterine synechiae and pregnancy. Obstet Gynecol 1965;26:710.

48. Friedman AJ, Rein MS, Atlas DH, et al: A randomized, placebo-controlled double-blind study evaluating leuprolide acetate depot treatment before myomectomy. Fertil Steril 1989;52:728.

49. Friedman AJ, Harrison-Atlas D, Barbieri R, et al: A randomized placebo-controlled double-blind study evaluating the efficacy of leuprolide acetate depot in the treatment of uterine leiomyomata. Fertil Steril 1989;51:251.

50. Friedman AJ, Barbieri R, Benacerraf BR, et al: Treatment of leiomyomata with intranasal or subcutaneous leuprolide, a gondadotropin-releasing hormone agonist. Fertil Steril 1987;48:560.

51. Friedman A, Defazio J, DeCherney AH: Severe obstetric complications following hysteroscopic lysis of adhesions. Obstet Gynecol 1986;67:864.

52. Fritsch H: Ein Fall von Volligem Schwund der Gebarmutterhohle nach Auskratzung. Zentralbl Gynaekol 1984;18:1337.

53. Garcia CR, Turock RW: Submucosal leiomyomas and infertility. Fertil Steril 1984;42:16.

54. Georgakopoulos P: Placenta accreta following lysis of uterine synechiae (Asherman's syndrome). J Obstet Gynecol Br Commonw 1974;81:730.

55. Gibbs E: Endometrial sclerosis. JAMA 1964;188:390.

56. Goldrath MH: Vaginal removal of the pedunculated submucous myoma: The use of laminaria. Obstet Gynecol 1987;70:670.

57. Goldzieher JW, Maqueom M, Ricaud L, et al: Induction of degenerative changes in uterine myomas by high-dosage progestin therapy. Am J Obstet Gynecol 1966;96:1078.

58. Goodman AL: Progesterone therapy in uterine fibromyoma. J Clin Endocrinol 1946;6:402.

59. Hallez JP, Perino A: Endoscopic intrauterine resection: Principles and technique. Acta Europ Fertil 1988;19:17.

60. Hamou J, Salat-Baroux J, Siegler AM: Diagnosis and treatment of intrauterine adhesions by microhysteroscopy. Fertil Steril 1983;39:321.

61. Haney AF, Hammond CB, Soules MR, et al: Diethylstilberstrol-induced upper genital tract abnormalities. Fertil Steril 1979;31:142.

62. Haning RV Jr, Harkins PG, Uehling DT: Preservation of fertility by transcervical resection of a benign mesodermal uterine tumor with a resectoscope and glycine distending medium. Fertil Steril 1980;33:209.

63. Hartwell SW: Surgical wounds in human beings. A histologic study of healing with practical applications. II: Fibrous healing. Arch Surg 1930;21:76.

64. Healy DL, Lawson SR, Abbott M, et al: Toward removing uterine fibroids without surgery: Subcutaneous infusion of a LHRH agonist commencing in the luteal phase. J Clin Endocrinol Metab 1986;63:619.

65. Ingersoll FM, Malone LJ: Myomectomy: an alternative to hysterectomy. Arch Surg 1970;100:557.

66. Jacobson BD: Abortion: its prediction and management. Obstet Gynecol 1956;7:206.

67. Jedeikin R, Olsfanger D, Kesslier I: Disseminated intravascular coagulapathy adult respiratory distress syndrome: Life-threatening complications of hysteroscopy. Am J Obstet Gynecol 1990;162:44.

68. Jewelewicz R, Khalof S, Neuwirth RS, et al: Obstetric complications after treatment of intrauterine synechiae (Asherman's syndrome). Obstet Gynecol 1976;47:701.

69. Joelsson IS: Hysteroscopy for delineating the intrauterine extent of endometrial carcinoma. In: Seigler AM and Lindemann HJ, eds. Hysteroscopy: principles and practice. Philadelphia: JB Lippincott, 1984.

70. John AH, Martin R: Growth of leiomyomata with estrogen-progesterone therapy. J Reprod Med 1971;6:49.

71. Katz VL, Dotters D, Droegemuller W: Complications of uterine leiomyomas in pregnancy. Obstet Gynecol 1989;73:593.

72. Kaufman RH, Binder GL, Gray PM Jr, et al: Upper genital tract changes associated with exposure in utero to diethylstilbestrol. Am J Obstet Gynecol 1977;128:51.

73. Kerr JMM: Wounds of the gravid and nongravid uterus: a study of uterine scars (Obstet Sect). Proc Rev Soc Med 1924;17:123.

74. Klein SM, Garcia CR: Asherman's syndrome: a critique and current review. Fertil Steril 1973;24:722.

75. Lancet M, Kessler I: A review of Asherman's syndrome, and results of modern treatment. Int J Fertil 1988;33:14.

76. Letterie GS, Coddington CC, Winkel C, et al: Efficacy of gonadotropin-releasing hormone agonist in the treatment of uterine leiomyomata: Long term follow-up. Fertil Steril 1989;5:951.

77. Levine RU, Neuwirth RS: Simultaneous laparoscopy and hysteroscopy for intrauterine adhesions. Obstet Gynecol 1973;42:441.

78. Loeffler FE, Noble AD: Myomectomy at Chelsea Hospital for Women. J Obstet Gynecol Br Common 1970;77:167.

79. Louros N, Danezis JM, Pontifix G: Use of intrauterine devices in the treatment of intrauterine adhesions. Fertil Steril 1968;19:509.

80. Maheux R, Guilloteau, Lemay A, et al: LHRH agonist and uterine leiomyoma. Am J Obstet 1985;152:1034.

81. Malone LJ, Ingersoll FM: Myomectomy in infertility. In: SJ Behrman, RW Kistner, eds. Progress in infertility, 2nd ed., Boston: Little, Brown & Co., 1975;86.

82. Malone LJ: Myomectomy: recurrence after removal of solitary and multiple myomas. Obstet Gynecol 1969;34:200.

83. Malone LJ, Ingersoll FM: Myomectomy. In: SJ Behrman, RW Kistner, eds. Progress in infertility, 1st ed. Boston: Little, Brown & Co., 1968; 115.

84. March CM, Israel R: Hysteroscopic management of recurrent abortion caused by septate uterus. Am J Obstet Gynecol 1987;156:834.

85. March CM, Israel R: Gestational outcome following hysteroscopic lysis of adhesions. Fertil Steril 1981;36:455.

86. March CM, Israel R, March AD: Hysteroscopic management of intrauterine adhesions. Am J Obstet Gyncecol 1978;130:653.

87. Massouras HG: Intrauterine adhesions: a syndrome of the past with the use of the Massouras duck's foot No. 2 intrauterine contraceptive device. Am J Obstet Gynecol 1973;116:576.

88. McCormick TA: Myomectomy with subsequent pregnancy. Am J Obstet Gynecol 1958:75:1128.

89. Miller HE, Tyrone CH: A survey of a series of myomectomies with a follow-up. Am J Obstet Gynecol 1933;26:575.

90. Milroy T: Traumatic uterine atresia. Minn Med 1963;46:761.

91. Munnell EW, Martin FW: Abdominal myomectomy. Advantages and disadvantages. Am J Obstet Gynecol 1951;62:109.

92. Musset R, Netter A: Synechies utérines. Encycylopedie Gynecol Paris 1972;10:140.

93. Musset R, Solomon Y: Traumatic menstrual disturbances after curettage. Rev Fr Gynecol Obstet 1953; 48:311.

94. Mussey RD, Randall LM, Doyle LW: Pregnancy following myomectomy. Am J Obstet Gynecol 1945; 49:508.

95. Netter A, Musset R, Lambert A, et al: Traumatic uterine synechiae: a common cause of menstrual insufficiency, sterility, and abortion. Am J Obstet Gynecol 1956;71:368.

96. Neuwirth RS: Hysteroscopic management of symptomatic submucous fibroids. Obstet Gynecol 1983;62:509.

97. Neuwirth RS, Hussein AR, Schuffman BM, et al: Hysteroscopic resection of intrauterine scars using a new technique. J Reprod Med 1982;60:111.

98. Neuwirth RS: A new way to manage fibroids. Contemp Obstet Gynecol 1978;12:101.

99. Novak ER, Jones GS, Jones HW: Novak's textbook of gynecology. Baltimore: Williams & Wilkins, 1975;361–362.

100. Novak ER, Woodruff JD: Myoma and other benign tumors of the uterus. In: Gynecologic and obstetric pathology, 8th ed. Philadelphia: WB Saunders 1979;260.

101. Oelsner G, David A, Insler V, et al: Outcome of pregnancy after treatment of intrauterine adhesions. Obstet Gynecol 1974;44:341.

102. Perino A, Mencaglia L, Hamou J, et al: Hysteroscopy for metroplasty of uterine septa: Report of 24 cases. Fertil Steril 1987;48:321.

103. Perino A, Cittidini E, Hamou J, et al: Hysteroscopic treatment of uterine septa. Acta Europ Fertil 1985;16:331.

104. Perl V, Marquez J, Schally AV, et al: Treatment of leiomyomata uteri with D-Tryp[6] leutinizing hormone-releasing hormone. Fertil Steril 1987; 48: 383.

105. Polishuk WZ, Siew FP, Gordon R, et al: Vascular changes in traumatic amenorrhea and hypomenorrhea. Int J Fertil 1977;22:189.

106. Rabau E, David A: Intrauterine adhesions: etiology, prevention and treatment. Obstet Gynecol 1963; 22:626.

107. Ranney B, Frederick I: The occasional need for myomectomy. Obstet Gynecol 1979;53:437.

108. Rice JP, Kay HH, Mahony BS: The clinical significance of uterine leiomyomas in pregnancy. Am J Obstet Gynecol 1989;160:1212.

109. Rock JA, Murphy AA, Cooper WH IV: Resectoscopic techniques for lysis of a Class V: complete uterine septum. Fertil Steril 1987;48:495.

110. Rock JA, Zacur HA: The clinical management of repeated early pregnancy wastage. Fertil Steril 1983;39:136.

111. Roopnarinesingh S, Suratsingh J, Roopnarinesingh A: The obstetric outcome of patients with previous myomectomy or hysterotomy. WI Med J 1985;34: 59.

112. Rosenberg SM, Bourque M, Riddick DH: Double uterine septa: A previously undetected entity. Obstet Gynecol 1981;58:250.

113. Rosenfeld DL: Abdominal myomectomy for otherwise unexplained infertility. Fertil Steril 1986; 46:328.

114. Ross RK, Pike MC, Jessey NP, et al: Risk factors for uterine fibroids: Reduced risk associated with contraceptives. Brit Med J 1986;293:359.

115. Rubin IC: Uterine fibromyomas and sterility. Clin Obstet Gynecol 1958;1:501.

116. Sanfillipo JS, Fitzgerald MR, Badaway SZ, et al: Asherman's syndrome: a comparison of methods. J Reprod Med 1982;27:328.

117. Schlaff WD, Zerhouni EA, Huth JA, et al: A placebo-controlled trial of depot GnRH analog (leuprolide) in the treatment of uterine leiomyomata. Obstet Gynecol 1989;74:856.

118. Siegler AM, Valle RF: Therapeutic hysteroscopic procedures. Fertil Steril 1988;50:685.

119. Siegler AM, Valle RF: Therapeutic hysteroscopic procedures. Fertil Steril 1988;50:685.

120. Siegler AM, Kontopoulos VG: Lysis of intrauterine adhesions under hysteroscopic control: a report of 25 operations. J Reprod Med 1981;26:372.

121. Siegler AM: Hysterography and hysteroscopy in the infertile patient. J Reprod Med 1977;18:143.

122. Siegler AM: Hysterosalpingography. New York: Medicom Press, 1974.

123. Siegel I: Scars of the pregnant and nonpregnant uterus. I: Histologic comparison of scars two weeks postoperatively. Am J Obstet Gynecol 1952;64:301.

124. Smith DC, Uhlir JK: Myomectomy as a reproductive procedure. Am J Obstet Gynecol 1990;162:1476.

125. Stevenson CS: Myomectomy for improvement of fertility. Fertil Steril 1964;15:367.
126. Sugimoto O, Ushiroyama T, Fukuda Y: Diagnostic and therapeutic hysteroscopy for traumatic intrauterine adhesions. In: Siegler AM, Lindemann HJ, eds. Hysteroscopy: principles and practice. Philadelphia: JB Lippincott, 1984.
127. Sugimoto O: Diagnostic therapeutic hysteroscopy for traumatic intrauterine adhesions. Am J Obstet Gynecol 1978;131:539.
128. Sweeny WF: Intrauterine synechiae. Obstet Gynecol 1966;27:284.
129. Toaff R, Ballas S: Traumatic hypomenorrhea-amenorrhea (Asherman's syndrome). Fertil Steril 1978;30:79.
130. Topkins PT: Traumatic intrauterine synechiae. Am J Obstet Gynecol 1962;83:1599.
131. Valle RF, Sciarra JJ: Intrauterine adhesions: hysteroscopic diagnosis, classification, treatment, and reproductive outcome. Am J Obstet Gynecol 1988;158:1459.
132. Valle RF: Hysteroscopic treatment of complete uterine septa with septate cervix. (Abstr.) Presented at the Third World Congress and Workshop on Hysteroscopy, Miami, Florida, January 16, 1987. Published by the American Association of Gynecological Laparoscopists in the preliminary program, p. 25.
133. Valle RF, Sciarra JJ: Current status of hysteroscopy in gynecologic practice. Fertil Steril 1979;32:619.
134. Wamsteker K: Hysteroscopy in Asherman's syndrome. In: Siegler AM, Lindemann JH, eds. Hysteroscopy: principles and practice. Philadelphia: JB Lippincott, 1984.
135. Weiss E: Treatment of fibroids of the uterus. Am J Obstet Gynecol 1926;11:343.
136. West CP, Lumsden MA, Lawson S, et al: Shrinkage of uterine fibroids during therapy with goserelin (Zoladex): a leutinizing-hormone releasing-hormone agonist administered as a monthly subcutaneous depot. Fertil Steril 1987;48:45.
137. Wider J, Marshall J: Hysterotomy and insertion of an intrauterine device for endometrial sclerosis: Importance of long-term follow-up. Fertil Steril 1970;21:240.
138. Wilson A, Yang F, Rees ED: Estradiol and progesterone binding in uterine leiomyomata and in normal uterine tissues. Obstet Gynecol 1980;55:20.
139. Wood J, Pena G: Treatment of uterine adhesions (Asherman's syndrome). Am J Obstet Gynecol 1969;105:862.
140. Yuen BH: Danazol and uterine leiomyomas. Can Med Assoc J 1981;124:963.
141. Zuanchong F, Yulian H: Hysteroscopic diagnosis and treatment of intrauterine adhesions: Clinical analysis of 70 cases. Symposium on Hysteroscopy, Shanghai, 1986, Family Planning Association.

RECONSTRUCTIVE SURGERY OF THE OVIDUCT

Ana Alvarez Murphy

INTRODUCTION

Several developments have made a significant impact on plastic surgery of the fallopian tube. The assisted reproductive technologies have radically changed our concept of the "appropriate" surgical candidate. Certainly, couples with severe tubal factor should be counseled about the dismal pregnancy rates seen after tuboplasty/neosalpingostomy, and should be offered extracorporeal fertilization. Additionally, operative laparoscopy for salpingolysis and neosalpingostomy has become an increasingly popular alternative to traditional microsurgical laparotomy. The significant decrease in morbidity and total cost of laparoscopic surgery have been well documented. Additionally, it appears that pregnancy rates are quite similar to those achieved by laparotomy (26,28). It is likely, however, that microsurgical tuboplasty by laparotomy, especially neosalpingostomy and tubal anastomosis, will continue to be used.

The following discussion of surgical technique is not intended to be an extensive review of the literature. Rather, this section will present the surgical techniques developed by the authors. The literature cited will bear directly on our observations and does not intend disrespect to other workers, whose contributions are well recognized.

TUBAL FACTORS IN INFERTILITY

The physiologic functions of the oviduct include ovum pickup, conduct of sperm and oocyte to the ampulla (where fertilization takes place), nourishment of the zygote, as well as transport to the uterine cavity. It appears that anatomic and pathologic alterations of the fallopian tube are associated with infertility. The anatomic relationship of the tubal infundibulum/fimbrica ovarica to the ovary appears to be important in ovum pickup. The ciliated lining of the fimbria embraces the ovary and transports the oocyte to the ampulla for fertilization.

Tubal infections generally alter the anatomy and function of the fallopian tube. Endosalpingitis may produce tubal occlusion along the entire course of the fallopian tube, but most commonly results in distal obstruction with formation of hydrosalpinx or fimbrial agglutination. Westrom (79) has estimated that 17.4% of patients will become infertile because of postpelvic inflammatory disease (PID) tubal damage. Multiple infection, increasing age at first infection, and severe infection are followed by more unfavorable fertility prognosis. PID can be divided into exogenous (sexually transmitted diseases) and endogenous agents. Sexually transmitted diseases account for 60–80% of PID in women below the age of 25. Gonococcal endosalpingitis is probably the best studied single cause; however, it has become increasingly clear that PID is more commonly polymicrobial. Furthermore, subclinical infections such as chlamydia may also cause irreparable damage to the tubal mucosa. Impairment of ciliary activity may interfere with tubal motility and ovum pickup. Peritubal adhesions with impaired tubal transport may also occur in association with endometriosis or from prior abdominopelvic surgery.

Diagnostic modalities to evaluate tubal function are discussed in detail in Chapter 2. The three currently available methods of observing tubal function include hysterosalpingography (HSG), laparoscopy, and salpingoscopy. The most complete evaluation may be accomplished with a combination of laparoscopy with either HSG or salpingoscopy. While laparosocopy is the most important method of assessing fallopian tubes, it cannot evaluate the endosalpinx. The presence of rugal folds on HSG is a favorable prognostic sign. Young (83) noted a significant decrease in pregnancy rates from 60.7% in patients with good rugal markings to 7.3% when none were seen. More recently, salpingoscopy has described adhesions, flattened mucosa, and agglutination. Preliminary studies suggest these findings correlate well with subsequent pregnancy success (18). A flexible bronchoscope at the time of laparoscopy may provide very useful information in delineating those patients who are likely to benefit from tubal surgery.

Microsurgery is a philosophy of gentle operative technique using delicate instruments, fine needles, and sutures only when absolutely necessary, minimal coagulation to achieve hemostasis, and magnification, traditionally using an operating microscope. A broadened definition of appropriate magnification would include the use of a hood, loupe, or laparoscope. It is understood that delicate and precise movements in a small operative field require skill and the appropriate instruments. Lasers have become popular to assist the microsurgeon at the time of tuboplasty. The CO_2 laser is the most widely used laser, although contact lasers such as the KTP 532 and Nd:Yag are gaining popularity. The reported advantages of lasers include precise lysis of adhesions with minimal tissue damage and bleeding. However, no evidence exists for a decrease in adhesion formation and subsequent increase in pregnancy rates (77). Microsurgical technique and lasers are discussed in separate chapters.

An important issue in plastic surgery of the reproductive tract is the lack of a generally accepted classification system for tubal surgery. The Ad Hoc Committee of the International Federation of Fertility and Sterility introduced a classification that was last modified in 1980 (27) (Table 8.1). International use of this classification may create some uniformity in

---

Table 8.1. Classification of Tubal Procedures[a]

1. Lysis of periadnexal adhesions (salpingolysis-ovariolysis): Classified according to adnexa with least pathology
   a. Minimal: 1 cm of tube or ovary involved
   b. Moderate: partially surround tube or ovary
   c. Severe: encapsulating peritubal and/or periovarian adhesions
2. Lysis of extraadnexal adhesions
   a. Minimal
   b. Moderate
   c. Severe
3. Tubouterine implantation
   a. Isthmic: implantation of isthmic segment
   b. Ampullary: implantation of ampullary segment
   c. Combination: different type implantation on right and left sides
4. Tubotubal anastomosis
   a. Interstitial (intramural)-isthmic
   b. Interstitial (intramural)-ampullary
   c. Isthmic-isthmic
   d. Isthmic-ampullary
   e. Ampullary-ampullary
   f. Ampullary-infundibular (fimbrial)
   g. Combination: different type anastomosis on right and left tubes
5. Salpingostomy (salpingoneostomy): Surgical creation of a new tubal ostium
   a. Terminal
   b. Ampullary
   c. Isthmic
   d. Combination: different type salpingostomy on right and left tubes
6. Fimbrioplasty: Reconstruction of existent fimbriae
   a. By deagglutination and dilatation
   b. With serosal incision (for completely occluded tube)
   c. Combination: different type fimbrioplasty on right and left tubes
7. Other reconstructive tubal operations (specify)
8. Combination of different types of operations
   a. Bipolar: for occlusion at both proximal and terminal end of tube (specify)
   b. Bilateral: different operations on the right and left sides (specify)

[a] From the Ad Hoc Committee of the International Federation of Fertility and Sterility.

reporting reliable success rates. The American Fertility Society has also proposed classifications for tubal procedures based on extent of disease. In addition, an inverse relationship exists between the grade of adhesions and the conception rate that is independent of the condition of the adnexa (7). Obviously, besides grade of adhesions and extent of disease, varying pathogenesis must be taken into account. Usefulness of these classification systems remains to be established, as there are few published studies using these new classifications.

In general, tubal surgery deals with four major areas of disease that dictate the type of surgery performed. Tubolysis or salpingolysis is performed for peritubal adhesion. Quite frequently, the ovary may be adhered to the sidewall, fixed to the fallopian tube, or enveloped in adhesions, and ovariolysis is performed as well. Neosalpingostomy or fimbrioplasty is performed for distal obstruction, depending on severity of disease. Segmental obstruction most commonly, but not exclusively secondary to previously ligated tubes, is treated with end-to-end anastomosis. Proximal obstruction is generally treated with tubocornual anastomosis. New nonsurgical therapies for proximal obstruction include hysteroscopic or fluoroscopic cannulation. Rarely is uterotubal implantation used, as pregnancy rates are lower than with anastomosis.

SALPINGOLYSIS

Patients with peritubular adhesions as a sole factor are uncommon. The infundibulum is by definition uninvolved. In our institutions, the incidence has remained fairly stable, at approximately 4–5% (13). Generally, these adhesions are secondary to salpingitis or previous abdominal (usually appendectomy) and gynecologic surgical procedures. Endometriosis frequently spares the infundibulum. However, endometriosis should not be included in this series because the pathogenesis of these adhesions is thought to be different.

Inspection of anatomic landmarks of the oviduct and ovary is necessary prior to undertaking adhesiolysis to avoid inadvertent incision of the fimbriated end, ovarian/mesosalpin-geal vasculature, or tubal serosa. Tubal surgery requires careful mobilization, elevation of the adnexa (at laparotomy for proper hand support), and excision of adhesions. If extensive adhesion formation is present, careful, painstaking removal of individual adhesions is required. This will prevent damage to underlying structures. Gentle dissection of a densely adherent adnexa with the finger will allow elevation to a platform made from lint-free laparotomy pads placed in the cul-de-sac. Once the adnexa are mobilized, the surgeon should carefully excise all adhesions at their origin and insertion. Plastic or insulated metal rods may be used to elevate adhesion so their insertion and origin are clearly identified. The adhesion should be placed on tension prior to excision, using fine-needle monopolar cautery or laser (Fig. 8.1). The adhesion should be completely lysed at the junction of adhesion and organ. Small adhesion "remnants" should not be left on the organ. Each adhesion should be removed from the pelvis using meticulous technique, avoiding trauma to serosal surfaces.

A variety of different types of adhesions to various locations may be identified. Large, fibrous, vascular adhesions between ovary, fallopian tube, and small bowel are particularly difficult to remove without damage to the serosal surface. An appropriately insulated manipulator may help prevent accidental damage secondary to electrocautery or laser. Once all adhesions are removed and the anatomy normalized, careful inspection of the fimbriae should be performed with magnification. Often, fine adhesions involving the infundibulum may be missed. Tear duct probes are often quite helpful in "combing" the fimbria for fimbrial adhesions.

Denuded areas may result, even with careful dissection. Careful consideration should be given to covering denuded areas with oxidized methylcellulose (Interceed, Johnson & Johnson, Raritan, NJ) or Gortex (W.L. Gore and Associates, Flagstaff, AZ) rather than reperitonealizing. Sutures are foreign substances that may cause anoxia if tied too tightly, and therefore increase the chances for adhesion formation. Moreover, peritoneum may be placed on tension and cause anatomic distortion.

Laparoscopy

Fertility-enhancing laparoscopic surgery was reported in 1977 by Gomel (29). Good results are dependent on the use of the microsurgical approach (34,60). As with laparotomy surgery, an adhesion should be incised at its attachment on both sides and removed from the pelvis entirely. This is best accomplished by placing the adhesion on traction by manipulating the uterus or using an ancillary puncture site to insert a probe or forcep. Excision may be accomplished with microscissors, fine-point needle cautery, knife, or laser. The scissors or knife may be combined with electrocautery as well. Once the adhesion is lysed, it may be grasped and rolled on a grasper to excise the other end (Fig. 8.1B). Multilayered adhesions should be lysed one layer at a time to prevent trauma to underlying structures, especially to ureter or bowel. The most important maneuver is countertraction on the tissues being separated and clear visualization of tissue planes. Vascular adhesions should be spot-coagulated prior to sharp lysis. Minimum coagulation with either cautery (preferably microbipolar) or laser should be used. Use of the laser, usually CO_2 but now more frequently the fiber lasers, has become popular. The techniques do not differ markedly. The laser beam with the smallest spot size possible and in superpulse mode is applied to the edge of the adherent surface with a sweeping motion to vaporize the tissue. Care must be taken to provide gentle traction, as tearing of the tissue is traumatic and causes bleeding. A reflective titanium probe, titanium suction irrigation cannula, or a pool of irrigant can serve as a backstop for the CO_2 laser.

Ovarian adhesions should also be lysed, as described above. However, a different technique may be needed for adhesions that encapsulate the ovary. If the adhesions cannot be dissected off, they may be vaporized using a defocused beam and low-power density. Copious irrigation to remove the carbonized tissue and other debris is necessary.

Hydrodissection is an alternative technique involving the application of irrigant at high pressure to develop cleavage planes between adherent structures (56). This is particularly effective at early second-look laparoscopic lysis of adhesions.

Results

Postoperative pregnancy rates are quite satisfactory following salpingolysis by laparotomy. Most series quote rates that range from 30–60% (3,39,68). Our experience has not

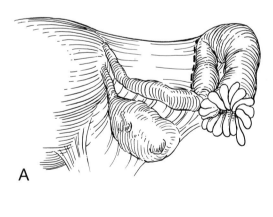

A

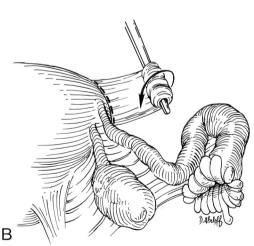

B

Figure 8.1. Salpingolysis. *A,* Adhesions are placed on tension and lysed at their insertion. A Teflon probe may facilitate exposure and protect underlying structure. *B,* Adhesions should be placed on tension to facilitate lysis. Adhesions should be removed from the pelvis in toto.

been different. Of 72 patients with bilateral adhesions treated by salpingolyis, 80% (58) conceived, and 68% delivered liveborn infants. Twelve ectopic pregnancies were seen (67).

Gomel (28) reported a series of 92 women who underwent laparoscopic salpingoovariolysis for moderate to severe adnexal adhesions; 57 (62%) achieved a term pregnancy. A 5% ectopic pregnancy rate was noted. Fayez (26) reported a 67% pregnancy rate with laparoscopic tubolysis, 72% with ovariolysis, and 50% with salpingoovariolysis. These results and others (6,24,56) are quite comparable to the intrauterine pregnancy rates following salpingoovariolysis via laparotomy (30–60%).

SALPINGOPLASTY

Salpingoplasty is a collective term that describes procedures that may be performed on the tubal infundibulum. The procedures include fimbrioplasty as well as neosalpingostomy. The normal anatomy must be restored prior to repairing the distal oviduct. Complete restoration of tuboovarian relationships should be the goal of reconstruction. In particular, the fimbria ovarica should be carefully identified, as it is an important landmark in the tuboovarian anatomy.

Fimbrioplasty

Fimbrioplasty is defined as the lysis of fimbrial adhesions or dilatation of fimbrial phimosis. On occasion, a peritoneal ring results in a relative obstruction of the distal portion of the fallopian tube such that simple lysis of this tissue will uncover normal-appearing fimbriae (Fig. 8.2). In most instances, periadnexal adhesions are also present. It is important to mobilize the shaft of the tube and ovary prior to attempting to establish patency by fimbriolysis.

If agglutination is found, a fine delicate mosquito forceps can be introduced into the phimotic opening of the tube and gently opened. With the forceps in the open position, they are gently withdrawn, causing dilatation of the tubal ostia. By repeating this procedure in several directions, even dilation of the fimbrial os is accomplished. In some instances, a small incision over scarred tissue may be necessary. Long-term patency may be aided by a few sutures of 8-0 polyglactic suture to maintain established eversion in some instances.

Laparoscopy

Phimotic or clubbed fimbria may be released through the laparoscope. The distal portion of the tube must be free of adhesions. The tube is distended to identify the lumen, and the fallopian tube is stabilized with atraumatic forceps. Occasionally, the anterior cul-de-sac may be used to provide a platform for dissection. It is understood that, as in laparotomy surgery, periadnexal adhesions are lysed and removed prior to fimbrial reconstruction. Fibrous tissue covering the terminal end of the tube is excised with fine-needle unipolar

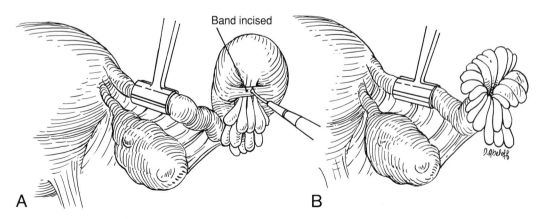

Band incised

A   B

Figure 8.2. Fimbrioplasty. *A,* Incomplete tubal obstruction resulting from a tubal band. *B,* When this scar is removed, normal fimbriae appear. One or two fine sutures will help maintain patency.

cautery, microscissors, or laser. If the fimbria are agglutinated, forceps or tongs may be introduced into the opening in the closed position and then gently withdrawn (Fig. 8.3). This may be repeated several times in different directions. Gentleness is necessary to avoid excessive trauma and bleeding.

The fimbriae should then be carefully explored for fimbrial adhesions. These may be freed with the fine-needle cautery, fine scissors, or laser. Care should be taken not to traumatize the fragile mucosa, as this may lead to complete fimbrial occlusion postoperatively.

Prefimbrial phimosis may be released by incising the fibrous band that constricts the infundibulum with laser or fine-needle cautery. A very shallow incision should be made along the avascular scarred area from the fimbriated end and extending just beyond the region of phimosis. If appropriate, the tubal mucosa can be everted with a defocused laser or very low-power cautery to the serosal surface.

Results

Recent series of microsurgical fimbrioplasty via laparotomy report intrauterine pregnancy rates of 30–70% (53,68). Similar intrauterine pregnancy rates of 20–50% have been reported for laparoscopic fimbrioplasty (26,28,43). A 5% ectopic pregnancy rate is reported for both laparotomy and laparoscopy series.

NEOSALPINGOSTOMY

Neosalpingostomy is the creation of a new tubal ostium where the fimbrial end is totally occluded. Terminal neosalpingostomy is the procedure of choice for establishing tubal patency in this case. Ampullary and isthmic salpingostomy are largely historical procedures that result in dismal pregnancy success rates.

A successful neosalpingostomy requires a complete understanding of the normal tubo-ovarian relationships, specifically, the fimbria ovarica and the relationship of the shaft of the oviduct to the ovary. Although there is some variation in the length of the fimbria ovarica, it is always present and provides a clue as to the normal axis of the oviduct. It should always be clearly identified before an ostium is created.

With a monopolar microelectrode, laser or fine, sharp scissors, adhesions are excised and the ovaries mobilized. The cul-de-sac may then be packed with lint-free laparotomy pads and the adnexa placed on an appropriate platform prior to establishing tuboovarian relationships. Once lysis of adhesions has established normal anatomy, attention is turned to the distal fallopian tube. The tubes are distended by

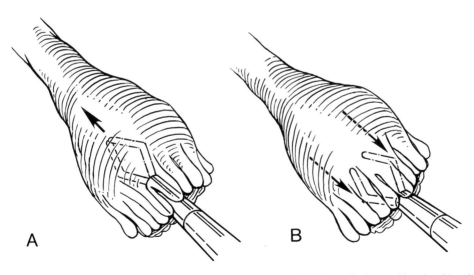

Figure 8.3. Fimbrial agglutination. *A,* The tongs, ampulla dilator, or small crile may be inserted into the phimotic tube in the closed position. *B,* The instrument is opened and carefully withdrawn in that position. This may be repeated at various angles to allow symmetric dilatation. The fimbriae should then be examined for interfimbrial adhesions, which should be carefully lysed.

injection of dilute methylene blue or indigo carmine dye through the fundus or cervix. Under magnification, a distinct vascular pattern with a white avascular area may sometimes be identified. As this scar is incised, the colored fluid will escape. It is our practice to insert a fine glass probe into the tube and explore the ampullary portion of the fallopian tube. A salpingoscope is inserted if available. Complete distal obstruction may occur without significant hydrosalpinx or fimbrial destruction (Fig. 8.4). In this case, normal-appearing fimbriae may protrude through the opening; however, more often than not, the fimbriae are severely damaged. In this case, an initial incision at 6 o'clock is performed in the direction of the fimbria ovarica and in a stellate pattern over areas of scar (Fig. 8.5). The mucosa is then carefully everted with a minimal number of sutures of 7-0 or 8-0. Tiny bleeding points may be visualized by irrigation and are coagulated with microtip bipolar forceps or laser.

Laparoscopy

The magnification of the laparoscope may be augmented by a loupe attachment to the laparoscopic eyepiece or via the video monitor. Neosalpingostomy requires that the end of the tube be free of adhesions. Two to three

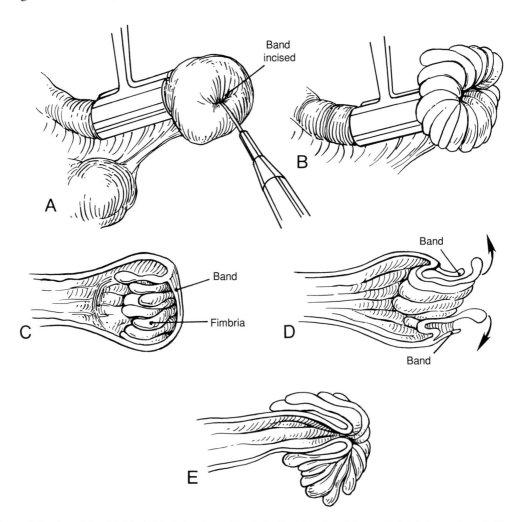

Figure 8.4. Complete distal fimbrial obstruction without significant hydrosalpinx or fimbrial destruction. *A,* The whitish scar is incised. *B,* Fimbrial strands are revealed. Some agglutination may be noted. A small forceps may be used to dilate the phimotic os. *C,* A cross-section reveals strands by peritoneal band. *D,* When the band is incised the fimbriae are released. *E,* Fimbriae assume their normal anatomic position.

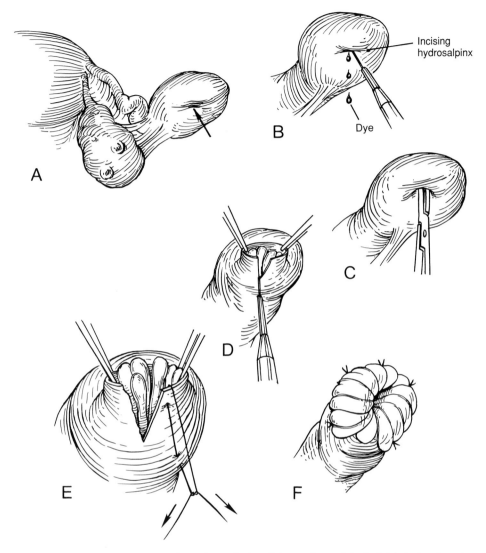

Figure 8.5.   Distal fimbrial obstruction with moderate hydrosalpinx and complete fimbrial destruction. *A* and *B*, Incision is made over the whitish scar on the distended hydrosalpinx. *C*, The ostium is dilated with a fine forcep. *D*, The incision is extended at 6 o'clock toward the fimbria ovarica. *E* and *F*, A cuff salpingostomy is achieved after eversion of the mucosa using 7-0 polyglactic suture.

ancillary puncture sites are necessary to properly manipulate the tube. Transcervical installation of dilute indigo carmine dye distends the hydrosalpinx and aids in the identification of the scarred ostium, fimbria ovarica, and adjacent structures. As with laparotomy microsurgery, it is important to reestablish the appropriate anatomy. The area of the dimple is incised with scissors, needle-point cautery, or laser (high-power density). The tube can be superficially scored with the laser or cautery prior to perforating the wall and collapsing the hy-

drosalpinx. This will facilitate completion of the dissection after collapse of the hydrosalpinx. The atraumatic forceps may then be repositioned to stabilize the margins of the incision. In cases where normal fimbriae are released, a single incision extended at 6 o'clock is usually sufficient to release the peritoneal band and allow eversion. In the majority of cases, two relaxing incisions to complete the shape of a "Y" may be necessary to achieve sufficient exposure of the residual fimbriae.

When using a CO_2 laser, great care is

necessary to avoid damage to the epithelum on the other side of the lumen. The "flowering" CO_2 laser technique consists of applying a defocused beam of low-power density to the serosal surface. The beam is moved continuously over the serosal area to limit damage to the tube. Absorption of water causes contraction of the serosal surface and a "flowering," thus exposing more mucosal area. The same technique can be accomplished using very low-power electrocoagulation or thermocoagulation. Eversion may also be accomplished by grasping the luminal surface gently and using another forcep to evert the edges. Sutures of 4-0 PDS may be placed using intraabdominal or extracorporeal endoscopic suture technique. This technique is particularly helpful for thick-walled sclerotic tubes where the serosal coagulation technique is not useful. An alternative technique involves placement of absorbable clips to everted edges of the tube (48).

Results

It is difficult to discuss results of surgery without an adequate description of the surgical technique as well as documentation of the degree of tubal disease and the amount of pelvic adhesion at the time of surgery. This information is usually inadequately provided. Differences in classification systems further confuse the issue. For instance, the 10th World Congress on Fertility and Sterility suggested that the term "salpingoneostomy" be used only for those procedures designed to relieve distally obstructed fallopian tubes where no identifiable fimbriae can be recovered. The condition of the fimbriae may vary widely once the obstruction is relieved. Thus, the condition of the fimbriae must be taken into account because it may be of prognostic value. The size of the hydrosalpinx appears to have prognostic value, as a hydrosalpinx larger than "Shirodkar's thumb" (2.5 cm) decreases pregnancy rates from 50 to 10% (69). In addition, Young (83) demonstrated an increase in pregnancy rate in patients noted to have rugae on postoperative hysterogram (HSG). The pregnancy rate decreased from 61% when rugae were noted to 7% when rugae were not demonstrated. Both size of hydrosalpinx and

rugae on HSG, probably reflect the condition of the fimbria. Boer-Meisel (5) has also analyzed the importance of additional factors for the prediction of subsequent conception. In addition to size of hydrosalpinx, extent of adhesions, and macroscopic aspects of the fimbria, the thickness of the tubal wall was analyzed. The combination of these four factors allowed the selection of three prognostic groups (good, intermediate, poor) with regard to pregnancy outcome. Vasquez (78), using scanning electron microscopy, demonstrated a significant reduction in ciliated cells from hydrosalpinx. With microbiopsy techniques, a correlation may be established with the condition of these cells and subsequent pregnancy rates. Preliminary evidence suggests that findings at salpingoscopy may mirror these changes and be of important prognostic value. Findings of adhesions, agglutination, and flattened mucosa correlated with poor pregnancy outcome. Puttemans (54) has introduced a classification of ampullary mucosa that will allow comparison of results in prospective studies. Hulka (35) stresses the importance of ovarian adhesions as prognosticators of pregnancy outcome.

Several classification systems have, therefore, been proposed to characterize prognosis following surgical repair of the hydrosalpinx (1,5,41,63). These usually incorporate the findings at laparoscopy, hysterosalpingogram, and the condition of fimbriae at definitive surgery (Table 8.2). In essence, women whose distal tubes had a diameter greater than 2.5 cm were found to have much lower pregnancy rates than those with smaller diameter hydrosalpinges. A significantly better outcome is seen when women have normal diameter tubes, rugation is seen on HSG, and pertitubular adhesions are absent.

Results of neosalpingostomy have been discouraging. Neosalpingostomy performed with a microscope has resulted in similar intrauterine pregnancy rates as compared with conventional techniques, although an increase in ectopic pregnancy rate has been observed (9, 30,32,50,72). The efficacy of the use of the microscope to perform this surgery remains to be established. Our own experience, using minimal magnification with the loupe, has not been dissimilar from pregnancy rates previously

Table 8.2.   Classification of the Extent of Tubal Disease with Distal Fimbrial Obstruction[a]

Extent of Disease	Findings
Mild	1. Absent or small hydrosalpinx < 15 mm diameter
	2. Inverted fimbriae easily recognized when patency achieved
	3. No significant peritubal or periovarian adhesions
	4. Preoperative hysterogram reveals a rugal pattern
Moderate	1. Hydrosalpinx 15–30 mm diameter
	2. Fragments of fimbriae not readily identified
	3. Periovarian and/or peritubular adhesions without fixation, minimal cul-de-sac adhesions
	4. Absence of a rugal pattern on preoperative hysterogram
Severe	1. Large hydrosalpinx > 30 mm diameter
	2. No fimbriae
	3. Dense pelvic or adnexal adhesions with fixation of the ovary and tube to either the broad ligament, pelvic sidewall, omentum, and/or bowel
	4. Obliteration of the cul-de-sac
	5. Frozen pelvis (adhesion formation so dense that limits of organs are difficult to define)

[a]Adapted from Rock and coauthors, 1978 (63).

reported (63). Schlaff and coauthors (67) have recently reported the Johns Hopkins experience with distal obstruction treated by neosalpingostomy using microsurgical technique (Table 8.3). The pregnancy rate in patients with mild disease was 80% (70% intrauterine and 10% ectopic), while those with severe disease had a pregnancy rate of 16% (12% intrauterine and 4% ectopic). With the classification systems proposed by Mage (41) and Boer-Meisel (5), patients in the better prognostic category had a 58.8% pregnancy rate (50% intrauterine, 8.8% ectopic) in Mage's series and 81% pregnancy rate (77% intrauterine and 4% ectopic) in Boer-Meisel's series. By comparison, those patients in the poor prognostic category had a 16.5% overall rate (7% intrauterine and 4% ectopic) and a 19% rate (3% intrauterine, 16% ectopic) in the two studies. These observations support the contention that the major determinant of successful outcome of distal tubal surgery is the severity of preexisting tubal pathology and the extent of adhesion formation.

Schlaff (67) compared the recent Johns Hopkins results with those reported in 1978 (Table 8.3). A similar number of patients was analyzed in both series using the identical classification system. Demographic characteristics and proportional distribution of extent of disease were similar. The sole significant difference between the two series was operative technique. When compared with the earlier

macrosurgical series in 1978, pregnancy rates with respect to extent of disease was similar, although the pregnancy rates were improved in the severe category with microsurgery. These findings suggest that the difference may be due to reduced adhesion formation using contemporary techniques. It appears that a clinically significant benefit to neosalpingostomy by microsurgery vs macrosurgery is not found when each technique is performed by an experienced reproductive surgeon.

It is difficult to compare laparoscopy and laparotomy for the treatment of distal tubal occlusion because of the relatively low number of published reports and small sample size. However, it appears that the overall intrauterine pregnancy rate achieved by laparoscopy approaches that of laparotomy. Laparoscopy series have ranged from 0 to 44% (15,26,43, 56). Donnez (20) reported 575 patients treated with CO_2 laser laparoscopy for adnexal adhesions and tubal occlusion. Three-hundred seventy-two patients had pelvic adhesions without tubal occlusion, and 203 patients had tubal occlusion. Postoperative pregnancy rates were 58% for patients with pelvic adhesions (64% for filmy and avascular adhesions, and 51% for dense and vascular "but not very thick adhesions"). This was similar to the rate obtained by the same group (56%) following microsurgical sapingolysis by laparotomy (21). After laparoscopic fimbrioplasty, the postoperative pregnancy rate was 61%. In a series with 142

Table 8.3. Pregnancy Outcome Following Neosalpingostomy with Respect to Extent of Disease[a]

Extent of disease and prognosis	Intrauterine Pregnancy Total Patients in Category		Ectopic Pregnancy Total Patients in Category	
	1989	1978	1989	1978
Mild	7/10 (70%)	12/15 (80%)	1/10 (10%)	1/15 (6%)
Moderate	5/29 (17%)	5/30 (16%)	4/29 (14%)	4/30 (13%)
Severe	7/56 (12%)	2/42 (4%)	2/56 (4%)	0/42 (0%)

[a]Adapted from Schlaff WD and Rock JA: Neosalpingostomy for distal tubal obstruction: prognostic factors in implact on surgical technique. Fertil Steril 1991;54:984.

patients undergoing fimbrioplasty by laparotomy microsurgery, a similar rate was obtained (20). After laparoscopic neosalpingostomy, Donnez (21) obtained a patency rate of 80%, with an intrauterine pregnancy rate of 20%. Dubuisson (25) observed a 27.7% intrauterine pregnancy rate with 18 months of follow-up in 65 women with "terminal tuboplasties" by laparoscopy. Women with severe adhesions corresponding to a "frozen" pelvis were excluded. The lower success rate in some series points out that successful endoscopic repair can be a technically difficult undertaking. It may also be related to severity of tubal damage and type and extent of adhesions rather than the surgical technique employed. This question cannot be answered without a randomized clinical trial of laparoscopy vs. laparotomy microsurgery for salpingolysis and distal tubal occlusion.

Patient selection is probably the most important determinant of success. Donnez (20) states that adhesiolysis of very dense and fibrous adhesions are better removed by open microsurgical procedures and so were not included in his series. Nezhat (48) reported a high conception rate (48%), but at salpingoscopy, a large number of patients had well-preserved cilia and fimbrial folds. This is in sharp contrast to the pregnancy rate (16%) in patients with severely damaged tubal lumens. Increasing severity of periadnexal adhesions lowered the conception rate further.

A poor operative prognosis might be expected in patients with evidence of proximal and distal tubal occlusion. Patton (52) reviewed the records of 295 patients in a 5-year period prior to the establishment of in-vitro fertilization (IVF-ET). Thirty-one patients had at least two distinct and separate anatomic sites of both proximal and distal occlusion. The probability of conception at 2.5 years after surgery was 12%, but there were no live births. The results of this study suggest that patients with multiple sites of oviductal occlusion have an extremely poor prognosis with surgical management. These patients are not candidates for tubal reconstruction.

The use of the CO_2 laser represents another generation of putative surgical breakthroughs in the treatment of distal tubal occlusion. The results of studies comparing the efficacy of the CO_2 laser and electrosurgery on adhesion formation in animal models vary among different centers. Unfortunately, Diamond (19a), in a multicenter study, found that reproductive surgery with the CO_2 laser was associated with significant adhesion formation. Tulandi (77) noted no significant difference in pregnancy rates in a randomized study comparing the CO_2 laser with electrosurgery in patients undergoing tuboplasty (24.3% laser vs. 20% electrocautery) after 2 years of follow-up. A decrease in surgery to pregnancy interval was noted in the CO_2 laser group. Mage (41) and Bruhat (6) also compared outcome of neosalpingostomy by laser to a group of historical controls treated with microcautery. No statistically significant difference was found between the two groups. Tulandi (76) also examined adhesion reformation after reproductive surgery with and without the CO_2 laser. The degree of periadnexal adhesions was significantly reduced after the first operation (laparotomy) in both groups of patients. No significant difference was found in the degree of periadnexal adhesions between the two groups. There was no difference between the occurrence of tubal reocclusion and fimbrial phimosis after laser surgery (12.9% and 6.4%, respectively) or electrocautery (21.2% and 12.1%). Although there were at least 30 patients in each arm, a larger study is required to exclude, with a low probability of error, a small but clinically significant benefit. These data do not support the contention that the use of the CO_2 laser provides any advantage over the other currently available surgical techniques.

Adjuvant therapy is designed to increase chances of pregnancy postoperatively. The search for the perfect adjuvant has been long and relatively unproductive. Adhesion formation and its treatment with adjuvants are discussed in detail in Chapter 1; however, a brief discussion will be offered here because of the possible importance of adjuvants in improving the high de novo and reformation rate of adhesions and generally disappointing pregnancy rates seen with surgery alone.

Early postoperative hydrotubation was popularized by Grant (32) in an attempt to increase postneosalpingostomy fallopian tube patency rates. However, in a multicenter, randomized, controlled clinical trial, a beneficial effect following postoperative hydrotubation with lactated Ringer's solution with or without hydrocortisone could not be demonstrated (61).

Over the last decade, a variety of medical and barrier adjuvants have been introduced to pelvic surgeons or have undergone animal studies with varying degrees of success. These include dextran, surgical barriers, corticosteroids, heparin, nonsteroidal anti-inflammatory drugs, fibrinolytics, hydrogels, and procoagulants. Few have been shown to be efficacious in randomized clinical trials.

Two studies have evaluated Dextran 70 in a prospective, randomized and double-blind fashion (66,75,76). Both evaluated adhesions at a primary laparotomy and then reevaluated them within 3 months at a second-look laparoscopy. The control consisted of saline in one and lactated Ringer's in the other. Both studies demonstrated a significant reduction in adhesions with the use of Dextran. The Adhesion Study Group noted the effect appeared to be limited to those patients with severe adhesions. They also noted that the effect was largely limited to "dependent" portions of the pelvis. Jansen (40), however, in a randomized clinical trial, was unable to show a decrease in the formation of adhesions. Moreover, it appeared that there were enough patients to exclude (with a very low probability of error) a small but perhaps clinically significant therapeutic benefit. Hyskon is less commonly used now.

The concept of using a physical barrier to prevent adhesion formation has long been attractive. Interceed (TC-7) is a fabric composed of oxidized regenerated cellulose specifically designed as a surgical adjuvant. In 13 investigational centers, infertility patients underwent elective laparotomy for lysis of bilateral pelvic sidewall adhesions (36). TC-7 was applied in an amount sufficient to completely cover all deperitonealized surfaces on the sidewall indicated by the randomization plan. The opposite sidewall was used as a control. A second-look laparoscopy was performed 1–14 weeks after the laparotomy. Interceed (Johnson & Johnson, New Brunswick, NJ) provided a 57% improvement in reducing the extent of adhesions over that provided by surgery alone. Although filmy adhesions were improved, a significant benefit was seen in reducing the number of "severe" adhesions. Interceed has also been placed through the laparoscope without difficulty (2). Other barriers such as Gortex (W.L. Gore and Assoc., Flagstaff, AZ) are currently undergoing randomized, controlled clinical trials. Although barriers appear promising, further research and clinical studies are necessary to fully evaluate this class of adjuvants.

CONGENITAL TUBAL ANOMALIES

Women with infertility may have congenital anomalies or anatomical distortion of otherwise healthy oviducts. Cohen (11) and others (4) have studied the derangements of the fimbrial-gonadal mechanisms related to congenital accessory ostia, elongated fimbria ovarica, and distal distortion caused by intervening paratubal cysts. Defects in cannalization of the Mullerian ducts may result in duplication of the ostia of the oviducts. The origins of paratubal cysts are described at length in the chapter on the ovary. Elongation of the fimbria ovarica has been reported in association with polycystic ovaries. Cohen and Katz (10) speculate that the larger heavier gonad may pull and stretch the supporting muscular ligaments.

The effects of these anomalies on fertility were studied in patients who were infertile for more than 3 years, and were observed for at least 1 year after laparoscopy before proceeding to microsurgical correction (11). All other infertility factors were normal. Patients who had bilateral accessory ostia greater than or equal to the diameter of their primary tubal ostia, elongation of the fimbria ovarica resulting in a tubal ostium greater than 4 cm from its fimbrial attachment to the ovary, and large paratubal cysts with fimbrial displacement were studied.

To repair congenital accessory tubal ostia, sutures of 8-0 nylon are placed in the proximal and distal ends of the ostia and held with delicate forceps. Elevation of angle sutures permits the "tucking in" of accessory endosalpingeal tissue into the lumen of the ampulla and defines their lateral seromuscular borders. These borders are then brought together with 8-0 interrupted nylon or Vicryl suture to close the gaps. Serosal sutures can be placed if desired.

Elongated fimbria ovarica are repaired after examination of the fimbria to ensure that there are no interfimbrial bridges or adhesions. The anatomy of the major arterial branch between the ovarian artery and anastomosing branch of the uterine artery are defined. The object is to reattach the fimbria ovarica to a chosen point on the outer surface of the ovary. Using 7-0 nylon or Vicryl suture, the anchor suture is placed on the upper surface of the ovary and inserted deep into the cortex. The suture is used to plicate the fimbria ovarica to a point approximately 2 cm distant from the ostium. This results in the relocation of the fimbria ovarica closer to the ovarian surface.

Cysts that result in gross distortion and displacement of the tubal ostium from the surface of the ipsilateral ovary are resected. The bipolar cautery is used to precoagulate any obvious large vessels traversing the mesosalpinx over the paratubal cyst along the intended lines of incision. The anterior mesosalpinx is preferred, so that the suture line is distant to the posterior ovarian and fimbrial side of the adnexa. The overlying peritoneum is elevated and divided. Once the correct plane is identified, the scissors are used to dissect the cyst in toto. Any attached vascular pedicles are coagulated. The mesosalpinx may be left open or repaired using fine sutures.

Results

Twenty-one patients underwent surgery after all infertility tests were normal and the patients had undergone ovulation induction for at least three cycles. A success rate of 46% was seen with repair of multiple congenital accessory tubal ostia. Forty-eight patients with elongated fimbria-ovarica were studied. The success rate for medical therapy was 10%. Forty-two patients underwent surgery, with a success rate of 57%. Seven patients with large paratubal cysts were studied. None responded to medical therapy. At 18 months of follow-up, two patients obtained viable pregnancies, for a success rate of 28%. The absence of ectopic pregnancy in this series is probably evidence for otherwise normal fallopian tubes. If these preliminary results are confirmed by other investigators, one could support surgical therapy for these otherwise "unexplained" infertility patients. The alternative modalities of in-vitro fertilization (IVF-ET) or gamete intra-fallopian transfer (GIFT) have a live birth rate of 15–20% (42).

TUBAL ANASTOMOSIS

Microsurgical technique received a great deal of interest as a result of the enhanced pregnancy rates reported following reversal of sterilization. Microsurgery appears to be an important technique in tubal reanastomosis. A comparison of Hellman's macrosurgical approach at Johns Hopkins and our microsurgical technique developed in 1976 resulted in an increased pregnancy rate (62). Other variables that may impact on subsequent pregnancy success following reversal of sterilization include type of sterilization procedure, segments anastomosed, tubal length, and time interval from sterilization.

Several types of sterilization procedures may

be reversed. Depending upon the extent of tubal destruction, different segments are anastomosed. It is therefore difficult to separate these variables when discussing sterilization procedures in general. In our experience, unipolar electrocautery is associated with destruction of a large amount of tube, especially when the triple-burn technique is used. As a result of the high variability in tubal destruction, preoperative laparoscopy is indicated in patients who have undergone sterilization by unipolar electrocautery to determine the amount of distal fallopian tube available for the anastomosis. The amount of proximal tube is known from the preoperative hysterosalpingogram (HSG). Proximal obstruction on HSG, however, is usually from tubal spasm and not from obstruction of the intramural portion of the fallopian tube.

It is extremely rare for the entire intramural portion of the fallopian tube to be destroyed by a sterilization procedure. Moreover, proximal pathological occlusions of the oviduct rarely affect the intramural segment. The proximal isthmus, the distal interstitial oviduct, or both, are usually the regions affected. Many diverse but relatively rare disease processes damage the proximal oviduct. Infections, such as endometritis or salpingitis, may precede obstruction. Cornual polyps, a manifestation of tubal polyposis, are less frequently recognized as a cause of obstruction. Salpingitis isthmica nodosa shows a predilection for the proximal oviduct. In such cases, a tubocornual anastomosis, as opposed to an implantation, is the procedure of choice (22,29,44,46,80). Although it is apparent that the uterotubal junction is not required for human intrauterine pregnancy, improved pregnancy success rates are seen with tubocornual anastomosis when compared with uterotubal implantation. Thus, attempts should be made to identify the amount of intramural obstruction before considering uterotubal implantation. Uterotubal implantation is undertaken only when tubocornual anastomosis or transcervical catheterization is not feasible. However, when necessary, we advocate the microsurgical approach to proximal obstruction and excise all pathologic tissue to effect an isthmic implantation and to minimize the operative injury to the tissues.

Technique of Tubal Anastomosis

A loupe, visor, or microscope may be used to obtain magnification. Magnification with loupes ranges from 1.5–6 ×, while the microscope may provide magnification from 3–40 ×. In a randomized trial, Rock (61) showed that pregnancy rates using loupe magnification or operating microscope were not different.

ISTHMIC-ISTHMIC ANASTOMOSIS

The proximal portion of the fallopian tube is identified and its distal tip resected from the mesosalpinx. The occluded tip is resected with straight Stevens scissors. A 2-0 nylon suture of 40″ may be introduced into the lumen with fine forceps, if desired. Its passage is facilitated by the distension of the uterine cavity and the interstitial portion of the oviduct with indigo carmine dye injected through the uterine fundus (with cervical obstruction by suitable instruments) as well as by stretching the tubal stump.

There should be no discrepancy in luminal size if the distal segment is truly part of the isthmus (Fig. 8.6). The proximal portion of the distal obstructed tube is resected in the same manner, and the nylon stent is passed through the oviduct and out the fimbriated end. The mesosalpinx is carefully approximated using 6-0 Vicryl to eliminate tension at the anastomotic site. The knot should be tied anteriorly to decrease the chances for adhesion formation involving the ovary. The lumina of the two ends are approximated with 7-0 or 8-0 Polygalactin (Vicryl) on a 3/8″ circle taper. Nylon may also be used. The needle is passed only through the muscularis of the proximal tube and distal segment. The sutures are tied securely but not tightly. Three to four sutures are usually necessary to approximate the muscularis. A second layer of three additional sutures may be placed to approximate the tubal serosa. The nylon stent is removed.

ISTHMIC-AMPULLARY ANASTOMOSIS

The proximal tube is prepared in a manner similar to that described above. A major difficulty is encountered in the isthmic-ampullary anastomosis because there is a large discrepancy in the diameter of the lumen in the

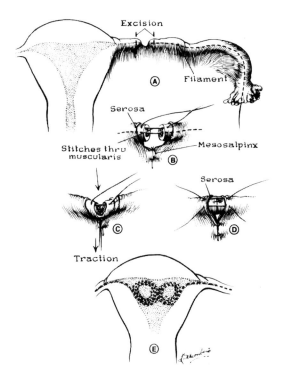

Figure 8.6. Isthmic-isthmic anastomosis. *A,* Patency of obstructed lumina established excision of obstructed segment. A 2-0 nylon suture is introduced into the lumen with fine forceps. *B,* The lumina may be approximated over a 2-0 nylon stent in two layers after the mesosalpinx is approximated. *C,* Three sutures are placed in the muscularis. *D,* The serosa is approximated. *E,* The stent is removed after the anastomosis is complete.

isthmus as compared with the ampullary portion of the tube. To prevent too large an opening in the ampulla, a needle technique for opening the ampulla has been described (Fig. 8.7). An obturator of an intravenous placement unit of Teflon (number 16) is introduced through the fimbriated end of the ampullary segment of the oviduct and advanced to the obstructed site. The needle is inserted through the Teflon obturator, and the obstructed end is perforated by the needle and the Teflon sheath. After the needle is removed, the 2-0 nylon is passed in a retrograde manner through the Teflon obturator. The mesosalpinx is approximated to reduce tension at the anastomotic site. Approximately three to four 7-0 or 8-0 Vicryl sutures are placed through the serosa and muscularis of the proximal oviduct and then through the distal tube. The tip of the needle may be introduced into the ampullary lumen by

being placed in the tip of the lumen of the Teflon obturator; then, the tip of the obturator is withdrawn into the ampullary portion of the tube. In some instances, a two-layer closure is possible. In those cases, an additional, second layer of suture is placed to approximate the tubal serosa. The nylon stents are removed intraoperatively.

Alternate methods of overcoming the tubal discrepancy have been described by others. Winston prefers to circumcise the very tip of the ampulla over the bulbous end of a probe inserted through the fimbrial ostia. Before cutting across the mucosa, he suggests stripping back the peritoneal coat to facilitate subsequent two-layer closure. A single-layer closure is necessary, however, in the rather large lumen of the distal ampullary portion of the oviduct. The wall in this area is quite thin, and if attempts are made to circumcise the fallopian tube, extensive bleeding occurs, as well as inadvertent widening of the oviductal lumen.

AMPULLARY-AMPULLARY ANASTOMOSIS

The muscularis of the ampullary region is relatively delicate. A single layer of suture easily approximates the tubal lumina. Four to eight sutures are placed around the circumference of the ampulla (Fig. 8.8). These sutures are placed through the serosa and muscularis. The endosalpinx is spared, if possible, when approximating the lumen. No stents are used.

INTERSTITIAL/AMPULLARY ANASTOMOSIS

Interstitial or cornual/ampullary anastomosis, on occasion, must be performed if a small proximal portion of the interstitial oviduct is occluded. A fine knife is necessary to core out the obstructed portion of the fallopian tube, creating a crater around the intramural tube (Fig. 8.9). The isthmic or ampullary (prepared so that the lumina are proportional) distal tube is then approximated to the intramural portion of the fallopian tube. This is the only procedure that requires high magnification and in which the microscope is most useful. These procedures are usually performed

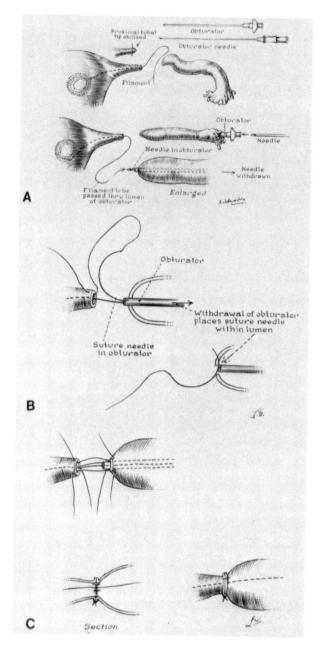

Figure 8.7. Isthmic-ampullary anastomosis. *A,* The proximal obstruction is excised. The Teflon obturator is inserted through the fimbriated end. Once appropriately placed, the needle is inserted to perforate the proximal portion of the distal tube. *B,* The obturator is slightly withdrawn to permit placement of the needle tip within the ampullary lumen. *C,* The stent is withdrawn after completion of the procedure.

at 10–20 X. If the distal portion is ampulla, the catheter technique previously described for an isthmic-ampullary anastomosis or the use of the circumcision technique is essential to obtain an ampullary lumen similar in size to the cornual lumen. Functional success of this procedure will be maximized if operative technique stresses an avoidance of lumen disparity. Good hemostasis must be achieved using either fine-needle electrocautery or laser. A two-layer closure is usually required for an interstitial/isthmic anastomosis.

Figure 8.8. Ampullary-ampullary anastomosis. Anastomosis of these lumina requires 6–8 sutures of 7-0 or 8-0 absorbable suture placed circumferentially, equidistant about the oviductal lumen.

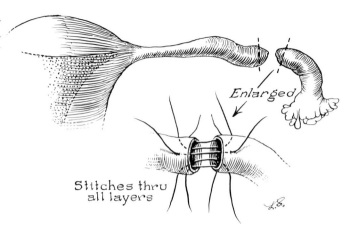

Enlarged

Stitches thru all layers

Uterotubal Implantation

Although this procedure is essentially obsolete, a brief description will be provided. Preparation of the distal oviduct for implantation consists of either slitting its antimesenteric border or performing bilateral incisions to "fish-mouth" the tube to help preserve patency. Preparation of the uterus has varied tremendously. The uterine incisions for implantation techniques include a sharp cornual wedge excision, a reamer, and the posterior fundal technique. Bonney (5a) incised the uterine fundus to implant the oviductal segments under direct vision. Holden and Sovak (34a) preferred to use a reamer to make a cornual passage. Von Csaba (79a) reported implantation through a posterior fundal incision between the uteroovarian ligaments. The fallopian tube (either isthmus or ampulla) is then inserted into the uterine cavity and a nonreactive absorbable suture is brought out through the uterus, superior and inferior to the incision, and tied securely. The myometrium is then closed in two layers.

Transcervical Fallopian Tube Catheterization

Relief of proximal obstruction not secondary to tubal ligation may be attempted by the transcervical approach. Failure of the transcervical approach would lead to a microsurgical tubointerstitial anastomosis. As noted previously, uterotubal implantation is rarely used.

Placement of the catheters may be performed under fluoroscopic guidance or hysteroscopic control (12,49). The catheter set consists of the coaxial catheters 9 F, 5.5 F, and 3 F in diameter. The catheters are introduced through the cervix with a vacuun adapter or hysteroscope. The 5.5 F catheter is wedged into the cornua, the 3 F catheter with wire guide is introduced, and the wire guide is advanced through the obstruction. The 3 F soft tube is then advanced over the wire. Balloon-tip catheters have also been developed, and dilate the proximal portion of the oviduct once cannalization is achieved.

Results

One may expect an overall pregnancy success rate of 60–80% live births; and 3–4% ectopic pregnancy rate (Table 8.5). Our own experience with microsurgical technique has been comparable to previously reported figures (Tables 8.4 and 8.5). In an attempt to find variables to predict pregnancy success, success rates after reversal of sterilization have been examined with respect to tubal length after anastomosis, the site of anastomosis, the sterilization procedure performed, and interval from sterilization procedure.

Fallopian tube length following anastomosis is widely agreed to be the most influential of all predicters of outcome. Silber and Cohen (70) have demonstrated pregnancy rates to be related to the length of the longest tube following repair. Gomel has observed that fallopian tubes of less than 3 cm in total length were associated with a long interval between

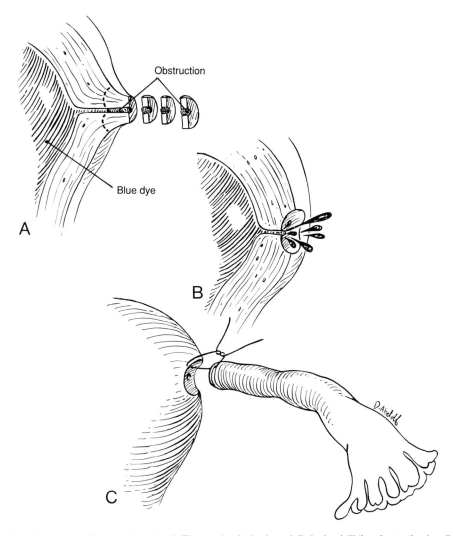

Figure 8.9. Tuboinsterstitial anastomosis. *A,* The proximal tube is serially incised till the obstruction is relieved and blue dye is seen. Incision of the cornual area may require a "crater" into the myometrium. *B,* Once absolute hemostasis is achieved, three sutures are placed through the muscular layer just within the serosal surface to the interstitial portion, avoiding the endosalpinx of the cornua. It is then continued through the muscularis of the distal segment. The serosa may be closed with approximated interrupted sutures or continuous sutures of 7-0 or 8-0 absorbable material.

reconstructive surgery and occurrence of pregnancy (27,82). Henderson (33a) and Hulka (35) have noted similar findings. Rock (60) determined that a significant decrease in pregnancy is associated with both tubes being less than 4 cm in length. Jansen (40), however, noted that tube length above 4 cm has no discernible effect on fallopian tube function when fimbrial access to the ovary is not compromised.

The site of anastomosis has been claimed to

be a predicter of success. Brosens and Winston (5b), Boeckx (4a), Henderson (90) and Chang (8) all claim that the less disparity between luminal sizes at the site of anastomosis, the better the pregnancy rate. They noted the highest pregnancy rate in isthmic-isthmic anastomosis or anastomosis without disparate lumens. Our own experience has not noted a reduced pregnancy rate among those patients requiring isthmic-ampullary anastomosis, although our procedure using the catheter tech-

8.4. Pregnancy Success Following Reversal of Sterilization at the Johns Hopkins Hospital, 1976–1983

Procedure	Number of Patients	Patients Pregnant	Live Births	Ectopic Pregnancy
Unipolar cautery	96	54%	35	8
Pomeroy	54	72%	32	1
Irving	12	58%	5	0
Partial salpingectomy	38	71%	22	1
Falope ring	45	86%	35	1
Clip	1	100%	1	0
Total	246	67%	130 (53%)	11 (4%)

Table 8.5. Pregnancy Success Following Tubal Anastomosis Using Microsurgical Technique

Author (Year)	Number of Cases	Percent Live Births	Percent Ectopic Pregnancy
Silber, Cohen (71)	25	56	4
Patterson (52)	50	40	4
Winston (82)	126	58	2
Gomel (27)	118	64	1
Grunert et al. (33)	40	57	3
Seiler (69a)	73	64	2
Paterson (52)	147	59	5
Rock (61)	246	53	4
Chang, Kim (8)	250	44	5
Total	1075	55%	3%

nique has resulted in an improved pregnancy rate over those achieved using macrosurgical techniques. It should be noted, however, that the univariate analysis performed in the above studies failed to show statistical significance. Rock (60) and Silber and Cohen (70) found the site of anastomosis to have no effect on outcome. Putman (54a) has recently attempted to adjust for confounding factors known or suspected to affect success rates with multiple logistic regression on the data set. They suggested that when confounding variables are resolved, the site of anastomosis does not affect the eventual pregnancy rate.

Pregnancy success rates after reversal of unipolar electrocautery appear to be diminished over those reported with the Falope ring and Hulka clip. Furthermore, bilateral partial salpingectomy or Pomeroy has a higher success rate (60). Others have not found this to be true (85). In our series, cautery also appears to have a higher ectopic pregnancy rate (61). Furthermore, associated pelvic pathology in the form of proximal hydrosalpinges and endometriosis is higher in patients following monopolar high-frequency diathermy (66). Donnez (23) has shown that oviduct deciliation may extend 2 cm from the site of cautery. When this question is examined using multivariate analysis and life-table comparisons, however, no significant difference is demonstrable (4a,54a). It appears that the choice of sterilization method per se does not affect chances of successful reversal, but that the poorer outcome following electrocautery, in some cases, is likely due to resulting tubal segments that are often less than 4 cm. Jansen (40) has shown that deleterious effects of endometriosis on fertility can be overcome surgically, provided precautions are taken to prevent formation of adnexal adhesions.

Vasquez et al. (78) have noted that the interval from sterilization to reversal has a significant impact on results, with a longer interval leading to lower pregnancy rates. This has been disputed by Silber (70), Boeckx (93), Hulka (35) and Rock (60). Recently, Putman (89) has also confirmed the lack of effect of sterilization interval on pregnancy rates.

The treatment of occlusion of the proximal

oviduct has been by tubouterine implantation with only recent use of microsurgical tubointerstitial anastomosis as an alternative. A life-table analysis of pregnancy success following uterotubal implantation reveals that the maximum cumulative rate of pregnancy is achieved after approximately 48 months. Pregnancy rates of 30–40% can be expected (58). The techniques of sharp cornual dissection by scalpel and cornual reaming have been compared by Rock and coworker. Based on uterotubal implantations performed from 1942 through 1976, cornual reaming appeared superior (38% vs. 12%).

Donnez and Casanas-Roux (22) report occlusion of the proximal oviduct treated exclusively by microsurgical tubointerstitial anastomosis with good results (44% term pregnancy rate). This corroborates the data of Gomel (29) and McComb (46), who noted a 57% term pregnancy rate. Winston (80) has found pregnancy success rates approaching 60%. With these improved pregnancy success rates, uterotubal implantation is indicated only when complete obliteration of the intramural portion of the fallopian tube is noted. Thus, attempts should be made to identify the amount of intramural obstruction before considering uterotubal implantation.

It is interesting to note that in Donnez's (21) series, patients with diverticular lesions and tubal obstruction achieved a lower pregnancy rate than those with obstruction alone. This was not seen in Gomel's (29) and McComb's (46) series. The diverticular pattern that is characteristic of salpingitis isthmica nodosa is often associated with infertility and ectopic pregnancy (14). However, in all three series, once the diseased segment is resected and the remainder of the tube anastomosed, there appears to be no greater risk for ectopic pregnancy than after tubointerstitial anastomosis for occlusion not associated with diverticular leasions.

There are no data to document pregnancy success rates after transcervical fallopian tube catheterization or cannalization procedures. However, patency of the proximal portion of the oviducts may be accomplished in approximately 60% of patients. These procedures are less invasive than the traditional exploratory laparotomy with anastomosis.

SECOND-LOOK LAPAROSCOPY

Second-look laparoscopy after reconstructive surgery refers to a laparoscopy that is performed usually but not necessarily after a laparotomy procedure. The interval from the initial surgery may vary from a few days to a year or more. These have traditionally been performed 1 year after "failed" reconstructive surgery. At that time, endoscopic lysis can be performed in an attempt to restore normal anatomy. Second tuboplasties by laparotomy have been shown to have a very poor success rate. Tulandi (76) has demonstrated that second tuboplasties through the laparoscope at 1 year do not significantly improve subsequent pregnancy rates.

Early second-look laparoscopy (1–12 weeks) after laparotomy or laparoscopic reconstructive surgery is controversial. Fibrosis of unlysed fibrin begins 3 days after serosal trauma and is completed by 21 days (37). Lysis of adhesion during the early period, especially before 21 days, is quite easy, as the adhesions are very filmy and avascular. The success of such a procedure in restoring normal anatomy and increasing subsequent pregnancy rate is widely debated.

Swolin (73) introduced the concept of second-look laparoscopy to evaluate the results of reproductive surgery. Daniell and Pittaway (17) suggested that early second-look may improve pregnancy rates. DeCherney and Mezer (19), in a cohort study, noted that 60% of early second-look patients had filmy adhesions, and 60% of the late second-look patients had thicker adhesions. Trimbos-Kemper (75) and Jansen (37) performed "third"-look laparoscopy on patients after early second-look laparoscopy (8–21 days). Using a cohort study design, Jansen suggested that early second-look laparoscopy is safe and effective in reducing adhesion formation (38). Trimbos-Kemper, in a prospective study (75), noted that there appeared to be a distinct relationship between the adhesions found at tubal surgery and the adhesions found at early second-look. In patients with no adhesions at tubal surgery or only slight ones, no adhesions had formed in 52% of cases. When moderate or severe adhesions had been treated at the time of fertility surgery, adhesions were present again in 70% of cases. In 73% of cases, the avascular adhesions removed at second-look did not recur. Of the vascular adhesions removed at second-look, 46% had not recurred at third-look. Of the dense adhesions removed with difficulty and bleeding at second-look, 17% were completely absent at follow-up laparoscopy.

A historical control group was used to rule out spontaneous resorption of adhesions and to assess a possible effect on pregnancy rate. The percentage of adnexa free of adhesions in the control group was 39%, vs. 63% in the study group. So it appears that a significant spontaneous resorption of adhesions does not occur. This suggests a beneficial effect of early second-look laparoscopy in diminishing permanent adhesions following tubal surgery. However, no difference was found between the intrauterine pregnancy rates in both groups, with a 33% and 34% pregnancy rate in both control group and study group, respectively, after 4 years. The surgery to conception interval, however, tended to be shorter in the study group. There was, also, a significant difference between the groups in ectopic pregnancy rates. In the study group, the cumulative ectopic pregnancy rate after 4 years was 11%, vs. 21% in the control group. This difference could be explained by the difference in ectopic pregnancy rate of the salpingostomy group. Surrey and Friedman (71) reported that the pregnancy rate after second-look at 6 weeks (52%) was much higher than after the same procedure done 6 months later (16.67%). Raj and Hulka (55) found that the optimal time for a second-look laparoscopy and salpingoovariolysis is 4–8 weeks after surgery. Indeed, in a randomized study, Tulandi (76) found that late second-look operative laparoscopy 1 year after reproductive surgery does not increase the pregnancy rate or decrease the incidence of ectopic pregnancy. Clearly, late second-look laparoscopy is ineffective. It remains to be seen with a randomized trial whether early second-look laparoscopy is effective in improving intrauterine pregnancy rate.

CONCLUSIONS

With refined technique and use of magnification, one can improve pregnancy success by reducing postoperative adhesion formation. This has been shown to be particularly true with reversals of sterilization. Microsurgery, whether by laparoscopy or laparotomy, is not a panacea for fallopian tubes with significant pathology. Although a reproductive surgeon can establish patency and minimize adhesion formation, this may be of no value in the oviduct where the mucosa has been severely damaged. In the future, the emphasis will be on better preoperative assessment of subsequent pregnancy success so we can limit surgical treatment by laparoscopy or laparotomy to those who will truly benefit from it. It must be remembered that the best that can be expected from IVF-ET at this time is 15–20% live birth (42). Those patients with poor prognosis should be encouraged to consider extracorporeal fertilization rather than distal neosalpingostomy unless practical, financial, or religious constraints render this unaccceptable. The experience of the surgeon will, of course, be a major factor in this decision, underscoring the importance of adequate training. Unfortunately, it is probably true that repair and rerepair of distal tubal closure is performed too often in current practice. Honest objectivity with respect to creating the most favorable situation leading to successful pregnancy should lead to referral for IVF-ET those patients presenting with absent or minimally preserved fimbriae.

References

1. American Fertility Society. The AFS classification of adnexal adhesions, distal tubal occlusion, tubal occlusion secondary to tubal ligation, tubal pregnancies, Mullerian anomalies and intrauterine adhesions. Fertil Steril 1988;49:944.
2. Azziz RA, Murphy AA, Rosenberg SM, et al: Use of Interceed (TC-7) absorable adhesion barrier at laparoscopy. J Reprod Med (in press).
3. Baibot S, Parent B, Dubuisson JB, et al: A clinical study of the CO_2 laser and electrosurgery for adhesiolysis in 172 cases followed by early second-look laparoscopy. Fertil Steril 1987;48:140.
4. Beyth Y, Kopolovic. Accessory tubes: a possible contributing factor in infertility. Fertil Steril 1982; 38:382–383.
4a. Boeckx W, Gordts S, Buysse K, et al: Reversibility after female sterilization. Br J Obstet Gynecol 1986; 93:839.
5. Boer-Meisel ME, teVelde ER, Habbena JDF, et al:

Predicting the pregnancy outcome in patients treated for hydrosalpinx: a prospective study. Fertil Steril 1986;45:23.

5a. Bonney V: The fruits of conservatism J Ob Gyn Br Commonwealth, 1937;44:1.

5b. Brosens J, Winston R: Reversibility of female sterilization. London: Academic Press, 1978.

6. Bruhat MA, Mage G, Manhes H, et al: Laparoscopic procedures to promote fertility. Ovariolysis and salpingolysis. Results of 93 selected cases. Acta Eur Fertil 113.

7. Caspi E, Halperin Y, Bukovsky I: The importance of periadnexal adhesions in tubal reconstructive surgery for infertility. Fertil Steril 1979;31:296.

8. Chang YS, Kim JG. Microsurgical reversal of tubal sterilization. Asia-Oceania J Obstet Gynecol 1986; 12:457.

9. Cognat M, Rochet Y: Salpingostomy. J Franc Gynecol Obstet Biol Repro 1977;6:839.

10. Cohen BM, Katz M. The significance of the convoluted oviduct in the infertil woman. J Reprod Med 1980;25:33–37.

11. Cohen BM. Microsurgical reconstruction of congenital tubal anomalies. Microsurgery 1987;8:68–77.

12. Confino E, Friberg J, Gleicher W: Preliminary experience with transcervical balloon tuboplasty. Am J Obstet Gynecol 1988;159:370.

13. Crane M, Woodruff JD: Factors influencing the success of tuboplastic procedures. Fertil Steril 1968; 19:810.

14. Creasy JL, Clarak RL, Cuttino JT, et al. Salpingitis isthmica nodosa: radiologic and clinical correlates. Radiology 1985;154:597.

15. Daniell JF, Herbert CM: Laparoscopic salpingostomy utilizing the CO_2 laser. Fertil Steril 1984;41:558.

16. Daniell JF, Miller W: Hysteroscopic correction of cornual occlusion with resultant term pregnancy. Fertil Steril 1987;48:490.

17. Daniell JF, Pittaway DE: Short-interval second look laparoscopy after infertility surgery: a preliminary report. J Reprod Med 1983;28:281.

18. DeBruyne F, Puttemans P, Boeckx W, et al: The clinical value of salpingoscopy in tubal infertility. Fertil Steril 1989;51:339.

19. DeCherney AH, Mezer HC: The nature of posttuboplasty pelvic adhesions as determined by early and late laparoscopy. Fertil Steril 1984;41:643.

19a. Diamond MP, Daniell JF, Martin DC, et al: Tubal patency and pelvic adhesions at early second-look laparoscopy following intraabdominal use of the carbon dioxide laser: initial report of the intraabdominal laser study group. Fertil Steril 1984;42:717.

20. Donnez J, Nisolle M, Casanas-Roux F: CO_2 laser laparoscopy in infertile women with adnexal adhesions and women with tubal occlusion. J Gynecol Surgery 1989;5:47–53.

21. Donnez J, Casanas-Roux F: Progostic factors of fimbrial microsurgery. Fertil Steril 1986;46:200.

22. Donnez J, Casanas-Roux F: Prognostic factors influencing the pregnancy rate after microsurgical cornual anastomosis. Fertil Steril 1986;46:1089.

23. Donnez J, Casanas-Roux F, Ferin J: Macroscopic and microscopic studies of fallopian tubes after laparoscopic sterilization. Contraception 1979;20:498.

24. Donnez J: CO_2 laser laparoscopy in infertile women with endometriosis and women with adnexal adhesions. Fertil Steril 1987;48:390.

25. Dubuisson JB, deJoliniere JB, Aubriot FX, et al: Terminal tuboplasties by laparoscopy: 65 consecutive cases. Fertil Steril 1990;54:401.

26. Fayez JA: An assessment of the role of operative laparoscopy in tuboplasty. Fertil Steril 1983;39:476.

27. Gomel V: Microsurgical reversal of female sterilization: a reappraisal. Fertil Steril 1980c;33:587.

28. Gomel V: Salpingo-ovariolysis by laparoscopy in infertility. Fertil Steril 1983;40:607.

29. Gomel V: Salpingostomy by laparoscopy. J Repro Med 1977;18:265.

30. Gomel V: Salpingostomy by microsurgery. Fertil Steril 1978;29:380.

31. Gomel V: Tubal reanastomosis by microsurgery. Fertil Steril 1977b;28:59.

32. Grant A: Infertility surgery of the oviduct. Fertil Steril 1971;22:496.

33. Grunert GM, Drake TS, Takaki NK: Microsurgical reanastomosis of the fallopian tubes for reversal of sterilization. Obstet Gynecol 1981;58:148.

33a. Henderson SR: The reversibility of female sterilization with use of microsurgery: A report on 102 patients with more than one year follow up. Am J Obstet Gynecol 1984;149:57.

34. Hesla JS, Rock JA: Laparoscopic tubal surgery and adhesiolysis. In: Azziz RA, Murphy AM, eds. Manual of operative laparoscopy. New York: Springer Verlag (in press).

34a. Holden FC, Sovak FW: Reconstruction of the oviduct: an improved technique with report of cases. Am J Obstet Gynecol 1932;24:684.

35. Hulka JF. Adnexal adhesions: a prognostic staging and classification system based on a five-year survey of fertility surgery results at Chapel Hill, North Carolina. Am J Obstet Gynecol 1982;144:141.

36. Interceed (TC-7) Adhesion Barrier Study Group. Prevention of post-surgical adhesion by Interceed, an absorbable adhesion barrier: a prospective randomized multicenter clinical study. Fertil Steril 1989; 51:933.

37. Jansen RPS: Failure of intraperitoneal adjuncts to improve the outcome of pelvic operations in young women. Am J Obstet Gynecol 1989;153:363.

38. Jansen RPS: Early laparoscopy after pelvic operations to prevent adhesions: safety and efficacy. Fertil Steril 1988;49:26.

39. Jansen RPS: Surgery-pregnancy time intervals after salpingolysis, unilateral salpingostomy, and bilateral salpingostomy. Fertil Steril 1980;34:222.

40. Jansen RPS: Tubal resection and anastomosis. Aust NZ J Obstet Gynecol 1986;26:300.

41. Mage G, Pouly JL, deJoliniere JB, et al: A preoperative classification to predict the intrauterine and ectopic pregnancy rates after distal tubal microsurgery. Fertil Steril 1986;46:807.

42. Medical Research International and the Society for Assisted Reproductive Technology, the American Fertility Society. In vitro fertilization and embryo transfer in the United States: 1988 results from the IVF-ET Registry. Fertil Steril 1990;53:13.

43. Mettler L, Giesel H, Semm K: Treatment of female infertility due to tubal obstruction by operative laparoscopy. Fertil Steril 1979;32:384.

44. McComb P, Gomel V. Cornual occlusion and its microsurgical reconstruction. Clin Obstet Gynecol 1980;23:1229.

45. McComb P. The determinants of successful surgery for proximal tubal disease. Fertil Steril 1986;46:1002.

46. McComb P: Microsurgical tubocornual anastomosis for occlusive cornual disease: reproductible results without the need for tubouterine implantation. Fertil Steril 1986;46:571.

47. Nezhat CR, Nezhat FR, Metzger DA, et al: Adhesion reformation after reproductive surgery by videolaseroscopy. Fertil Steril 1990;53:1008.

48. Nezhat C, Winer WK, Cooper JD, et al: Endoscopic infertility surgery. J Reprod Med 1989;34:127.

49. Novy MJ, Thurmond AS, Patton P, et al: Diagnosis of cornual obstruction by transcervical fallopian tube cannulation. Fertil Steril 1988;50:434.

50. O'Brien JR, Arronet GH, Eduljee SY: Operative treatment of fallopian tube pathology in human fertility. Am J Obstet Gynecol 1969;103:520.

51. Patterson PJ: Factors influencing the success of microsurgical tuboplasty for sterilization reversal. Clin Reprod Fertil 1985;3:57.

52. Patterson P: Reversal of sterilization. Population Reports, Population Information Program 1980;Vol 8, No. 5.

53. Patton PE, Williams TJ, Coulam CB: Results of microsurgical reconstruction in patients with combined proximal and distal tubal occlusion: double obstruction. Fertil Steril 1987;48:670.

54. Patton GW: Pregnancy outcome following microsurgical fimbrioplasty. Fertil Steril 1982;37:150.

54a. Putman JM, Holden AEC, Olive DL: Pregnancy rates following tubal anastomosis: Pomeroy partial salpingectomy vs electrocautery. J Gynecol Surg 1990;6:173.

55. Puttemans P, Brosens I, Dlahin P, et al: Salpingoscopy vs. hysterosalpingography in hydrosalpinges. Human Reproduction 1987;2:535.

56. Raj SG, Hulka JF: Second look laparoscopy after reconstructive pelvic surgery for infertility. Fertil Steril 1982;38:325–329.

57. Reich H: Laparoscopic treatment of extensive pelvic adhesions, including hydrosalpinx. J Reprod Med 1987;32:736.

58. Rock JA, Katayama KP, Martin EJ, et al: Uterotubal implantation and obstetric outcome after previous sterilization. Am J Obstet Gynecol 1977;128:665.

59. Rock JA: Pregnancy success following salpingolysis. The Johns Hopkins Hospital (personal series) 1989.

60. Rock JA: Reconstruction of the fallopian tube. In: Thompson J, Rock J, eds. TeLinde's operative gynecology. Philadelphia: JB Lippincott & Co. (in press).

61. Rock JA, Guzick DS, Katz E, Zacur HA, King TM: Tubal anastomosis: pregnancy success following reversal of Falope ring or monopolar cautery sterilization. Fertil Steril 1987;48:13.

62. Rock JA, Bergquist CA, Kimball AW Jr, et al: Comparison of the operating microscope and loupe for microsurgical tubal anastomosis—a randomized clinical trial. Fertil Steril 1984;41:229.

63. Rock JA, Katayama PK, Jones HW Jr: Tubal reanastomosis: a comparison of Hellman's approach without magnification and a microsurgical technique. Microsurgery in gynecology. In: Phillips JM, ed. Microsurgery in gynecology, ed 32, 176. Los Angeles: American Association of Gynecologic Laparoscopists, 1981c.

64. Rock JA, Katayama P, Martin EJ, et al: Factors influencing the success of salpingostomy techniques for distal fimbrial obstruction. Obstet Gynecol 1978; 52:591.

65. Rock JA, Katayama KP, Martin EJ, et al. Uterotubal implantation and obstetric outcome after previous sterilization. Am J Obstet Gynecol 1977;128:665.

66. Rock JA, Parmley TH, King TM, et al: Endometriosis and the development of tuboperitoneal fistulas after tubal ligation. Fertil Steril 1981d;35:16.

67. Rosenberg SM, Board JA: High molecular weight dextran in human infertility surgery. Am J Obstet Gynecol 1984;148.

68. Schlaff WD, Hossiokos D, Damewood MD, et al: Neosalpingostomy for distal tubal obstruction: Prognostic factors and impact of surgical technique. Fertil Steril 1991;54:984.

69. Schoysman R: Tubal microsurgery versus in vitro fertilization. Acta Eur Fertil 1984;15:5.

69a. Seiler JC: Factors influencing the outcome of microsurgical tubal ligation reversals. Am J Obstet Gynecol 1983;146:292

70. Shirodkar VN: Factors influencing the results of salpingostomy. Int J Fertil 1966;2:361.

71. Silber SJ, Cohen RS: Microsurgical reversal of female sterilization. Fertil Steril 1980;33:598.

72. Surrey MW, Friedman S: Second look laparoscopy after reconstructive pelvic surgery for infertility. J Reprod Med 1967;27:234–267.

73. Swolin K: Electromicrosurgery and salpingostomy: long-term results. Am J Obstet Gynecol 1975;121:418.

74. Swolin K. 50 Fertilitatsoperationen. Acta Obstet Gynecol Scandinav 1967;46:234–267.

75. The Adhesion Study Group: Reduction of postoperative pelvic adhesions with intraperitoneal 32% dextran 70: a prospective randomized clinical trial. Fertil Steril 1983;40.

76. Trimbos-Kemper TCM, Trimbos JB, van Hall EV: Adhesion formation after tubal surgery: results of the eight-day laparoscopy in 188 patients. Fertil Steril 1985;43:395.

77. Tulandi T, Falcone T, Kafka I: Second-look operative laparoscopy 1 year following reproductive surgery. Fertil Steril 1989;52:421.

78. Tulandi T, Vilos GA: A comparison between laser surgery and electrosurgery for bilateral hydrosalpinx: A 2 year follow-up. Fertil Steril 1985;44:846.

79. Vasquez G, Winston RML, Boeckx W, et al: Tubal lesions subsequent to sterilization and their relation to fertility after attempts at reversal. Am J Obstet Gynecol 1980;138:86.

79a. Von Csaba I, Keller G, Magi P, et al. Chirurgiche behandbling der weiblichen Steriletat tubenimplantation. Zentralbl Gynaekol 1974;96:490.

80. Westrom L: Pelvic inflammatory disease: bacteriology and sequelae. Contraception 1987;36:111.

81. Winston RML: Microsurgical tubocornual anastomosis for reversal of sterilization. Lancet 1977;1:284.

82. Winston RML: Reversal of sterilization. Clin Obstet Gynecol 1980c;23:1261.

83. Winston RML: Microsurgery and the fallopian tube: from fantasy to reality. Fertil Steril 1981;34:521.

84. Young PE, Egan JE, Barlow JA, et al: Reconstructive surgery for infertility at the Boston Hospital for Women. Am J Obstet Gynecol 1970;108:1092.

ECTOPIC PREGNANCY

Alan H. DeCherney and Alan S. Penzias

INTRODUCTION

Ectopic pregnancy is hardly a new phenomenon, but it has received special attention lately because of better diagnostic techniques. As a result, earlier diagnosis and change in management are possible.

Ninety-seven percent of ectopic pregnancies are located in the fallopian tube with about 2.5% located in the cornua. The remainder consist of ovarian, cervical, and abdominal pregnancies. Ectopic pregnancies are divided equally between the left and right tubes, with some reports showing a slight preponderance on the right side (9). Where the ectopic pregnancy is located within the tube is critical because the location dictates management. Older reports suggest that ectopics are located in the ampullary portion of the tube. A recent report by Smith (26) however, shows that ampullary ectopic pregnancy represents only 69% of the total with isthmic ectopics, representing 19.7% of the total (Fig. 9.1).

Statistics regarding future reproductive success in patients with ectopic pregnancies are often confusing and difficult to apply to the individual patient. It is helpful to consider two characteristics when considering the various therapeutic options and later in counseling the patient. These catagories are: (*a*) the number of prior ectopic pregnancies; and (*b*) the patient's reproductive history (Fig. 9.2).

Patients who have had two or more ectopic pregnancies have a much different reproductive potential from those who have had less than two. In the former group, about two-thirds will be unable to achieve spontaneous pregnancy,

and of the one-third who do conceive, one-quarter will have another ectopic pregnancy, for an overall viable pregnancy rate of roughly 25%.

Patients with ectopic pregnancies come from two groups, the general population and the infertile population. If one looks at ectopic pregnancy in the general population, the subsequent intrauterine pregnancy rate is approximately 85%, with a 15% ectopic pregnancy rate. On the other hand, if the patient has a history of infertility, the patient has only a 50% chance of spontaneous pregnancy with a 20% chance of having a repeat ectopic pregnancy. In counseling patients, keep in mind that sometimes these figures are mixed. The physician must tailor the information to the patient at hand.

DIAGNOSIS

The diagnosis of ectopic pregnancy can be made accurately by culdocentesis, hCG assay,

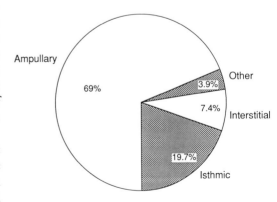

Figure 9.1. Ectopic pregnancy distribution by location.

ultrasound, doppler flow studies, serum progesterone, and laparoscopy, but none can rest as a single test at this time. The goal of these tests is not only accuracy but early diagnosis, to facilitate less invasive therapy.

Signs and Symptoms

Clinical symptoms and physical findings vary greatly and depend in part upon: (*a*) when in gestation the diagnosis is made; (*b*) the location of the pregnancy; and (*c*) whether it is in the ruptured or unruptured state (Table 9.1) (27). Abdominal pain, the most common symptom of ectopic pregnancy, is generally localized to the lower abdomen and may be accompanied by complaints of rectal pain. The presence of shoulder pain is an ominous if infrequent finding and represents diaphragmatic irritation by intraperitoneal blood. Signs of peritoneal irritation may be absent, despite the presence of blood in the abdominal cavity. Abnormal vaginal bleeding is noted in 50–80% of patients, though some series report amenorrhea in 75–95% of patients.

The physical exam may reveal unilateral adnexal tenderness with or without an appreciable mass, and uterine size may or may not be appropriate for expected gestational age. All of these findings are nonspecific, and the diagnosis is made in conjunction with additional diagnostic studies.

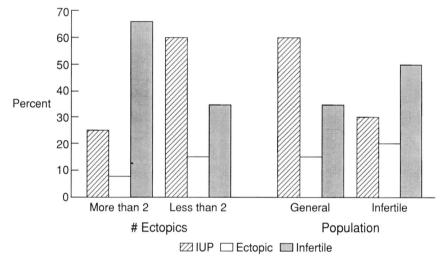

Figure 9.2.   Expected future reproductive performance of patients with ectopic pregnancy categorized by number of prior ectopic pregnancies and prior reproductive performance.

Table 9.1.   Clinical Findings in Proven Ectopic Pregnancy[a]

Number of Patients	Abdominal Pain (%)	Shock (%)	Mass (%)	Rebound Tenderness (%)	Normal-Sized Uterus (%)
130		15.3			
224		8.9	32.6		
300	90.7	23.3	38.3	33.7	75
481	92.7	26.6	67.3	40.1	
50	98	20	64	74	70
268	37.7	7.8	56.7		
699	93.5		50		
654		48.7	49	52	
284	83.5	1.4	29.9	41.2	74.3
191			17.3	42.9	85.9
300			53.7		70.7

[a]Modified from Stabile I, Grudzinskas JG: Ob Gyn Survey 1990;45:335.

Culdocentesis

Culdocentesis, an older test, still provides superior information with regard to diagnosing an ectopic pregnancy. The combination of a positive pregnancy test and a positive culdocentesis strongly suggests that the patient has an ectopic pregnancy. Romero (22) reported that in 158 patients with positive culdocentesis where the pregnancy tests were not evaluated, 132 (86%) had an ectopic pregnancy. When used in conjunction with a positive pregnancy test, the specificity for ectopic pregnancy of a positive culdocentesis rises to 99%. Culdocentesis is also helpful in that it allows for quantitation of blood; greater than 10 cc of free-flowing blood represents an ominous situation, where further evaluation and treatment should not be delayed. A positive culdocentesis does not indicate rupture, however, since 65% of ectopic pregnancies in the unruptured state will have a positive culdocentesis as well. This is due to sudulation of blood out the distal end of the tube between the layers of luminal epithelium and serosa.

hCG

The cornerstone of diagnosis that revolutionized the management of ectopic pregnancy was the isolation of the β subunit of hCG. The hCG assay initially measured the entire hormone, both α and β subunits.

To standardize the measurement of hCG around the globe, a group of 11 laboratories from eight countries agreed on an international reference preparation of purified human chorionic gonadotropin (IRP). This preparation was studied using various in-vivo and in-vitro bioassays and receptor assays. It was finally agreed that the IRP was suitable to serve as an international standard for immunmoassay, and it was assigned a unitage of 650 IU/ampule (28). A change in the IRP for immunoassay resulted in a change of the international standard (IS), and this accounts for the difference in values for first and second IS.

The homology between hCG and endogenous luteinizing hormone (LH), however, forced a sacrifice in sensitivity so that a positive test was not caused by endogenous LH production. The older tests had sensitivities between 750–1500 mIU/ml. As a result, only about 50% of patients with ectopic pregnancies had a positive pregnancy test.

This was soon replaced by the radioreceptor assay (RRA) with a sensitivity of 200 mIU/ml. Today, most laboratories use the radioimmune assay (RIA) for β-hCG with a sensitivity of 10 mIU/ml or less. The recently developed specific two-site "sandwich" immunofluorometric assay (IFMA) is capable of detecting hCG concentrations as low as 0.01 ng/ml (<1mIU/ml). In addition, the new monoclonal enzyme-linked immunosorbent assay (ELISA) with sensitivities of 40 mIU/ml have a false-negative rate of only 1.6%. The ready accessibility of these tests makes it easier to diagnose an ectopic pregnancy.

The absolute value of β-hCG is not helpful in determining whether a patient has an abnormal pregnancy. It is the pattern of production that is critical because the range of normal values at any fixed time in gestation can be quite varied. This clearly correlates strongly to the dating of the pregnancy; however, there are significant individual variations. It also must be stressed that abnormal β-hCG production patterns are not pathognomonic for ectopic pregnancy but are also associated with inevitable abortions.

Four patterns of β-hCG production emerge in patients with ectopic pregnancies: (*a*) a normal slope of rise; (*b*) an abnormal slope of rise; (*c*) a plateauing value; and (*d*) a falling value (Fig. 9.3) (21). Plateauing or falling values are easy to interpret and have high predictive value for an ectopic pregnancy. Certainly, after two or three measurements of the hormone, failure of the β-hCG production to show an increase is a serious finding and dictates further diagnostic workup. The doubling time of the serum β-hCG level in a normal intrauterine pregnancy varies from 1.3–3.5 days (Table 9.2). The rate of rise is dependent upon the time in gestation that the β-hCG is obtained. Most clinicians use 3 days to cover any discrepancies in the doubling time and to avoid premature intervention. Serum β-hCG levels should double every 3 days during the window from 5–9 weeks' gestation. If it continues on that path, one must use other diagnostic tests, particularly ultrasound, to aid in diagnosing an ectopic pregnancy. There is no correlation between the absolute value of β-hCG and the ectopic pregnancy as far as clinical findings are concerned. One cannot predict a ruptured or an unruptured ectopic pregnancy based on this value, nor can one predict its size (8).

Progesterone

Yeko and Stovall have reported that a single serum progesterone level is an excellent test for diagnosing an ectopic pregnancy. Yeko (32) reported that a serum progesterone level of less than 15 ng/ml was highly predictive of an abnormal pregnancy (Fig. 9.4). Stovall (29) subsequently showed that 54 of 67 (81%) patients with an ectopic pregnancy had a serum progesterone less than 15 ng/ml, while only 11% of patients with an intrauterine pregnancy had a progesterone level below this value. The addition of progesterone adds to the diagnosis of ectopic pregnancy, but does not supplant the use of β-hCG.

Other Biochemical Markers

The search for other biochemical markers of ectopic pregnancy continues. The role of substances such as CA-125, plasma renin activity, pregnancy-associated plasma protein-A (PAPP-A), pregnancy-specific β-1 glycoprotein (PSBG), relaxin, and schwangerschaft protein

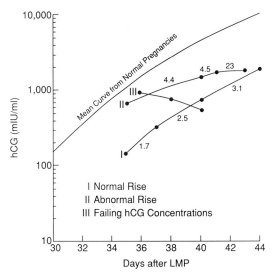

Figure 9.3. Patterns of hCG production from three surgically proven ectopic pregnancies. The numbers indicate the calculated doubling times based on hCG production rates during the marked intervals. (From Pittaway, et al: Am J Obstet Gynecol 1985;152:299. Reproduced with permission.)

Table 9.2.   Doubling Times of Serum β-hCG in Viable Pregnancies Over a Sampling Period (Days) from Time (0). For this table, BBT = basal body temperature, LMP = last menstrual period[a]

Time (0)	Sampling Period (days)	No. of Patients	Doubling Time (days)
LH Peak	8–20	22	1.3
BBT Nadir	10–22	57	1.4
Administration of hCG	11–21	7	1.7
Insemination	11–32	27	1.9
Detection of hCG	0–20	4	2.0
LMP	29–64	26	2.0
BBT Shift	12–30	189	2.2
LMP	28–60	20	3.3
LMP	28–60	57	3.5
BBT Shift	13–20	18	1.5
BBT Shift	13–25	26	1.9
BBT Shift	13–30	30	2.2
BBT Shift	13–39	35	2.7
LMP	28–35	17	1.4
LMP	28–42	35	2.2
LMP	28–49	40	2.5
LMP	28–56	42	2.9

[a]Modified from Pittaway, et al. Am J Obstet Gynecol 1985;152:299. Reproduced with permission.

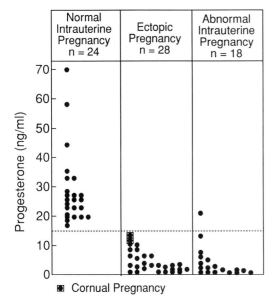

Figure 9.4. Serum progesterone concentrations categorized by outcome group. (From Yeko, TR, et al: Timely diagnosis of early ectopic pregnancy using a single blood progesterone measurement. Fertil Steril 1987;48:6. Reproduced with permission of the American Fertility Society.)

has yet to be defined but may provide new insight into the early diagnosis of ectopic pregnancy.

Ultrasound

Ultrasound has two functions in diagnosing an ectopic pregnancy. First, it allows the clinician to see the ectopic pregnancy directly by noting hematosalpinges or fetal parts, and occasionally fetal heart tones in the tube itself. This is an uncommon finding, and using an abdominal sector scanner is seen only 10% of the time. Kadar's (15) definition of a discriminatory zone was critical. The discriminatory zone is that level of β-hCG at which an intrauterine pregnancy must be seen. Utilizing the abdominal scanner and the first international standard for β-hCG, this discriminatory zone seemed to be 6500 mIU/ml. Romero, Kadar and associates (23) reported a prospective study of 383 patients with clinically suspected ectopic pregnancy. The absence of an intrauterine gestational sac at an hCG level above 6500 mIU/ml had a sensitivity of 100% and specificity of 96% for ectopic pregnancy.

Utilizing the second international standard, the discriminatory zone is roughly 3500 mIU/ml.

The introduction of the transvaginal ultrasound probe has changed some of these parameters. Ectopic pregnancies can now be seen directly about 20% of the time (6). Shapiro (24) reported a series of 22 patients with surgically proven ectopic pregnancy. The majority (77%) of them had hCG titers below the discriminatory zone level of 6500 mIU/ml, which was characterized as the level below which visualization of a sac would not be expected in a normal intrauterine pregnancy. The transvaginal ultrasound scan was able to identify the ectopic pregnancy before the expected appearance of an intrauterine gestational sac in 92% of patients with titers below 3600 mIU/ml. In a prospective study of 10 women, Fossum (12) reported that transvaginal sonography can identify an intrauterine sac, on average, at a serum β-hCG concentration of 1398 mIU/ml (first international standard) or 914 mIU/ml (second international standard).

Doppler flow studies of the ovarian artery as described by Taylor (31) are also extremely helpful. A characteristic trophoblastic flow with a slow ascent and slow descent is noted in 40% of ectopic pregnancies and is a significant finding. Another important characteristic is impedance to flow. Impedance is markedly increased in threatened abortions, as compared with either ectopic or normal intrauterine pregnancies (Fig. 9.5).

PATHOLOGY OF ECTOPIC PREGNANCIES

Budowick (5) reported that an ampullary ectopic pregnancy propagates primarily between the serosa and epithelium of the fallopian tube. This work was later corroborated by Pauerstein (20). They used a cross-sectional approach and demonstrated that ampullary ectopic pregnancies were confined to the extralumenal portion of the tube 75% of the time. This is a contradistinction to isthmic ectopic pregnancies, which propagate in and then destroy the tubal lumen. Hence, the pathology dictates the surgical approach. When one removes an ampullary ectopic pregnancy with

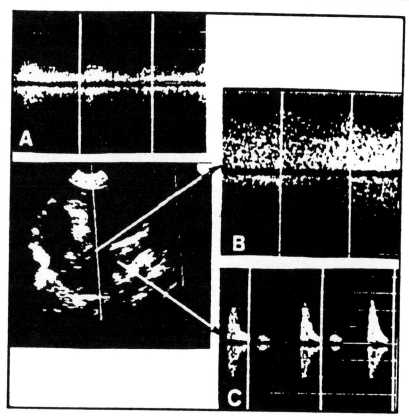

Figure 9.5. Examination of ovaries with pulsed Doppler. *A,* Flow characteristics in corpus luteum. *B,* Placental flow at site of trophoblastic invasion. *C,* High impedance main uterine signal. (From Taylor K, et al: Ectopic pregnancy: duplex Doppler evaluation. Radiology 1986;173:93 Reproduced with permission.)

conservative surgery, the normal tubal epithelium rapidly comes together. On the other hand, in an isthmic ectopic pregnancy, the epithelium is destroyed by the trophoblastic tissue (Fig. 9.6), and therefore, recanalization is not usually seen.

Earlier diagnosis and modern surgical technique have altered the management of ectopic pregnancy. In 1986, Breen (3) reported a series of 654 ectopic pregnancies of which 79.3% were ruptured at the time of diagnosis. Today, the inverse is true, and approximately 80% of ectopic pregnancies are diagnosed in the unruptured state. As we begin to diagnose ectopic pregnancies in the unruptured state, conservative surgery becomes a more realistic option. It is difficult to determine exactly what percentage of ampullary ectopic pregnancies are treated conservatively by linear salpingostomy each year, yet the trend nationally seems to be on the rise.

SURGICAL MANAGEMENT

Linear Salpingostomy

When performing a linear salpingostomy for an ampullary ectopic pregnancy, an incision is made on the antimesenteric side of the tube over the point of maximal bulge, and the products of conception are removed. The surgical principles involved in linear salpingostomy include achieving hemostasis at the incision line and at the bed of the ectopic pregnancy. Vigorous removal of tissue and excessive probing of the tubal lumen should be avoided. Leaving residual trophoblastic tissue in the tube has become an area of increasing concern. Kamrava and associates (16) reviewed 12 ectopic pregnancies that were treated by linear salpingostomy and an equal number that were treated by salpingectomy. They found that in both cases, the β-hCG was positive up to 12

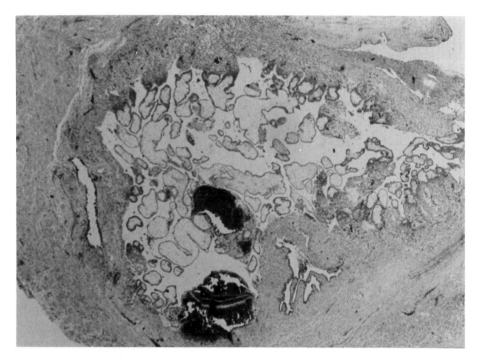

Figure 9.6. Trophoblastic tissue is seen within the isthmic lumen and has destroyed its epithelial lining.

days after the original procedure. This indicates that the presence of β-hCG reflects incomplete clearance of the hormone rather than the persistence of trophoblastic tissue (Fig. 9.7). It is for that reason that patients should be followed 2 weeks after conservative surgery and those 12% who continue to have a positive β-hCG should be followed over a longer period of time until the β-hCG reverts to zero.

Another area of controversy is whether the surgical site of the ectopic pregnancy should be closed by primary or secondary intention. Nelson (18), utilizing a rabbit model, clearly demonstrated that there is no difference with regard to adhesion formation, nidation index, pregnancy rate, or fistula rate if closure was by secondary intention. This, of course, facilitates linear salpingostomy and introduces the possibility of a laparoscopic approach.

An interesting study (10) looked at patients with a single patent fallopian tube who had linear salpingostomies to evaluate their subsequent pregnancy rate. The pregnancy rate in this group of patients was 50%, with a repeat ectopic pregnancy rate of approximately 15%. This indicates that subsequent intrauterine

pregnancies in patients treated conservatively don't all occur through the contralateral tube. It also demonstrates that conservative surgery is successful in helping the patient achieve a pregnancy without increasing her risk of repeat ectopic pregnancy beyond that incurred by more radical treatment.

The approach to laparoscopic linear salpingostomy includes positioning the patient to your advantage. Positioning the patient prior to beginning operative laparoscopy requires the cooperation of the operating room staff and the anesthesiologist. Taking the time to position the patient properly will allow the surgeon greater mobility and access to the pelvic organs. This, in turn, will optimize the surgical conditions and permit the surgeon to perform to the best of his or her abilities. The two key elements are tucking the patient's arms and lowering her legs. With the arms safely tucked by the patient's side, the surgeon can maneuver up to the patient's shoulders, allowing greater visualization of the pelvis with less neck flexion and bodily contortions.

Second, the patient's knees should be lowered so that the abdomen and thighs lie in

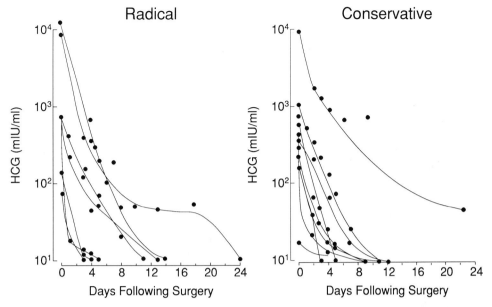

Figure 9.7. Disappearance curve of β-hCG in patients treated by salpingectomy (radical) and linear salpingostomy (conservative). (From Kamrava MM, et al: Obstet Gynecol 1983;62:487. Reproduced with permission of the American College of Obstetricians and Gynecologists.)

nearly the same plane. This allows greater mobility of the suprapubic and lower abdominal instrumentation.

The patient is prepared for surgery with a combined abdominal/vaginal wash with betadine solution. The bladder is emptied by straight catheterization. A single-toothed tenaculum is placed on the anterior lip of the cervix, and the Jarcho cannula is placed in the external cervical os. The patient is then draped so that the area from the umbilicus to the suprapubic region is left exposed. A sterile towel is placed around the vaginal instrumentation and secured with a sterile rubberband.

The operating table is placed in the Trendelenburg position. A small intraumbilical incision is made either in the vertical direction of an umbilical fold or transversely along the inferior rim of the umbilicus. The verres needle is inserted into the abdomen with the stopcock in the open position. After the surgeon senses that the peritoneum has been entered, 10 cc of saline are injected, and aspiration is attempted. If there is resistance while injecting, the tip of the verres needle may be in an enclosed space rather than the peritoneal cavity. Similarly, if the saline can be aspirated, the verres needle should

be repositioned. Aspiration of bright red blood or bowel contents suggests the need for exploratory laparotomy.

If the saline is injected with ease and none is aspirated, a small drop of saline is placed on the open Luer lock of the verres needle, and the abdomen is tented upward. The disappearance of the drop suggests that the verres needle is in a potential space in which negative pressure has been created by tenting the abdomen. These quick tests do not absolutely confirm needle position but are highly suggestive of proper placement.

The abdomen is insufflated with 3–4 liters of CO_2 at a pressure not to exceed 15 mmHg. The incision is then enlarged to accommodate the trochar and laparoscope. We prefer the 12-mm operating channel laparoscope for pelviscopy. The abdominal cavity and pelvis are visualized. A beam-splitting video camera is attached to the laparoscope, while a small suprapubic incision is made with the scalpel. A 5-mm trochar and sheath are placed approximately 3 cm above the symphysis pubis under direct vision, and a blunt probe is placed. The Trendelenburg angle is steepened, and the bowel is swept cephalad with the blunt probe.

We are now able to clearly visualize all pelvic structures including an ampullary ectopic pregnancy and are ready to proceed (Fig. 9.8). A second lower abdominal 5-mm trochar is placed just lateral to the inferior epigastric vessels. An atraumatic grasping forceps is placed through this port to stabilize the fallo-

pian tube. A 10-cc syringe containing a solution made up of 20 units of pitressin in 20 cc of Ringer's lactate is attached to a laparoscopic needle, which is inserted under direct vision through the suprapubic port. The solution is injected on the antimesenteric border of the fallopian tube along the prospective incision

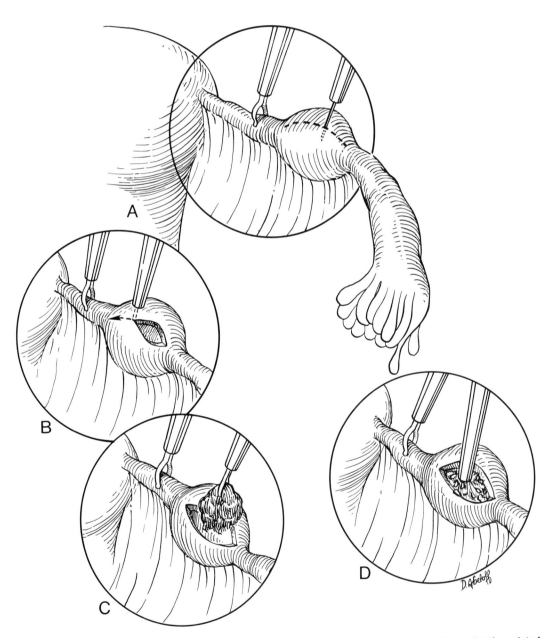

Figure 9.8. *A,* The atraumatic forceps are used to stabilize the fallopian tube, and pitressin is injected at the point of maximum bulge. *B,* The CO_2 laser is used to incise the fallopian tube at the point of maximum bulge. *C,* The tissue is gently removed from its bed. Gentle irrigation of the ectopic bed is performed, and the wound is allowed to heal by secondary intention.

line. The needle is removed and exchanged for the suction/irrigation wand.

The CO_2 laser is attached to the operating channel, and an incision is made on the antimesenteric border of the fallopian tube over the point of maximum bulge. The products are often spontaneously extruded. The suction/irrigation wand is used to remove smoke generated by the laser from the abdomen. It is removed and replaced by grasping forceps.

The ectopic pregnancy is gently teased from its bed and held in view. The laser is detached from the operating channel to allow passage of the 10-mm specimen scoop. The products are then removed from the abdominal cavity. The bed of the ectopic pregnancy is then copiously irrigated and inspected for hemostasis. The tube is allowed to heal by secondary intention.

The gas is permitted to escape, and the instrumentation is removed from the abdomen and vagina. The incisions are closed with subcuticular 4-0 vicryl and dressed with steri-strips.

There are no hard and fast rules that determine whether treatment should be by laparoscopy or laparotomy. Ectopic pregnancies that are surrounded by lots of pelvic adhesions with anatomical distortion or those greater than 4 cm are more difficult to do with a laparoscopic approach. Operative laparoscopy requires some special instrumentation and surgical skill. When the necessary instruments are unavailable and clinical experience is limited, laparoscopy should not be performed. If laparotomy is elected, the patient is prepped and draped in the supine position, and the abdominal cavity is entered. The hemoperitoneum is cleared, bowel packed into the upper abdomen, and the pelvic structures are visualized. The surgeon can elevate the affected fallopian tube into the field with gentle traction (Fig. 9.9). Moist laparotomy packs can be placed beneath the tube on either side to maintain its elevation and isolation. The tissue should be handled gently to avoid undue serosal trauma and subsequent adhesion formation.

Twenty units of pitressin should be diluted in 20 cc of Ringer's lactate or normal saline. A 22-gauge needle should be used to inject the solution on the antimesenteric border of the fallopian tube along the prospective incision line. A microelectrocautery is used to open the serosa over the point of maximum bulge (Fig. 9.10). The products will frequently extrude

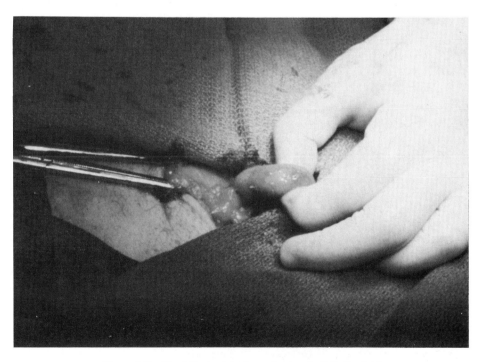

Figure 9.9. The fallopian tube is gently elevated into the field.

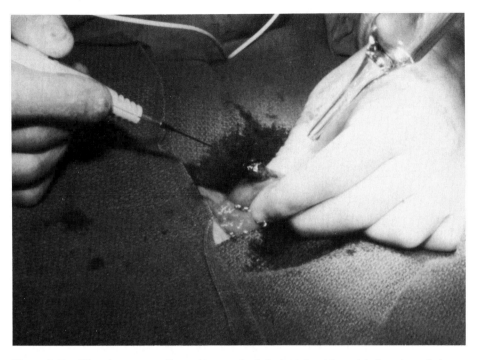

Figure 9.10. Microelectrocautery is used to open the fallopian tube at the point of maximum bulge.

spontaneously at this point. The ectopic tissue is gently teased from its bed with smooth tissue forceps. The bed of the ectopic pregnancy is then copiously irrigated and inspected for hemostasis (Fig. 9.11). It is also important to understand that postoperative success rates for laparoscopic procedures, as measured by subsequent fertility, are not superior but equivalent to those obtained at laparotomy.

Segmental Resection

The surgical approach to an isthmic ectopic pregnancy differs from that of the ampullary ectopic because of their different histopathology. Linear salpingostomy here often leads to complications such as tubal occlusion, fistula formation, and recurrent ectopic pregnancy. One surgical option is segmental resection, which can be performed either via laparoscopy or laparotomy. If a segmental resection is performed, the patient is left with a discontinuous, patent, distal segment. The options are immediate intraoperative anastomosis, anastomosis at a later date, and no further surgical treatment. Immediate and delayed anastomosis are both successful where subsequent intrauter-

ine pregnancy is concerned, with a somewhat better rate after delayed closure. If one plans to delay or decline anastomosis, the patient must be cautioned about the chance of having an ectopic pregnancy in the blind duct that's been created.

The laparoscopic approach described for linear salpingostomy can be applied to segmental resection as well. The fallopian tube is stabilized at the distal resection margin (Fig. 9.12). The Kleppinger bipolar electrocautery forceps are then applied to the proximal resection margin, and the tube, mesosalpinx and blood vessels are fulgurated. The hook scissors then transect the coagulated area. The grasping forceps are moved proximal to grasp the leading edge of the segment to be resected, and it is tented anteriorly. Electrocautery followed by transection is performed in a serial manner along the mesosalpinx to the distal resection margin, at which point the segment is removed.

If the decision has been made to proceed with segmental resection with immediate intraoperative anastomosis, the fallopian tube is positioned as in a linear salpingostomy at laparotomy. The microelectrocautery is used to carefully excise the affected portion of the tube.

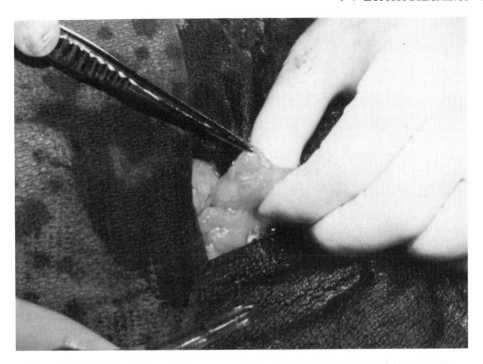

Figure 9.11. The bed of the ectopic pregnancy is then irrigated and inspected for hemostasis.

Hemostasis can be achieved as needed by a combination of electrocautery and selective ligation of mesosalpingeal vessels with 4-0 vicryl suture.

A 00-lacrimal duct probe is passed retrograde through the fimbria to the proximal end of the distal tubal segment (Fig. 9.13). An epidural catheter is wedged on the end of the probe, and it is drawn through the tube. A #2 nylon is inserted into the center of the epidural catheter and drawn through the tube to remain in place as a stent. This nylon is then passed into the proximal tubal segment. A 6-0 vicryl is placed in the mesosalpinx at the 6 o'clock position to secure the tubal segments in place for anastomosis. The operating microscope is then brought into the field.

Under magnification, the tubal anatomy is revealed, and the stent is visualized in the lumen. Seven-0 or 8-0 vicryl sutures are placed in the muscularis first at the 6 o'clock then at the 9, 3, and 12 o'clock positions. The serosa can be closed with interrupted 6-0 vicryl sutures. Defects in the mesosalpinx are similarly closed with 6-0 vicryl suture. Tubal patency can be assessed by chromopertubation with indigo carmine dye. The suture line can be covered

with TC-7 (Interceed) just prior to abdominal closure.

Salpingectomy

If the patient has completed her childbearing, the procedure of choice, regardless of location or rupture, is salpingectomy. Salpingectomy should also be considered if hemostasis cannot be achieved during conservative surgery, if an ectopic pregnancy recurs in a tube, or if the tube is irreparably damaged. The laparoscope allows an effective approach to salpingectomy. A number of procedures have been described for laparoscopic salpingectomy, all of which adhere to two basic principles: (*a*) interruption of the tubal blood supply without compromising ovarian perfusion; and (*b*) resection of the specimen.

One form of laparoscopic salpingectomy employs a sterile prefabricated 0-chromic catgut loop (Fig. 9.14). The fallopian tube is stabilized, as previously described. The endoloop is introduced into the abdomen, and the distal end of the tube is regrasped through the suture. The loop is then cinched down proximal to the ectopic pregnancy. A second loop is

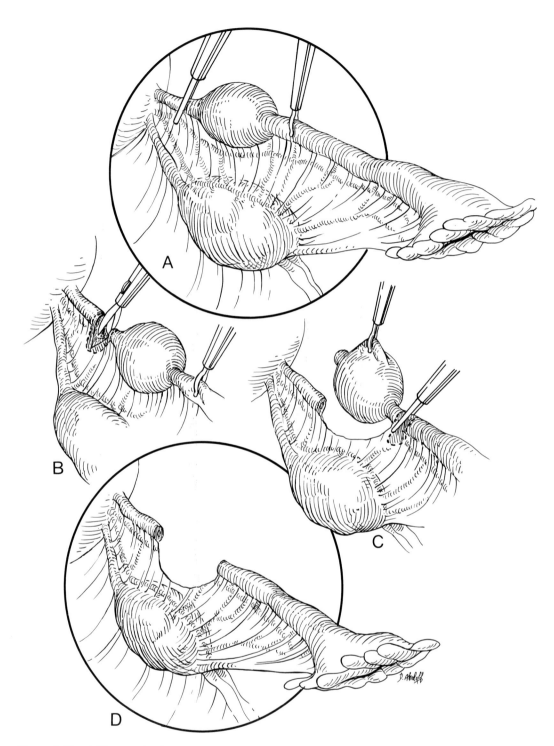

Figure 9.12. *A,* The grasping forceps are placed distal to the ectopic pregnancy and used to stabilize the fallopian tube. The bipolar cautery is then used to fulgurate the fallopian tube proximal to the ectopic pregnancy. *B,* The hook scissors are then used to transect the fulgurated area. *C,* Serial electrocautery and transection are used to undermine and free the area containing the ectopic pregnancy. *D,* The final appearance of the fallopian tube following segmental resection.

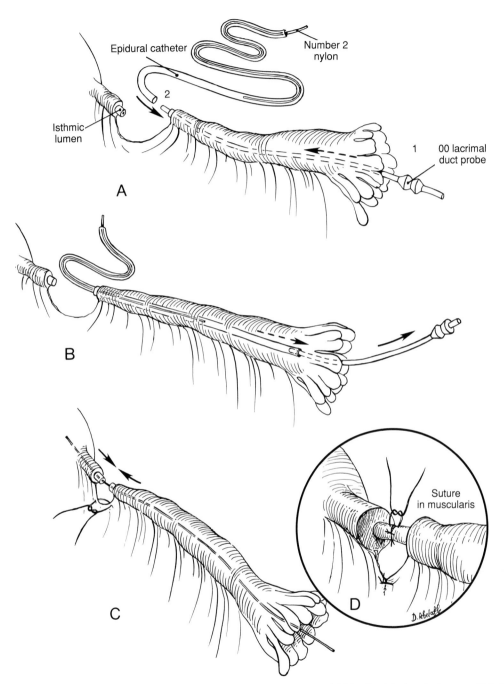

Figure 9.13. *A,* A #2 nylon is loaded into the end of an epidural catheter. A 00 lacrimal duct probe is passed into the distal segment of the fallopian tube. *B,* The epidural catheter is then wedged onto the lacrimal duct probe and drawn through the length of the tube. *C,* The epidural catheter is removed, and the nylon is passed into the proximal segment of the fallopian tube to serve as a stent. *D,* The muscularis of the fallopian tube is then sutured closed with 7-0 or 8-0 polyglycolic acid suture over the nylon stent. The nylon stent is removed following completion of the anastomosis.

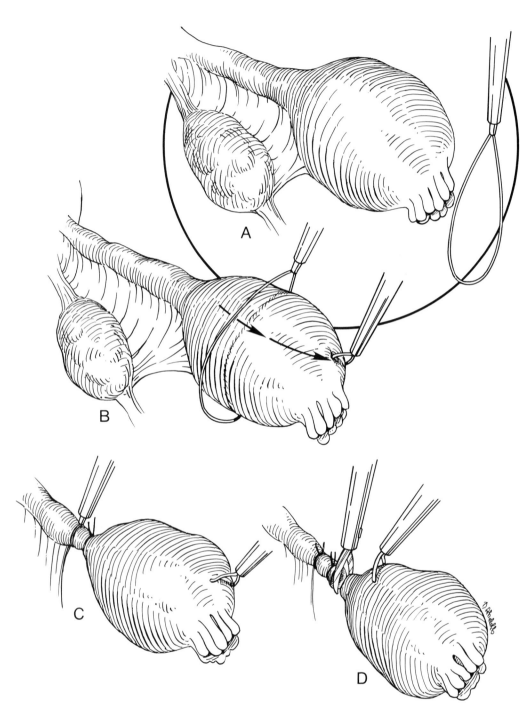

Figure 9.14.   *A,* The endoloop is placed near the ectopic pregnancy. *B,* The fallopian tube is grasped through the endoloop, and the ectopic pregnancy drawn through it. *C,* The loop is tightened proximal to the ectopic pregnancy. *D,* After placing a second endoloop tie, the specimen is resected with hook scissors and removed from the pelvis.

placed just distal to the first for added hemostasis, and the specimen is excised with the hook scissors. The pedicle is lavaged and observed for hemostasis. If additional hemostasis is required, it can be achieved by bipolar electrocautery.

An alternate method of laparoscopic salpingectomy uses the bipolar electrocautery and hook scissors (Fig. 9.15). Kleppinger bipolar electrocautery forceps fulgurate the fallopian tube at the uteroisthmic junction. The hook scissors are used to transect the coagulated region. The grasping forceps are moved proximal to grasp the leading edge of the tube and is tented anteriorly. Electrocautery followed by transection is performed in a serial manner along the mesosalpinx to the fimbria, at which point the tube is removed. Care must be taken when coagulating near the ovary to avoid compromising its vascular supply.

Relative success rates with respect to subsequent pregnancy for conservative and radical surgery were summarized by Oelsner (19) (Table 9.3). Women desiring pregnancy who underwent radical surgery achieved a cumulative intrauterine pregnancy rate of 40.9% and an ectopic pregnancy rate of 14.2%. This is in contrast to those who underwent conservative surgery, who achieved intrauterine and ectopic pregnancy rates of 45.5 and 11.5%, respectively.

Cornual Resection

Treatment of cornual ectopic pregnancy depends upon the condition of the ipsi- and contralateral fallopian tubes as well as the patient's desire for future pregnancy. If tubal reimplantation is planned for a later date, the tube is conserved. If no such operation will occur, the operation begins by mobilizing the fallopian tube from the mesosalpinx to the cornua. The electrocautery is used to excise the cornua in a V-shaped wedge. Figure-of-eight sutures of 0-vicryl are placed in the myometrium in one or two layers. Finally, a 3-0 vicryl running suture is placed in the serosa. If the round ligament was disrupted by the resection, it can be reincorporated with the serosal layer. Once adequate hemostasis is achieved, the suture line is covered with TC-7 (Interceed).

Tubal Abortion

Tubal abortion represents a distinct entity where the products of conception are removed by gentle suction or teasing as they exit the fimbrial portion of the tube. These patients seem to have a better prognosis (4), with pregnancy rates being as high as 75%. A tubal abortion is not to be confused with milking the fallopian tube. Although some studies (25) show that this is an excellent way to manage ampullary ectopic pregnancies, with 92% of the patients achieving intrauterine pregnancy, actually, milking anything other than an infundibular pregnancy or a tubal abortion is quite detrimental to the tube. The process of milking causes the products of conception to dissect their way through the loose adventitial tissue between the serosa and the tubal epithelium. This destructive technique increases the risk of excessive bleeding.

Second-Look Laparoscopy

Surgical procedures, whether performed laparoscopically or at laparotomy, carry a risk of postoperative adhesion formation. Lundorff (17) performed second-look laparoscopy on 102 women, who desired future pregnancy, 6–10 weeks after surgery for ectopic pregnancy. They discovered that 40% of these women had developed peritubal adhesions that were not present at the initial surgery for the ectopic pregnancy. Laparoscopic lysis of adhesions was performed during the second-look procedure in 42 women, 13% were offered tubal microsurgery, and 14% were recommended for in-vitro fertilization (IVF). This study suggests that patients who desire subsequent pregnancies are good candidates for second-look surgery. Although these findings are interesting, second-look laparoscopy has not consistently improved pregnancy rates in this population.

MEDICAL MANAGEMENT

Chemotherapy

In 1982, Tanaka (30) reported the use of the chemotherapeutic agent methotrexate in treat-

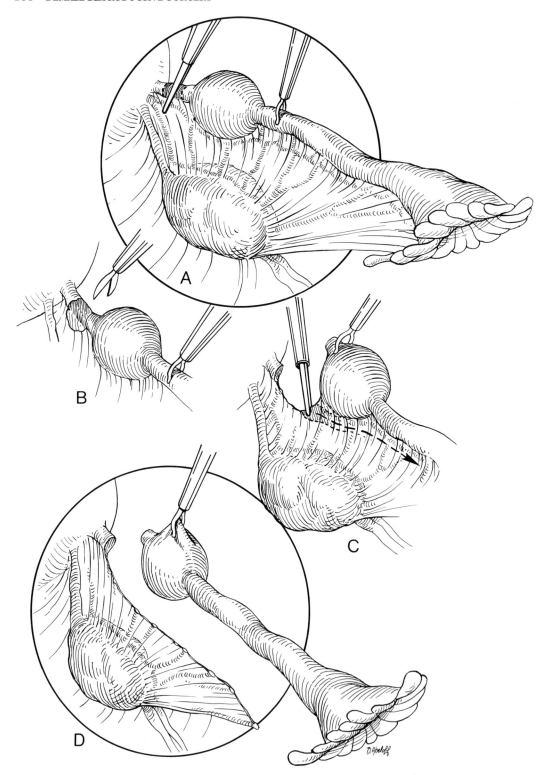

Figure 9.15. *A,* The grasping forceps are used to stabilize the fallopian tube distal to the ectopic pregnancy, and electrocautery is applied proximally. *B,* The hook scissors are used to then transect the fulgurated region. *C,* Serial fulguration and transection are then used to free the entire length of the fallopian tube. *D,* The final appearance of the fallopian tube and ovary following removal.

Table 9.3.   Relative Success Rates with Respect to Subsequent Pregnancy for Radical and Conservative Surgery: Review of the Literature[a]

	Women Desiring Pregnancy	Women with Intrauterine Pregnancy (%)	Women with Repeat Extrauterine Pregnancy (%)
Radical Surgery	1,630	667 (40.9)*	231 (14.2)*
Conservative Surgery	442	201 (45.5)*	51 (41.5)*

*$P > 0.05$
[a]From Oelsner, G: Clin Obstet Gynecol 1987;30:225. Reproduced with permission.

ing a patient with a cornual ectopic pregnancy. This was a success, and heralded a new area in the treatment of ectopic pregnancy. The regimen and route of administration of methotrexate varies greatly. Most studies, however, recommend 1 mg/kg intramuscularly per day for a course of 5 days, with citrovorum rescue factor. One must be cautioned, though, that methotrexate can have severe side effects, including profound leukopenia, liver enzyme elevation, pleuritis, dermatitis, and stomatitis.

There are three instances in which methotrexate can be used: (*a*) to treat every ectopic pregnancy; (*b*) to treat only abdominal, cervical, and cornual ectopic pregnancies; and (*c*) to treat patients with persistent trophoblastic tissue after surgical management of ectopic pregnancy.

Certainly, in small cervical pregnancies, abdominal pregnancies, and cornual pregnancies, methotrexate is ideal since the surgical ramifications of these are often profound. Nowhere is that clearer than in the management of a cornual ectopic pregnancy in which lumenal integrity is impossible to achieve under any circumstance, and en-bloc resection actually weakens the uterine wall for future pregnancies.

The option of using methotrexate to treat all ectopic pregnancies has not yet been proven effective with regard to subsequent pregnancy rates. Although the majority of these patients will do well with regard to tubal patency and rapid resolution of the β-hCG hormone, no large series has yet looked at subsequent pregnancy rates and demonstrated that they are comparable to the surgical approach. At present, an absolute contraindication to the use of methotrexate in tubal ectopic pregnancies is the presence of fetal heart tones.

In cases of persistent trophoblastic tissue manifested by a positive β-hCG more than 2 weeks after the original surgery, these cases can be treated with chemotherapy, or they can be observed. A small number of these patients will require repeat surgery (2).

Recently, there have been reports of local methotrexate injection into the ectopic pregnancy by an ultrasound-guided or laparoscopic approach. Actinomycin-D, another chemotherapeutic agent used to treat trophoblastic disease, has also been used to treat ectopic pregnancy (1). So far, these represent anecdotal reports, and no large series documenting subsequent pregnancy rates is yet available.

Prostaglandins

Prostaglandin $F_{2\alpha}$ has been simultaneously injected into the ectopic pregnancy and the corpus luteum at the time of laparoscopy. Reports of this method are few, and data to support its routine use are lacking at present.

Antiprogestational Agents

RU-486 has been described as a possibly effective method of terminating an early gestation via its antiprogestational effect. Success rates decline with advancing gestational age. Recently, Frydman (13) reported the development and use of a monoclonal hCG antibody in three patients with ectopic pregnancy. These two new forms of medical therapy represent interesting and exciting prospects on the horizon of ectopic pregnancy management.

Expectant Management

It must also be kept in mind that many ectopic pregnancies, as reported by Garcia (14), will resolve on their own. He studied 15 ectopic pregnancies serially without intervention and found that only three of them required surgical intervention. A similar report (11) was published involving the nonsurgical management of 12 ectopic pregnancies. Carson and associates (7) reported that a rising human chorionic somatomammotrophin reflects continued syncytiotrophoblast activity. In 21 patients treated with methotrexate for ectopic pregnancy, two required surgery for rupture. Both of these patients had rising hCS levels despite a decline in both hCG and progesterone. They suggest that patients with an hCS level of <10 ng/ml may safely be managed expectantly. These reports would suggest that observation may be an acceptable form of management in certain carefully selected cases.

CONCLUSION

In conclusion, ectopic pregnancy is a dynamic disease changing in many ways, both surgically and diagnostically. Certainly, the future aim is to diagnose them earlier and smaller so that they can be treated effectively and safely with chemotherapy alone. Today, however, the surgical approach seems best in managing these patients. A problem has arisen in that roughly 5% of patients operated on in a conservative fashion, either laparoscopically or by laparotomy, have a β-hCG pattern consistent with persistent trophoblastic disease. These patients can be treated with chemotherapy, although occasionally, a repeat surgical procedure is required. Rapid positive gains have been made by the early, conservative treatment of ampullary ectopic pregnancy with linear salpingostomy. The subsequent intrauterine pregnancy rate for certain patients approaches 85%, thus achieving some positive goals in the treatment of ectopic pregnancy.

References

1. Altaras M, Cohen I, Cordoba M, et al: Treatment of an interstitial pregnancy with actinomycin-D. Case report. Br J Obstet Gynecol 1988;95:1321.
2. Bell OR, Awadalla SG, Mattox JH. Persistent ectopic syndrome: a case report and literature review. Obstet Gynecol 1987;69:521.
3. Breen J. A 21-year survey of 654 ectopic pregnancies. Am J Obstet Gynecol 1986;106:1004.
4. Bruhat MA, Manhes H, Mage G, et al: Treatment of ectopic pregnancy by means of laparoscopy. Fertil Steril 1980;33:411.
5. Budowick M, Johnson TRB Jr, Genadry R, et al: The histopathology of the developing tubal ectopic pregnancy. Fertil Steril 1980;34:169.
6. Cacciatore B, Ylostalo P, Stenman U-H, et al: Suspected ectopic pregnancy: ultrasound findings and hCG levels assessed by an immunofluorometric assay. Br J Obstet Gynecol 1988;95:497.
7. Carson SA, Stovall T, Umstot E, et al: Rising human chorionic somatomammotropin predicts ectopic pregnancy rupture following methotrexate chemotherapy. Fertil Steril 1989;51:593.
8. Cartwright PS, Herbert CM, Maxson WS. Operative laparoscopy for the management of tubal pregnancy. J Reprod Med 1986;31:589.
9. Chez R, Moore J: Diagnostic errors in the management of ectopic pregnancy. Surg Gyn Ob 1963;589.
10. DeCherney AH, Maheux R, Naftolin F. Salpingostomy for ectopic pregnancy in the sole patent oviduct: reproductive outcome. Fertil Steril 1982;37:619.
11. Dericks-Tan JSE, Scholz C, Taubert H-D. Spontaneous recovery of ectopic pregnancy: a preliminary report. Eur J Obstet Gynecol Reprod Biol 1987;25:181.
12. Fossum GT, Davajan V, Kletzky O. Early detection of pregnancy with transvaginal ultrasound. Fertil Steril 1988;49:788.
13. Frydman R, Fernandez H, Troalen F, et al: Phase I clinical trial of monoclonal anti-human chorionic gonadotropin antibody in women with an ectopic pregnancy. Fertil Steril 1989;52:734.
14. Garcia AJ, Aubert JM, Sama J, et al: Expectant management of presumed ectopic pregnancies. Fertil Steril 1987;48:395.
15. Kadar N, DeVore G, Romero R. The discriminatory hCG zone. Its use in the sonographic evaluation of ectopic pregnancy. Obstet Gynecol 1980;50:156.
16. Kamrava MM, Taymor ML, Berger MJ, et al: Disappearance of human chorionic gonadotropin following removal of ectopic pregnancy. Obstet Gynecol 1983;62:486.
17. Lundorff P, Thorburn J, Lindblom B. Second-look laparoscopy after ectopic pregnancy. Fertil Steril 1990;53:604.
18. Nelson LM, Margara RA, Winston RML. Primary and secondary closure of ampullary salpingostomy compared in the rabbit. Fertil Steril 1986;45:292.

19. Oelsner G. Ectopic pregnancy in the sole remaining tube and the management of the patient with multiple ectopic pregnancies. Clin Obstet Gynecol 1987; 30:225.

20. Pauerstein CJ, Croxatto HB, Eddy CA, et al: Anatomy and pathology of tubal pregnancy. Obstet Gynecol 1986;67:301.

21. Pittway DE, Reish MS, Wentz AC. Doubling times of human chorionic gonadotropin increase in early viable intrauterine pregnancies. Am J Obstet Gynecol 1985; 152:299.

22. Romero R, Copel JA, Kadar N, et al: Value of culdocentesis in the diagnosis of ectopic pregnancy, Obstet Gynecol 1985;65:519.

23. Romero R, Kadar N, Jeanty P, et al: Diagnosis in ectopic pregnancy: value of the discriminatory human chorionic gonadotropin zone. Obstet Gynecol 1985; 66:357.

24. Shapiro BS, Cullen M, Taylor KJW, et al: Transvaginal ultrasonography for the diagnosis of ectopic pregnancy. Fertil Steril 1988;50:425.

25. Sherman D, Langer R, Herman A, et al: Reproductive outcome after fimbrial evacuation of tubal pregnancy. Fertil Steril 1987;47:420.

26. Smith HO, Toledo AA, Thompson JD. Conservative surgical management of isthmic ectopic pregnancies. Am J Obstet Gynecol 1987;157:604.

27. Stabile I, Grudzinskas JG. Ectopic pregnancy: A review of incidence, etiology and diagnostic aspects. Obstet Gynecol Survey 1990;45:335.

28. Storring PL, Gaines-Das RE, Bangham DR. International reference preparation of human chorionic gonadotropin for immunoassay: potency estimates in various bioassay and protein binding assay systems; and international reference preparations of the α and β subunits of human chorionic gonadotropin for immunoassay. J Endocrin 1980;84:294–310.

29. Stovall TG, Ling FW, Cope BJ, et al: Preventing ruptured ectopic pregnancy with a single serum progesterone. Am J Obstet Gynecol 1989;160:1425.

30. Tanaka T, Hayashi H, Kutsuzawa T, et al: Treatment of interstitial ectopic pregnancy with methotrexate: report of a successful case. Fertil Steril 1982;37:851.

31. Taylor K, Ramos I, Feyock A, et al: Ectopic pregnancy: duplex doppler evaluation. Radiology 1986; 173:93.

32. Yeko TR, Gorrill MJ, Hughes LH, et al: Timely diagnosis of early ectopic pregnancy using a single blood progesterone measurement. Fertil Steril 1987; 48:1048.

10

RECONSTRUCTIVE SURGERY OF THE OVARY

Ana Alvarez Murphy

GENERAL CONSIDERATIONS

Ovarian surgery for the treatment of infertility is limited to the resection of benign cysts, paraovarian cysts, wedge resection, and laparoscopic ovarian cautery for the induction of ovulation in women with polycystic ovarian disease (PCO). A very common indication for ovarian surgery is endometriosis. In addition, the lysis of periovarian adhesions resulting from previous surgery, pelvic inflammatory disease, or endometriosis may be performed in an effort to enhance fertility. These will be considered separately.

Extensive periovarian and peritubular adhesions may result from ovarian surgery and cause infertility or pelvic pain. In ovarian reconstructive surgery, atraumatic technique cannot be overemphasized. A detailed discussion of microsurgical technique and adhesion prevention is provided elsewhere in this book; however, a short discussion as it applies to the ovary will be presented.

The weight of experimental and clinical evidence suggests that ischemia, trauma, coagulation, or foreign material leads to adhesion formation. In an animal model, two studies suggest that external sutures are significantly more adhesiogenic than nonclosure of the ovarian cortex. Oelsner (32) compared three methods of ovarian reconstruction in New Zealand white rabbits. The Buxton stitch is a horizontal mattress through the base of the ovarian defect, with a second layer approximat-

ing the cortex. This was compared to hemostasis achieved with either bipolar electrocautery or internal sutures and the same microsurgical closure of the cortex with 8-0 suture. The former caused a significant increase in adhesion formation and a decrease in nidation index (number of embryos in each lateral horn of the uterus divided by the number of corpora lutea on the same side). No difference was seen between the latter two methods, bipolar electrocautery, and internal sutures, with microsurgical closure of the cortex. They concluded that mattress sutures may cause vascular compression and promote ischemia as well as promote a foreign body reaction. The decrease in nidation index that reflects the efficacy of the tuboovarian-uterine unit demonstrates the detrimental effect of the mattress sutures in reconstructive surgery. Since the number of corpora lutea was unchanged, endocrine function did not appear compromised.

Wiskind (43) compared closure to nonclosure of the cortex in rabbit ovaries, where hemostasis was obtained by bipolar electrocautery in both cases. Using microsurgical technique at laparotomy, a significantly higher adhesion score was seen in the ovaries that were closed compared with nonclosure. Most of the adhesions in the closure group involved the incision line. Consistent with multiple studies, a foreign body tissue reaction with subsequent adhesiogenesis was noted. It is probable that a subcapsular closure that is possible in human ovaries but not in rabbit ovaries may be less adhesiogenic than the continuous suture through the ovarian capsule used in this study. It should also be noted that the ovaries were bivalved for this study and so naturally fell together, restoring normal anatomy. In contrast, ovarian procedures in humans may result in a markedly distorted, thin, elongated shell. It remains to be established whether normal tuboovarian relationships can be established by closure or nonclosure of this distorted ovary. Every effort should be made to make incisions in the axis of the ovary and in its most dependent portion so that normal ovarian anatomy may be reestablished.

Trauma to the tissue during the operative procedure also appeared to be a significant adhesiogenic factor. Most of the adhesions in the nonclosure ovaries involved the lateral and medial surfaces of the ovary and were most likely due to trauma from manipulation of the ovarian surface. Thus, gentle, atraumatic tissue handling is of paramount importance. Marked atrophy of an ovary was noted in 18% of animals at second-look, evenly distributed between the two groups. Thus, compromise of the blood supply can result from surgical closure or excessive electrocautery. The use of minimal suturing or coagulation consistent with good hemostasis is a goal of microsurgical technique.

Whether removing a benign ovarian cyst in a woman of reproductive age or performing surgery for induction of ovulation in patients with PCO, the conservation of ovarian cortex, where primordial follicles are present, is of obvious importance. Women of childbearing age should have the most conservative procedure possible performed.

The value of paradoxical oophorectomy has been debated. Jeffcoate (23) suggested that in a patient with one functional tube, removing the opposite normal ovary should improve fertility with repeated ovulations from the ovary alongside the patent tube. Scott (35) reported a series of 24 patients with unilateral tubal patency and contralateral oophorectomy or salpingooophorectomy, noting a 67% pregnancy rate. Randomized controlled clinical trials should be performed to assess the efficacy of this procedure before it is used. Increased pregnancy rates following in-vitro fertilization correlate with the number of embryos placed in the uterus. The number of oocytes retrieved for fertilization is a reflection of the number of ovaries available for superovulation. Normal ovaries should not be removed until more data are available on this issue.

ANATOMY

The human ovaries are approximately 3–5 cm long, 2–3 cm wide, and 1–2 cm thick, with a wrinkled pearly white appearance. The surface and size may vary with the stage of the menstrual cycle and age. Prepubertal ovaries are usually smooth, resembling the smooth, thick-capsuled ovaries sometimes seen with polycystic ovarian disease. The ovary is covered with a single layer of flattened cells, called the germinal epithelium, which is continuous with the peritoneum of the hilum and broad ligament. A layer of condensed ovarian stroma lies beneath the epithelium and is referred to as the tunica albuginea. The cortex contains the germ cells and stroma. The medulla is afollicular and consists of fibrous stroma, blood vessels, and the rete ovarii, which in the male develop into testes.

Typically, the ovary lies on the side wall in a shallow fossa between the external iliac vein and ureter. The importance of identifying the ureter prior to dissection of the ovary from the sidewall is obvious. The ovary is attached to the sidewall by the infundibulopelvic ligament. The vasculature and nerves enter and exit the ovary along the hilum. The uteroovarian ligament connects the ovary to the uterus. The infundibulum of the fallopian tube extends to the ovary and is termed the fimbria ovarica. Preservation and restoration of these anatomic relationships should be the goal of reconstructive surgery of the ovary (Fig. 10.1).

The ovarian artery arises from the aorta just below the renal arteries. It courses downward, crosses the ureter, and enters the infundibulopelvic ligament, where it gives rise to the tubal and ovarian branches and anastomoses with the uterine artery to form an arcade. The ovarian veins give rise to the pampiniform plexus in the mesosalpinx, which coalesces to

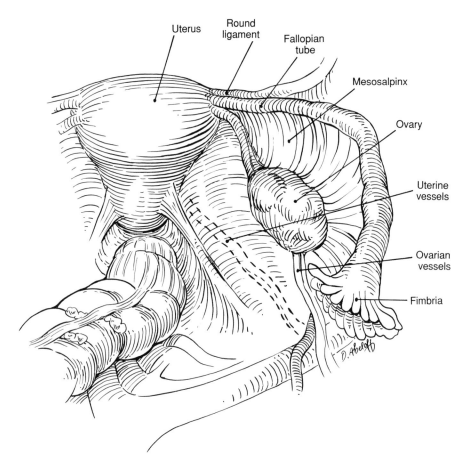

Figure 10.1.   Normal anatomy.

form the ovarian vein. The ovarian vein accompanies the artery and empties into the inferior vena cava on the right and the renal vein on the left. Lymphatic drainage accompanies the ovarian vessels and reaches the periaortic nodes near the kidneys. Additionally, the ovaries communicate with lymphatic vessels traversing through the uteroovarian ligament and uterine fundus. Some channels reach the superficial inguinal nodes through the round ligaments. The segmental nerves from T10 and T11 supply the motor and sensory nerves to the ovary through the hilum.

A clear understanding of embryology is important to the reproductive surgeon. Supernumerary, accessory, and malpositioned ovaries are more easily understood with this knowledge (45). The propensity of dermoids to occur in the midline can also be understood. Germ cells originate in the wall of the yolk sac and migrate along the midline to enter the coelomic cavity (44). The germ cells then migrate laterally to the gonadal ridge. A thickening on the medial aspect of the coelomic cavity adjacent to the mesonephros is termed the gonadal ridge. This tissue develops at approximately 4–5 weeks and projects into what will develop into the peritoneal cavity. Medullary or testicular differentiation is first noted at 6 weeks. Onset of meiosis at the end of the first trimester is the first distinctive sign of cortical/ovarian differentiation. Just prior to this, the primitive germ cells undergo mitosis and become oogonia. A progressive entry into meiosis is seen from the innermost cortex to the periphery. By late gestation, differentiation is arrested, and the oocytes remain in the diplotene stage. It appears that ovarian hormone production is not required for the differentiation of the female reproductive tract. Agonadal embryos develop along normal female lines.

Deviations from normal embryologic development give rise to supernumerary, accessory, and malpositioned ovaries (Fig. 10.2). The former is a structure containing ovarian tissue that has no connection to the normally placed ovary. A supernumerary ovary is most commonly found in the midline or laterally between the kidney and normally placed ovary, although ovaries have been found in liver and spleen. Such structures are thought to develop from a separate primordium arising from arrested migrating gonadocytes. An accessory ovary is close to the normally placed ovary and is connected to the uteroovarian or infundibulopelvic ligament. Ovarian malposition may result from abnormal descent of the ovary. The ovary is attached to the uterus by the uteroovarian ligament and to the fallopian tube by the fimbria ovarica. Consequently, uteroovarian

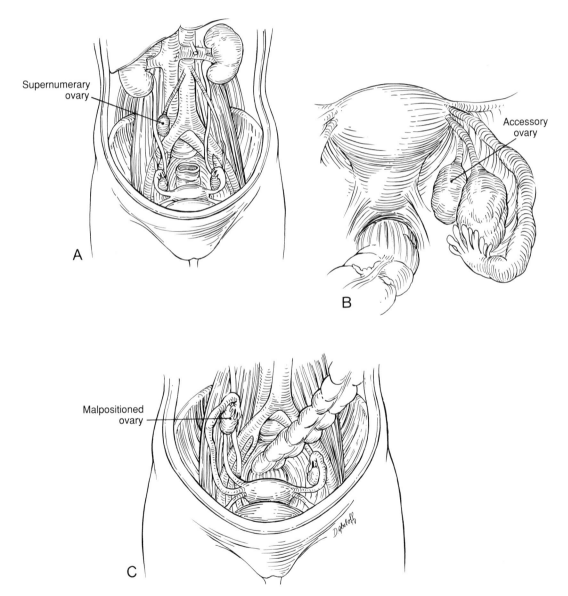

Figure 10.2. Deviations from normal embryologic development. *A,* Supernumerary ovary. Ovarian tissue that has no connection to the normally placed ovary. *B,* Accessory ovary. The ovary is close to the normally placed ovary and is connected to the uteroovarian or infundibulopelvic ligament. *C,* Ovarian malposition. Results from abnormal descent of the ovary. The anatomic relationships are normal, but the uteroovarian ligament and/or the fallopian tube is very long.

ligaments and/or fallopian tubes may be very long. Fallopian tubes have been described that measure 20–26 cm in length (33). The reproductive consequences of these anomalies is unknown.

The paraovarian cyst has been so designated in most texts because of its location in the broad ligament, approximating both the ovary and the oviduct. It is often confused with an ovarian cyst preoperatively. Gardner (14) and Genadry (15) have discussed in detail the origin of these cystic and solid tumors. Genadry studied 132 benign paraovarian cysts and eight paraovarian neoplasms and demonstrated that the majority were of paramesonephric (Müllerian duct) or mesothelial origin and not of mesonephric origin (Wolffian duct).

Embryologically, the mesodermal components of the urogenital system include the mesonephric duct, and paramesonephric duct, the nephric structures, and the gonad. The mesonephric duct contributes to the development of the ureter, the trigone of the bladder, and the adjacent urethra. The cranial part of the duct and its tubules may be preserved, and in the female adult are regularly found in the broad ligament region, lateral portions of the cervix, and adjacent vagina. The paramesonephric duct appears as an invagination of the coelomic mesothelium at approximately 5–6 weeks embryonic life. The opening of the duct into the coelomic cavity becomes the future ostium of the fallopian tube, and the production of fimbria is accomplished by compression of this ostium between the receding pronephros and the large mesonephric body. This compression favors the development of multiple lumina, one of which predominates as the fallopian tube. Nevertheless, one or more of the folds may remain as accessory lumina or diverticula. It is possible that the dilatation of occluded accessory lumina could produce a small hydrosalpinx, or occlusion of a diverticulum could develop into a hydatid cyst. The presence of paramesonephric epithelium and/or adjacent circular musculature identifies the origin of the cyst.

In the study by Genadry, paraovarian cysts were rarely of mesonephric origin. Small hydrosalpinx-like structures and mesothelial inclusions were the lesions most frequently suggested by the histologic features. Samaha (34) confirmed that the majority of the lesions represented accessory lumina of the fallopian tube. A reflection of its embryologic potential, "metaplasia" of the mesothelium, frequently reproduces müllerian duct-type epithelium.

RESECTION OF BENIGN OVARIAN CYSTS/TUMORS

Physiologic enlargement of the ovary may occur as a result of failure of either follicular or corpus luteum regression. The majority of these cysts regress, but they may persist and on occasion become excessively large. Occasionally, surgery is necessary because of intraperitoneal bleeding resulting from rupture of the cyst wall, persistence, symptoms, or size. At times, they may be adhered to the pelvic sidewall or may markedly distort the fallopian tube.

Pain, a mass, abdominal enlargement, and pressure on the rectum or bladder are common to all ovarian lesions. There are few specific symptoms that distinguish one ovarian cyst or mass from another histologic type. Benign ovarian tumors include epithelial tumors, such as serous, mucinous, and endometrioid, as well as functioning and nonfunctioning stromal tumors. Hormone-producing tumor may become symptomatic while still quite small and cause symptoms of androgen excess.

Dermoids or benign cystic teratoma are among the most common ovarian tumors (19). The interior is usually composed of multiloculated cysts filled with sebum, hair, bone, or teeth. Derivatives of any of the three germ layers may be evident microscopically. Pelvic pain is common despite the fact that the ovary has no peritoneal cover. Cystic teratomas tend to expand, producing a large quantity of sebum. They tend to be heavy, pedunculated, and ballotable anterior to the uterus. Occasionally, the cells have the capacity to produce chorionic gonadotropin that is readily identifiable in blood or urine. Approximately 10–25% of these tumors are bilateral, so the contralateral ovary should be carefully examined. Malignant change in cystic teratomas is rare, and the highest incidence is in women in the fourth or fifth decades of life. The incidence of malignancy in an ovarian teratoma is 1–3% (26). Malignant teratomas contain immature and embryonal types of tissue, while benign teratoma show adult tissue of all varieties.

Very seldom, if ever, is the diagnosis of paraovarian cyst or tumor made preoperatively. Only 3% are bilateral. These cysts and tumors are usually incidental findings at operation. Very few are symptomatic since few reach 10 cm or more. As dilatation of simple paraovarian cysts is probably due to the secretory products of the tubal type of epithelium, it is not surprising that the largest clinically symptomatic paraovarian cysts are seen in the postpubertal years after onset of functional activity.

Acute adnexal torsion is a rare but important cause of abdominal pain in girls and women. Classic clinical findings include lower abdominal pain and a palpable adnexal mass. In the majority of cases, adnexal torsion is associated with a preexisting cystic adnexal mass (41). Rarely is the diagnosis made preoperatively. The difficulty of diagnosing adnexal torsion may lead to the loss of the adnexa. The classic surgical approach to torsion has been aimed at curing the torsion and preventing a sudden massive embolization of necrotic tissue. Most authors recommend lateral entry into the retroperitoneum, with immediate cross-clamping and division of the infundibulopelvic ligament after identification of the ureter. The torsed adnexa may then be mobilized and the torsion corrected. Oophorectomy or adnexectomy is then performed. Untwisting torsed, necrotic adnexal tissue as a primary surgical procedure is a relatively new concept, although it was originally proposed by Way (41a). Numerous authors have since suggested untwisting ovaries that have undergone torsion or attempting wedge removal of associated necrotic tissue to salvage the residual ovarian tissue. Others advocate untwisting and simply observing torsed and necrotic ovarian tissue that appears to have no salvageable component on initial gross inspection. Opponents point out that this procedure may allow embolization of necrotic tissue, and that the patient will also continue to experience pain. There is currently no consensus on the appropriate management for adnexal torsion. Elkins (13) suggests that in young patients who plan to have children, a more conservative procedure aimed at preserving ovarian tissue would be reasonable. This would be particularly reasonable for patients whose other adnexa was lost previously or who appear prone to torsion as well.

Obviously, the laparoscope will be used often to confirm the diagnosis of ovarian or pelvic mass. However, there is currently much debate about what ovarian lesions can reasonably be approached with the laparoscope. Benign ovarian lesions can be removed through the laparoscope; however, it is difficult to predict which are benign prior to pathologic examination. Ovarian cancer occurs in one out of 95 women with an ovarian cyst between the ages of 20–35. Although recent evidence suggests that peritoneal spill does not change the prognosis of Stage IA ovarian cancer, definitive data are not available (11). Dembo presented evidence that the only factors influencing the ultimate rate of relapse and survival were tumor grade, the presence of dense adhesions, and the presence of large-volume ascites. When these factors were accounted for in a logistic regression, multivariate analysis, the rate of relapse and prognosis was not influenced by rupture of the tumor. Thus, the theoretic potential for tumor dissemination by rupture of a malignant cyst remains conjectural. A recent study by Parker (32a) in postmenopausal women discussed the management of selected cystic adnexal masses by operative laparoscopy. Using the screening criteria of cystic adnexal mass <10 cm with distinct borders and no evidence of solid parts, thick septae, ascites, or matted bowel, and a normal CA-125, 88% of patients were successfully managed by operative laparoscopy and adnexectomy.

Nezhat (31) reported laparoscopic removal of unilateral or bilateral dermoid cysts in nine women of reproductive age. There were no immediate or long-term complications. Four patients had repeat laparoscopy for evaluation of possible pelvic adhesion formation; one had mild periovarian adhesions; and the pelvis appeared normal in the other three. There were no malignant changes in this very small series.

The issue of laparoscopic cystectomy has generated intense debate. Endometriomas are almost always predictably benign, although a few cases of malignancy have been reported. Perfectly smooth cysts that are echolucent are almost always also predictably benign. However, these cysts are relatively rare as a reason for laparoscopic surgery since they are usually functional and resolve with observation. The majority of laparoscopic surgeons are comfortable approaching these two entities through the laparoscope. Ovarian cysts with solid components or superficial excrescences should be approached with caution until more data are available.

SURGICAL TECHNIQUE

Laparotomy

At laparotomy, an elliptical incision is made above the thin ovarian cortex (Fig. 10.3A). The incision should be made in the axis of the ovary and in its most dependent area. This will facilitate reconstruction of the ovary and ensure a more "anatomic" closure. The end of the knife handle may then be inserted and a plane developed over the cyst wall (Fig. 10.3B). After the cyst wall has been completely separated from its adhesive attachments to the ovarian cortex, it may be shelled out without rupture. On occasion, however, because of friability of the cyst wall, rupture may occur even with the gentlest technique. It is of utmost importance prior to shelling out the cyst to surround the ovary with moist lint-free packs so that if rupture occurs, spillage will not contaminate the rest of the pelvis. After the cyst is removed, the dead space may be obliterated with internal sutures placed as a purse-string, running lock, or interrupted of #4-0 or #5-0 nonreactive suture (Fig. 10.3C). The ovarian cortex may be approximated with subcuticular sutures of #5-0 or #6-0 nonreactive suture (Fig. 10.3D). Suture on the ovarian surface should be avoided if at all possible.

In some instances, there may be excessive redundant thin cortex, which may present a special problem in ovarian reconstruction. Cortex generally should not be trimmed unless it is extremely thin. At second-look procedures, ovaries that were distorted because of redundant cortex generally resume normal shape and anatomic relationships if the appropriate incision has been made. A careful study of the ovary

prior to making the initial incision is necessary. Incision of the ovarian cortex should allow a symmetric reconstruction when possible.

Resection of large or multiple endometriomas may present a difficult problem to the surgeon. Regardless of the extent of scarring or the size of the endometrioma, certain surgical principles apply. The ovarian cortical incision should be placed so as to preserve the anatomic relationship of the uteroovarian ligament and the fimbria ovarica. The least number of incisions should be made. If any sutures are placed, they should all be internal. Occasionally, a major portion of the ovarian substance may be completely destroyed by endometriosis. After resection, only a small portion of the ovarian cortex may be present; however, this should not be an indication for oophorectomy. Pregnancies have been noted in women who have had less than one-quarter of an ovary remaining.

When a normal fallopian tube is distorted over an enlarged ovarian or paraovarian mass, great care must be taken not to traumatize or injure the fallopian tube. Most often, an ovarian incision can be made away from the fallopian tube. Decompression of the ovary by cystectomy generally restores anatomic relationships. Paraovarian cysts are generally not removed unless they reach great size and distort anatomy. An incision in the broad ligament away from the fallopian tube, which allows access to the cyst, is made. Gentle dissection and removal of an intact cyst or cyst wall can then be accomplished with less trauma to the fallopian tube. The peritoneum is usually not closed.

Laparoscopic Cystectomy

Under general anesthesia and after induction of a pneumoperitoneum, the operating laparoscope is inserted intraumbilically. Second-puncture sites are placed in the midline and on either side of the midline approximately 3 inches laterally. The midline site is cephalad to the uterus. The midline site is generally used to puncture and irrigate the cyst as well as aspirate plume and debris if the laser is used. The lateral ancillary sites are used to stabilize the ovary and grasp the cyst wall lining.

The pelvis and the abdominal cavity are inspected carefully to ensure that the ovary does

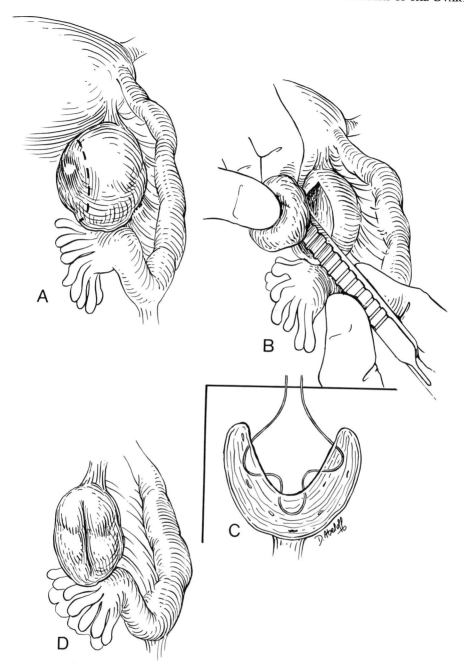

Figure 10.3. Resection of ovarian cyst at laparotomy. *A,* An elliptical incision is made along the horizontal axis of the ovary and its most dependent portion, if possible. *B,* The cyst is shelled out with a knife handle, in most instances, without rupture. *C,* Internal sutures are placed to close the dead space. *D,* The ovarian cortex is approximated with a subcuticular nonreactive suture of 7-0 or 8-0.

not have excresences or areas suspicious for malignancy. Peritoneal washings should be sent for cytology. The cyst is aspirated and irrigated as much as possible, using a 16-gauge needle. A small incision is made (approximately .5 cm), and the large suction/irrigator is used to aspirate and irrigate the cyst thoroughly. Minimal spillage will occur using this technique (30). Copious lavage of the peritoneal cavity is then performed if spillage has occurred. The incision is then extended. The ovarian cyst should be opened on its axis and in the most dependent portion (Fig. 10.4A). The cyst wall lining is closely inspected. If the cyst wall is not suspicious, the cystectomy proceeds. If the cyst wall is suspicious, multiple biopsies may be obtained and sent for frozen section.

A relaxing incision may be made to help identify the capsule. Atraumatic grasping forceps are used to hold the ovary at the uteroovarian ligament. The Hasson ovarian grasper is quite helpful if the ovary needs to be grasped anywhere else. An atraumatic forcep provides countertraction (Fig. 10.4B). The cyst wall is grasped, and dissection is carried out with laser, scissors, or bluntly. The forcep grasping the cyst wall can be rotated to bluntly dissect the wall from ovarian tissue (Fig. 10.4C). Incompletely resected areas may be further dissected, coagulated, or vaporized. Extreme care must be taken when working near the hilum of the ovary. Traumatic injury to these blood vessels may result in excessive bleeding that is difficult to stop without possibly compromising the blood supply to the ovary.

An alternate method involves coagulation or vaporization of the lining rather than resection of the cyst wall. Some argue that resection of the cyst wall may be very traumatic to the ovary, particularly with very large endometriomas, and that all modalities (laser, cautery, thermocoagulation) have enough depth of penetration to destroy the cyst wall lining. While this may be quite appropriate with an endometrioma, other cyst walls should be sent to pathology to rule out malignancy.

Although laparoscopic suturing can be performed to close the ovary, it is rarely done unless the cyst removed is quite large or the anatomy distorted (Fig. 10.4D). Careful placement of the initial incision should obviate the need for closure with suture. Internal sutures of #4-0 PDS may be placed to approximate the edges. Again, suture placement on the ovarian surface should be strongly discouraged.

SURGERY FOR OVULATION INDUCTION IN PCO

Polycystic ovarian disease (PCO) was described by Stein and Leventhal in 1935 (36) as an association of enlarged ovaries with amenor-

rhea, obesity, and evidence of androgen excess. Although the definition of PCO has broadened, chronic oligoanovulation and hirsutism have remained the hallmarks of this syndrome. The initiation of the cycle that perpetuates the hormonal milieu of PCO patients is unknown, but it is clear that elevated levels of androgens and estrogens maintain the chronic anovulatory state (3,4,7,46,47). The stigmata of PCO may also be seen in patients with virilizing ovarian or adrenal tumors as well as congenital adrenal hyperplasia.

The histologic findings in a polycystic ovary cover a broad spectrum. The spectrum extends from the typical Stein-Leventhal ovary with large numbers of follicular cysts, few atretic cysts, and marked stromal hyperplasia or hyperthecosis, to a smaller ovary with a few follicular cysts. Between these endpoints, there is a continuum bearing numbers of follicular cysts, atretic follicles, and stromal hyperplasia. Occasionally, the polycystic ovary may exhibit microscopic islands of luteinized thecal cells scattered in the stroma. Usually, there is a thickened fibrosed tunica with a large number of cystic follicles beneath this thickened capsule.

Patients with chronic anovulation because of PCO generally respond to clomiphene citrate for induction of ovulation (7). However, 10–15% of patients remain anovulatory despite increasing amounts of clomiphene and the addition of hCG. Remaining medical options includes human menopausal gonadotropins or pure human FSH therapy. These are costly and require careful hormonal and ultrasound monitoring to prevent the hyperstimulation syndrome that occurs with increased frequency in patients with PCO.

Surgical therapy for the induction of ovulation has long been used to induce long-term resumption of ovulation in patients with PCO. The mechanism by which ovarian wedge resection can induce ovulation is unclear. However, dramatic changes are seen in androgen, estrogen, and gonadotropin levels, which result in ovulation (24,25). Reduction in androgens and estrogens theoretically allows the normalization of the gonadotropin ratio, resulting in ovulation.

There is debate as to the amount of ovarian

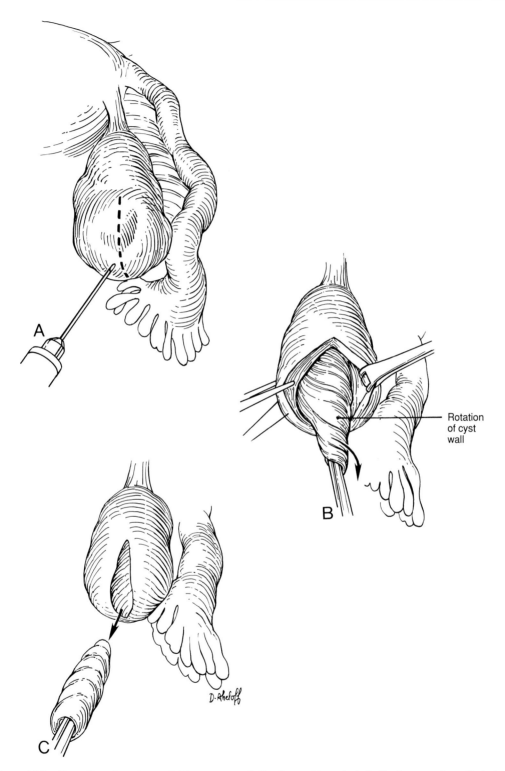

Figure 10.4.   Resection of ovarian cyst at laparoscopy. *A,* Ovarian cyst is aspirated with sharp needle and irrigated. *B,* Atraumatic forceps are used to grasp the ovary and provide countertraction so the cyst wall can be inspected and grasped by another forcep. The cyst wall is sharply or bluntly dissected. The grasper may be rotated to separate the cyst wall from the ovarian tissue. *C,* The ovary is left to heal by secondary intention.

mass that should be removed at the time of wedge resection. Halbe et al. (20) attempted to clarify this question by removing different amounts of ovarian substances from a random selection of patients with PCO. Thirty-eight of 62 patients were interested in conception. The patients were divided into three groups that had 20%, 33%, and 50–75% of the original ovarian mass removed. Resumption of ovulatory cycles was 53%, 71%, and 91%, respectively. These authors concluded that removal of at least 50% of the ovarian medulla would provide the best ovulatory results.

Stein and Leventhal thought that the size of the ovary was an important factor in patient selection for a wedge resection. Others have found no relationship between the results following surgery and the size of the ovaries (17). As the size of the ovary may vary with the spectrum of disease, this probably has no bearing on patient selection.

Adashi et al. (2) observed a resumption of ovulation in 91% of patients treated with bilateral ovarian wedge resection. Furthermore, within the ovulatory group, patients characterized by oligoovulation had a reduced conception rate of 29%, as compared with 60% in normoovulatory patients. Persistent oligoovulation and anovulation, as well as the presence of concurrent tuboperitoneal adhesions, were the most important determinants of the likelihood of conception.

There has been much concern over adhesion formation following wedge resection (5,42). Toaff et al. (38) noted extensive peritubular and periovarian adhesions in seven patients who did not conceive after bilateral wedge resection. Four of these patients had reconstructive surgery, and three conceived subsequently. Bilateral ovarian atrophy was noted in one patient, while unilateral ovarian atrophy was noted in two patients. Recent studies examined the application of microsurgical techniques for ovarian wedge resection and have provided conflicting data regarding adhesion formation (12). It is still unclear whether microsurgical technique will make a significant difference. The operation is presently infrequently performed because of the potential development of pelvic adhesions and infertility.

Surgical Technique for Wedge Resection

An incision is made in an elliptical manner with a knife, laser, or cautery (Fig. 10.5A). Note that it is made in the axis of the ovary. Through the elliptical incision, a portion of the medulla and cortex is removed. Care is taken to avoid the hilus of the ovary, as excessive bleeding may occur. Approximately 50% of the ovary or less is removed. The ovarian defect is then closed with one to two layers of internal interrupted sutures of #4-0 nonreactive suture (Fig. 10.5B and C). The last layer is a subcuticular suture of #6-0 to approximate the ovarian cortex (Fig. 10.5D). External sutures are avoided.

LAPAROSCOPIC SURGERY FOR OVULATION INDUCTION IN PCO

Laparoscopic techniques for ovulation induction in patients with PCO include ovarian biopsy, resection, and cautery. Gjonnaess (16) was the first to report laparoscopic ovarian cautery for the induction of ovulation in women with PCO. Endocrine changes after laparoscopic ovarian cautery have been examined. It is similar to wedge resection (1,6,18). A dramatic fall in testosterone and androstenedione levels are seen in the early postoperative period (18). A fall in estradiol levels is also observed, with a subsequent rise in FSH levels. Long-term (up to 1 yr) follow-up in 58 women with PCO revealed testosterone, androstenedione, and dihydrotestosterone levels that were significantly reduced. Mean serum levels of LH and FSH remained in the normal range for 1 year after ovarian cautery, suggesting that these results may persist in some patients.

Gjonnaess (16) reported that 92% of 62 PCO patients treated with laparoscopic ovarian cautery ovulated immediately after surgery. Those who did not spontaneously ovulate generally responded to clomiphene citrate. An overall pregnancy success rate of 69% was seen, with the rate increasing to 80% after the addition of clomiphene. This has been subsequently confirmed. Others have reported similar results ranging from 45–66% at 6–12 months of follow-up (1,18,40). Similar techniques utilizing laser vaporization of the ova-

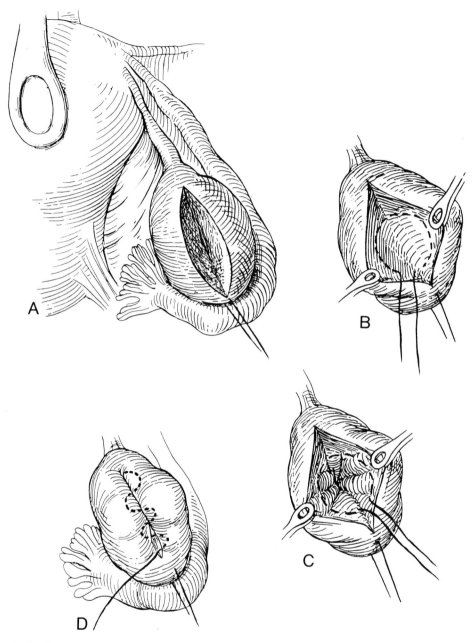

Figure 10.5. Ovarian wedge resection by laparotomy. *A*, An elliptical incision is made in the most dependent portion of the ovary and on its axis. *B*, A portion of the cortex and medulla is removed. *C*, The defect is closed with subcortical, internal, interrupted sutures or horizontal mattress sutures. *D*, The cortex is not closed or closed with subcuticular sutures of 7-0 absorbable material.

ries note a 70–80% spontaneous ovulation rate. Those who do not ovulate almost always respond to clomiphene citrate. These patients had previously failed therapy with this medication. Pregnancy rates of 60% have been reported with laser surgery (9,21,28).

No serious complications have been re-

ported with laparoscopic ovarian cautery. Of concern is the issue of postoperative adhesion formation, which has not been addressed with this modality. One preliminary study suggests that laparoscopic surgery is also complicated by adhesion formation (29). Second-look laparoscopy was performed on six women approximately 4 weeks after surgery. All patients were noted to have adhesions, which were extensive in some cases. At this time, adhesions are easily lysed. Jansen (22) has suggested that early second-look laparoscopy is followed by a decrease in adhesion formation. Lyles et al. suggest that second-look laparoscopy may be needed to prevent permanent adhesion formation with this technique (29).

Surgical Technique

After appropriate pneumoperitoneum is established, the typically enlarged ovaries are visualized. The ovary is stabilized with atraumatic forceps placed on the uteroovarian ligament. Using a third puncture site or the operating channel of the laparoscope, a sharp instrument such as the fine-tip needle monopolar cautery is used to penetrate the cortex of the ovary and make approximately 10 holes about 4 mm in diameter and 5 mm in depth (Fig. 10.6). The monopolar knife or scissors as well as thin bipolar paddles may also be used. Others have suggested the Palmer drill forceps. The holes are made at random or on superficial follicles. It is imperative that care is taken to avoid the area of the hilar vessels. Tissue

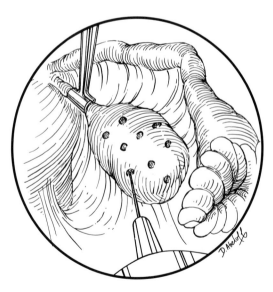

Figure 10.6. Laparoscopic cautery for ovulation induction in patients with PCO. Using monopolar needlepoint cautery or laser, 10–15 holes are made at random or on superficial follicles. The holes are approximately 4 mm in diameter and 5 mm in depth.

damage secondary to monopolar cautery may be seen as far as 2–3 cm, depending on the amount of current used and whether it is applied as cutting or coagulating current.

The CO_2, KTP, argon, and Nd:YAG lasers have also been used. The procedure is identical. The CO_2 laser can be used even though it is generally a cutting as opposed to a coagulating laser. Rarely must unipolar or bipolar be used to obtain hemostasis. The fiber lasers (KTP and argon) have further increased the ease of the procedure since these lasers coagulate better than the CO_2 and produce no smoke. The use of the fiberoptic delivery system with sapphire tips with the Nd:YAG laser enhances its applicability for this procedure, producing photocoagulation.

CONCLUSION

It appears that ovarian surgery, whether accomplished by laparotomy using microsurgical technique or by laparoscopy, is complicated by adhesion formation in many cases. Concern over adhesions after ovarian surgery for ovarian cysts was voiced by Van der Wat (39), who noted 45% infertility at a later date. Van der Wat made a plea for surgeons not to interfere with functional cysts in normal ovaries, as resulting adhesion formation may compromise fertility. Such advice should be heeded.

It is imperative that surgeons consider the untoward effects that may be seen with removal of ovaries for benign processes. Often, these benign processes are bilateral, such as dermoid cysts, and recurrent, such as endometriomas, follicular cysts, and patients with a propensity for torsion. These patients are at increased risk for surgical castration. Paradoxical oophorectomy should not be performed because its efficacy has not been established. Ovarian conservation is also desirable, as pregnancy rates with assisted reproductive technologies are dependent on the number of follicles obtained. The most conservative ovarian procedure consistent with good surgical judgment should be the goal of all reproductive surgeons.

References

1. Aakvagg A, Gjonnaess H: Hormonal response to electrocautery of the ovary in patients with polycystic

ovarian disease. Br J Obstet Gynaecol 1985;92:1258–1264.

2. Adashi E, Rock JA, Wentz A, et al: Fertility following bilateral ovarian wedge resection: a critical analysis of 90 consecutive cases of polycystic ovarian disease. Fertil Steril 1981;36:320.

3. Barnes RB, Lobo RA: Central opioid activity in polycystic ovary syndrome with and without dopaminergic modulation. J Clin Endocrinol Metab 1985; 61:779–782.

4. Barnes RB, Mileikowsky GN, Cha KY, et al: Effects of dopamine and metoclopramide in polycystic ovary syndrome. J Clin Endocrinol Metab 1986;63:506–509.

5. Buttram V, Vaquero C: Post-ovarian wedge resection adhesive disease. Fertil Steril 1975;26:874–876.

6. Casper RF, Greenblatt EM: Laparoscopic ovarian cautery for induction of ovulation in women with PCO. In: Reid R, ed. Seminars in reproductive endocrinology, vol 8. New York: Thieme Medical Publishers, 1990;208.

7. Coney P: Polycystic ovarian disease: current concepts of pathophysiology and therapy. Fertil Steril 1984; 42:667–682.

8. Daniell JF, Pittaway DE: Short interval second-look laparoscopy after infertility surgery: a preliminary report. J Reprod Med 1983;28:281–283.

9. Daniell JF, Miller W: Polycystic ovaries treated by laparoscopic laser vaporization. Fertil Steril 1989; 51:232–236.

10. DeCherney AH, Kase N. In: Tovell HMM, Dank LD, eds. Gynecologic operations. New York: Harper & Row, 1978:60.

11. Dembo AJ, Davy M, Stenwig AE, et al: Prognostic factors in patients with stage I epithelial ovarian cancer. Obstet Gynecol 1990;75:263.

12. Eddy CA, Asch RH, Balmaceda JP: Pelvic adhesions following microsurgical and macrosurgical wedge resection of the ovaries. Fertil Steril 1980;33:557–561.

13. Elkins TE: Adnexal torsion. Female Patient 1990; 15:43.

14. Gardner GH, Greene RL, Peckham BM: Tumors of the broad ligament. Am J Obstet Gynecol 1957;73:536.

15. Genadry R, Parmley T, Woodruff JD: The origin and clinical behavior of the paraovarian tumor. Am J Obstet Gynecol 1977;129:873.

16. Gjonnaess H: Polycystic ovarian syndrome treated by ovarian electrocautery through the laparoscope. Fertil Steril 1984;41:20–25.

17. Goldzieher JA, Lehrman SJ, Kistner RW: Polycystic ovarian disease. In: Behrman SJ, Kistner RW, eds. Progress in infertility. Boston: Little, Brown & Co., 1975;325.

18. Greenblatt EM, Casper RF: Endocrine changes after laparoscopic ovarian cautery in polycystic ovarian syndrome. Am J Obstet Gynecol 1987;156:279–285.

19. Gutenberg I: Benign cystic teratoma of the ovary: a 10 year review. J Am Osteopath Assoc 1971;71:147.

20. Halbe HW, da Fonseca AM, Silva P deP, et al:

Stein-Leventhal syndrome. Am J Obstet Gynecol 1972;114:280.

21. Huber J, Hosmann J, Spona J: Polycystic ovarian syndrome treated by laser through the laparoscope. Lancet 1988;2:215.

22. Jansen RPS: Early laparoscopy after pelvic operations to prevent adhesions: safety and efficacy. Fertil Steril 1988;49:26.

23. Jeffcoate TA: Principles of gynecology. London: Butterworth, 1975.

24. Judd HL, Riggs LA, Anderson DC, et al: The effects of ovarian wedge resection on circulating gonadotropin and ovarian steroid levels in patients with polycystic ovary syndrome. J Clin Endocrinol Metab 1976;43:346–355.

25. Katz M, Carr PJ, Cohen BM, et al: Hormonal effects of wedge resection of polycystic ovaries. Obstet Gynecol 1978;51:437.

26. Kelley RR, Scully: Cancer developing in dermoid cysts of the ovary. A report of 8 cases, including a carcinoid and a leiomyosarcoma. Cancer 1961;14:989–1000.

27. Kistner RW, Patton GW: Surgery of the ovary. In: Atlas of infertility surgery. Boston: Little, Brown & Co. 1975.

28. Kojima E, Yanagibori A, Otaka K, et al: Ovarian wedge resection with contact ND: YAG laser irradiation used laparoscopically. J Reprod Med 1989;34:444–446.

29. Lyles R, Goldzieher JW, Betts JW, et al: Early second look laparoscopy after the treatment of polycystic ovarian disease with laparoscopic ovarian electrocautery and/or ND: YAG laser photocoagulation. (Abstract 0-061) 45th Annual Meeting of the American Fertility Society, San Francisco, November 13–16, 1989.

30. Murphy AA: Diagnostic and operative laparoscopy. In: Thompson JD, Rock JA, eds. TeLinde's operative gynecology. Philadelphia: JB Lippincott, 1991;361–384.

31. Nezhat C, Winer WK, Nezhat F: Laparoscopic removal of dermoid cysts. Ob Gyn 1989;73:279.

32. Oelsner G, Graebe RA, Boyers SP, et al: A comparison of three techniques for ovarian reconstruction. Am J Obstet Gynecol 1985;154:569.

32a. Parker WH, Berek JS: Management of selected cystic adnexal masses in postmenopausal women by operative laparoscopy: a pilot study. Am J Obstet Gyn 1990;163:1574.

33. Rock JA, Parmley TP, Murphy AA, et al: Malposition of the ovary associated with uterine anomalies. Fertil Steril 1986;45:561.

34. Samaha M, Woodruff JD: Paratubal cysts: Frequency, histogenesis and associated clinical features. Obstet Gynecol 1985;65:691–693.

35. Scott JS, Lynch EM, Anderson JA: Surgical treatment of female infertility: value of paradoxical oophorectomy. Br Med J 1976:631.

36. Stein IF, Leventhal ML: Amenorrhea associated with bilateral polycystic ovaries. Am J Obstet Gynecol 1935;29:181–191.

37. TeLinde RW and Mattingly RF, eds. Operative gynecology. Philadelphia: JB Lippincott, 1970.

38. Toaff R, Toaff ME, Peyser MR: Infertility following wedge resection of the ovaries. Am J Obstet Gynecol 1976;124:92–96.

39. Van der Wat JJ: The mutilated ovary syndrome. S Afr Med J 1970;44:687.

40. van der Weiden RM, Alberda AT: Laparoscopic ovarian electrocautery in patients with polycystic ovarian disease resistant to clomiphene citrate. Surg Endosc 1987;1:217–219.

41. Warner MA, Fleischer AC, Edell SL, et al: Uterine adnexal torsion: sonographic findings. Radiology 1985;154:773.

41a. Way S: Ovarian cystectomy of twisted cysts. Lancet 1946;2:47.

42. Weinstein D, Polishuk WZ: Role of wedge resection of the ovary as a cause for mechanical sterility. Surg Gynecol Obstet 1975;141:417.

43. Wiskind AK, Toledo AA, Dudley AG, et al: Adhesion formation after ovarian wound repair in New Zealand while rabbits: a comparison of ovarian microsurgical closure with ovarian nonclosure. Am J Obstet Gynecol 1990;163:1674.

44. Witschi E: Migration of the germ cells of human embryos from the yolk sac to the primitive gonadal folds. Contrib Embryol 1948;32:69.

45. Witschi E: Embryology of the ovary. In: Grady HG, Smith DE, eds. The ovary. Baltimore: Williams & Wilkins, 1963;1–10.

46. Yen SSC: The polycystic ovary syndrome. Clin Endocrinol 1980;12:177–207.

47. Zumoff B, Freeman R, Coupey S, et al: A chronobiologic abnormality in luteinizing hormone secretion in teenage girls with the polycystic ovary syndrome. N Engl J Med 1983;309:1206–1209.

11
ENDOMETRIOSIS

John S. Hesla and John A. Rock

INTRODUCTION

Endometriosis has been extensively investigated since its original description by von Rokitansky in 1860 (184). Nevertheless, it remains an enigmatic disease process. The data available are inconclusive to support many of the hormonal and surgical therapies that have been proposed for the disease. In addition, the frequently subtle and varied appearances of endometriosis may make recognition and surgical staging difficult, thereby casting doubt on the utility of the current classification systems. Nevertheless, the findings of well-designed clinical trials and recent studies that have elucidated the pathogenesis of endometriosis have enabled a more rational approach to the medical and surgical management of this disease.

HISTOGENESIS

Endometriosis usually effects women in their reproductive years. It is defined as the presence of functioning endometrial glands and stroma outside of their usual location lining the uterine cavity. A complete understanding of the histogenesis of endometriosis has been compromised due to the variations of disease presentation. The widely accepted transplantation theory of Sampson (154) suggests that viable endometrial cells reflux through the fallopian tubes during menstruation and implant on surrounding pelvic structures (161). The anatomic distribution of endometriosis as noted at laparoscopy is consistent with this pattern of development (83). In addition, women with anomalies of the müllerian tract have an in-creased occurrence of endometriosis (128). Epidemiologic data suggest that women who menstruate more frequently, more heavily, or for longer duration have an increased likelihood of developing the disease (66). Nevertheless, bloody peritoneal fluid has been observed in 90% of women with patent fallopian tubes undergoing laparoscopy during the perimenstrual time period (68), a figure much higher than the estimated 2–5% prevalence of endometriosis in reproductive age women (75). Alterations in cellular immunity may facilitate the successful implantation of translocated endometrial cells in this patient population (40).

Endometrial cells also may be transported to extrauterine sites via blood vessels, the lymphatic system, or by contamination of the pelvis or abdominal wall incision if the uterine cavity is surgically entered (67). Retroperitoneal endometriosis is hypothesized to arise from lymph vascular spread (110); 29% of patients with pelvic endometriosis documented on autopsy had pelvic lymph nodes that contained endometriosis. Coelomic metaplasia of the cells lining the pelvic peritoneum has been proposed as a possible etiology for endometriotic lesions in unusual locations (64,106,122).

The role of steroid hormones in the initiation and maintenance of endometriosis was investigated in primates by diZerega et al. (36). They demonstrated that endometriosis required no steroidal supplementation to become established; nevertheless, survival of the experimentally induced endometrial plaques appeared to require continuous exposure to ovarian steroids. This concept fails to explain the 10% of cases of bowel endometriosis that occur in the hypoestrogenic, postmenopausal age group.

The possibility of a familial tendency to endometriosis has been reported by several investigators (90,140,167). No studies have confirmed an HLA linkage for the disease; a polygenic, multifactorial mode of inheritance has been suggested (107,168).

PREVALENCE

Although the exact prevalence of endometriosis in the general female population of reproductive age is not precisely known, it is believed to lie within the range of 2–5% (169). Endometriosis was noted in as many as 50% of gynecologic laparotomies by Williams and Pratt (193). Jeffcoate (82) reported that endometriosis was found in 10–25% of women undergoing laparotomy by gynecologists in the United Kingdom and the United States. Twenty to forty percent of infertile women are diagnosed with the disease (96). Of 459 consecutive patients with primary infertility investigated at The Johns Hopkins Hospital, 114 (25%) were found to have endometriosis (84). Verkauf (182) prospectively identified endometriosis in 38.5% of infertile women and 5.2% of fertile women. Other studies have confirmed the odds that infertile women are 7–10 times more likely to have endometriosis than their fertile counterparts (65).

NATURAL HISTORY

The natural history of endometriosis is not clearly understood. The disease appears to progress in the majority of untreated patients, although spontaneous regression has been described in milder cases. Surgical and medical therapies may prevent a temporal regression but may not effectively eliminate microscopic, retroperitoneal, and hormonally resistant disease. Dmowski and Cohen (38) described persistent disease in 15% of patients treated with danazol, while Henzl and associates noted a progression of disease during the course of treatment in 4–8% of patients receiving danazol or GnRH analog (GnRHa). When conservative surgery was combined with danazol or GnRHa therapy, the overall recurrence rate at 36 months was between 13.5–33% (96).

The effect of pregnancy on the clinical course of endometriosis is uncertain. Although Sampson (153) suggested that pregnancy induces involution of implants, more recent authors have proposed a variable response to the condition. Walton (185) studied endometriosis patients after pregnancy and found that the presenting symptoms and sites of endometriotic involvement were unchanged. It is possible, however, that the endometriosis was temporarily suppressed during the pregnancy. McArthur and Ulfelder (95) analyzed the clinical effect of pregnancy on endometriosis in 24 patients. They found that the behavior of endometriosis during the gravid state was extremely variable and that the regression of disease appeared to be more likely due to decreased tissue responsiveness to hormonal stimulation than actual necrosis of the lesions. More patients in their series experienced disease persistence than permanent regression. Monkey studies have confirmed these findings; the response of endometrial implants to pregnancy varied from total regression to significant progression (158).

PATHOPHYSIOLOGY

When extensive pelvic scarring or large endometriomas are present in the patient with endometriosis, the associated infertility may be clearly attributed to anatomic distortion. However, the pathophysiology of infertility in patients with less advanced disease is more controversial (Table 11.1) (175).

Endometriotic implants within the fallopian tube or ovary may promote a local inflammatory response that may have a direct deleterious effect on tubal function. Oocyte pickup by the fallopian tube may be prevented despite the normal process of oocyte maturation and ovulation (127). Chronic salpingitis was detected in 29 of 87 (33%) of fallopian tubes of patients undergoing laparotomy for ovarian endometriosis; tubal obstruction could be demonstrated in only one of these cases (29). Tuboovarian adhesions were found in 15 patients (17%), although only seven had the adhesions associated with salpingitis. Endometriosis has been identified in the resected segments of fallopian tubes in patients undergoing tubal-cornual

Table 11.1.   Proposed Mechanisms for Infertility in Endometriosis[a]

Mechanical Factors
  Adhesions
  Tubal pathology
Alterations in Peritoneal Fluid and Local Immune
    Response
  Direct toxic effects
  Macrophage activation
  Cellular secretory products
Alterations in Systemic Immune Response
  Enhanced cell-mediated immune response
  Antiendometrial antibodies
Ovulatory Dysfunction
  Abnormal gonadotropin secretion
  Prolactin hypersecretion
  Abnormal follicular growth
  Luteinized unruptured follicle syndrome
  Luteal phase abnormalities
Abnormalities of Fertilization
Early Pregnancy Loss
  Implantation defects
  Spontaneous abortion

[a]From Surrey ES, Halme J: Endometriosis as a cause for infertility. Obstet Gynecol Clin N Am 1989;16:79, with permission.

anastomosis for proximal tubal obstruction when there was no evidence of endometriosis elsewhere in the pelvis (138). Although other investigators have reported tubal endometriosis and chronic salpingitis in similar cases, Forrest et al. (56) found no relationship between tubal inflammatory changes and endometriosis.

Several published studies have described altered folliculogenesis or ovulation in endometriotric patients. Doody et al. (47) sonographically evaluated follicular development in 20 patients with mild endometriosis previously treated with diathermy or conservative surgery, 46 patients who received clomiphene citrate, and a control of 20 fertile women. Linear regression analysis of increasing follicular diameter demonstrated a lower rate of growth in all endometriotic patients. They speculated that an abnormal follicular growth rate and total growth period may disturb the normal synchronization of oocyte maturation, uterine receptivity, and ovulation. Tummon et al. (180) reported that women with minimal endometriosis had more yet smaller follicles and lower preovulatory estradiol levels at the time of luteinizing hormone (LH) surge.

Luteinized unruptured follicle syndrome (LUF), a condition of normal ovulatory hormone secretion and luteinization of the follicle without ovulation taking place, has been reported to exist more commonly in patients with endometriosis. Donnez and Thomas (45) were able to identify stigmata of ovulation in only 28 and 49% of patients with moderate and severe endometriosis, respectively, at the time of laparoscopy. These figures were significantly lower than the 91% and 85% stigma formation in cases of normal controls and mild endometriosis, respectively. Schenken et al. (155) also noted an increased rate of LUF and associated luteal phase deficiency in monkeys with surgically induced moderate to severe endometriosis. Other studies have confirmed and refuted these findings. Sonographic evidence of failure of midcycle follicular collapse in patients with mild endometriosis has ranged from 4–34% in the literature (39,96,178).

Luteal phase function has been evaluated by endometrial biopsy and peripheral progesterone concentrations. There is insufficient evidence to conclusively link endometriosis with a deficiency of corpus luteum activity, although some studies have suggested the existence of a shortened luteal phase and delayed rise in progesterone secretion following ovulation (13,181). Conversely, measurement of estradiol and progesterone levels in the peripheral and ovarian veins of women with endometriosis during the early follicular phase has suggested an increased frequency of inadequate luteolysis and prolongation of corpus luteum function into the subsequent menstrual cycle (7).

The effect of endometriosis on fertilization and preimplantation development is widely debated. Sueldo et al. (171) reported that peritoneal fluid from patients with endometriosis had a deleterious effect on sperm-oocyte interaction in a homologous mouse fertilization assay. Exposure of two cell mouse embryos to peritoneal fluid or serum of patients with endometriosis has resulted in a decreased rate of cleavage and development to the blastocyst and hatching stages as compared with control, nonendometriotic specimens (30,112). In addition, women with severe endometriosis have reduced fertilization and conception rates through in-vitro fertilization (IVF) as compared with controls, although the impact of lesser stages of disease on IVF outcome appears to be less significant. A high frequency of abortions in infertile women with endometriosis has been reported (188), although the relationship has been questioned due to potential control group bias (105,135).

Because of the uncertain etiology of infertility and pelvic pain in patients with minimal and mild endometriosis, many investigators have attempted to identify specific alterations in the peritoneal environment that would explain these symptoms. Significant increases or decreases in peritoneal fluid volume due to increased production by the ovaries, altered mesothelial permeability, or increases in the colloid osmotic pressure have been hypothesized to inhibit ovum capture by the fallopian tube or adversely affect tubal transport. Koninckx et al. (89) reported elevations in peritoneal fluid volume during cycle days 1–5 in patients with mild and moderate endometriosis. The quantity of fluid was comparable to control subjects during the remainder of the follicular phase. This study described reduced volumes in the early luteal phase, which directly contrast with that reported by Oak (124). Rock et al. (148) studied patients during cycle days 8–12 and measured no difference in fluid volumes in patients with endometriosis as compared with control subjects. Similar findings were noted by Rezai and associates (146). Hence, it appears unlikely that fluid volume alone plays a role in the establishment of infertility.

Peritoneal fluid from patients with minimal and mild endometriosis has been shown to increase macrophage proliferation in vitro. In addition, several studies have described increases in total macrophage number in the peritoneal fluid of patients with endometriosis. Hill et al. (76) measured significant elevations in total leukocytes, macrophages, helper T cells, lymphocytes, and natural killer cells in women with stages I and II endometriosis. Activated macrophages may affect the reproductive process by altering sperm motility, fimbrial ovum capture, sperm oocyte interaction, and early embryonic growth in vitro. Increased sperm phagocytosis by macrophages has been demonstrated by in-vivo animal and in-vitro human

studies (116). Suginami et al. (172) suggested that an ovum capture inhibitor is present in higher concentrations in endometriosis patients. This macromolecule may prevent contact between the fimbrial cells and cumulus oophorus. Halme et al. (69) have proposed that macrophage-derived growth factor enhances the ectopic growth of endometrial cells in the peritoneal cavity.

Prostaglandins, interleukins, and other substances produced by macrophages may be harmful to reproduction. Fakih et al. (52) demonstrated that interleukin-1 was present in the peritoneal fluid of almost all patients with endometriosis but not in the fertile control group. Interleukins have been shown to adversely affect mouse embryo growth in vitro. In addition, interleukin-1 stimulated fibroblast proliferation, collagen deposition, and fibrinogen formation; hence, elevated concentrations of such lymphokines may explain the development of fibrosis and adhesions in advanced stages of endometriosis. Nevertheless, not all studies have confirmed the existence of a difference in interleukin activity between endometriosis patients and control groups (6). A decreased plasminogen activator activity in endometriotic implants may also be a cause for increased adhesion formation (126).

Chronic elevation in levels of peritoneal prostaglandins have been hypothesized to interfere with ovulation (87), alter tubal mobility such that the embryo may arrive in the uterus at a suboptimal time for implantation (192), or diminish corpus luteum function (142). Drake and associates (49) measured the metabolites of PGI_2 and thromboxane A_2 in peritoneal fluid and noted a 10-fold increase in these levels in patients with endometriosis. Ylikorkla et al. (194) confirmed these observations, although the increase of the prostanoid metabolites in the patients with endometriosis was less than twice the controls. When cycle stage is controlled, Rock et al. (148) and Rezai and associates (146) failed to demonstrate a significant change in prostaglandin levels in peritoneal fluid from patients with endometriosis as compared with control groups. Similarly, Sgarlata et al. (165), Dawood et al. (34), and Chacho et al. were unable to show an alteration in prostaglandin levels with endometriosis.

Dawood et al., however, did measure an elevated concentration of a prostacycline metabolite in endometriosis patients. No significant differences in prostaglandin concentrations were noted between the follicular and luteal phase in either endometriosis patients or controls (22,35). Variations in collection of samples during the menstrual cycle, control group selection, and collection techniques have compromised the interpretation of data regarding the relative importance of prostanoid content in peritoneal fluid.

Systemic immune response in patients with endometriosis may be altered, leading to decreased fertility. Dmowski et al. (40) reported that rhesus monkeys with spontaneous endometriosis have a decreased lymphocytic reaction to intradermal injections of autologous endometrial antigens and a decreased blastogenic transformation of in-vitro lymphocytes in response to the same autologous antigens. This finding suggests that translocated endometrial cells may implant only in those patients with an inherent deficit in cell-mediated immunity.

Weed and Arquembourg (187) suggested that aberrant endometrium that responds to hormonal stimuli will undergo hyperplasia and shedding as does normal endometrium. Menstrual fluid that contains endometrial proteins may be recognized by the host as foreign and trigger an autoimmune response. The authors note that the host reaction is variable, thus explaining why some women with a weak autoimmune response and varying extent of disease may conceive with no difficulty. Since this initial report, other investigators have confirmed the high frequency of autoantibodies against endometrial and ovarian tissues in the sera as well as in cervical and vaginal secretions of women with endometriosis. Badawy et al. (8) reported an increase in the concentration of T cells, B cells, and the ratio of CD4/CD8 lymphocytes in patients with endometriosis compared with control patients in both the peritoneal fluid and peripheral blood. This suggests that activated B cells may regulate increased immunoglobulin production.

Gleicher et al. (61) reported that in a study of 59 patients with endometriosis, 29% had positive antinuclear antibody (ANA) titers, 46% had positive lupus anticoagulant assays,

and almost 50% demonstrated IGM and IGG antibodies. However, others have noted no change in IGG, IGM, and IGA in patients with endometriosis as compared with healthy control subjects. Hence, the above studies suggest but do not conclusively identify the precise role of the immune system in causing the sequelae of endometriosis.

SYMPTOMS

Dysmenorrhea, dyspareunia, and pelvic, back, and rectal pain, the more common symptoms of endometriosis, have been assumed to be caused by the presence of endometrial implants. However, the development of such symptoms is not diagnostic of the disease state. Greater than 60% of women questioned in one random survey reported dyspareunia at some point in their lives, and 33% had persistent discomfort (60). The prevalence of laparoscopically diagnosed endometriosis in patients with chronic pelvic pain has ranged from 4–52% of published series (132).

Some authorities have suggested that the patient's symptoms may be dependent upon the location of the implants, presence of adhesions, distortion of ovarian anatomy by endometriosis, and involvement of other organs such as the ureter or rectum. Deep infiltration of the fibromuscular tissue of the pelvis has been strongly correlated with pelvic pain (25). Nevertheless, Fedele and colleagues (53) found no significant association in AFS disease stage and the presence and severity of dysmenorrhea, pelvic pain, and dyspareunia in their prospective study of 160 women. The pain profile of the patients with ovarian lesions were similar to that of the patients with peritoneal or ovarian and peritoneal disease.

There is no universally accepted hypothesis that explains how endometriosis can cause these symptoms. The symptoms generally correlate with the fluctuation of steroid hormones. In response to the cyclic stimulation by ovarian estradiol and progesterone, endometriotic lesions undergo epithelial and stromal proliferation, variable secretory changes, stromal pseudodecidual reaction, and periodic regression in the manner similar to normal endometrium. Surgical castration and ovarian suppressive therapy results in pain relief in the majority of patients.

DIAGNOSIS OF ENDOMETRIOSIS

Awareness of the wide range of visual appearances of endometriosis is necessary for accurate diagnosis and appropriate surgical therapy of the disease (37). Although darkly pigmented lesions are readily recognizable and are considered a classic presentation of endometriosis, less discernible yet common forms of implants have been described as early as the 1920s, when Sampson noted "red raspberries, purple raspberries, blueberries, blebs, and peritoneal pockets" (154). The black or blue puckered "powder burn" implant is a late consequence of cyclic growth and regression of the lesion, to the point where bleeding and hemosiderin staining of the tissue has occurred. Biopsy of such areas reveals inactive endometrial glands and fibrous stroma.

Distinctive morphologic variations and endometriosis include vesicles, flat plaques, raised lesions, polypoid structures, areas of fibrosis and adhesion formation, and peritoneal defects (81) (Table 11.2). Yellow, brown, blue, and black coloration is proportional to the amount of hemosiderin deposition. Red polypoid lesions share the closest histologic characteristics with native endometrium and are thought to have the greatest metabolic activity, as suggested by their high concentrations of prostaglandin metabolites (183). Biopsy of nonpigmented implants reveals the presence of active endometriotic glands and stroma. Conversely, white lesions are predominantly fibromuscular scarring with scattered glandular and stromal elements. Peritoneal defects and subovarian adhesions contain endometriosis in 40–50% of cases (183).

Other peritoneal lesions share similar morphologic features with endometriosis. Hence, the differential diagnosis may include old suture, epithelial malignancies, hemangioma, inflammatory reaction to infection or oil-based hysterosalpingogram dye, and carbon deposition from laser surgery (183). The ability to detect subtle lesions of endometriosis increases with the experience of the surgeon and is reinforced by histological confirmation (101) (Table 11.3).

Small endometriotic lesions become more visible during the premenstrual and menstrual phases of the cycle, for during this time, microfoci of peritoneal disease become congested with blood and debris. In addition, vascular dilatation, superficial hemorrhage, and ecchymosis formation cause an accentuation of the more typical features of endometriosis. Performance of laparoscopy at a time when ovarian steroidogenesis is suppressed by medications such as danazol or GnRH analogs may lead to inaccuracies in the assessment of extent of disease (50).

Jansen and Russell (183) reported the presence of nonpigmented lesions in 38% of their 202 patients with biopsy-proven endometriosis; 15% had only nonpigmented implants. Most areas of pigmented endometriosis are surrounded by nonpigmented endometriosis. These subtle lesions may represent the first stage of development of peritoneal disease; appropriate diagnosis and initiation of surgical therapy may prevent long-term sequelae. Recognition of nonpigmented endometriosis may be enhanced by "painting" the peritoneum with the patient's blood (143).

Although depth perception is impaired when the pelvic cavity is viewed through the monocular optics of the laparoscope, its magnification ability when closely approximated to the peritoneum may allow identification of subtle surface irregularities present in occult disease (144). Magnification up to 8× power may be obtained with the laparoscope, depending on the working distance (Table 11.4).

Table 11.2. Atypical Appearances of Endometriosis

White opacification	Jansen and Russell, 1986
Red flame-like lesion	Jansen and Russell, 1986
Glandular excrescences	Jansen and Russell, 1986
Endometriosis in adhesions	Jansen and Russell, 1986
Yellow-brown peritoneal patches	Jansen and Russell, 1986
Peritoneal defect	Chatman, 1981
Petechial peritoneum	Donnez and Nisolle, 1988
Hypervascularization	Donnez and Nisolle, 1988
Retroperitoneal disease	Martin and Diamond, 1986
	Moore and coauthors, 1988
	Cornillie and coauthors, 1990

Table 11.3. Histologic Confirmation of Lesions Categorized by Appearance

Author, Year	Black	White	Red	Glandular	Subovarian Adhesions	Patches	Yellow-Brown Pockets
Jansen, 1986	ns	81%	81%	67%	50%	47%	47%
Stripling, 1988	97%	91%	75%	ns[a]	ns	33%	ns
Martin, 1989	94%	80%	75%	66%	39%	22%	39%

[a]ns = not stated.

Table 11.4. Powers of Magnification Obtained with Operating Laparoscopes[a]

Operating Laparoscope Working Distance (mm)	Magnification Rate
3	8.2
5	5.7
10	3.2
15	2.2
20	1.7
30	1.2
50	0.7

[a]From Murphy AA, Guzick DS, Rock JA: Microscopic peritoneal endometriosis (Letter to the Editor). Fertil Steril 1989;51:1072. Reprinted with permission.

Nevertheless, microscopic implants of endometriosis have been documented by scanning electron microscopy in peritoneal biopsies of patients with unexplained infertility, who had no evidence of disease at the time of laparoscopy (14). Similarly, a scanning electron microscopic study of samples of supposedly normal tissue from endometriosis patients documented the presence of endometriotic foci in 25% of cases (113,170). Lesions as small as 200 μm have been documented (114). Hence, surgical treatment of all visible disease is more accurately described as cytoreductive rather than ablative.

Recognition of deep ovarian endometriosis is necessary for correct staging of the disease. Candiani et al. (19) described the presence of small endometriomas in 48% of infertile women who had mildly enlarged ovaries (3.5–5.0 cm in diameter) when the ovaries were punctured with a 16-gauge needle. The ovarian surfaces were without gross disease. Preoperative sonographic evaluation may be a useful screening test for the presence of these small endometriomas; their identification may affect the disease categorization of the patient.

CA-125, a high molecular weight glycoprotein expressed on the cell surface of some derivatives of embryonic coelomic epithelium, is frequently elevated in patients with AFS stage II-IV endometriosis. Barbieri et al. (9) reported that a value of >35 U/ml had positive predictive value of 0.58 and a negative predictive value of 0.96 in establishing the presence of endometriosis. Many other conditions have been associated with an elevated CA-125 concentration, including acute pelvic inflammatory disease, adenomyosis, uterine leiomyoma, menstruation, pregnancy, epithelial ovarian cancer, pancreatitis, and chronic liver disease. In contrast to the above finding, Pittaway (134) reported that 80% of women with pelvic pain and endometriosis had a CA-125 titer > 16 U/ml, whereas only 6% of patients with pelvic pain and without endometriosis had an increased serum concentration of this cell-surface antigen.

CLASSIFICATION OF DISEASE

Many endometriosis classification systems have been introduced in an attempt to allow direct comparison of patient response to medical and surgical treatments as well as to identify factors predictive of disease outcome.

One of the earliest classifications was proposed by Wick and Larsen (191), who recommended a survey of the pelvis to correlate clinical symptomatology and physical findings with the histologic grading of endometriosis. Riva et al. (147) presented a classification system based upon scalar criteria of the location of disease as noted at the time of culdoscopy. They recommended assessment based on the bulk of the endometriotic lesions and any associated disturbance of normal pelvic anatomy. Although this classification did not accurately describe the extent of endometriosis

The American Fertility Society*†

Birmingham, Alabama

Patient's Name _____ Date_____

| Stage I (Minimal) · 1-5 |
| Stage II (Mild) · 6-15 |
| Stage III (Moderate) · 16-40 |
| Stage IV (Severe) · >40 |
| Total_____ |

Laparoscopy_____ Laparotomy_____ Photography_____
Recommended Treatment_____

Prognosis_____

PERITONEUM	ENDOMETRIOSIS		<1cm	1-3cm	>3cm
	Superficial		1	2	4
	Deep		2	4	6
OVARY	R	Superficial	1	2	4
		Deep	4	16	20
	L	Superficial	1	2	4
		Deep	4	16	20
	POSTERIOR CULDESAC OBLITERATION		Partial		Complete
			4		40
	ADHESIONS		<1/3 Enclosure	1/3-2/3 Enclosure	>2/3 Enclosure
OVARY	R	Filmy	1	2	4
		Dense	4	8	16
	L	Filmy	1	2	4
		Dense	4	8	16
TUBE	R	Filmy	1	2	4
		Dense	4*	8*	16
	L	Filmy	1	2	4
		Dense	4*	8*	16

*If the fimbriated end of the fallopian tube is completely enclosed, change the point assignment to 16.

Figure 11.1. The Revised American Fertility Society Classification of Endometriosis (1985).

present, these investigators did demonstrate a direct relationship between the number of pelvic organs involved and the response to hormonal pseudopregnancy.

Acosta et al. (1) proposed a concise classification of endometriosis based on the sites and amount of disease present at the time of surgery. Each case was characterized as mild, moderate, or severe, according to precise criteria. This classification was noteworthy for ascribing importance to the presence of periovarian and peritubal adhesions in differentiating mild and moderate stages of endometriosis.

The Acosta classification was further modified by Buttram (16) to include laterality of disease; however, the classification was primarily descriptive and did not quantitate endometriosis sites. Kistner et al. (88) based their classification system on the geographic dissemination of implants rather than apparent severity of disease.

The American Fertility Society organized a panel of experts in 1979 (4) to develop a classification system that might serve as a basis for evaluating various therapies. By attempting to quantify the location and extent of endometriosis in a scalar rather than numerical terminology, the Committee devised an innovative scheme based upon the natural progression of disease. Three anatomic areas, the peritoneum, ovary, and fallopian tube, were examined for the presence of endometriosis or adhesions, with allowances made for unilateral involvement. However, no weight system was incorporated to factor in the depth of infiltration of peritoneal implants. An arbitrary point system was assigned to each area of disease involvement that was based on a presumption that implant size and adhesion characteristics were associated with disease prognosis. The stage of disease was determined by the cumulative score of the assigned points.

The classification system by Buttram, Kistner, and coauthors, and the American Fertility Society Committee were compared in a retrospective study of 214 infertile women with proven endometriosis treated only by conservative surgery (150). Application of the Kistner classification revealed a significant decline of fecundity rates as the stage of disease increased; however, no association was found with pain relief or the risk of recurrence and subsequent surgery. Using the AFS classification, no statistically significant decrease in unadjusted pregnancy rates or fecundity was established as the stage of disease increased, unless patients in the mild and moderate groups were combined and compared with the severe and extensive degree groups. In addition, no association was found between pain relief or the risk of recurrence and the need for subsequent surgery and the stage of disease assigned at the time of initial laparotomy. Hence, the above classification systems were criticized for their arbitrary division of endometriosis categories that did not necessarily reflect the true relative risk of sequelae of disease.

The American Fertility Society classification was revised in 1985 to provide a more standard assessment of endometriosis for correlation of surgical treatment with distribution and severity of implants (Fig. 11.1) (3). The point range of mild disease was expanded, and greater weight was given to deep endometriosis, dense adhesions, and cul-de-sac obliteration by adhesive disease. While the revised staging system appropriately acknowledges the importance of adhesive disease and endometriomas, a majority of women with extensive peritoneal disease in the absence of ovarian involvement may receive a very low score on laparoscopic inspection of the lesions.

This revised AFS classification has been widely utilized by investigators to categorize disease states. Nevertheless, direct comparison of treatment outcome is compromised by persistent inconsistencies in the application of various staging criteria. The evaluation of the extent of disease by laparoscopy may be limited by a lack of recognition of atypical implants, particularly if the patient is hypoestrogenic due to recent discontinuation of medical therapy for endometriosis. The great variations in medical and surgical therapeutic options being applied in the management of the disease compromise an analysis of disease outcome. Furthermore, the division between stages of endometriosis re-

mains arbitrary, and this classification does not address extrapelvic endometriosis. A staging system to account for distant disease has been proposed by Markham et al. (97), (Table 11.5).

The revised American Fertility Society classification system is oriented towards infertility patients, since the stage and location of endometriosis have not been associated with the frequency and severity of dysmenorrhea, pelvic pain, and dyspareunia. Our limited knowledge of the specific pathophysiological alterations by which endometriosis can cause these symptoms prevents a precise categorization of disease based upon response to conventional therapies.

THERAPY

Expectant

Treatment of mild and moderate endometriosis with hormonal preparations may not offer any advantage over expectant management in promoting conception. In studies by Seibel et al. (163), Hull et al. (77), and Telimaa (177), patients assigned to expectant management conceived earlier than the medically treated group, and the cumulative pregnancy rate was not higher for women receiving progestogens or danazol. Perhaps this lack of enhancement of fecundability may be related to the lower number of estrogen, progesterone, and/or androgen receptors in endometriotic lesions, as compared with normal endometrium (80,176). Nevertheless, patients with minimal or mild disease who have pelvic pain or dysmenorrhea may benefit from hormonal therapy. Certainly, the age and duration of infertility of the patient are important factors in determining appropriate therapy for the symptomatic individual. Laser laparoscopic ablation of milder stages of endometriosis appears to lessen the interval to conception, although the cumulative pregnancy rate may not be greater than that for women who are managed expectantly. Surgical therapy for more advanced disease results in a higher pregnancy rate than mere expectant management or hormonal treatment, due at least in part to correction of mechanical factors that may be inhibiting ovulation or tubal function.

Androgens

Methyltestosterone temporarily alleviates symptoms of endometriosis without necessarily

---

Table 11.5.   Classification and Stages of Extrapelvic Endometriosis[a]

Classification of Extrapelvic Endometriosis
   Class I: Endometriosis involving the intestinal tract
   Class U: Endometriosis involving the urinary tract
   Class L: Endometriosis involving the lung and thoracic cage
   Class O: Endometriosis involving other sites outside the abdominal cavity
Staging of Extrapelvic Endometriosis
   Stage I   No organ defect
        1. Extrinsic: surface of organ (serosa, pleura)
          a. $<$1 cm lesion
          b. 1 to 4 cm lesion
          c. $>$4 cm lesion
        2. Intrinsic: mucosal, muscle, parenchyma
          a. $<$1 cm lesion
          b. 1 to 4 cm lesion
          c. $>$4 cm lesion
   Stage II Organ defect[b]
        1. Extrinsic: surface of organ (serosa, pleura)
          a. $<$1 cm lesion
          b. 1 to 4 cm lesion
          c. $>$4 cm lesion
        2. Intrinsic: mucosal, muscle, parenchyma
          a. $<$1 cm lesion
          b. 1 to 4 cm lesion
          c. $>$4 cm lesion

---

[a]From Markham SM, Carpenter SE, Rock JA: Extrapelvic endometriosis. Obstet Gynecol Clin North Am 1989;16:193.
[b]Organ defect would depend on the organ of involvement and would include but not be limited to obstruction and partial obstruction of the urinary tract and the intestinal tract and hemothorax, hemoptysis, and pneumothorax resulting from pulmonary involvement.

---

affecting either ovulation or menstrual cyclicity (85). The regressive action of androgens on the endometrium are minor, and the side effects of acne, hirsutism, clitoromegaly, and deepening of the voice may be significant at higher doses. Because ovulation is not impaired, masculinization of a female fetus may occur when androgens are ingested during an unrecognized pregnancy. As a result, other hormonal therapies have supplanted the use of androgens in most cases of endometriosis.

Progestogens

High-dose combination estrogen-progestogen regimens were introduced in the late 1950s for the symptomatic relief of endometriosis. The rationale for this therapy was based on the observation that pregnancy provided subjective and objective improvement in many patients with extensive pelvic endometriosis. As occurs in pregnancy, high doses of estrogens and progestogens are thought to transform endometrial tissue into decidua that ultimately undergoes necrosis and involution. Oral contraceptives with strongly progestational properties have been traditionally used. Typical regimens include an initial dose of two tablets daily; the dose is increased by one-two tablets at biweekly intervals until the patient is amenorrheic and/or is receiving the equivalent of 20 mg of norethynodrel. This is continued for 6–9 months. Although this combination therapy does relieve pelvic pain and dysmenorrhea in 50–80% of patients, significant side effects are encountered, including weight gain, mastalgia, nausea, headaches, and irregular bleeding (121). As a result, the discontinuation rate has been high.

Because of the above side effects and potential risks of high-dose administration of estrogen in some patients, progestogen only regimens have gained favor over the continuous high-dose oral contraceptive schedule in creating a pseudopregnancy state. Progestogens inhibit the pituitary release of LH and thereby suppress ovarian steroidogenesis as well as promote secretory changes in the glandular epithelium and decidualization of the endometrial stroma. Progestogens also oppose the growth-promoting effects of estrogens on the endometrial tissue by altering the clearance of the nuclear estrogen receptor and inducing 17β hydroxysteroid dehydrogenase, which converts estradiol to the weaker estrone. Moreover, by eliminating cyclic bleeding and suppressing uterine contractility, progestogens prevent reflux menstruation, a potential stimulus for continued endometriosis development.

Luciano and colleagues (94) administered medroxyprogesterone acetate 50 mg/day for 4 months to symptomatic women with moderate to severe endometriosis. Improvement of pain, pelvic nodularity, and tenderness on examination occurred in 80% of patients. Twenty percent of women experienced breakthrough bleeding, and an additional 10% reported persistent cyclic bleeding. Minor weight gain, edema, and increased irritability were other described side effects that were generally well tolerated. A lower daily dosage (such as 30 mg) may provide equivalent relief of symptoms. The low cost of this medication as compared with danazol or GnRH analogs is a notable advantage.

Schlaff et al. (159) reported a similar response rate with the use of megestrol acetate. Doses of 40 mg/day for up to 24 months resulted in significant relief of dysmenorrhea, noncyclic pelvic pain, and dyspareunia in 86% of subjects.

The rate of recurrence of symptomatic endometriosis after progestogen therapy appears to be related to the length of follow-up. Riva et al. (147) reported an 18% recurrence rate after an average of 11 months, while Moghissi and Boyce (108) described a 42% recurrence rate during a 2-year interval following discontinuation of medication.

Danazol

Danazol, a synthetic (2,3-isoxazole) derivative of 17α-ethinyl testosterone, was introduced into clinical practice by Greenblatt and colleagues in 1971 (63). The drug gained rapid acceptance due to its effectiveness in relieving pain associated with endometriosis and in enhancing fertility, as suggested by uncontrolled trials. Its pharmacologic action is complex (10). By directly inhibiting GnRH secretion, the midcycle LH surge is ablated, although basal gonadotropin concentrations are maintained. Danazol interacts with endometrial androgen and progesterone receptors, suppresses the activity of multiple enzymes necessary for ovarian and adrenal steroidogenesis, and displaces androgens from sex hormone-binding globulin, thereby augmenting androgen action on endometrial receptors. The decline in sex hormone-binding globulin induced by danazol lowers estradiol binding, increases estradiol clearance, and promotes a fall in the circulating level of this hormone. Hence, the derivative has direct androgenic and antiprogestational action on endometrial implants and creates a hypoestrogenic, hypoprogestational environment antagonistic to endometriosis. Moreover, by producing amenorrhea, danazol prevents peritoneal seeding of refluxed endometrial tissue.

The adverse effects of danazol reflect its anabolic, androgenic, and antiestrogenic properties and may be dose-related. Weight gain, muscle cramps, decreased breast size, and vasomotor symptoms are noted in 50% or more of patients maintained on doses of 400–800 mg/day. In Buttram's 1985 series, 41% of patients treated with 800 mg/day, the standard dose, gained more than 10 pounds during the course of therapy (18). The threefold increase in free testosterone may cause acne, oily skin, and deepening of the voice in a small percentage of recipients. HDL cholesterol declines by 50% or more in response to the altered steroid concentrations (93). Most series have reported a concomitant increase in LDL cholesterol. Because danazol is metabolized by the liver, modest elevations in SGOT and SGPT may arise. Significant side effects occur in as many as 85% of patients, and at least 10% of women receiving danazol discontinue pharmacologic treatment because of intolerable adverse effects (94). Combining danazol therapy with aerobic exercise appears to reduce the incidence of many of these androgenic side effects (20).

The amenorrhea induced by danazol has been found to benefit patients with dysmenorrhea, dyspareunia, and cyclic pelvic pain associated with endometriosis. Young and Blackmore (195) reviewed the effects of different dosages of danazol with respect to relief of symptoms in 452 patients. At the 800 mg dosage, 95% noted relief of dysmenorrhea, while 89% of the patients reported relief of pelvic pain. At the

400 mg dosage, posttherapeutic relief was reduced by 10%. Moore et al. (109) reported that pain associated with minimal and moderate pelvic endometriosis appeared to respond well to doses of danazol less than or equal to 400 mg/day, whereas severe endometriosis was best treated with doses greater than 400 mg/day. Unfortunately, recurrence of symptoms within 4–12 months after discontinuation of therapy approaches 50% in most studies. Lower daily doses of medication and courses of treatment less than 4 months in duration may result in a shorter symptom-free interval (41).

Danazol has been extensively prescribed as therapy of endometriosis-associated infertility; however, there are no well-controlled studies to support any medical approach to the treatment of infertility. Pregnancy rates following danazol as single therapy have ranged from 30.9–52.6% in mild endometriosis, 23.1–50% in moderate disease, and 0–100% in severe stages (160). Monthly fecudity rates range from 1.6–6.8% (127). The findings of many early studies have been questioned due to the lack of randomization, failure to include an expectant management control group, and failure to account for the presence of other infertility factors. Recent data concerning medical therapy of minimal, mild, and moderate stages of disease refute any therapeutic benefit in enhancing conception (77,163,177). Furthermore, attempts at conception are delayed while the patient is receiving the medication.

GONADOTROPIN-RELEASING HORMONE AGONIST

Gonadotropin-releasing hormone agonists (GnRHa) have recently become available for use in the treatment of estrogen-dependent diseases such as endometriosis. Some of the more frequently studied analogs include leuprolide, nafarelin, buserelin, and goserelin. Alteration of the amino acid at position 6 and ethylamide replacement of the C-terminal amino acid of the native decapeptide hormone results in a GnRH analog with increased resistance to lysosomal degradation. Pituitary receptor binding is enhanced, resulting in a decline in the number of receptors available for further occupancy. Continued administration of the GnRHa leads to a desensitization of the pituitary gonadotrope receptor and a reversible down-regulation of the pituitary-ovarian axis (103). Ovarian estrogen secretion may reach castrate levels.

The initial response to GnRHa administration is a markedly increased secretion of pituitary stores of FSH and LH. If therapy is begun in the follicular phase of the menstrual cycle, the developing follicle may respond to the flare in circulating gonadotropin levels with a rapid rise in estradiol production. Estradiol levels may remain elevated for 3 weeks before declining. GnRHa administration in the luteal phase leads to a more rapid decline in estrogen secretion, although FSH and LH levels remain elevated for 1 and 4 weeks, respectively.

GnRHa treatment results in an improvement or resolution of pain symptoms in all stages of disease. Lemay et al. (91) reported resolution of pain in 70% and improvement in discomfort in 15% of 24 subjects after 2–4 months of treatment with the agonist buserelin. Dyspareunia improved in 9% and disappeared in 91% of patients studied. Henzl and associates, in a double-blind, multicenter study, treated 213 patients with either danazol or one of two doses of nafarelin (73). After 6 months of treatment, over 80% of patients in all groups experienced a significant reduction in visible implants. A 43% reduction in AFS score was noted for each treatment group; there was no difference in response among patients receiving the 400 mcg and 800 mcg daily dose of nafarelin. Most patients continued to demonstrate some visible implants at the time of follow-up laparoscopy, and, as with danazol, there was some diminution in size of endometriomas but no effect on preexisting adhesions.

Response to therapy may be dependent upon route of administration. Donnez et al. (44) have reported that buserelin administration by a long-acting subcutaneous implant led to a greater reduction in endometriosis score, mitotic index, and endometrial cyst diameter than when given in an intranasal form. This may have been due to a greater consistency in hormonal release by the injected preparation.

As occurs with danazol and progestogen regimens, symptoms recur at variable time periods following discontinuation of GnRHa therapy. Franssen and colleagues (57) noted a lasting and significant amelioration of dysmenorrhea and dyspareunia 6 months after completion of treatment; however, scores for pelvic pain had nearly reached their pretreatment level after this time interval had elapsed.

The effect of GnRH analogs on endometriosis-associated infertility is difficult to assess due to a lack of an expectant management control group in most clinic studies. The preliminary pregnancy rates, which range from 0–60%, are derived from trials that do categorize response based upon stage of disease.

Most of the side effects associated with GnRHa therapy are related to hypoestrogenism. Hot flushes are common and may lead to sleep disturbances and chronic fatigue in extreme cases. Vaginal dryness, superficial dyspareunia, headaches, and depression have been reported. In general, these adverse effects are better tolerated than those experienced with danazol use. In addition, there are no undesirable changes in total, HDL, and LDL cholesterol throughout the prolonged period of hypoestrogenism induced by GnRHa as compared to that experienced with danazol intake (73,91). A decline in trabecular bone mineral content and rise in urinary calcium excretion to menopausal levels occurs during the course of GnRHa therapy in approximately two-thirds of patients (73). Restoration of normal estrogen production following cessation of therapy appears to reverse these bone changes.

Concomitant administration of a progestogen during the course of GnRHa therapy has been examined in an attempt to ameliorate vasomotor symptoms and retard both urinary calcium excretion and radiologic evidence of loss of bone mineral density. Cedars et al. (21) reported a diminution in the above side effects when medroxyprogesterone acetate was administered at a dose of 20–30 mg/day during the 6-month course of agonist therapy; however, review laparoscopy following completion of therapy failed to reveal any improvement or suppression of active endometriosis with the combination regimen. Conversely, Surrey et al. (174) described a significant resolution of laparoscopic evidence of nonadhesive endometriosis when GnRHa was combined with norethindrone 0.35–3.5 mg/day (mean 1.4 mg/day)

to an extent equivalent to that achieved with GnRHa alone. Hot flushes and bone mineral loss were retarded. The cause for the difference in effect between norethindrone and medroxyprogesterone acetate is not clear, but may be related to the relative potency in inducing endometrial atrophy as well as the potential estrogenic action of the metabolic products of the progestogen.

CONSERVATIVE SURGERY

Endoscopic assessment of the pelvis allows determination of the appropriate treatment of patients with endometriosis. Conservative resection of disease by laparotomy is most valuable in cases of extensive pelvic adhesions or endometriomas greater than 3 cm in diameter. In addition, deep involvement of the rectovaginal septum with fibrotic extension into the perirectal fossa, invasion of the bowel muscularis, and endometriotic infiltration in the region of the uterine vessels are best approached through the open abdomen. The objective of the microsurgical procedure is complete excision of all endometriosis and associated adhesive disease in an attempt to restore normal functional anatomy of the reproductive tract.

GENERAL CONSIDERATIONS

As with all pelvic reconstructive procedures, the fundamental tenets of microsurgery must be followed, including adequate exposure of the operating field, gentle tissue handling, use of atraumatic instruments, precise hemostasis, and, when necessary, reperitonealization with fine suture. Continuous irrigation with heparinized Ringer's lactate solution and dissection with fine scissors, microelectrode, or laser are recommended. Loupe magnification or use of the operating microscope may aid in reconstruction.

The surgical approach is usually through a transverse suprapubic incision. A Maylard approach may offer greater access to the pelvic structures than the Pfannenstiel technique. A longitudinal incision is necessary if a presacral neurectomy is planned or if there are very large ovarian masses.

Prior to proceeding with pelvic dissection, a

thorough exploration of the pelvic and abdominal organs should be routinely performed. The ovaries are frequently adherent to the posterior broad ligaments and must be carefully displaced from these sites before resection of endometriomas is possible. Immobilizing adhesions may be merely divided during the preparatory phase of the procedure; precise excision is more easily accomplished after the involved organs are freed. Prior to dissection of the pelvic sidewall, the ureter must be identified and isolated, as it is frequently displaced by endometriotic adhesive disease. Vital structures may be protected during adhesiolysis by isolating the adhesion band with a glass rod or titanium probe.

PERITONEAL ENDOMETRIOSIS

Small lesions of superficial endometriosis <5 mm in diameter are easily treated with bipolar coagulation or laser while under a constant stream of irrigation (Fig. 11.2). Deep lesions or more extensive peritoneal disease must be excised with at least a 2-4-mm tissue margin, for, as noted previously, microscopic lesions are commonly present in tissue adjacent to visible implants. Reliance on monopolar microdiathermy or CO_2 laser vaporization to ablate rather than excise deep disease may result in inadequate resection and a greater amount of ischemic damage to the tissue, heightening the propensity toward adhesion formation. Peritoneal defects may be reapproximated with fine nonreactive absorbable suture, such as 5-0 polyglactin, and covered with an adhesion barrier. Suture placement should be avoided if the defect is small and hemostatic, for it may promote tissue anoxia and resultant fibrosis.

OVARIAN ENDOMETRIOSIS

Superficial endometriosis of the ovary usually presents as small, dark, punctate lesions immediately beneath the cortical surface. This disease may be readily treated with laser or bipolar forceps under constant irrigation. However, on occasion, the small, visible lesion may be merely the tip of a large endometrial cyst. If there is any doubt, the implant should be excised and the ovary explored to determine the extent of disease.

Extensive ovarian endometriosis is frequently associated with periovarian and peritubal adhesions. Filmy adhesions are elevated with delicate tissue forceps and may be resected with fine-needle cautery or the laser. Care must be taken to maintain the integrity of the ovarian capsule. After the appropriate adhesiolysis is accomplished, the posterior cul-de-sac is packed with moist, lint-free packs and the silicon surgical platform may be placed to stabilize the adnexae. The ovary should be carefully examined for extent of disease involvement prior to creation of the initial incision. Peritoneal spillage of the contents of the endometrioma can be avoided by placement of a lint-free pack around the platform.

The cortical incision should be made so as to preserve the normal anatomic relationships of the ovary with the uteroovarian ligament and fimbria ovarica (Fig. 11.3). This is best accomplished by making a shallow longitudinal incision over the endometrioma with the monopolar microneedle or laser. The surgeon should attempt to remove the endometrioma in an intact state; however, if the cyst cavity is inadvertently entered, an elliptical incision around the site of rupture is useful for exposure. The intact endometrioma is transfixed with a traction suture of 2-0 nylon to facilitate creation of a cleavage plane between the cyst and the normal ovarian tissue. Blunt, curved scissors or a knife handle is used for dissection. Particular care must be taken in dissecting the hilar region in order to maintain hemostasis. An attempt should be made to preserve as much of the normal ovarian cortex as possible; pregnancies have been achieved with only a small fraction of remaining ovary.

The ovary is reconstructed by placement of 1–2 purse-string sutures of 4-0 polyglactin, polyglycolic acid, or polydioxanone suture to eliminate the dead space and maximize hemostasis followed by a running subcortical 5-0 suture of the same delayed absorbable material (Fig. 11.3). In some circumstances, less tissue distortion can be achieved by placing a deep layer of interrupted mattress suture followed by additional layers of running suture (Fig. 11.4). Few knots should extrude beyond the ovarian surface.

After the ovary has been carefully approxi-

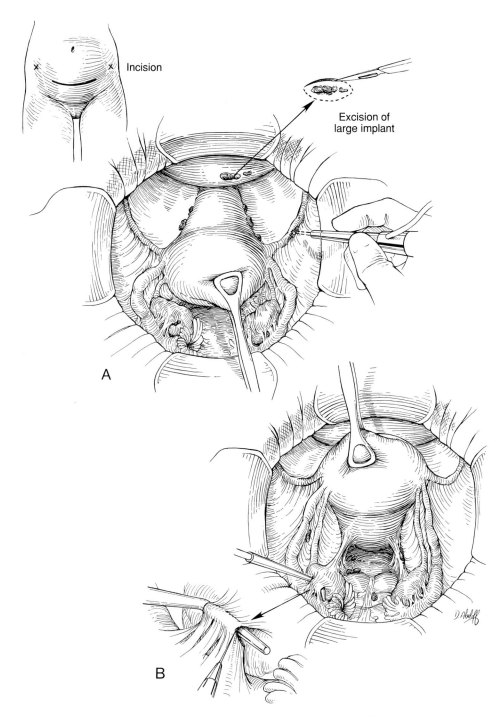

Figure 11.2.   Excision or CO_2 laser vaporization of peritoneal implants. *A,* Superficial implants are vaporized using power densities between 1000–3000 W/cm², with a spot size of 0.8–1.0 mm or are cauterized with fine bipolar forceps. More extensive peritoneal disease is excised. Large defects may be closed with 5-0 or 6-0 polyglactin or polydioxanone. *B,* Endometriosis may be associated with extensive adnexal adhesions. Wide adhesion bands may be retracted with a glass rod and excised with microtip monopolar microelectrode.

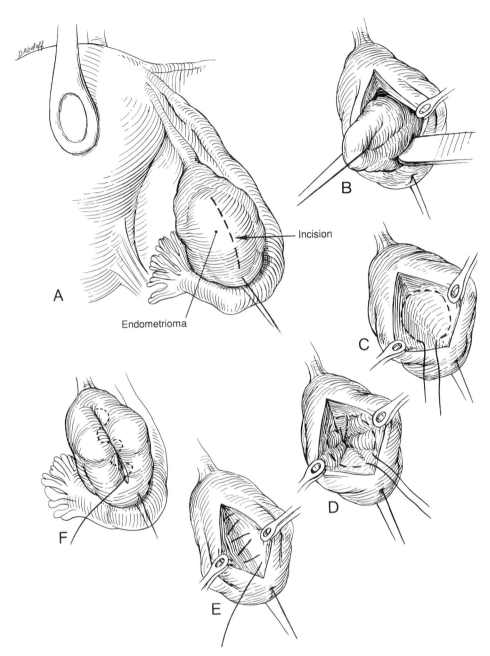

Figure 11.3. Excision of ovarian endometrioma through the open abdomen. *A,* The ovarian cortex is gently incised so as not to enter the endometrial cyst. The incision is made along the longitudinal axis of the ovary. *B,* The endometrioma is then peeled out with the blunt knife handle. *C,* and *D,* The ovarian defect is obliterated with two layers of purse-string sutures of 4-0 absorbable nonreactive material. *E,* In the case of a deep defect, a more superficial running suture may be necessary before approximating the cortical edges with 5-0 nonreactive, delayed absorbable suture (F).

mated, the posterior surface of the uterus and broad ligament are inspected for hemostasis, where the ovary was previously adherent. Bipolar cauterization may be necessary. Placement of an adhesion barrier may be useful in separating raw peritoneal surfaces.

INTESTINAL ENDOMETRIOSIS

Intestinal involvement has been estimated to occur in 3–37% of women with endometriosis. Symptoms that should arouse suspicion of colorectal involvement include constipation alternating with diarrhea, hematochezia, rectal pain, tenesmus, dyspareunia, and dysmenorrhea (27). Bowel resection should be undertaken in the symptomatic patient or when there is a suspicion of malignancy; however, the incidence of such indications is small. In a series of 1573 consecutive patients diagnosed with endometriosis, only 11 women (0.7%) required bowel resection (139). Appendiceal endometriosis is an uncommon finding and is unlikely to be of clinical significance. Thus, the appendix should not be removed unless absolutely indicated.

Preoperative preparation for bowel resection should include danazol or GnRHa therapy for at least 3 months prior to surgery. In addition, full mechanical and antibiotic bowel preparation are necessary preoperatively. Serosal and superficial muscularis lesions may be carefully resected with scissors. However, all cases of deep colorectal involvement should undergo wedge or segmental bowel resection with end-to-end anastomosis by a surgeon with such expertise. If the uterosacral ligaments are also significantly infiltrated with endometriosis, they may be removed en block while attached to the rectosigmoid colon. It may be necessary to remove a portion of the vaginal muscularis with the bowel specimen to completely excise the endometriosis. Coronado et al. (27) reported a complete relief of pelvic symptoms in 38 patients (49.4%) and an improvement in 30 patients (39%) who underwent full-thickness resection of the colon; 13 of 33 women (39.4%) achieved a term pregnancy.

URINARY TRACT ENDOMETRIOSIS

Endometriosis involving the urinary tract is relatively rare. The spectrum of disease severity varies from incidental findings at laparoscopy, laparotomy, or cystoscopy to more significantly associated hematuria, flank pain, hypertension, and ureteral obstruction (111). Cystoscopy and intravenous pylography are helpful studies in documenting the extent of disease. Vesical endometriosis may be treated by hormonal suppressive therapy or partial cystectomy. Extrinsic ureteral compression by endometriosis presents four times more frequently than intrinsic involvement and is most likely to occur in the region of the ovarian fossa (166). Patients with paracervical and extensive uterosacral ligament disease are also at risk. The preferred treatment for ureteral obstruction is ureterolysis or resection of the involved segment, followed by ureteroneocystostomy or ureteroureterostomy (166).

UTERINE SUSPENSION

Uterine suspension techniques have been devised in an effort to prevent adhesion formation of denuded peritoneal surfaces of the posterior cul-de-sac, uterine serosa, and/or broad ligament. Furthermore, elevation of the adnexa may prevent adhesion reformation of the ovary or fallopian tube to a site where existing adhesions have been excised. This procedure may be particularly useful in the case of a posterior or retroflexed uterus. There is no evidence to suggest that uterine suspension is detrimental to subsequent pregnancies. The modified Gilliam procedure offers certain advantages over other uterine suspensions due to its maintenance of normal anatomical relationships. By shortening the round ligament through the internal inguinal ring, no opening is made lateral to the point of the ligament's attachment to the abdominal wall, as occurs in the Olshausen suspension.

When performing a modified Gilliam suspension, the uterus is elevated, and a 2-0 chromic suture is placed around each round ligament approximately 3–4 cm from its insertion into the uterus (Fig. 11.5). The edge of the rectus fascia is grasped by a Kocher clamp at the level of the anterosuperior spine of the ileum. The adjacent peritoneal edge is grasped with a Kelly clamp. The rectus fascia is separated from the underlying musculature via blunt dissection. A long Kelly clamp is inserted between the fascia and muscle to the level of the inguinal

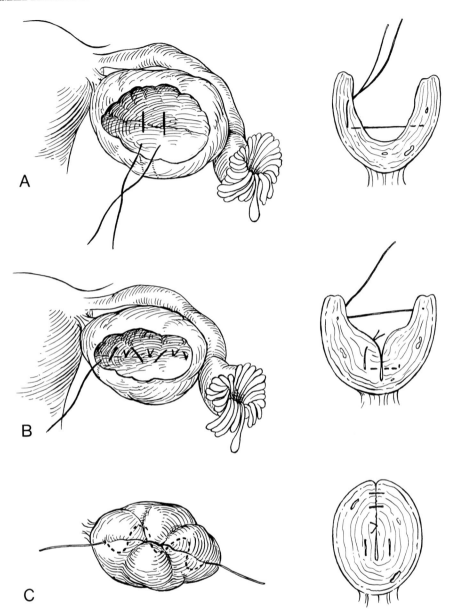

Figure 11.4. Ovarian reconstruction following endometrioma resection. *A,* Approximation of hilar region with interrupted mattress sutures of 4-0 nonreactive absorbable suture. *B,* Placement of more superficial running suture. *C,* Running, subcortical suture of 5-0 delayed absorbable material.

ring, while displacing the peritoneum superiorly. This clamp is inserted through the ring and along the round ligament by gently opening and closing the instrument. The insertion is facilitated by placing traction on the chromic suture to stabilize the round ligament. The peritoneum overlying the ligament is then incised adjacent to where the chromic suture has been placed, and the suture is grasped by the Kelly clamp. By withdrawing the clamp, the round ligament is brought through the internal ring and outside of the peritoneal cavity, where it may be sutured to the rectus sheath using 2-0 interrupted delayed absorbable sutures. These sutures must be placed through the round ligament so as not to encircle the ligament and thus occlude its blood supply. This procedure is repeated on the opposite side.

At the termination of the suspension, the surgeon's hands should be introduced into the abdomen to ascertain whether there is a loop of round ligament lateral to the point where the ligament has been withdrawn from the peritoneal cavity. If so, this should be corrected to prevent strangulation of the involved segment lying between the ligament and abdominal wall. In addition, the fallopian tube should be inspected to ensure that its course has not been disturbed. This may occur if the traction suture has been placed through a segment of round ligament too close to the uterus.

PRESACRAL NEURECTOMY

Presacral neurectomy is frequently useful as an adjunctive procedure to eliminate the uterine component of dysmenorrhea caused by endometriosis. There is no evidence that this procedure enhances fertility (74,136,149). A significantly greater relief of midline pelvic pain is achieved when endometriosis resection is combined with presacral neurectomy over conservative resection alone (179). Lateralizing adnexal pain is not affected by this procedure.

The hypogastric plexus consists of fine strands of nerves embedded in a delicate areolar tissue and is formed as a continuation of the aortic and inferior mesenteric plexuses. The plexus passes over the bifurcation of the aorta and continues below the promontory of the sacrum before dividing into the right and left inferior hypogastric nerves.

The presacral neurectomy procedure should be performed through a longitudinal incision (Fig. 11.6). This allows a proper exposure of the region of the bifurcation of the aorta and facilitates adequate displacement of the intestine. The descending colon is packed superiorly and to the left to expose the left margin of the hypogastric plexus. The posterior peritoneum overlying the sacrum is elevated and incised with the scalpel. The incision is extended caudally with scissors for approximately 5 cm to the 3 or 4 sacral vertebra and cranially to just below the bifurcation of the aorta. The margin of the posterior peritoneum may be drawn upward and outward by a stay suture or an Allis clamp. A Kitner sponge is then used to dissect the areolar tissue and associated nerve fibers off of the posterior aspect of the peritoneal flap. The right ureter is readily visible and may be retracted laterally, while the areolar tissue is dissected from it without disturbing its blood supply. The common iliac artery, which lies just below the ureter, is freed superiorly from the adjacent tissue. A right-angle clamp or probe may be introduced medially next to the promontory to elevate the sheath and allow blunt dissection underneath it. Care must be taken to avoid the middle sacral vessels that may be left intact on the surface of the promontory. Injury to the middle sacral vein can result in significant blood loss.

The areolar tissue is then taken off the left flap of peritoneum until the superior hemorrhoidal vessels are exposed. These vessels should remain on the peritoneum but are bluntly freed from the overlying tissue. By elevating the sheath, a small number of branches that feed into the left common iliac vein may be identified. These branches are isolated, clamped, and tied as they are visualized. When the plexus has been isolated, a Babcock clamp may be used to elevate the sheath. A suture of #2-0 chromic or silk is placed around the proximal and distal aspect of a 5-cm segment of plexus and is loosely tied. The tonsil clamp is applied to each end of the nerve bundle. As the clamps are removed, the sutures are slipped down over the crushed areas and tied securely. The intervening portion of the plexus is then excised. The procedure is terminated by approximating the peritoneum with absorbable suture. Black (12) and Hamod and Rock (71) noted that 60–70% of patients with secondary dysmenorrhea may have complete relief of symptoms. In a more recent series, all 17 patients undergoing presacral neurectomy noted a complete resolution of midline pelvic pain, and only two of these had a recurrence of pain within the 42-month follow-up period (179).

Two common side effects of the presacral neurectomy procedure have been observed. Constipation requiring laxatives or stool softeners for a period of 3–4 months has been described. Vaginal dryness may occur in as many as 10–15% of patients; this is transient and usually resolves within 6 months. Difficulties with micturition are an infrequent compli-

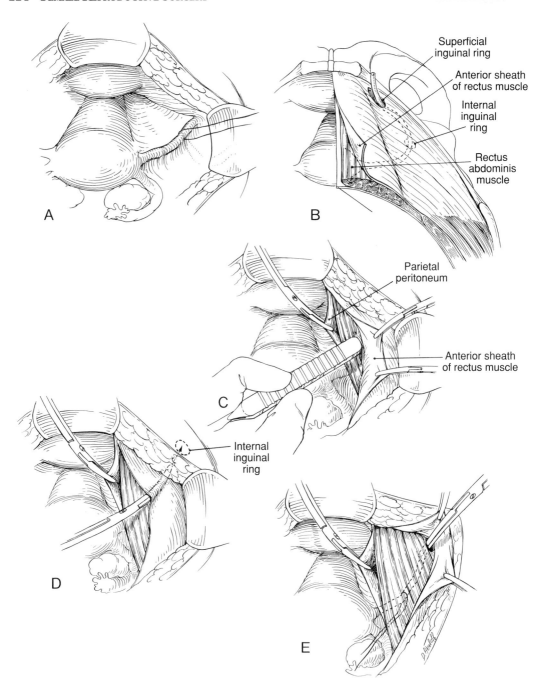

Figure 11.5. Modified Gilliam suspension. *A,* A chromic catgut suture is placed around the round ligament approximately 3–4 cm from the uterine cornu. *B,* Anatomic landmarks should be identified to assist instrument placement. *C,* The rectus fascia is grasped with Kocher clamps and separated from the belly of the rectus muscle bluntly with the index finder or a knife handle. *D,* The parietal peritoneum is grasped with a Kelly forceps. *E,* A long Kelly forceps is introduced through the internal inguinal ring as it passes over the belly of the rectus *F,* The Kelly clamp is brought through the internal inguinal ring and along the round ligament to a point adjacent to the chromic stay suture. A knife is used to open the peritoneum. *G,* The ends of the chromic suture are grasped by the Kelly clamp. *H,* As traction is applied to the suture, a knuckle of the round ligament passes through the internal ring. *I,* and *J,* Three sutures of 2-0 delayed absorbable or silk suture are placed, fixing the ligament to the rectus fascia in a manner so as to not interfere with the blood supply.

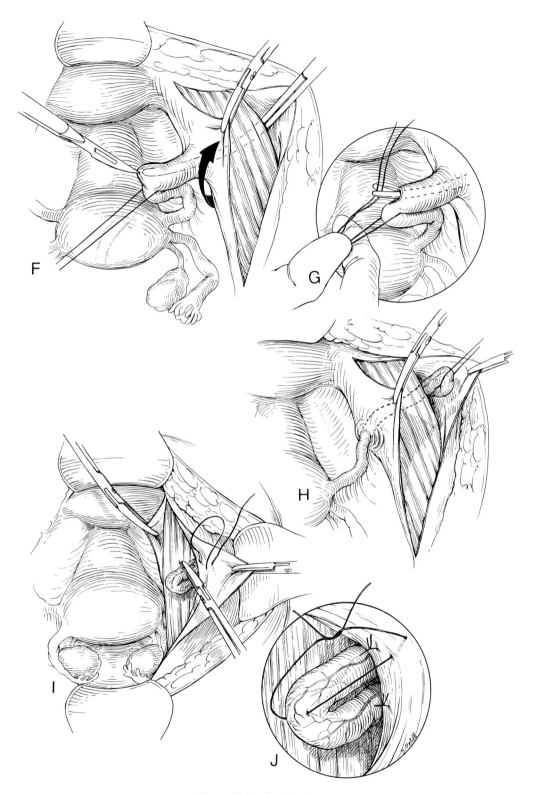

Figure 11.5.   *Continued.*

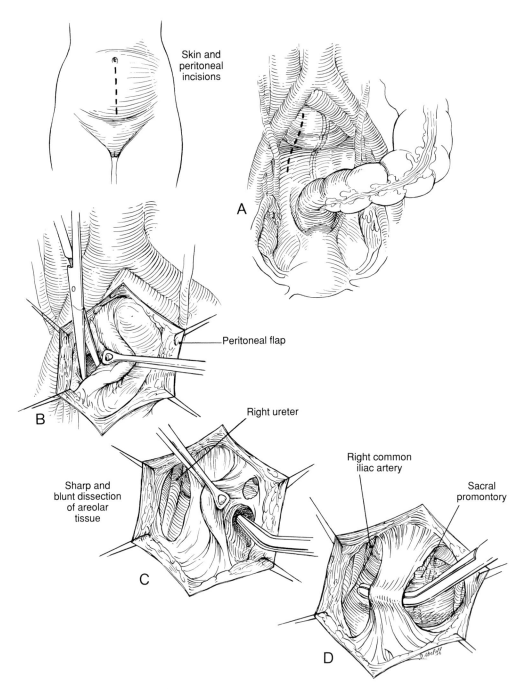

Figure 11.6. Presacral neurectomy. *A,* Location of incision in relation to anatomic landmarks. The descending colon is displaced superiorly and to the left for good exposure of the left margin of the hypogastric plexus. *B,* A Kitner sponge is used to dissect the areolar tissue medially and off the posterior aspect of the peritoneal flap. The right ureter may be easily identified. *C,* The areolar nerve-bearing tissue is dissected from the peritoneum on the left side, exposing the left internal iliac vessels and superior hemorrhoidal vessels. *D,* The plexus is isolated and elevated off the sacral promontory. *E,* An approximate 5-cm segment of plexus is isolated with 2-0 silk suture and excised. *F,* Relationship of pedicles of the excised nerve bundle with adjacent structures. *G,* Reperitonealization with 4-0 nonreactive, absorbable suture.

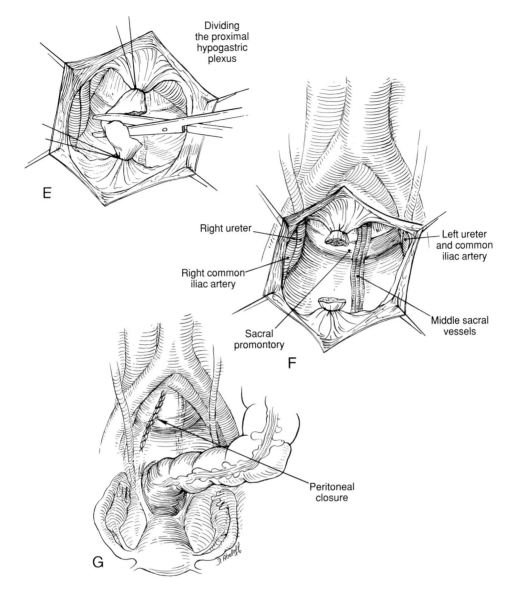

Figure 11.6. *Continued.*

cation of this procedure. The bladder dysfunction rarely lasts for more than 1 or 2 months.

LAPAROSCOPIC THERAPY

The advent of operative laparoscopy represents an advance in the treatment of endometriosis. The advantages of endoscopic therapy over traditional laparotomy include a decrease in patient morbidity, reduction in length of hospital stay and expenses, the opportunity to treat at the time of diagnosis, and possibly a reduction in postoperative adhesion formation and increased rate of pregnancy (120). Perhaps the progression of disease may be impeded with laparoscopic treatment of early stages of endometriosis at the time of diagnosis.

The decision whether to perform surgical resection of endometriosis through the laparoscope or open abdomen is not necessarily dependent upon the stage of disease encountered. Laparoscopy may be considered for all cases except when there is difficulty in establishing the appropriate tissue planes of dissection or if improved access is necessary for atraumatic manipulation of the involved organs.

Specific endoscopic procedures include ablation of endometriotic implants, adhesiolysis, ovarian cystectomy, oophorectomy, and salpingectomy. Laparotomy is necessary for bowel resection, complete resection of the presacral nerve plexus, and excision or ablation of deep endometriosis that cannot be safely isolated from vital structures.

Several basic techniques are available for the endoscopic ablation of endometriosis, including excision, coagulation, and vaporization (102). Coagulation may be achieved by monopolar or bipolar cautery, thermocoagulation, or in some circumstances laser, depending upon the wave length of energy applied. The extent of tissue penetration in electrocautery is related to the power and type of current, duration of application, and size of electrode. Less tissue damage is achieved with bipolar than monopolar cautery.

Endocoagulation, or thermocoagulation, arises from direct application of a probe heated to 100–120°C. Coagulation is achieved to a depth of 1–2 mm. Although the superficial spread of energy results in limited tissue injury, deep endometrial implants are not adequately ablated with this technique.

The zone of thermal necrosis is minimal with the CO_2 laser, particularly when applied in the super pulse mode. As a result, it is quite effective when used to vaporize tissue. The beam may be passed through the open channel of the operative laparoscope or through an ancillary sleeve. The use of the wave guide for the CO_2 laser eliminates the need for centering the beam down the operative channel; articulation has been a problem with some laser equipment. The decreased capacity for coagulation and high degree of smoke production associated with the CO_2 laser are avoided with fiber lasers of lower wave length, such as Nd:YAG, KTP, and Argon (28). Nevertheless, these laser energy sources are associated with increased tissue damage (Fig. 11.7).

PERITONEAL ENDOMETRIOSIS

Superficial implants may be destroyed by bipolar cauterization; however, 25% of pa-

tients have lesions >5 mm in depth (100). Deep (>5 mm) and very deep (>10 mm) represent a very active form of the disease (25). Estimation of the depth of endometrial implants at the time of laparoscopic resection correlate well with histologic measurements. These very deep implants are typically found in the posterior cul-de-sac region near the uterosacral ligaments and have been demonstrated to occur almost exclusively in patients who complain of pain. Their destruction requires greater current penetration, best achieved with a pointed monopolar electrode or with carbon dioxide or fiber lasers. It is difficult to evaluate the depth of tissue damage with electrocauterization; laser vaporization allows visualization of the 3-dimensional boundaries of every lesion. The laser beam should be applied until the bubbling of retroperioneal areolar tissue is noted. CO_2 laser spot sizes from 0.4–2.5 mm, power settings of 5–20 W, and power densities of 2500–15,000 W/cm² may be used. In the region of the ureter, the urinary bladder, colon, or large blood vessels, single or repeat pulse mode of 0.05–0.1 seconds allows a depth of penetration of 100–200 μm. Irrigation of the pelvis will wash off debris and carbon deposition so as to better expose the base of the site of laser impact. An alternative technique is to excise the involved peritoneum. The lesions are isolated along with an island of peritoneum, lifted from the underlying structures, undermined, and excised (33,119).

In addition to direct visualization, the diagnosis of retroperitoneal endometriosis is suggested by preoperative digital rectovaginal palpation and laparoscopic blunt probe palpation. The laparoscopic treatment of this disease is often complicated by the close proximity of implants to vital structures such as the ureter, bladder, and vessels. The diseased peritoneum may be separated from the underlying tissue by a technique called hydrodissection, where irrigant is forcefully injected retroperitoneally through a small defect created in the peritoneum. This retroperitoneal placement of fluid acts to dissipate CO_2 laser energy, and in doing so, promotes safer dissection or vaporization of the peritoneal surface. Dissection of retroperitoneal disease may be facilitated by placing a bougie in the rectum and sponge forceps in the

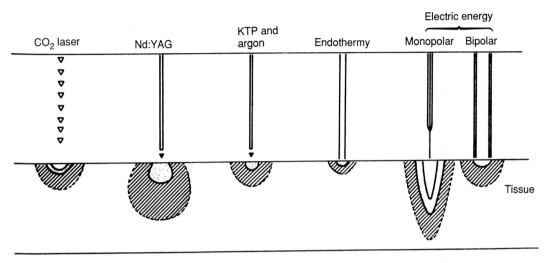

Irreversible thermal damage (tissue temperature of 60°-80°C)

Reversible thermal damage (tissue temperature of 40°-60°C)

Figure 11.7.   Relative tissue damage created by various energy sources.

vagina (Fig. 11.8). Traction in either direction will open the rectovaginal and perirectal spaces. Coagulation or vaporization of disease in the ovarian fossa or near the uterosacral ligament should be undertaken only after clear identification of the ureter (Fig. 11.9).

As noted previously, defects in the peritoneal surface are frequently associated with endometriosis and may be found in the posterior cul-de-sac region (24). The margins of the defect should be explored and vaporized even if they appear grossly normal, due to the frequency of microscopic disease. Injection of irrigant retroperitoneally will serve as a buffer for safe CO_2 laser vaporization. Superficial invasion of the muscularis of bowel or bladder may be ablated by laser vaporization. The minimal spread of the carbon dioxide laser energy makes it well suited for treatment of this disease.

ADHESIOLYSIS

The range of adhesions encountered in patients with endometriosis varies from transparent, avascular bands, to dense, cohesive adhesions that obliterate the tissue planes (133). The basic surgical maxim, to operate with minimal tissue trauma, applies to laparoscopic lysis of adhesions. Forceful blunt dissection should be avoided.

Transparent, avascular adhesions that approximate two structures may be lysed with scissors, laser, or forceful pressure of irrigant. Dense, cohesive adhesions must be treated by a combination of blunt and sharp dissection. Hemostasis is accomplished with bipolar or thermal coagulation. The use of surgical laser for adhesiolysis does offer the advantage of simultaneous coagulation of small capillaries during the tissue dissection.

As in the case of laparotomy, vital structures involved in the adhesion complex must be clearly identified prior to dissection. Ancillary suprapubic instruments may be necessary in order to optimally orient the tissue planes. Irrigant or a backstop may be used to absorb the beam energy and protect adjacent structures.

OVARIAN ENDOMETRIOMA RESECTION

Surgical treatment of endometriosis <3 cm in diameter may be accomplished with relative ease; however, endoscopic resection of larger lesions may be compromised due to the presence of concomitant adhesions as well as the difficulty encountered in removal of the entire cyst wall.

The endometrioma may be excised in an

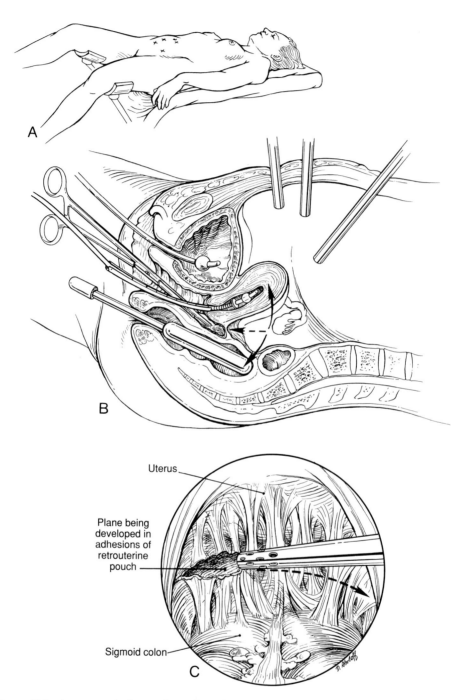

Figure 11.8. Laparoscopic therapy for endometriosis. *A,* Dorsal lithotomy positioning for surgery, with multiple puncture sites marked for placement of ancillary instruments. *B,* Traction on bougie in rectum and sponge forceps in vagina to mobilize rectovaginal and perirectal spaces. Uterine manipulation cannula, bladder drainage, and multiple transabdominal instruments facilitate safe dissection. *C,* CO_2 laser division of endometriosis-associated adhesions extending from lower uterus to rectal serosa, using laser wave guide.

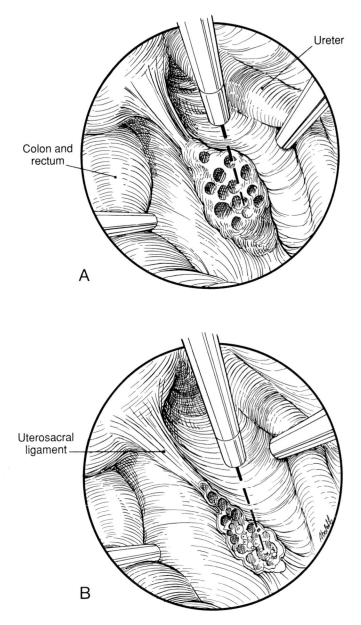

Figure 11.9. *A* and *B,* Laser vaporization of endometriotic implant of uterosacral ligament. The beam is applied until the lesion has been completely destroyed. The course of the ureter must be traced before initiation of surgical ablation.

intact or ruptured state. In either case, the procedure is initiated by incising the capsule overlying the endometrioma (Fig. 11.10). The cyst is drained, and the cavity is irrigated and inspected for papillary structures or other suspicious features. Small endometriomas may be effectively treated by laser vaporization of the mucosal lining. With larger endometriomas, the normal ovarian cortex is stabilized with atraumatic forceps, and the cyst wall is grasped with biopsy forceps and stripped from the bed of normal ovarian tissue with a twisting "corkscrew" maneuver. If difficulty is encountered in removal of the endometrioma due to friability or fibrosis, blunt and sharp dissection of the cyst from the ovarian capsule may be necessary. Remaining fragments of the cyst wall should be vaporized with laser or fulgurated with electro-

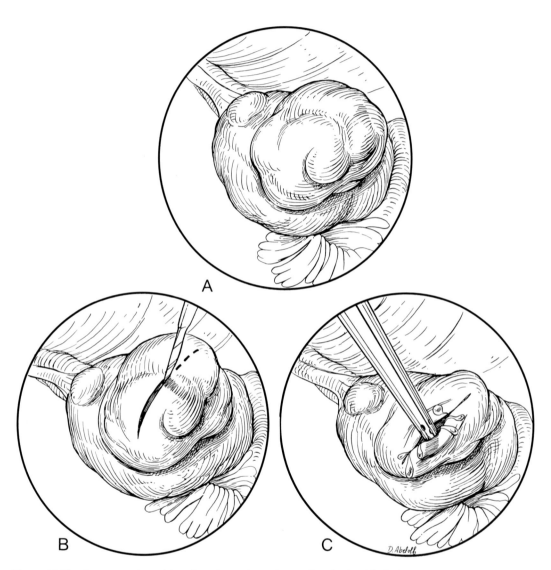

Figure 11.10. Laparoscopic excision of ovarian endometrioma <3 cm in size (*A*). *B*, A linear incision is made in the cortex overlying the cyst with the knife electrode or laser. *C*, The contents of the cyst are aspirated and the cavity is copiously irrigated. *D*, Vaporization of the mucosal lining of the endometrioma is carried out with a power setting of 25–30 W in a continuous mode application. *E*, and *F*, In the case of large cysts, interrupted sutures of 4-0 polydioxanone may be placed, using laparoscopic instruments to reapproximate the margins of the incision. Suturing is not required if the edges spontaneously overlap or lay in close approximation.

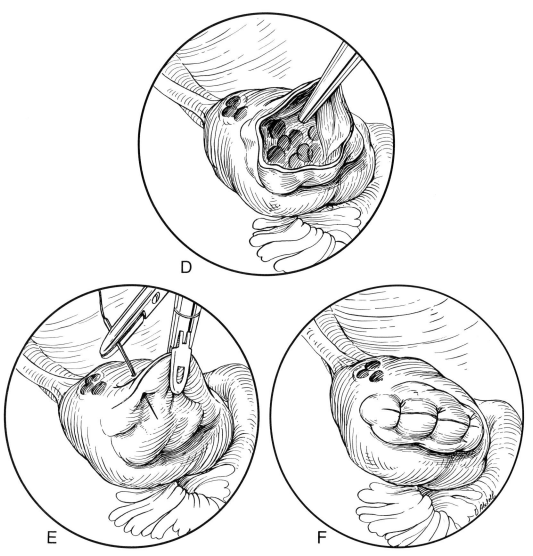

D

E

F

Figure 11.10. *Continued.*

cautery. Hemostasis may be achieved with bipolar cautery.

An alternative technique involves the use of sharp and blunt dissection to remove the cyst in an intact state. Hydrodissection may aid in separation of the tissue planes. The contents then may be drained in order to facilitate removal from the peritoneal cavity.

The ovarian defect may be left to heal spontaneously or may be reapproximated with interrupted sutures of 4-0 polydioxanone (Fig. 11.10E). An absorbable adhesion barrier may be applied to minimize the chance of postoperative adhesions to adjacent organs. Most authors have reported excellent results with this nonsuture technique (15).

If there is evidence of functional destruction of the ovary, or if the patient has chronic, incapacitating pelvic pain secondary to ovarian endometriosis and has completed her family, appropriate therapy may consist of oophorectomy. The infundibulopelvic and uteroovarian ligaments may be ligated with Roeder loop suture, bipolar coagulation, or surgical staples prior to excision of the structure. The ovary is retrieved by morcellation or via posterior colpotomy.

UTERINE NERVE ABLATION

Although the presacral neurectomy is highly successful in relieving midline pelvic pain in appropriately selected cases, the procedure requires a laparotomy and does not usually interrupt the nerve supply to the cervix. The technique of uterosacral neurectomy, initially described by Ruggi (151) and later popularized by Doyle (48), has been adapted for performance during laparoscopic procedures for the alleviation of dysmenorrhea.

Sympathetic fibers T10-L1, contained within the inferior hypogastric plexus, course along the inferior vena cava and sacrum to enter the uterus through the nerves of the uterosacral ligaments and accompanying uterine arteries. The parasympathetic components of the paracervical nerves originate from S1–S3 or S4, travel within the nervi erigentes, and emerge in the lateral pelvis to form Frankenhauser's ganglia lateral to the cervix. Division of the uterosacral ligaments at the point of their attachment to the cervix should lead to an interruption of most of the sensory nerve fibers of the cervix and some of the sensory fibers to the uterine corpus.

In general, laser uterine nerve ablation is preferred over an electrocautery technique due to the greater possibility of increased thermal damage with the latter. The course of the ureters and adjacent vasculature should be noted prior to commencement of dissection. The uterosacral ligaments are exposed by manipulating the uterine cannula to anteflex the corpus and by applying pressure to the posterior cervix with an ancillary laparoscopic probe.

The CO_2 laser is employed at 5,000–15,000 W/cm^2 to vaporize the uterosacral ligaments immediately adjacent to their attachments to the cervix. A 2–5 cm segment of each ligament should be vaporized to a depth of approximately 1 cm. The posterior aspect of the cervix between the insertion of the uterosacral ligaments may be superficially vaporized to interrupt the sensory fibers crossing to the contralateral side (31). Extension of the beam too far laterally or posteriorly may result in considerable bleeding; therefore, the surgeon should have immediate access to bipolar cautery, endocoagulation, and/or hemostatic clips. Deaths have occurred due to unrecognized hemorrhage following this procedure. Fiber lasers such as the KTP/532 offer the advantages of increased hemostasis and lack of carbon plume, as compared with the CO_2 instrument. If bipolar diathermy is used to fulgurate the uterosacral ligament, laparoscopic scissors are employed to excise the segment of ligament in question.

Feste (54,55) reported significant improvement in symptoms of primary dysmenorrhea or dysmenorrhea associated with endometriosis in 71% of his series of 42 women who underwent the procedure. In a similar series of 100 patients by Donnez (46), 50% experienced complete relief, 41% had mild-moderate relief, and 9% described no relief. Lichten and Bombard (92) published the only randomized, prospective double-blind study of laparoscopic uterosacral nerve ablation for treatment of severe or incapacitating dysmenorrhea unresponsive to oral contraceptives and nonsteroidal anti-inflammatory agents. None of the control patients noted improvement, whereas 9 of 11 in the treated group had almost complete relief at 3 months and 5 of 11 described complete relief from dysmenorrhea 1 year after surgery. This success is achieved via a procedure that takes 5 minutes to perform.

COMBINATION HORMONAL - SURGICAL THERAPY

Both preoperative and postoperative medical therapies have been proposed to enhance fertility in patients undergoing conservative resection of endometriosis (18,32,86). Preoperative suppression of disease with hormonal agents may facilitate the surgical procedure due to reduced tissue vascularity; moreover, the greater ease in tissue dissection may decrease adhesion formation during the postoperative period (26). Initiation of medical therapy following the surgical procedure may inhibit the activity of any residual disease. Nevertheless, the use of medications as part of the treatment of endometriosis-associated infertility results in a time span of several months during which the patient is unable to attempt conception. The utility of such combined therapy has not been shown to be efficacious in less advanced stages of disease (130).

Danazol and GnRHa therapy may decrease the size of larger endometriomas, but they do not cause a complete resolution of such disease (11). Wheeler and Malinak (189) demonstrated an improved pregnancy rate with danazol treatment in the immediate postlaparotomy period in patients with severe endometriosis as compared with patients who were treated with surgery alone. Nevertheless, in Buttram's 1985 (18) series, the conception rate

Table 11.6.   Conservative Surgery for Mild Endometriosis[a]

Author, year[b]	No. Pregnant/ No. Treated	%	Cycle Fecundity Rate
Acosta et al., 1973	6/8	75%	
Hammond et al., 1976	2/3	67%	
García, David, 1977	2/3	67%	
Schenken, Malinak, 1978	11/34	32%	
Buttram, 1979	61/88	69%	
Rock et al., 1981b[c]	28/45	62%	0.022
Schenken, Malinak, 1982	32/42	76%	
Rantala et al., 1983	26/44	59%	
Gordts et al., 1984[c]	8/20	40%	
Olive, Lee, 1986	5/11	46%	0.039
Totals	181/298	61%	

[a]Adapted from Olive DL: In: Schenken RS, ed. Conservative surgery in endometriosis. Philadelphia: JB Lippincott 1989;239.
[b]All used staging system of Acosta et al., except where indicated.
[c]AFS staging system.

for severe disease treated with conservative surgery followed by a 6-month course of danazol was only 32% (7 of 22); this compared with a 40% rate when surgery alone was used (historical control). Andrews and Larsen (5) have noted that the best chance for postsurgical conception occurs within the first 6 months after conservative surgery via laparotomy. Thus, suppressing ovulation during that critical period may actually reduce the chance of pregnancy. Preoperative danazol therapy has been shown to lead to a slight improvement in fecundity rates as compared with sole surgical therapy (18), although these results have been questioned due to the lack of randomization of subjects into treatment groups. Hence, the efficacy of combination therapy in the treatment of endometriosis-associated infertility remains controversial.

SURGICAL OUTCOME

Although the older classification schedules for endometriosis do not provide an accurate correlation between extent of disease and pregnancy rate, and the utility of the revised AFS classification is still being determined, such categorization does provide a framework in which to report the outcome of therapy. The crude pregnancy rate following conservative surgery for mild endometriosis via laparoscopy is 61% (Table 11.6); this approximates the 74% rate derived from an accumulated series of patients with minimal and mild endometriosis treated by CO_2 laser laparoscopy (Table 11.7). The results of electrical thermal coagulation of all stages of disease are presented in Table 11.8.

Table 11.7. CO_2 Laser Laparoscopy: Endometriosis As an Isolated Factor[a]

Author	All Patients		Minimal/Mild		Moderate		Severe/Extensive	
	Number	Pregnant	Number	Pregnant	Number	Pregnant	Number	Pregnant
Feste	60	42 (70%)	44	31 (70%)	14	10 (71%)	2	1 (50%)
Martin	34	23 (67%)	13	9 (69%)	11	6 (55%)	10	8 (80%)
Nezhat	102	65 (64%)	24	18 (75%)	51	32 (63%)	27	15 (56%)
Paulsen	228	169 (74%)	140	109 (78%)	88	60 (68%)	0	0 (%)
Gast	27	7 (26%)	NA[b]		NA		0	0 (%)
Adamson	60	39 (65%)	47	31 (66%)	11	7 (61%)	2	0 (%)
Nezhat	243	168 (69%)	39	28 (72%)	86	60 (70%)	118	80 (68%)
Total	754	513 (68%)	307	226 (74%)	261	175 (67%)	159	104 (65%)

[a]Adapted from Martin DC: Laparoscopic appearance of endometriosis, vol. I, second edition, Memphis: The Resurge Press, with permission.
[b]NA = not available.

Murphy et al. (115), using life-table analysis and the two parameter exponential method, studied 72 patients with Stage I or Stage II endometriosis who underwent laparoscopic electrocoagulation of endometrial implants. They reported a crude pregnancy rate of 74% for Stage I and 57% for stage II during an average follow-up period of 7.9 months. The estimated cure rates using the two parameter model were 98.2% for Stage I and 76.6% for Stage II; however, the monthly fecundity rates for these treated subjects was only 10.3% for Stage I and 7.59% for Stage II. Expectant management of mild to moderate endometriosis after its diagnosis by laparoscopy yields a crude pregnancy rate of approximately 50%; hence, surgical therapy of lesser stages of disease may not promote fertility, although the interval to conception may be possibly shortened. The lack of a definitive, prospective, randomized controlled study that includes an expectant management group impairs data interpretation. Certainly, the value of conservative surgery via laparotomy for milder stages of disease is suspect.

The operative treatment of more extensive disease does result in a greater likelihood of conception than expectant management (129) (Tables 11.9 and 11.10). This may be due in part to a correction of mechanical factors, such as adhesions. Only a small number of series (Table 11.9) have been published regarding the

use of laser laparoscopy in this patient population. Expert endoscopists have reported results that appear to be as good as those obtained through the open abdomen, although there are no data available that directly compare the two surgical modalities. The lack of difference in pregnancy rates among the various stages of

Table 11.9.   Conservative Surgery for Moderate Endometriosis[a]

Author, Year[b]	No. Pregnant/ No. Treated	%	Cycle Fecundity Rate
Acosta et al., 1973	30/60	50%	
Hammond et al., 1976	3/5	60%	
García, David, 1977	7/19	37%	
Sadigh et al., 1977	17/23	74%	
Schenken, Malinak, 1978	12/36	33%	
Buttram, 1979	28/50	56%	
Rock et al., 1981b[c]	48/88	55%	0.020
Rantala et al., 1983	22/39	56%	
Gordts et al., 1984[c]	42/99	42%	
Olive, Lee, 1986	22/43	51%	0.039
Totals	231/462	50%	

[a]Adapted from Olive DL: In: Schenken RS, ed. Conservative surgery in endometriosis. Philadelphia: JB Lippincott 1989;239.
[b]All used staging system of Acosta et al. except where indicated.
[c]AFS staging system.

Table 11.10.   Conservative Surgery for Severe Endometriosis[a]

Author, Year	No. Pregnant/ No. Treated	%	Cycle Fecundity Rate
Acosta et al., 1973	13/39	33%	
Hammond et al., 1976	0/2	0%	
García, David, 1977	14/49	29%	
Sadigh et al., 1977	20/42	48%	
Schenken, Malinak, 1978	6/21	29%	
Buttram, 1979	32/68	47%	
Rock et al., 1981b[b]	39/81	48%	0.020
Rantala et al., 1983	18/46	39%	
Gordts et al., 1984[c]	20/57	35%	
Olive, Lee, 1986	10/34	29%	0.039
Totals	127/439	39%	

[a]Adapted from Olive DL: In: Schenken RS, ed. Conservative surgery in endometriosis. Philadelphia: JB Lippincott 1989;239.
[b]All used staging system of Acosta et al. except where indicated.
[c]AFS staging system.

Table 11.8.   Laparoscopic Electrical Thermal Coagulation[a]

Author	Patients	Follow-up	Pregnancies
Eward, 1978	25	1–2 yrs	14 (56%)
Hasson et al., 1979	8	1–4 yrs	6 (75%)
Mettler et al., 1979	90	1–6 yrs	22 (24%)
Sulewski et al., 1980	100	1–5 yrs	40 (40%)
Daniell and Christianson, 1981	60	1–2 yrs	34 (57%)
Seiler et al., 1986	45	7 mos	20 (44%)
Reich and McGlynn, 1986	20	1–7 yrs	12 (60%)
Nowroozi et al., 1987	69	8 mos	42 (61%)
Pouly et al., 1987	52	4–30 mos	30 (57.7%)
Murphy et al., 1990	53	1–14 yrs	31 (58%)
Total	530		251 (47%)

[a]Adapted from Martin DC: Laparoscopic appearance of endometriosis, vol. 1, second edition. Memphis: Resurge Press, with permission.

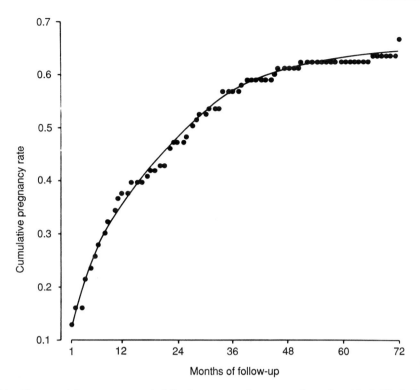

Figure 11.11. The cumulative pregnancy rate following conservative surgery for endometriosis (Rock et al., 1981).

endometriosis treated through laser laparoscopy is noteworthy.

Results of life-table analysis have demonstrated that pregnancy will most likely occur within the first 36 months following surgery (Fig. 11.11). Disease progression is possible in those who remain infertile. Rock et al. (150) have shown that 13.5% of patients initially treated with conservative surgery required subsequent operative procedures. Furthermore, Wheeler and Malinak (190) noted a cumulative recurrence rate at 3 and 5 years of 13.5 and 40.3%, respectively, after conservative surgery. Neither the initial staging nor the ability to conceive following the initial surgery had a significant effect on the recurrence.

Surgery offers a more prompt, complete, and long-term relief of pain symptoms associated with endometriosis than the various medical regimens available. Definitive surgery for endometriosis in patients with persistent symptoms involves removal of the uterus with or without the adnexae. The chance of pain recurrence following hysterectomy with conservation of normal ovaries is only approximately 3%.

ASSISTED REPRODUCTIVE TECHNOLOGIES

If spontaneous conception is not achieved within 3 years of surgical resection of endometriosis or within 1 year following repair of tubal obstruction associated with endometriosis, the odds are poor that it will ever occur (150,162). Techniques in assisted reproduction have been widely employed during the past decade for the management of endometriosis-associated infertility unresponsive to cytoreductive surgical and/or hormonal therapy. Twenty-five to 35% of women undergoing in-vitro fertilization/embryo transfer (IVF/ET) have endometriosis as their sole identifiable cause for infertility. Oehninger et al. (125), in a review of the IVF/ET experience of the Jones Institute for Reproductive Medicine, noted that the responses to gonadotropin stimulation, numbers of preovulatory oocytes, fertilization and cleavage rates, and clinical pregnancy rates in endometriosis patients were comparable to those of patients with tubal disease and unexplained infertility. However, the miscarriage rate was significantly higher in women with moderate or severe endometriosis, perhaps due to poor embryo quality. Consequently, the per cycle and per transfer ongoing pregnancy rates were lower in the more advanced stages of disease, although the differences did not attain statistical significance.

In a 1986 study by Wardle et al. (186), oocyte fertilization rates were reduced markedly in women with untreated endometriosis, as compared with endometriosis patients treated with danazol for 6–9 months prior to IVF attempt and tubal infertility controls. Nevertheless, requirement of prior endometriosis therapy before resorting to assisted reproductive technologies remains controversial. Hulme et al. (78) performed gamete intrafallopian transfer (GIFT) on 46 infertile patients with minimal to moderate active endometriosis who had not been treated by medical or surgical methods. The only prerequisite of the investigators was patency of at least one fallopian tube. The pregnancy rate per GIFT cycle was 30.5% (18/59); this compared with a clinical pregnancy rate of 25.8% for *all* patients undergoing the procedure at their unit. In 11 patients, one or more endometriomas were aspirated from the ovaries at the time of follicle aspiration; four of these patients achieved live births from the GIFT. GIFT may overcome impairment of sperm transport to the fallopian tube, failed ovum capture, or abnormalities in the peritoneal environment associated with endometriosis.

Controlled ovarian stimulation with exogenous gonadotropins in conjunction with intrauterine insemination (hMG/IUI) has been proposed as a method to increase cycle fecundity of patients with endometriosis (42), although few series have been published to date. By increasing the number of oocytes released at the time of ovulation and introducing a high concentration of spermatozoa into the female reproductive tract, the chance for conception may be improved merely due to the larger number of gametes available for fertilization. In addition, subtle abnormalities of folliculogenesis, corpus luteum function, tubal motility, or sperm function may be corrected with this therapy. Dodson et al. (42) reported the occurrence of six pregnancies in 15 cycles initiated in women with AFS Stage I endometriosis, yielding a fecundity rate of 0.40. Results were less favorable for women with advanced stages of disease. Hurst et al. (79) achieved four pregnancies in 17 cycles (fecundity 0.24) through hMG/IUI in this treatment group. The overall cycle fecundity of couples undergoing hMG/IUI with infertility associated with endometriosis in the absence of obstructed oviducts was 0.17 in Dodson's series (42), a figure greater than that previously reported in studies of untreated couples with endometriosis or that described following hormonal or surgical therapy (127).

CONCLUSION

Many factors must be considered in selecting the appropriate therapy for the patient with endometriosis, including the symptoms, physical signs of disease, age of the individual, and desire for future childbearing. Surgery is indicated in cases of large endometriomas, symptomatic adhesions, and partial obstruction of the bowel or urinary tract. A greater range of options is available for the management of lesser amounts of disease.

All other potential factors for infertility should be excluded in the woman with endometriosis. Young patients with minimal and mild disease may be followed expectantly if the time interval of attempting conception has been brief. At present, operative laparoscopy, conservative laparotomy, and hormonal suppression are empiric treatments, since there are no well-controlled studies that conclusively justify their use. Assisted reproductive technologies should be considered in those patients who remain infertile.

Surgical therapy of advanced stages of disease in the infertile population does improve the conception rate over mere observation; the outcome may be enhanced by preoperative hormonal therapy. In-vitro fertilization and, in some circumstances, gamete intrafallopian transfer are important treatment options in the woman who has failed to conceive, despite surgical reconstruction.

Pain treatment unresponsive to analgesics may be treated medically or surgically. Conservative resection of disease via laparoscopy or laparotomy leads to a more prolonged course of remission than medical therapy; in addition, the presacral neurectomy procedure effectively relieves midline pelvic pain. A hysterectomy with or without oophorectomy may be considered, depending upon the patient's age and desire for future childbearing.

Significant progress has been made during the past decade in our understanding of the pathophysiology of endometriosis. Future therapies may arise as additional insights are gained into the role of the immune system in the development of endometriosis and its effect on factors that may influence fecundity.

References

1. Acosta AA, Buttram VC, Bresch PK, et al: A proposed classification of pelvic endometriosis. Obstet Gynecol 1973;42:19.
2. Adamson GD, Lu J, Suback LL: Laparoscopic CO_2 laser vaporization of endometriosis compared with traditional treatments. Fertil Steril 1989;51:237.
3. American Fertility Society: Revised American Fertility Society Classification of Endometriosis: 1985. Fertil Steril 1985;43:351.
4. American Fertility Society. The Classification of Endometriosis. Fertil Steril 1979;32:633.
5. Andrews WE, Larsen GD: Endometriosis: treatment with hormonal pseudopregnancy and/or operation. Am J Obstet Gynecol 1974;118:643.
6. Awadalla SG, Friedman CI, Haq AU, et al: Local peritoneal factors: their role in infertility associated with endometriosis. Am J Obstet Gynecol 1987;157:1207.
7. Ayers JWT, Birenbaum DL, Menon KMJ: Luteal phase dysfunction in endometriosis elevated progesterone levels in peripheral and ovarian veins during the follicular phase. Fertil Steril 1987;47:925.
8. Badawy SZA, Cuenca V, Kaufman L, et al: The regulation of immunoglobulin production by B cells in patients with endometriosis. Fertil Steril 1989;51:770.
9. Barbieri RL, Niloff JM, Bast RC Jr, et al: Elevated serum concentrations of CA-125 in patients with advanced endometriosis. Fertil Steril 1986;45:630.
10. Barbieri RL, Ryan KJ: Danazol—Endocrine pharmacology and therapeutic applications. Am J Obstet Gynecol 1981;141:453.
11. Biberoglu KO, Behrman SJ: Dosage aspects of danazol therapy in endometriosis: short term and long term effectiveness. Am J Obstet Gynecol 1981;138:645.
12. Black WT, Jr: Use of presacral sympathectomy in the treatment of dysmenorrhea. Obstet Gynecol 1964;9:16.
13. Bronsens IA, Konickx PR, Corveleyn PA: A study of plasma progesterone, oestradiol-17 β, prolactin and LH levels and of the luteal phase appearance of the ovaries in patients with endometriosis and infertility. Br J Obstet Gynaecol 1978;85:246.
14. Bronsens I, Vasquez G, Gordts S: Scanning electron microscopy study of the pelvic peritoneum in unexplained infertility and endometriosis. Fertil Steril 1984;41:215.
15. Brumsted JR, Deaton J, Lavigne E, et al: Postoperative adhesion formation after ovarian wedge resection with and without ovarian reconstruction in the rabbit. Fertil Steril 1990;53:723.
16. Buttram VC Jr: Surgical treatment of endometriosis in the infertile female: a modified approach. Fertil Steril 1979;32:635.
17. Buttram VC Jr: Conservative surgery for endometriosis in the infertile female: a study of 206 patients with implications for both medical and surgical therapy. Fertil Steril 1979;31:117.
18. Buttram VC Jr, Reifer RC, Ward S: Treatment of endometriosis with danazol: report of a 6 year prospective study. Fertil Steril 1985;43:353.
19. Candiani GB, Vercellini P, Fedele L: Laparoscopic ovarian puncture for correct staging of endometriosis. Fertil Steril 1990;53:994.
20. Carpenter SE, Markham SM, Rock JA: Exercise may reduce side effects of danazol. Infertility 1988;2:259.
21. Cedars MI, Lu JKH, Meldrum DR, et al: Treatment of endometriosis with a long-acting gonadotropin releasing hormone agonist plus medroxyprogesterone acetate. Obstet Gynecol 1900;75:641.
22. Chacho KJ, Andreson PJ, Scommegna A: The effect of peritoneal macrophage incubates on the spermatozoa assay. Fertil Steril 1987;48:694.
23. Chatman DL: Pelvic peritoneal defects and endometriosis; Allen-Masters syndrome revisited. Fertil Steril 1981;36:751.
24. Chatman DL, Zbella EA: Pelvic peritoneal defects and endometriosis: further observations. Fertil Steril 1986;46:711.
25. Cornillie FJ, Oosterlynck D, Lauweryns JM, et al: Deeply infiltrating pelvic endometriosis: histology and clinical significance. Fertil Steril 1989;53:978.
26. Corfman RS, Grainger DA: Endometriosis-associated infertility. Treatment options. J Reprod Med 1989;34:135.
27. Coronado C, Franklin RR, Lotze EC, et al: Surgical treatment of symptomatic colorectal endometriosis. Fertil Steril 1990;53:411.
28. Corson SL, Unger M, Kwa D, et al: Laparoscopic laser treatment of endometriosis with the Nd:YAG sapphire probe. Am J Obstet Gynecol 1989;160:718.
29. Czernobilsky B, Silverstein A: Salpingitis in ovarian endometriosis. Fertil Steril 1978;30:45.
30. Damewood M.D, Hesla JS, Schlaff WD, et al: Effect of serum from patients with minimal to mild endometriosis on mouse embryo development in vitro. Fertil Steril 1990;54:917.
31. Daniell JF: Fiberoptic laser laparoscopy. Baillieres Clin Obstet Gynaecol 1989;3:545.

32. Daniell JF, Christianson C: Combined laparoscopic surgery and danazol therapy for pelvic endometriosis. Fertil Steril 1981;35:521.

33. Davis GD, Brooks RA: Excision of pelvic endometriosis with the carbon dioxide laser laparoscope. Obstet Gynecol 1988;72:816.

34. Dawood MY, Kahn-Dawood FS, Wilson L Jr: Peritoneal fluid prostaglandins and prostanoids in women with endometriosis, chronic pelvic inflammatory disease, and pelvic pain. Am J Obstet Gynecol 1984; 148:391.

35. DeLeon FD, Vijayakumar R, Brown M, et al: Peritoneal fluid volume, estrogen, progesterone, prostaglandin, and epidermal growth factor concentrations in patients with and without endometriosis. Obstet Gynecol 1896;68:189.

36. diZerega G, Hodgen G: Endometriosis: role of ovarian steroids in initiation, maintenance, and suppression. Fertil Steril 1980a;33:649.

37. Dmowski WP: Pitfalls in clinical, laparoscopic and histologic diagnosis of endometriosis. Acta Obstet Gynecol Scand Suppl 1984;123:61.

38. Dmowski WP, Cohen MR: Treatment of endometriosis with an antigonadotropin, danazol. A laparoscopic and histologic evaluation. Obstet Gynecol 1975; 46:147.

39. Dmowski WP, Radwanska E, Binor Z, et al: Mild endometriosis and ovulatory dysfunction: effect of danazol treatment on success of ovulation induction. Fertil Steril 1986;46:784.

40. Dmowski WP, Steele RW, Baker GF: Deficient cellular immunity in endometriosis. Am J Obstet Gynecol 1981;141:377.

41. Döberl A, Berquist A, Jeppson S, et al: Regression of endometriosis following the shorter treatment with, or lower dose of danazol. Acta Obstet Gynecol Scand Suppl 1984;123:51.

42. Dodson WC, Whitesides DB, Hughes CL Jr, et al: Superovulation with intrauterine insemination in the treatment of infertility: a possible alternative to gamete intrafallopian transfer and in vitro fertilization. Fertil Steril 1987;48:441.

43. Donnez J, Nisolle-Pochet M: Appearance of peritoneal endometriosis. In: Proceedings of the Eleventh International Laser Surgery Symposium. Brussels, 1988.

44. Donnez J, Nisolle-Pochet M, Clerckx-Braun F, et al: Administration of nasal buserelin as compared with subcutaneous buserelin implant for endometriosis. Fertil Steril 1989;52:27.

45. Donnez J, Thomas K: Incidence of luteinized unruptured follicle syndrome in fertile women and in women with endometriosis. Eur J Obstet Gynecol Reprod Biol 1982;14:187.

46. Donnez J, Nicolle M: CO$_2$ laser laparoscopic surgery. Adhesiolysis, salpingostomy, laser uterine nerve ablations and tubal pregnancy. Baillieres Clin Obstet Gynaecol 1989;3:525.

47. Doody MC, Gibbons WE, Buttram VC: Linear regression analysis of ultrasound follicular growth series: evidence for an abnormality of follicular growth in endometriosis patients. Fertil Steril 1988; 49:47.

48. Doyle JB: Paracervical uterine denervation by transection of the cervical plexus for the relief of dysmenorrhea. Am J Obstet Gynecol 1955;70:11.

49. Drake TS, O'Brien WF, Ramwell PW, et al: Peritoneal fluid thromboxane B$_2$ 6-keto-prostaglandin F$_{1\alpha}$ in endometriosis. Am J Obstet Gynecol 1981;140:401.

50. Evers, JLH: The second look laparoscopy for evaluation of the results of medical treatment of endometriosis should not be performed during ovarian suppression. Fertil Steril 1987;47:502.

51. Eward RD: Cauterization of stage I and II endometriosis and resulting pregnancy rate. In: Phillips JM, ed. Endoscopy and gynecology. American Association of Gynecologic Laparoscopists, Downey, California, 1978;276.

52. Fakih H, Baggett B, Holtz G, et al: Interleukin-1: a possible role in the infertility associated with endometriosis. Fertil Steril 1987;47:218.

53. Fedele L, Parazzini F, Bianchi S, et al: Stage and localization of pelvic endometriosis and pain. Fertil Steril 1990;53:155.

54. Feste JR: Endoscopic laser surgery in gynecology. In: Reproductive Surgery. Postgraduate Course Syllabus. American Fertility Society, Chicago, 1985.

55. Feste JR: Laser laparoscopy. A new modality. J Reprod Med 1985;30:413.

56. Forrest J, Buckley CH, Fox H: Pelvic endometriosis and tubal inflamatory disease. Int J Gynecol Pathol 1984;3:343.

57. Franssen AMHW, Kaver FM, Rolland R, et al: The effect of LHRH agonist therapy in the treatment of endometriosis (Dutch experience). Prog Clin Biol Res 1986;225:201.

58. García C-R, David SS: Pelvic endometriosis: Infertility and pelvic pain. Am J Obstet Gynecol 1977; 129:740.

59. Gast MJ, Tobler R, Strickler RC, et al: Laser vaporization of endometriosis in an infertile population: the role of complicating infertility factors. Fertil Steril 1988;50:704.

60. Glatt AE, Zinner SH, McCormack WM: The prevalence of dyspareunia. Obstet Gynecol 1990;75:433.

61. Gleicher N, El-Roeiy A, Confino E, et al: Is endometriosis an autoimmune disease? Obstet Gynecol 1987; 70:115.

62. Gordts S, Boeckx W, Brosens I: Microsurgery in endometriosis in fertile patients. Fertil Steril 1984; 42:520.

63. Greenblatt RB, Dmowski WP, Mahesh VB, et al: Clinical studies with an antigonadotropin danazol. Fertil Steril 1971;22:102.

64. Gruenwald P: Origin of endometriosis from the mesenchyme of the coelomic walls. Am J Obstet Gynecol 1942;44:470.

65. Guzick DS: Clinical epidemiology of endometriosis and infertility. Obstet Gynecol Clin N A 1989;16:43.

66. Guzick DS, Rock JA: Estimation of a model of cumulative pregnancy following infertility therapy. Am J Obstet Gynecol 1981;140:573.

67. Halban J: Hysteroadenosis metastatica: die lymphongene genese der sog. adenofibromatosis heterotopica. Archiv Gynakologie 1925;124:457.

68. Halme J, Hammond MG, Hulka JF, et al: Retrograde menstruation in healthy women and in patients with endometriosis. Obstet Gynecol 1984;64:151.

69. Halme J, White C, Kauma S, et al: Peritoneal macrophages from patients with endometriosis release growth factor activity in vitro. J Clin Endocrinol Metab 1988;66:1044.

70. Hammond CB, Rock JA, Parker RT: Conservative treatment of endometriosis: the effects of limited surgery and hormonal pseudopregnancy. Fertil Steril 1976;27:756.

71. Hamod K, Rock JA: Pain relief following presacral neurectomy in women with endometriosis. Unpublished data, 1982.

72. Hasson HM: Electrocoagulation of pelvic endometriotic lesions with laparoscopic control. Am J Obstet Gynecol 1979;132:115.

73. Henzl MR, Corson SL, Moghissi K, et al: Administration of nasal nafarelin as compared with oral danazol for endometriosis. N Engl J Med 1988;318:485.

74. Hernandez E, Sapp K, Rock JA: Danazol in the treatment of recurrent or persistent endometriosis: a preliminary report. Infertility 1981;4:29.

75. Houston DE, Noller RL, Melton LJ, III, et al: Incidence of pelvic endometriosis in Rochester, Minnesota, 1970–1979. Am J Epidemiol 1987;125:959.

76. Hill JA, Faris HMP, Schiff I, et al: Characterization of leukocyte subpopulations in the peritoneal fluid of women with endometriosis. Fertil Steril 1988;50:216.

77. Hull ME, Moghissi KS, Magyar DF, et al: Comparison of different treatment modalities of endometriosis in infertile women. Fertil Steril 1987;47:40.

78. Hulme VA, van der Merwe JP, Kruger TF: Gamete intrafallopian transfer as treatment for infertility associated with endometriosis. Fertil Steril 1990;53:1095.

79. Hurst BS, Tjaden BL, Kimball A, et al: Superovulation with or without intrauterine insemination for the treatment of infertility. Pacific Coast Fertility Society 38th Annual Meeting, 1990 (abstr).

80. Jänne O, Kauppila A, Kukko E, et al: Estrogen and progestin receptors in endometriosis lesions: comparison with endometrial tissue. Am J Obstet Gynecol 1981;141:562.

81. Jansen RP, Russell P: Nonpigmented endometriosis: clinical, laparoscopic, and pathologic definition. Am J Obstet Gynecol 1986;155:1154.

82. Jeffcoate TA: Principles of gynecology. London: Butterworth, 1975.

83. Jenkins S, Olive DL, Haney AF: Endometriosis: pathogenetic implications of the anatomic distribution. Obstet Gynecol 1986;67:335.

84. Jones HW, Jr, Rock JA: Regulation of female infertility. In: E. Diczfalusy, ed. Regulation of human fertility. Moscow: WHO Symposium, 1976. Scriptor, Copenhagen, 1977;181.

85. Katayama KP, Manuel J, Jones HW Jr, et al: Methytestosterone treatment of infertility associated with pelvic endometriosis. Fertil Steril 1976;27:83.

86. Kettel LM, Murphy AA: Combination medical and surgical therapy for infertile patients with endometriosis. Obstet Gynecol Clin N Amer 1989;16:167.

87. Killick S, Elstein M: Pharmacologic production of luteinized unruptured follicles by prostaglandin synthetase inhibitors. Fertil Steril 1987;47:773.

88. Kistner RW, Siegler AM, Behrman SJ: Suggested classification for endometriosis: relation to infertility. Fertil Steril 1977;28:1008.

89. Koninckx P, Ide P, Vandenbroucke W, Brosens I: New aspects of the pathophysiology of endometriosis and associated infertility. J Reprod Med 1980;24:257.

90. Lamb K, Hoffman RG, Nichols TR: Family trait analysis: a case-control study of 43 women with endometriosis and their best friends. Am J Obstet Gynecol 1986;154:596.

91. Lemay A, Maheux R, Faure N, et al: Reversible hypogonadism induced by a luteinizing hormone-releasing hormone (LH-RH) agonist (Buserelin) as a new therapeutic approach for endometriosis. Fertil Steril 1984;41:863.

92. Lichten EM, Bombard J: Surgical treatment of primary dysmenorrhea with laparoscopic uterine nerve ablation. J Reprod Med 1987;32:37.

93. Luciano AA, Hauser KS, Davis WA, et al: Effects of danazol on plasma lipids and lipoprotein levels in healthy women and in women with endometriosis. Am J Obstet Gynecol 1983;145:422.

94. Luciano AA, Turksoy RN, Carleo J: Evaluation of oral medroxyprogesterone acetate in the treatment of endometriosis. Obstet Gynecol 1988;72:323.

95. McArthur JW, Ulfelder H: The effect of pregnancy upon endometriosis. Obstet Gynecol Survey 1965;20:709.

96. Mahmood TA, Templeton A: Pathophysiology of mild endometriosis: review of literature. Hum Reprod 1990;5:765–784.

97. Markham SM, Carpenter SE, Rock JA: Extrapelvic endometriosis. Obstet Gynecol Clin North Am 1989;16:193.

98. Martin DC: CO_2 laser laparoscopy for endometriosis associated with infertility. J Reprod Med 1986;31:1089.

99. Martin DC, Diamond MP: Operative laparoscopy: Comparison of lasers with other techniques. Curr Prob Obstet Gynecol Fertil 1986;9:564.

100. Martin DC, Hubert GD, Levy BS: Depth of infiltration of endometriosis. J Gynecol Surg 1989a;5:55.

101. Martin DC, Hubert GD, Vander Zwaag R, et al: Laparoscopic appearances of peritoneal endometriosis. Fertil Steril 1989b;51:63.

102. Martin DC, Vander Zwaag R: Excisional techniques for endometriosis with the CO_2 laser laparoscope. J Reprod Med 1987;32:753.

103. Meldrum DR, Chang RJ, Lu J, et al: "Medical oophorectomy" using a long-acting GnRH agonist—a possible new approach to the treatment of

endometriosis. J Clin Endocrinol Metab 1982; 54:1081.

104. Mettler L, Giesel H, Semm K: Treatment of female infertility due to obstruction by operative laparoscopy. Fertil Steril 1979;32:384.

105. Metzger DA, Olive DL, Stohs GF, et al: Association of endometriosis and spontaneous abortion: effect of control group selection. Fertil Steril 1986;45:18.

106. Meyer R: Uber entzundliche neterotope epithelwucherungen im weiblichen genetalgibrete under uber eine bis in die wurzel des mesocolon ausgedehnte benigne wurcherung dis darmepitheb. Virchow's Arch Pathol Anat 1909;195:487.

107. Moen M, Bratlie A, Moen T: Distribution of HLA antigens among patients with endometriosis. Acta Obstet Gynecol Scand Suppl 1984;123:25.

108. Moghissi KS, Boyce CRK: Management of endometriosis with oral medroxyprogesterone acetate. Obstet Gynecol 1976;47:265.

109. Moore EE, Harger JH, Rock JA, et al: Management of pelvic endometriosis with low-dose danazol. Fertil Steril 1981;36:15.

110. Moore JG, Binstock MA, Growdon WA: The clinical implications of retroperitoneal endometriosis. Am J Obstet Gynecol 1988;158:1291.

111. Moore JG, Hibbard LT, Growdon WA, Schifrin BS: Urinary tract endometriosis: enigmas in diagnosis and management. Am J Obstet Gynecol 1979; 134:162–172.

112. Morcos RN, Gibbons WE, Findlay WE: Effect of peritoneal fluid on in vitro cleavage of 2-cell mouse embryos: possible role in infertility associated with endometriosis. Fertil Steril 1985;44: 678.

113. Murphy AA, Green WR, Bobbie D, et al: Unsuspected endometriosis documented by scanning electron microscopy in visually normal peritoneum. Fertil Steril 1986;46:522.

114. Murphy AA, Guzick DS, Rock JA: Microscopic peritoneal endometriosis. (Letter to the Editor). Fertil Steril 1989;51:1072.

115. Murphy AA, Schlaff WD, Hassiakos D, et al: Laparoscopic cautery in the treatment of endometriosis-related infertility. Fertil Steril 1991;55:246.

116. Muscato JJ, Haney AF, Weinberg JB: Sperm phagocytosis by human peritoneal macrophages: a possible cause of infertility in endometriosis. Am J Obstet Gynecol 1982;144:503.

117. Nezhat C, Crowgey SR: Surgical treatment of endometriosis via laser laparoscopy. Fertil Steril 1986;45:778.

118. Nezhat C, Crowgey SR, Nezhat F: Videolaseroscopy for the treatment of endometriosis associated with infertility. Fertil Steril 1989;51:237.

119. Nezhat C, Nezhat FR: Safe laser endoscopic excision or vaporization of peritoneal endometriosis. Fertil Steril 1989;52:149.

120. Nezhat CR, Nezhat FR, Metzger DA, et al: Adhesion reformation after reproductive surgery by videolaseroscopy. Fertil Steril 1990;53:1008.

121. Noble AD, Letchworth AT: Medical treatment of endometriosis: a comparative trial. Postgrad Med J 1979;55:37.

122. Novak E: Significance of uterine mucosa in fallopian tubes with discussion of origin of aberrant endometrium. Am J Obstet Gynecol 1926;12:484.

123. Nowroozi K, Chase JS, Check JH, et al: The importance of laparoscopic coagulation of mild endometriosis in infertile women. Int J Fertil 1987; 32:442.

124. Oak MK, Chantler EN, Williams CA, et al: Sperm survival studies in peritoneal fluid from infertile women with endometriosis and unexplained infertility. Clin Reprod Fertil 1985;3:297.

125. Oehninger S, Acosta AA, Kreiner D, et al: In vitro fertilization and embryo transfer (IVF/ET): an established and successful therapy for endometriosis. J Vitro Fert Embryo Transfer 1988;5:249.

126. Ohtsuka N: Study on pathogenesis of adhesions in endometriosis. Nippon Sanka Fujinka Gakkai Zasshi 1980;32:1758.

127. Olive DL, Haney AF: Endometriosis-associated infertility: a critical review of therapeutic approaches. Obstet Gynecol Survey 1986;41:1.

128. Olive DL, Henderson DY: Endometriosis and müllerian anomalies. Obstet Gynecol 1987;69:412.

129. Olive DL, Lee KL: Analysis of sequential treatment protocols for endometriosis-associated infertility. Am J Obstet Gynecol 1986;154:613.

130. Olive DL, Martin DC: Treatment of endometriosis-associated infertility with CO_2 laser laparoscopy: The use of one- and two-parameter exponential models. Fertil Steril 1987;48:18.

131. Paulsen JD, Asmar P: The use of CO_2 laser laparoscopy for treating endometriosis. Int J Fertil 1987; 32:237.

132. Pittaway DE: CA-125 in women with endometriosis. Obstet Gynecol Clin N Am 1989;16:237.

133. Pittaway DE, Daniell JF, Maxson WS: Ovarian surgery in an infertility patient as an indication for a short-interval second-look laparoscopy: a preliminary study. Fertil Steril 1985;44:611.

134. Pittaway DE, Douglas JW: Serum CA-125 in women with endometriosis, and chronic pelvic pain. Fertil Steril 1989;51:68.

135. Pittaway DE, Vernon C, Fayez JA: Spontaneous abortions in women with endometriosis. Fertil Steril 1988;50:711.

136. Polan ML, DeCherney A: Presacral neurectomy for pelvic pain in infertility. Fertil Steril 1980;34:557.

137. Pouly JL, Mankes H, Mage G, et al: Laparoscopic treatment of endometriosis (laser excluded). Contr Gynecol Obstet 1987;16:280.

138. Punnonen R, Soderstrom P, Alanen A: Isthmic tubal occlusion: Etiology and histology. Acta Eur Fertil 1984;15:39.

139. Prystowsky JB, Stryker SJ, Ujiki GT, et al: Gastrointestinal endometriosis. Incidence and indications for resection. Arch Surg 1988;123:855–858.

140. Ranney B: Endometriosis IV: hereditary tendency. Obstet Gynecol 1971;37:734.

141. Rantala ML, Kahanpaa KV, Koskimies AI, et al:

Fertility prognosis after surgical treatment of pelvic endometriosis. Acta Obstet Gynecol Scand 1983; 62:11.

142. Rao B, Darim SMM: In vitro effects of ICI 81008, a PGF$_{2\alpha}$ analogue on the human corpus luteum. IRCS Med Sc Endocrinol Syst 1985;3:339.

143. Redwine DB: Peritoneal blood painting: An aid in the diagnosis of endometriosis. Am J Obstet Gynecol 1989;161:865.

144. Redwine DB: The distribution of endometriosis in the pelvis by age groups and fertility. Fertil Steril 1987;47:173.

145. Reich H, McGlynn F: Treatment of ovarian endometriosis using laparoscopic surgical techniques. J Reprod Med 1986;31:557.

146. Rezai N, Ghodgaonkar RB, Zacur HA, et al: Cul-de-sac fluid in women with endometriosis: fluid volume, protein and prostanoid concentration during the periovulatory period—days 13 to 18. Fertil Steril 1987;48:29.

147. Riva HL, Kawasaki DM, Messinger AJ: Further experience with norethynodrel in treatment of endometriosis. Obstet Gynecol 1962;19:111.

148. Rock JA, Dubin NH, Ghodgaonkar RB, et al: Cul-de-sac fluid in women with endometriosis: fluid volume and prostanoid concentration during the proliferative phase of the cycle-days 8–12. Fertil Steril 1982;37:747.

149. Rock JA, Guzick DS, Jones HW Jr: The efficacy of accessory surgical intervention in conjunction with resection and fulguration of endometriosis. Infertility 1981a;4:193.

150. Rock JA, Guzick DS, Sengos C, et al: Evaluation of pregnancy success with respect to extent of disease as categorized using contemporary classification systems. Fertil Steril 1981b;35:131.

151. Ruggi G: Della sympatectamia al collo ed ale ad ome. Policlinico 1899;193.

152. Sadigh H, Naples JD, Batt RE: Conservative surgery for endometriosis in the infertile couple. Obstet Gynecol 1977;49:562.

153. Sampson JA: Benign and malignant endometrial implants in peritoneal cavity, and their relation to certain ovarian tumors. Surg Gynecol Obstet 1924; 38:287.

154. Sampson JA: Peritoneal endometriosis due to menstrual dissemination of endometrial tissue into the peritoneal cavity. Am J Obstet Gynecol 1927; 14:422.

155. Schenken RS, Asch RH, Williams RF, et al: Etiology of infertility in monkeys with endometriosis: luteinized unruptured follicles, luteal phase defects, pelvic adhesions and spontaneous abortions. Fertil Steril 1984;41:122.

156. Schenken RS, Malinak LR: Re-operation after initial treatment of endometriosis with conservative surgery. Am J Obstet Gynecol 1978;131:426.

157. Schenken RS, Malinak LR: Conservative surgery versus expectant management for the infertile patient with mild endometriosis. Fertil Steril 1982;37:183.

158. Schenken RS, Williams RF, Hodgen GD: Effect of

159. Schlaff WD, Dugoff L, Damewood MD, et al: Megestrol acetate for treatment of endometriosis. Obstet Gynecol 1990;75:646.

160. Schmidt CL: Endometriosis: a reappraisal of pathogenesis and treatment. Fertil Steril 1985;44:157.

161. Scott RD, TeLinde RW: External endometriosis: the scourge of the private patient. Ann Surg 1950; 131:697.

162. Schroysman R: Tubal microsurgery versus in vitro fertilization. Acta Eur Fertil 1984;15:5.

163. Seibel MM, Berger MJ, Weinstein FG, et al: The effectiveness of danazol on subsequent fertility in minimal endometriosis. Fertil Steril 1982;38:534.

164. Seiler JC, Gidwani G, Ballard L: Laparoscopic cauterization of endometriosis for fertility: a controlled study. Fertil Steril 1986;46:1098.

165. Sgarlata CS, Hertelendy F, Mikhail G: The prostanoid content in peritoneal fluid and plasma of women with endometriosis. Am J Obstet Gynecol 1983;147:563.

166. Shook TE, Nyberg LM: Endometriosis of the urinary tract. Urology 1988;31:1–6.

167. Simpson JL, Elias S, Malinak LR, et al: Heritable aspects of endometriosis I. Genetic studies. Am J Obstet Gynecol 1980;137:327.

168. Simpson JL, Malinak LR, Elias S, et al: HLA associations in endometriosis. Am J Obstet Gynecol 1984;148:395.

169. Strathy JH, Molgaard CA, Coulam CB, et al: Endometriosis and infertility. A laparoscopic study of endometriosis among fertile and infertile women. Fertil Steril 1982;38:667.

170. Stripling MC, Martin DC, Chatman DL, et al: Subtle appearance of pelvic endometriosis. Fertil Steril 1988;49:427.

171. Sueldo CE, Lambert H, Steinleitner A, et al: The effect of peritoneal fluid from patients with endometriosis or murine sperm-oocyte interaction. Fertil Steril 1987;48:697.

172. Suginami H, Yano K, Watanabe K, et al: A factor inhibiting ovum capture by the oviductal fimbriae present in endometriosis peritoneal fluid. Fertil Steril 1986;46:1140.

173. Sulewski J, Curcio F, Bronitsky C, et al: The treatment of endometriosis at laparoscopy for infertility. Am J Obstet Gynecol 1980;138:128.

174. Surrey ES, Gambone JC, Lu JKH, et al: The effects of combining norethindrone with a gonadotropin-releasing hormone agonist in the treatment of symptomatic endometriosis. Fertil Steril 1990;53:620.

175. Surrey ES, Halme J: Endometriosis as a cause of infertility. Obstet Gynecol Clin N Am 1989;16:79.

176. Tamaya T, Motoyama T, Ohono Y, et al: Steroid receptor levels and histology of endometriosis and adenomyosis. Fertil Steril 1979;31:396.

177. Telimaa S: Danazol and medroxyprogesterone ace-

tate inefficacious in the treatment of infertility in endometriosis. Fertil Steril 1988;50:872.

178. Thomas EJ, Lenton EA, Cooke ID: Follicle growth patterns and endocrinological abnormalities in infertile women with minor degrees of endometriosis. Br J Obstet Gynaecol 1986;93:852.

179. Tjaden B, Schlaff WD, Kimball A, et al: The efficacy of presacral neurectomy for the relief of midline dysmenorrhea. Obstet Gynecol 1990;76:89–91.

180. Tummon IS, Maclin VM, Radwanska E, et al: Occult ovulatory dysfunction in women with minimal endometriosis and unexplained infertility. Fertil Steril 1988;50:716.

181. Vaughan Williams CA, Oak MK, Elstein M: Cyclical gonadotrophin and progesterone secretion in women with minimal endometriosis. Clin Reprod Fertil 1986;4:259.

182. Verkauf BS: The incidence, symptoms, and signs of endometriosis in fertile and infertile women. J Fla Med Assoc 1987;74:671.

183. Vernon MW, Beard JS, Graves K, et al: Classification of endometriotic implants by morphologic appearance and capacity to synthesize prostaglandin F. Fertil Steril 1986;46:801.

184. von Rokitansky C: Ueber uterusdrusen-neubildung in uterus and ovarialsarcomen. Zkk Gesellsch d Aerzte zu Wien 1860;37:577.

185. Walton LA: A reeexamination of endometriosis after pregnancy. J Reprod Med 1977;19:341.

186. Wardle PG, Foster PA, Mitchell JD: Endometriosis and IVF: Effect of prior therapy. Lancet 1986;1:276.

187. Weed JC, Arquembourg PC: Endometriosis: Can it produce an autoimmune response resulting in infertility? Clin Obstet Gynecol 1980;23:885.

188. Wheeler JM, Johnston BM, Malinak LR: The relationship of endometriosis to spontaneous abortion. Fertil Steril 1983;39:656.

189. Wheeler JM, Malinak LR: Postoperative danazol therapy in infertility patients with severe endometriosis. Fertil Steril 1981;36:460.

190. Wheeler JM, Malinak LR: Recurrent endometriosis: incidence, management, and prognosis. Am J Obstet Gynecol 1983;146:247.

191. Wick MJ, Larsen CD: Histologic criteria for evaluating endometriosis. Northwest Med J 1949;48:611.

192. Wilhemsson L, Lindblom B, Wiqvist N: The human uterotubal junction: contractile patterns of different smooth muscle layers and the influence of prostaglandin E_2, prostaglandin $F_{2\alpha}$ and prostaglandin I_2 in vitro. Fertil Steril 1979;32:303.

193. Williams T, Pratt JH: Endometriosis in 1000 consecutive celiotomies: incidence and management. Am J Obstet Gynecol 1977;129:245.

194. Ylikorkla O, Koskimies A, Laatkainen T, et al: Peritoneal fluid prostaglandins in endometriosis, tubal disorders, and unexplained infertility. Obstet Gynecol 1984;63:616.

195. Young MD, Blackmore WP: The use of danazol in the management of endometriosis. J Int Med Res (Suppl 3)1977;5:86.

Section 3.
Congenital Anomalies

12

RECONSTRUCTION OF CONGENITAL UTEROVAGINAL ANOMALIES

Howard W. Jones, Jr.

INTRODUCTION

A simple classification of müllerian anomalies comprises three groups:

1. Agenesis (Rokitansky-Kuster-Hauser syndrome)
2. Problems of lateral fusion
   a. Obstructive
   b. Nonobstructive
3. Problems of vertical fusion
   a. Obstructive
   b. Nonobstructive

Agenesis of the uterus and vagina (Rokitansky-Kuster-Hauser syndrome) is a defect with reasonably constant findings. It is often referred to as congenital absence of the vagina.

Problems of lateral fusion of the two müllerian ducts are especially noteworthy in that obstructive lesions seem to have been observed clinically only when the obstruction was unilateral. This observation is of considerable embryological interest because unilateral obstruction is almost invariably accompanied by absence of the ipsilateral kidney. It is therefore likely that bilateral obstruction would be associated with bilateral kidney agenesis, with consequent nonviability of the developing embryo.

Attention to obstructive lesions is often urgently necessary to prevent deterioration of reproductive capacity from retained mucus or menstrual blood. On the other hand, attention to nonobstructive malformations is seldom of an emergency nature, but may be required before reproduction is possible.

Problems of vertical fusion may be considered to represent faults in the function between the down-growing müllerian ducts (müllerian tubercle) and the up-growing derivative from the urogenital sinus.

ROKITANSKY-KUSTER-HAUSER SYNDROME

Patients with congenital absence of the vagina usually also have absence of the uterus. It is for this reason that the eponym is used to describe the condition, although many times it is referred to in the literature as congenital absence of the vagina. Perhaps a more accurate term might be aplasia or dysplasia of the müllerian ducts. Such patients may have a normally developed lower vagina of a very few centimeters. The usual lesion includes absence of the middle and upper third of the vagina and the uterus, although as will be described, the fallopian tubes generally are normally developed.

Some reported series of congenital absence of the vagina have included patients with the uterus and absence of various lengths of the vagina. In view of the homogeneity and specificity of the syndrome under discussion, that is, no uterus and high incidence of urinary tract anomalies, we have preferred to consider patients with a uterus and absent vagina under the category of transverse vaginal septum.

It is uncommon for a diagnosis of this

condition to be made in the newborn. Indeed, it cannot be made except by a very careful examination that includes some procedure to determine the vaginal length by sound and rectal examination to identify the presence or absence of the uterus. It is difficult to justify such a routine examination in the newborn, since therapy should be delayed until much later.

Such patients usually seek the physician at puberty or later because of failure of menstruation to appear. The general growth and development of such patients is quite normal, including the secondary sex characteristics; and the external genitalia are quite normal, but as noted, the vagina is absent or there may be only a shallow vaginal dimple (Fig. 12.1).

Individuals with an imperforate hymen may be suspected of having no vagina. This is particularly true in infancy and prior to the menarche. After the onset of menses, the diagnosis of imperforate hymen is easier due to the bulging of the accumulated blood (Figs. 12.2 and 12.3). Sometimes in infancy, mucus

accumulates in the vagina and causes bulging (Fig. 12.4).

Prior to the menarche, the differential diagnosis between an imperforate hymen and the Rokitansky syndrome may be difficult and depends on the ability to determine the presence or absence of a uterus.

A careful examination by ultrasonography or magnetic resonance imaging may be very helpful in ascertaining the presence of a uterus. However, a negative finding must be interpreted with a degree of skepticism.

A hymen with a tiny opening may be a source of confusion (Fig. 12.5).

A possible difficulty in the differential diagnosis is to distinguish the condition from the testicular feminization syndrome, in which situation there may be a shallow vagina with no uterus palpable on rectal examination. It is commonly said that patients with the testicular feminization syndrome have little or no hair. This is often true, and therefore, the differential diagnosis may be made on this basis. On the other hand, some patients with testicular feminization have an amount of pubic and axillary hair that approaches normal, and mistakes can be made. If there is the slightest doubt, the differential diagnosis can easily be made by a karyotype, as there are generally no karyotypic

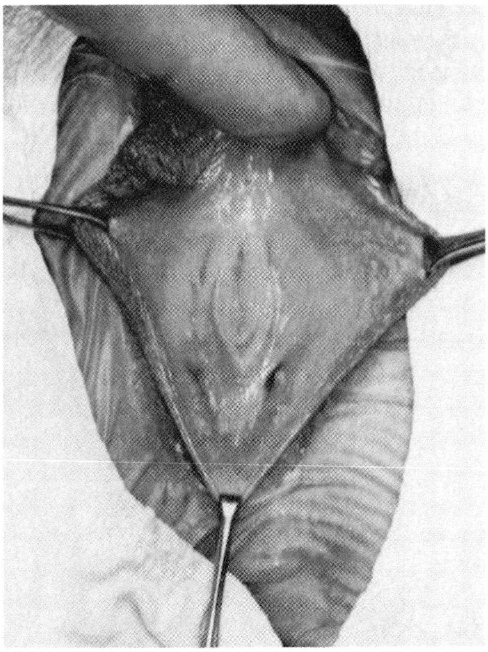

Figure 12.1. External genitalia of a patient without a vaginal opening. Note that the urethral meatus seems to be unusually patulous. This is a fairly common observation in this condition.

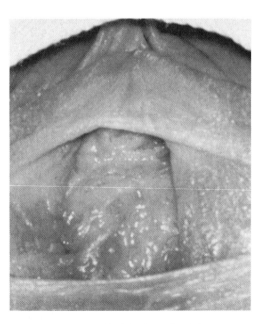

Figure 12.2. A bulging imperforate hymen.

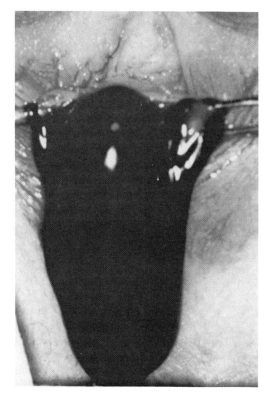

Figure 12.3. Large amounts of chocolate blood obtained on incision of an imperforate hymen.

abnormalities in either the testicular feminization syndrome or in the Rokitansky syndrome.

Congenital absence of the uterus and vagina with internal pelvic findings exactly as in the Rokitansky syndrome have been found to be associated with shortness of stature, severe bony abnormalities involving the spine, and sometimes deafness. This syndrome was originally described by Park and Jones et al. (14) and has been seen seven times since the description of the original case (Fig. 12.6). Curiously, the deafness in this syndrome, when it is present, is associated with bony anomalies of the small bones of the middle ear (Fig. 12.7). This seems to fit with the disturbance of bony development in the spine in these cases and with the occasional bony defects seen in patients with the Rokitansky syndrome, as noted below.

Generally, it is not necessary to perform a laparotomy, or indeed a laparoscopy, for the treatment of these conditions. However, the laparotomies that have been done make it possible to describe the internal findings. The tubes and ovaries are generally quite normal. However, the uterus is represented by small rudimentary structures, suggesting a very immature bicornuate uterus (Fig. 12.8). It is normally not necessary to remove these rudimentary structures, but if this is done, microscopic examination has shown whirls of what appear to be typical uterine myometrium and at the center a few scraps of endometrium made up entirely of basalis, as generally they exhibit not the slightest response to ovarian hormones (Fig. 12.9). In very unusual circumstances, in the order of 1% of all cases, such a rudimentary structure may contain functioning endometrium, so that the patient will complain of cyclic abdominal pain due to the retention of blood in the rudimentary structure. The amount of blood retained may be quite small. Obviously, if a patient seems to have Rokitansky syndrome and complains of cyclic abdominal pain, this is an indication for a laparoscopy. However, the amount of blood may be so small that it might be difficult or impossible to determine by laparoscopic examination that blood has accumulated in the rudimentary structure. In other cases, the functioning endometrium is of sufficient quantity to cause considerable unilateral enlargement. In either case, excision of the rudimentary structure is indicated and results in the alleviation of the patient's cyclic abdominal pain (Fig. 12.10).

In the usual situation, the laterally placed

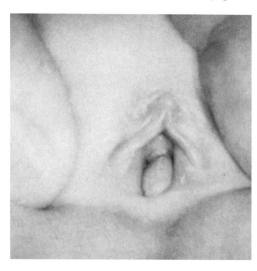

Figure 12.4. Imperforate hymen in an infant. Note the bulging due to a hydromucocolpos.

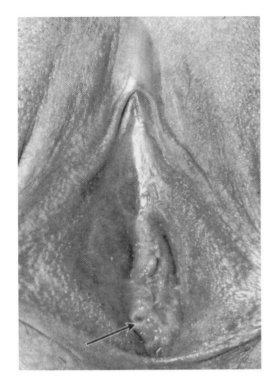

Figure 12.5. A hymen with a pinpoint opening. This patient was pregnant, indicating the ability of sperm to traverse the vagina.

rudimentary structures fade off below but fuse in the midline to become a continuous structure that measures 2 or 3 mm in diameter. This is apparently the undeveloped anlage of the uterus. Actually, this structure can sometimes be felt on rectal examination in a cooperative patient or under anesthesia. When this can be identified, it tends to confirm the diagnosis of the Rokitansky syndrome, as in the testicular feminization syndrome, this structure is not present and therefore not palpable.

Anomalies in the urinary tract are present in a significant number of patients. The percentage of anomalies depends entirely on the strictness with which one defines the anomalous situation. If anomalies are limited to major defects, such as congenital absence of the kidney on one side or the presence of a pelvic kidney, which sometimes happens unilaterally, the percentage of anomalies would be in the neighborhood of about 15%. On the other hand, if more trivial anomalies are included, such as malrotation of the kidney, a partial double collecting system on one side, or

malposition of the kidney, the percentage of anomalies rises to about 40%.

Generally, anomalies of the urinary tract have little clinical significance. However, in rare circumstances, a pelvic kidney will be located so that the normal vaginal position is compromised, and the surgical construction of the vagina must be done with great care.

Obviously, an intravenous pyelogram should be part of the routine workup of all patients with congenital absence of the uterus and vagina.

Anomalies of the bony structures are also not uncommon. It is usually stated that such anomalies occur in about 5% of patients. However, it is likely that this is a minimal figure because examination of the bones is generally quite limited. It is not at all unusual in the routine intravenous pyelogram to observe anomalies of the lumbar spine such as sacralization of L5 or the presence of six lumbar vertebrae. Fusion of the cervical vertebrae can occur, and in the special syndrome of Park and

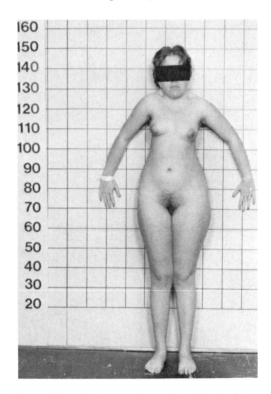

Figure 12.6. Photograph of a patient with a body type suggestive of the Turner syndrome. However, her amenorrhea is due to the Rokitansky syndrome associated with bony abnormalities, including deafness.

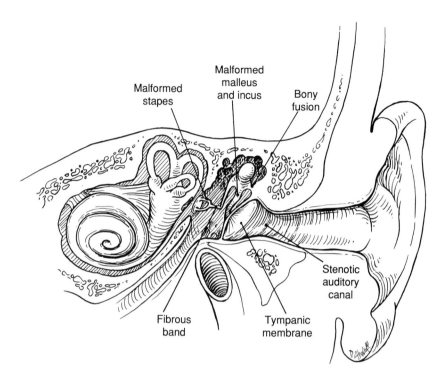

Figure 12.7.   A drawing of the deformity of the bones of the middle ear in a patient with the Park-Jones syndrome.

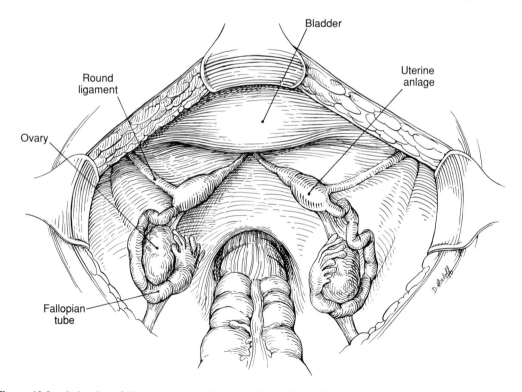

Figure 12.8.   A drawing of the internal genitalia of a patient with the Rokitansky syndrome. The abnormality as shown is the usual finding.

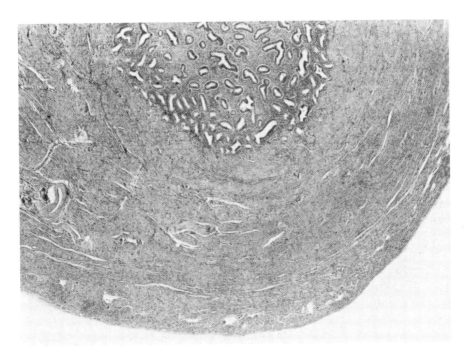

Figure 12.9. Photomicrograph of a cross-section of a uterine anlage showing uterine muscle and nonresponsive endometrium.

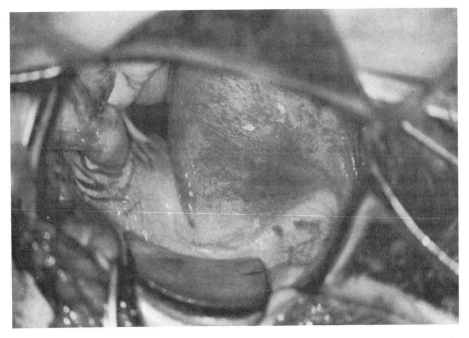

Figure 12.10. The internal genitalia of a patient with the Rokitansky syndrome with some functioning endometrium in one of the uterine anlagen.

Jones (14), fusion of the cervical vertebrae is the rule. This has occasionally been so troublesome that anesthesia is difficult, in that intubation is almost impossible because of the rigidity of the neck.

If a systematic search is made for bony abnormalities, they turn out to be quite frequent; for example, Strubbe et al. (15), in a routine radiographic examination of the hands of 40 patients with the Rokitansky syndrome, found that when accurately measured, the phalanges in all patients were too short. Furthermore, there were serious abnormalities in the hands of two patients.

Thus, widespread bony abnormalities seem to be far more common than generally appreciated. Fortunately, many of these have little or no clinical significance.

The etiology of the Rokitansky syndrome has not been satisfactorily elucidated.

There have been numerous cytogenetic studies, beginning with a study of Azoury and Jones (2), but except for rare and probably coincidental associated karyotypic anomalies, the rule is that such patients are 46,XX.

Jones and Mermut (10) recorded five examples of sisters with this disorder. Such a finding raises the possibility that the disorder is due to a very rare autosomal recessive disorder. However, the evidence of this is not persuasive.

Shokeir (16) has reported several sibships in which the disorder seems to be transmitted to a sex-linked autosomal dominant. However, there have been no confirmatory reports.

It is perhaps significant that an occasional patient exposed to thalidomide during embryogenesis has been found to have the Rokitansky syndrome. This is particularly suggestive as an etiologic agent because thalidomide affects bony development. It is curious that in one instance we observed a patient with phocomelia and the Rokitansky syndrome, even though this patient had not been exposed to thalidomide (Fig. 12.11). While such evidence can be no more than suggestive, it may be that the disorder is caused by some as yet unidentified toxic agent to which the embryo is exposed during intrauterine life.

While the exact cause of the disorder is not known, the timing of it probably occurs during embryogenesis. The state of development of the müllerian ducts at 7 weeks after fertilization, or about 9 weeks after the last menstrual period, reaches the state that is very similar to the state

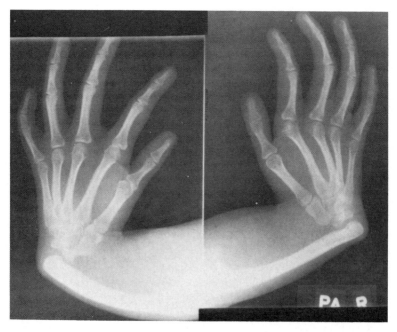

Figure 12.11. X-rays of the upper extremities of a patient with the Rokitansky syndrome associated with phocomelia.

seen in the müllerian ducts in the Rokitansky syndrome (Fig. 12.12). This would suggest that development is arrested about 9 weeks after the last menstrual period. An epidemiological study of very large proportions would be required to study this problem, as the incidence of the Rokitansky syndrome is quite low and indeed cannot be stated with any precision.

Suggested treatments have varied from the so-called Frank technique, involving the prolonged use of dilators to develop a vagina, to the use of small and large intestine and other materials to line a surgically created vaginal space. Our experience through the last 25 years with the use of a split-thickness graft to line a neovaginal cavity has been so satisfactory that this operative procedure can be highly recommended. This is not to say that a trial with the Frank technique in suitable circumstances should not be used. On the contrary, if there is adequate time, a motivated patient, and an anatomical situation that seems favorable, it is more sensible to attempt to create a vagina by manual dilatation. A graduated set of rectal dilators is quite suitable. Plastic centrifuge tubes of increasing size are usually generally available and make an inexpensive and adequate substitute.

Even when there is a favorable anatomical situation, such as a small vaginal dimple, and there is adequate time, patients are sometimes unsuccessful in using this technique. Many times there are specific reasons to prefer operation. For example, if there has been a previous operation attempt and there is scar tissue in the position of the neovagina, it is unlikely that vaginal dilatation will be helpful. A very odd but practical indication is the sudden realization that a young girl, because of age, will no longer be covered by parental insurance. Many times, such a patient has come in with only 4–6 remaining weeks of insurance coverage, with the request to solve the problem promptly. In addition, surgery may be selected when a functioning vagina is required for whatever reason in a few weeks' time, or in the older patient, say above the age of 30, where the tissues are less elastic than they are in the teens.

The selection of the proper age to perform the operation is a very important consideration. There is a certain amount of discomfort associated with the postoperative care revolving around the self-manipulation of the vaginal form for a period of a few weeks after the operation. If the procedure is performed before the patient is sufficiently motivated to wish to have a vagina, the stent is apt to be left out for prolonged periods with unfortunate results. In the only two unsatisfactory results that we have had with this operation over a period of years, the operation was carried out before the patients were 16 years of age. Even in this era of sexual revolution, it is our observation that teenagers are not sufficiently motivated to wish to have a vagina prior to about the age of 17 or even later.

While the McIndoe procedure is certainly easier to perform in a patient who has not previously been operated on, it is certainly possible to use the procedure in patients with previously failed operation. However, by far, the most common indication for secondary operation has resulted from a missed diagnosis where there has been an unwise exploration of the space between the rectum and bladder in the search for a vagina through what was expected to be an imperforate hymen. A differ-

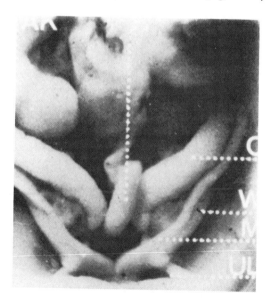

Figure 12.12. The embryonic development of the müllerian ducts at 7 weeks gestation; i.e., 9 weeks after the last menstrual period. Note that the development of the müllerian ducts is more or less the same as found in the Rokitansky syndrome. This suggests that the insult to patients with the Rokitansky syndrome occurred at about 9 weeks after the last menstrual period.

ential diagnosis between an imperforate hymen, a transverse vaginal septum, and the Rokitansky syndrome is difficult to make prior to the onset of puberty, as mentioned previously. There is really no reason to hurry the diagnosis, and it is far better to wait for a little blood to accumulate in the vagina than to inadvertently open the rectovesicle space. In the event the procedure should be done, it is best to allow the area to heal primarily rather than to attempt to maintain a cavity by using gauze packs, cigarette drains, or similar devices, or even a suitable vaginal stent, as the mistake is usually made about the age of puberty, and the patient will not be cooperative enough to expect to have a functioning vagina.

One of the most important steps in the operation is obtaining a satisfactory split-thickness graft. This can be done with any suitable instrument, but it is very important to use a technique that will secure a graft which is about 4 inches, i.e., 10 cm wide, and long enough to be twice the vaginal depth. For many years, we used the Reese drum dermatome with satisfactory results. However, within the last few years, an electric model has become available. This model is preferable in that it is no longer necessary to use dermatome cement, and

it is quite infrequent not to get a most satisfactory graft. For the vaginal cavity, a relatively thick graft is desirable. A thickness of about 18/1000″ is quite satisfactory. A thicker graft will sometimes remove so much dermis that healing of the donor site may be delayed (Fig. 12.13).

To render the donor site invisible, it is convenient to remove the split-thickness graft from the buttock. It is useful to determine from the patient ahead of time the upper and lower limits of her bathing trunks and to stay within bounds. Either buttock may be used (Fig. 12.14).

With the patient in the Sims' position, the upper most thigh and knee must be secured on the table firmly by tape or other device. The donor site must be carefully shaved and the skin prepared with any favorite preoperative technique. As mentioned above, the graft should be at least 22 or 24 cm long and 10 cm wide.

The remainder of the operation is performed with the patient in the lithotomy position. A transverse incision at the site of the vaginal orifice is desirable, and this should tend to be more posterior than anterior to assure maximum protection of the urethra by any available vaginal flap. The development of the vaginal

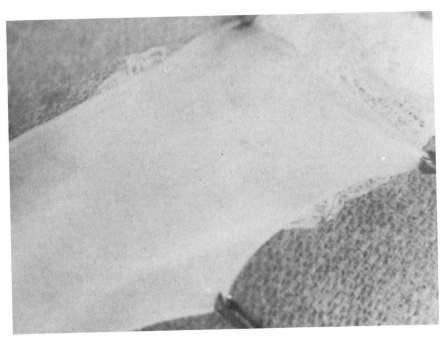

Figure 12.13. A satisfactory split-thickness graft measuring about 10 cm wide and 25 cm long.

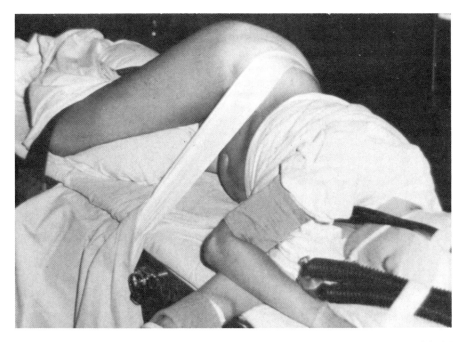

Figure 12.14. A patient positioned on the table to take a split-thickness graft from the area of the hip.

cavity is usually not too difficult in patients who have not previously been operated upon. The dissection is most easily developed on one or another or both sides of the median raphe where the tissue between the bladder and rectum seems to be condensed almost enough to warrant the designation of a rectourethralis ligament. If, however, the spaces are developed by blunt dissection with the fingers on either side of this condensed tissue band, the latter may be conveniently removed by dissection with the scissors. The dissection should be carried up to the peritoneum, but care must be exercised so as not to expose too large an area of the peritoneum, lest an enterocele develop several months after the vaginal cavity has been made (Fig. 12.15). The cavity must be reasonably dry, and often it is possible to develop the neovagina without the necessity of clamping and tying a single vessel. However, the most frequent bleeding vessels are around the edge of the vaginal epithelium at the site of the initial incision. There are other troublesome bleeding vessels from time to time deep in the lateral aspect of the vagina about two-thirds of the way to the apex. These can be caught with long Kelly clamps if necessary and tied with a free tie (Fig. 12.16).

A suitable material for the prosthesis is desirable. This should be resilient but should have sufficient substance to maintain the vaginal cavity. Ordinary foam rubber, available from any upholstery shop, has a very desirable consistency and can be readily sterilized in blocks of about 10x10x20 cm. Such a large block has the advantage of furnishing sufficient material to cut the prosthetic device to a suitable size for a particular patient. The form should be cut about twice the desired size and further compressed by the covering of two rubber sheaths, which are ordinary condoms. These are tied so that just the proper amount of air is trapped with the foam rubber to give the proper vaginal size.

After it is determined that the foam rubber form covered by the two condoms is a satisfactory size, the skin graft can be sewed to the form using very fine material such as 5-0 synthetic absorbable suture. Interrupted vertical mattress sutures are used so that the exteriorized undersurface of the graft is approximated to the exteriorized undersurface at the suture edges (Fig. 12.17). When all is ready, the mold covered by the graft is inserted into the newly created space (Fig. 12.18).

After the graft has been inserted into the

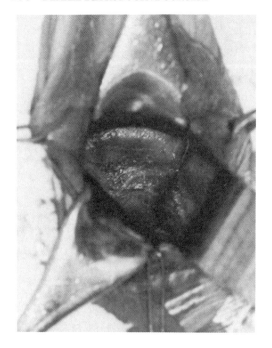

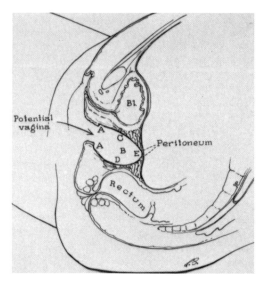

Figure 12.16. A diagram showing important points in the dissection. *A* and *B,* Potential bleeding points from the edge of the original vaginal epithelium. *C* and *D,* Potential bleeding points. *E,* A button of peritoneum.

Figure 12.15. A satisfactory dissection of the space between the bladder and rectum. The bladder is anterior, the rectum posterior, and a button on peritoneum is showing at the depth of the dissection.

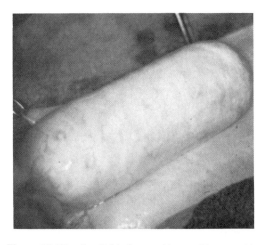

Figure 12.17. A suitable foam rubber mold covered by a condom in position to be enclosed with the split-thickness graft.

cavity, the edges of the graft may be sutured to the cut edges of the original vaginal epithelium. However, if this is inconvenient, these extra stitches may be dispensed with. In fact, it is important not to make this contact too tight since if there is any serum that collects under the graft, it is important for it to have a route of escape.

Although various types of straps and harnesses have been suggested for holding the vaginal form in place, it is our experience that none of these is completely satisfactory. We therefore now use rather large braided silk sutures though the labia to prevent extrusion of the form. These stitches may be uncomfortable for a day or two, but they have been so satisfactory in holding the form in place that this has been considered an overriding point.

A suprapubic catheter is recommended to prevent pressure on a transurethral catheter, which could conceivably result in necrosis of the urethra.

Postoperatively, the patient is kept on a low-residue diet, antibiotics, and a position in bed that is quite flat. This is desirable for a period of approximately 1 week, after which the labial stitches can be cut, the vaginal form carefully removed, the suprapubic catheter withdrawn, and the vaginal cavity irrigated. It is desirable to have previously prepared a second vaginal form so that this can be reinserted (Figs. 12.19 and 12.20).

About 24 or more hours after the removal of the original mold, the patient is instructed in

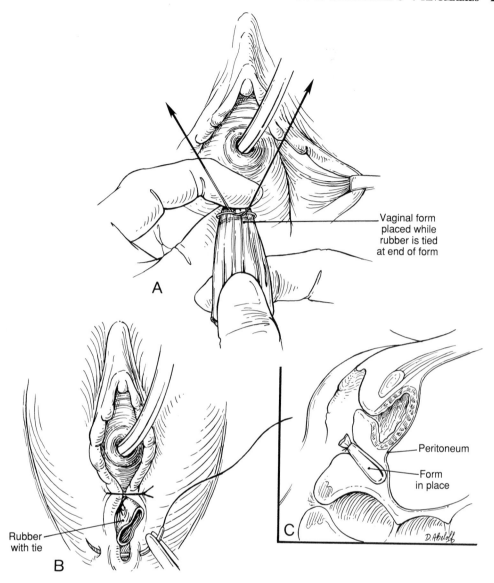

Figure 12.18. *A,* The graft-covered stent has been placed in the neovaginal space. *B,* Stitches are being placed to hold the form secure. *C,* Vaginal section showing the relative position of the bladder, peritoneum, and rectum to the neovagina with the form in place.

self-removal of the mold. The first time this is done, it may be desirable to administer 50 mg of demerol or its equivalent. After that, the patient can usually do it herself without any difficulty. At the time of the daily removals, a low pressure clear warm water douche is desirable. The mold is cleaned, covered with a new condom, if necessary, and reintroduced with neutral vaginal lubricant. As soon as she is able to do this, she is ready for discharge from the hospital.

After about 6 weeks, a silastic form or one of similar material is much easier for the patient to handle, as she can wash it off with tap water and does not have to replace condoms (Fig. 12.21). With the use of prophylactic antibiotics for the prevention of infections, it is now the rule to expect a 100% take of the graft. The vagina should be comfortable and functional in a period of 6–10 weeks after the operation. As reported by Garcia and Jones (7), a very high rate of success can be expected.

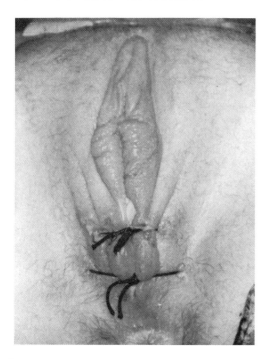

Figure 12.19. Appearance of the external genitalia 1 week after the operation and just prior to cutting the labial stitches and removal of the vaginal form.

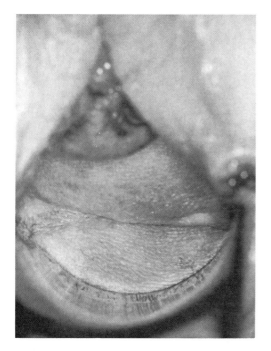

Figure 12.20. The appearance of the graft immediately after the vaginal form has been removed and the vagina irrigated. One hundred percent take of graft can be expected.

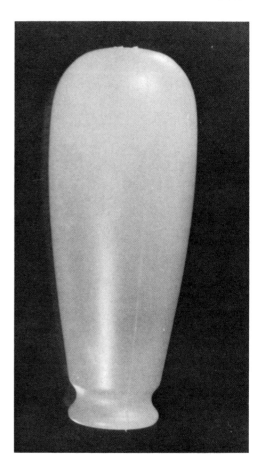

Figure 12.21. A silastic form that may be used with convenience by a patient in decreasing lengths of time for a period of about 4 months after her operation.

PROBLEMS OF LATERAL FUSION

Vertical Septa: Obstructive

This section will consider problems that result from failure of lateral fusion of the two müllerian ducts. One-sided failure of the lumen to communicate with the outside will also be discussed. Failure to recognize and relieve these problems can destroy any residual potential reproduction.

The point of obstruction may vary from low in the vagina to the region where the normal corpus of the uterus should develop. The resulting symptoms are very much related to the site of obstruction.

When there is the development of what is essentially a uterus didelphys with a double vagina but with an obstruction low in the vagina on one side, a large amount of blood may accumulate, and the condition may go unrecognized for a number of years after the onset of menstruation. This is apparently due to the fact that the distensible vagina can accommodate to the increments of blood resulting from each menstrual period with absorption of enough fluid between menstrual periods so that succeeding menstrual periods add to the accumulated blood without the production of excruciating pain. When this unfortunate situation occurs, retrograde involvement of the tubes and the development of a rather large tuboovarian accumulation of menstrual blood with endometriosis may also occur (Fig. 12.22).

If the septum is removed before the tubes and ovaries are compromised by infection or endometriosis, reproduction may occur consistent with the uterine duplication.

A special situation exists when, in addition to the low vaginal obstruction, there is a lateral communication between the two horns of the uterus. This communication is usually through the cervix (Fig. 12.23). Under this circumstance, the obstructive symptoms are not so pressing, and patients often complain of a disappearing mass at the vaginal outlet. From

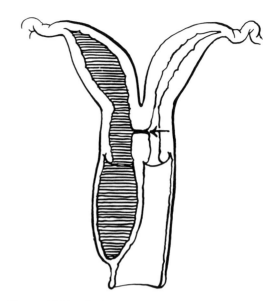

Figure 12.23. A diagram of a patient with double vagina with unilateral obstruction, but with a lateral communicating uterus.

the history, one might suspect a large Bartholin gland cyst, but on examination, such cannot be found. It is significant that the diagnosis is often difficult, largely because it is not considered. In a series of 11 patients collected by Toaff (17), the age at which the first symptom appeared was 15.5 years, but the age at which a definitive diagnosis was made and therapy carried out was 23.7 years, indicating the problem of diagnosis. These patients complain very often not only of a vaginal mass that disappears, but also of intermenstrual vaginal discharge, sometimes bloody. If the patient has been instrumented in an attempt to make a diagnosis, a low-grade infection of the obstructed vagina may occur with an increase in the patient's discharge.

Treatment of this particular special situation involves only the removal of the vaginal septum. No treatment is needed for the lateral communication of the uterus and reproduction is consistent with the duplicated uterus, unless neglect of the original condition has destroyed tubal function.

If obstruction occurs in the region of the cervix, the reservoir-like action of the vagina to accommodate the cyclic menstrual blood is lost, and symptoms are often very acute from the retention of the blood within the endometrial

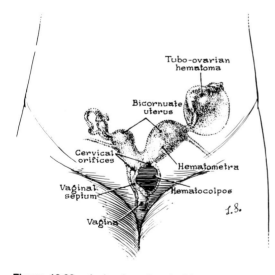

Figure 12.22. A drawing of a double uterus with a double vagina, with a unilateral obstruction. Because of the distensibility of the vagina, the symptoms were not acute, and the patient did not come to medical attention until 6 years after the onset of her menstrual periods.

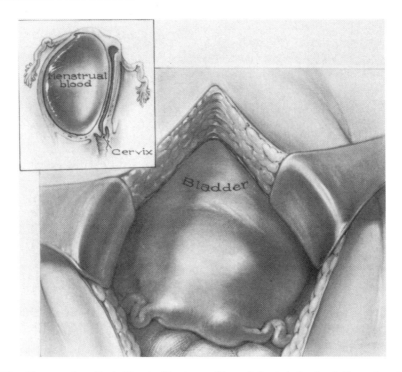

Figure 12.24. Diagram of a patient with a double uterus with a unilateral obstruction in the region of the cervix.

cavity. Such patients will seldom have more than three or four periods before the excruciating pain demands attention (Fig. 12.24). If the cervix is well formed on the unobstructed side, consideration may be given to anastomosing the obstructed side to the unobstructed one. In anomalies of this type, it is sometimes technically impossible to remove the obstructed side and leave a functioning uterus (Fig. 12.25).

At times, the obstruction involves what amounts to an isolated horn of the uterus with minimal connection to the unobstructed side. When this occurs, early removal is desirable so that retrograde menstruation will not cause endometriosis and compromise subsequent reproduction.

Fortunately, in some instances of a rudimentary horn with obstruction, there is also a failure of communication of the cavity of the uterus with the fallopian tube so that there is no opportunity for the spill of menstrual blood. Excision of these horns gives a very satisfactory result (Fig. 12.26).

A few examples of pregnancy in an obstructed rudimentary horn have been observed. Essentially, all of these have been in very young individuals who were exposed to pregnancy

before the monthly accumulation of trapped menstrual blood had had an opportunity to "gum up" the function of the obstructed horn. In these instances, by necessity, sperm ascended through the unobstructed side. All such patients have presented with symptoms of an ectopic pregnancy (Fig. 12.27). In most of these cases, the rudimentary horn was surgically excised, but in others, this was difficult because of the attachment of the rudimentary horn to the functioning side.

When there is failure of lateral fusion of the müllerian ducts with unilateral obstruction, absence of the ipsilateral kidney is the rule. Thus, an intravenous pyelogram is a very useful diagnostic tool and may clarify the diagnosis in obscure circumstances (Fig. 12.28).

The epithelium of an obstructed vagina is almost always composed of cuboidal cells. This testifies to the müllerian origin of the epithelium. If the obstruction is incomplete, even if the communication with the unobstructed side is extremely small, the cuboidal epithelium seems to have been replaced by the squamous epithelium of the vagina, presumably by a process of metaplasia, which may be the normal embryological process in the development of

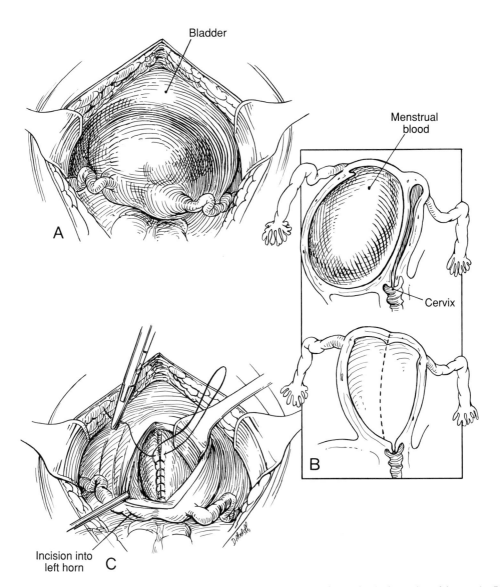

Bladder

Menstrual
blood

Cervix

A

B

Incision into
left horn   C

Figure 12.25. *A,* Diagram of a patient with a double uterus with a unilateral obstruction in the region of the cervix. *B,* Section through the anomaly as it originally was (upper). Diagram of the reconstructed uterus (lower). The dotted line is the posterior incision. The cavity has not yet been closed anteriorly. *C,* The septum has been excised and the posterior incision is being closed with a continuous stitch. A small incision had originally been made in the left horn with the passage of a uterine sound down through the cervix to help in the identification of the details of the anomaly.

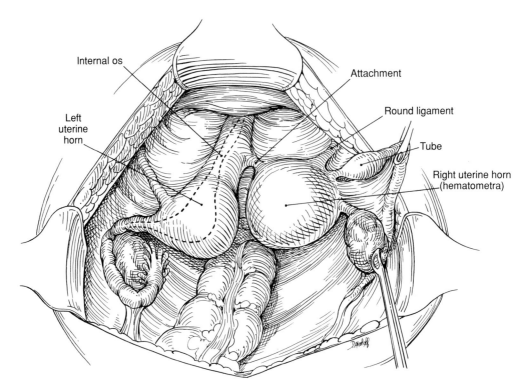

Figure 12.26. A drawing of a noncommunicating rudimentary horn. The fallopian tube was congenitally obstructed and there was no endometriosis. Treatment consisted of excision of the rudimentary horn.

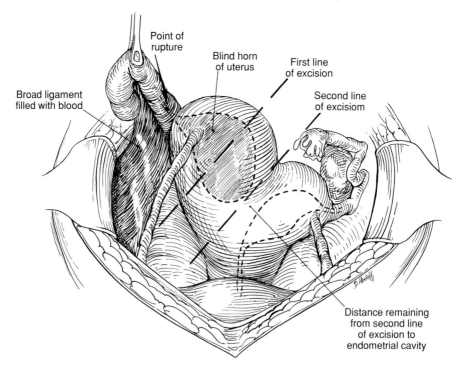

Figure 12.27. Drawing of a patient with a rudimentary horn with a pregnancy in the rudimentary horn. Although the horn was broadly attached to the relatively more normal side, it was possible to remove the horn without damaging the myometrium of the opposite side. Subsequent to the operation, the patient has had two normal term deliveries.

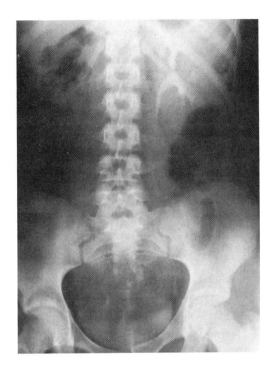

Figure 12.28. Intravenous pyelogram of patient with unilateral müllerian obstruction. The kidney abnormality is invariably on the side with the greatest müllerian deformity.

the vagina. Thus, when the vaginal septum is removed in obstructed circumstances, the newly opened vagina is lined with adenomatous epithelium (Fig. 12.29). In effect, the patient has vaginal adenosis. This adenomatous epithelium is slowly replaced by metaplasia, but if the area involved is of any size, as it might be when the obstruction is low in the vagina, the metaplastic process will require 2 or 3 years, or even more, before the vagina has attained its normal adult squamous composition.

A rare situation may occur when there seems to be both a problem of lateral fusion and a problem of vertical fusion (Fig. 12.30).

Vertical Septa: Nonobstructed

In nonobstructed failure of lateral fusion involving the uterus and vagina (uterus didelphys), there are no symptoms related to menstruation (Fig. 12.31). However, due to narrowness of the vagina, dyspareunia may be a problem (Fig. 12.32). If so, removal of the septum may be required and is not particularly difficult, although sometimes it is very thick and

and contains a large number of blood vessels that must be secured. At times, there is asymmetry of the two vaginal cavities so that vaginal function is normal and satisfactory with one side but quite impossible with the other.

Although exact data are lacking, overall reproduction seems to be modestly compromised in patients with didelphic uteri. Information is almost anecdotal and consists of case reports or small series recording examples of primary infertility, pregnancy wastage, and premature labor. A number of examples of simultaneous pregnancies in each have been reported. Several of these have had a happy outcome for both pregnancies. The older literature contains examples of deliveries from below with sequential labor with remarkable intervals between the birth of each child. An interval of 24 hours is not unusual, and intervals of several days have been reported. Cesarean section would doubtless be used almost routinely at present.

There is no indication for surgical intervention in a didelphic condition except for the removal of the vaginal septum, which might cause dyspareunia, or for uterine unification if prematurity is a problem.

Information about reproduction in a unicornuate uterus is not too different from that of the didelphic situation. Perhaps this is not too surprising, as a didelphic uterus is a symmetrical duplication of a unicornuate uterus (Fig. 12.33).

A unicornuate uterus may also be obstructed (Fig. 12.34).

As judged by the report of small series, reproduction is somewhat compromised by infertility, pregnancy wastage, and premature labor. However, pregnancies seem to result in a viable child.

Treatment for problems of pregnancy wastage in the unicornuate uterus is not standardized. In some instances, for patients with repeated miscarriages, the author has removed the contralateral müllerian remnant that seemed to attach high on the developed side. Term children followed. Andrews and Jones (1) reported the details of reproductive performance in five cases.

Cerclage has also been favorably reported in cases of repeated miscarriage and premature labor.

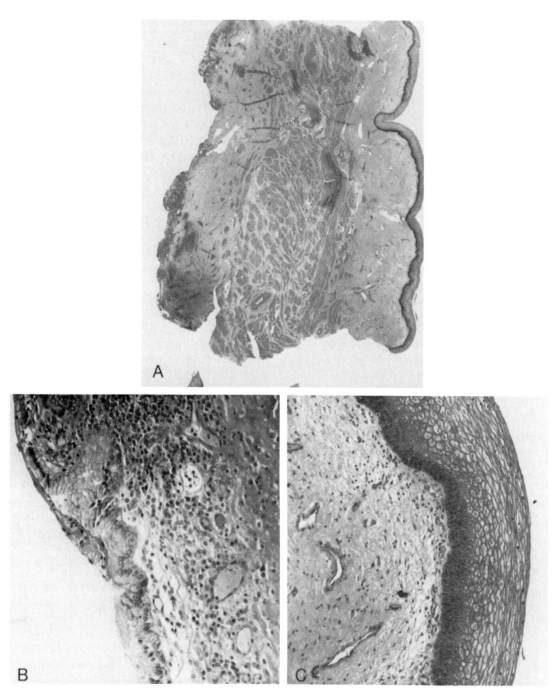

Figure 12.29. Photomicrograph of excised septum of a patient with a unilateral vaginal obstruction. *A,* Low-power view of the septum showing columnar epithelium on the obstructed side and adult vaginal epithelium on the unobstructed side. *B,* High-power view showing adenomatous epithelium. *C,* High-power view showing normal vaginal epithelium on unobstructed vaginal septum.

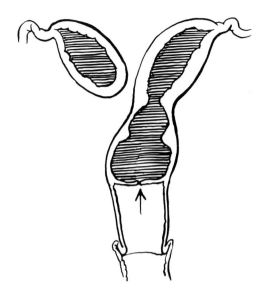

Figure 12.30. Diagram of a patient who had an isolated uterine horn on the right and a unicornuate uterus on the left with a pinpoint opening in a transverse vaginal septum.

There is a need for a comprehensive study of reported material on both unicornuate and didelphic uterus, although existing data are probably biased because of reports of only abnormal situations.

THE BICORNUATE AND SEPTATE UTERUS

A symmetrical nonobstructed double uterus of a special type may cause a problem in reproduction. Generally, there is no problem in becoming pregnant, but the difficulty arises from abortion, which is often repeated, or from premature labor. In the event pregnancies are carried to term, obstetrical malpresentation and difficulties in delivery are not unusual. Primary infertility in a patient with a symmetrical double uterus is sometimes observed, but the etiological relationship between the infertility and the anomaly is an unresolved problem.

Classification

In symmetrical double uterus without obstruction, the type of uterus is of great importance (Fig. 12.31). It is crucial to distinguish between the bicornuate uterus and the septate uterus because the bicornuate uterus gives only minimal problems with reproduction, whereas the septate uterus is almost always the type that is involved with reproductive failure. The distinction between these two types of uteri cannot be made by an examination of a hysterogram, as the image of the cavities may be the same (Fig. 12.35). In the bicornuate uterus, two distinct horns may be felt. In the septate uterus, the exterior configuration of the uterus may be essentially normal, and many of these uteri cannot be recognized, even at laparotomy (Fig. 12.36). However, there may be the slightest indentation where a midline raphe may be and sometimes on pelvic examination one can suspect a septate uterus because of the broadness of the organ. The external configuration of the uterus is such an important consideration in the diagnosis that if there is any uncertainty about this point on simple pelvic examination, an examination under anesthesia or even laparoscopy may be indicated to be certain. Ultrasonography may be helpful, and can often make the critical distinction between a bicornuate and a septate uterus. As may be inferred from the above comments, it is seldom that a bicornuate uterus needs surgical reconstruction. Accordingly, if a double uterus gives reproductive problems that require surgical attention, it is usually the septate uterus that will be involved.

A special situation pertains to the anomalies associated with and probably caused by exposure in utero to diethylstilbestrol (DES). Kaufman et al. (11) called attention to a uterus shaped like a T with some variations in many DES-exposed patients (Figs. 12.37 and 12.38). Haney et al. (8a) have described the lesion in detail. Barnes et al. (3) and others have pointed out the unfavorable outcome of pregnancies in DES-exposed women. Treatment for this special situation is difficult, but in selected circumstances, surgical reconstruction seems to be helpful, as reported by Muasher et al. (13).

DIAGNOSIS

The diagnosis of a reproductive problem due to a double uterus is essentially by exclusion. Because reproduction in a double uterus, particularly of the bicornuate type, may be essentially normal, it is necessary to determine whether a particular uterus is responsible for the reproductive problem. As indicated above,

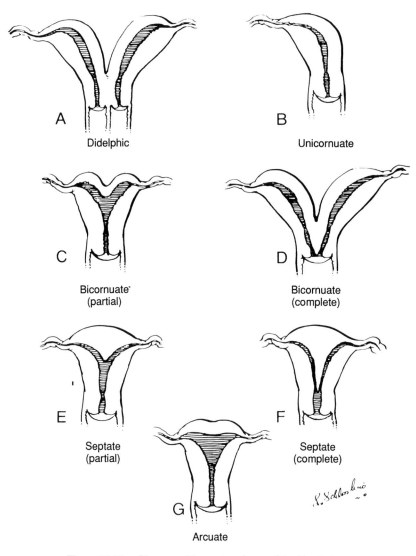

A — Didelphic

B — Unicornuate

C — Bicornuate (partial)

D — Bicornuate (complete)

E — Septate (partial)

F — Septate (complete)

G — Arcuate

Figure 12.31. Diagram of the various forms of double uteri.

there is considerable uncertainty about the relationship of primary infertility to a double uterus. Most often, the problem revolves around repeated miscarriage. It is essential in making the diagnosis of pregnancy wastage due to the double uterus that all other causes of repeated miscarriage be excluded. This would include male factors and would include such female factors as cervical incompetence, chronic illness, luteal defects, and other endocrine disorders of the adrenal and thyroid that are sometimes encountered in this circumstance. In addition, it would require the exclusion of fetal factors, immunological causes, and particularly

karyotypic anomalies in one or the other of the potential parents with the resulting genetically defective zygote. Furthermore, it might involve placental endocrine factors that cannot be identified except by a study of placental hormones during a test pregnancy.

The history of the miscarriage is particularly significant. The characteristic story is that of an early midtrimester loss associated with what amounts to a mini-labor, starting with cramps, followed by bleeding. In a primigravida, the labor may last up to 6 hours or even more, resulting in the delivery of a well-formed, but not viable fetus. In miscarriages that occur in

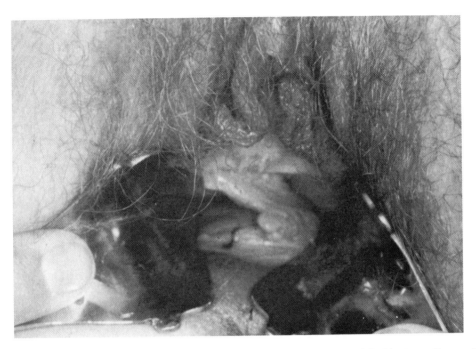

Figure 12.32.   Photograph of external genitalia of a patient with a double vagina and double uterus. Her condition is an example of uterus didelphys.

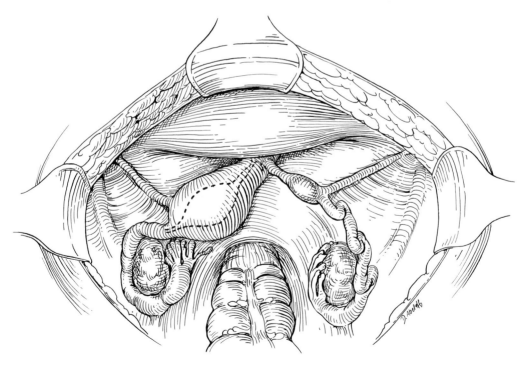

Figure 12.33.   Unicornuate uterus. Note the contralateral müllerian anlage. This latter situation exists bilaterally in the Rokitansky-Kuster-Hauser syndrome.

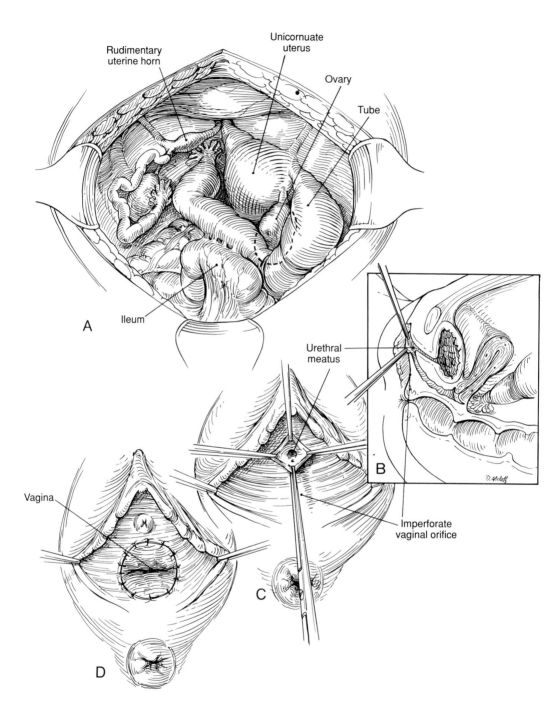

Figure 12.34. *A,* A patient with a unicornuate uterus with an obstruction in the low vagina. A drawing of internal genitalia. On the left may be seen the typical finding of the Rokitansky syndrome. On the right there is a unicornuate uterus and tube with ovary. Because of the obstruction in the low vagina, there is a hematosalpinx with obstruction. *B,* A sagittal diagram showing the relationship of the vagina to the urethra. *C,* The external genitalia showing a pinpoint opening into the vagina. *D,* The final situation with the vagina exteriorized.

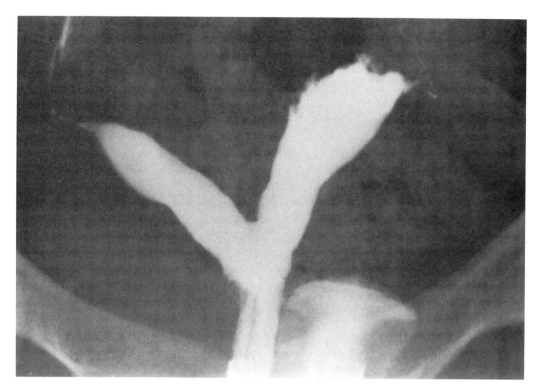

Figure 12.35. Hysterogram of a septate uterus. It is impossible to tell from the hysterogram whether one is dealing with a septate uterus or a bicornuate uterus.

the first trimester or where there is a history of lack of recognition of an embryo, it is necessary to suspect that the cause is other than an anatomical defect of the uterus. On the other hand, histories that differ from the typical one described above are sometimes encountered. In the absence of other causes of miscarriage, such patients may deserve surgical attention because some of these patients have subsequently had term delivery after reconstruction of the uterus.

THE PATHOGENESIS OF REPRODUCTIVE FAILURE

Why some septate uteri (including uteri that have a T-shaped cavity, regardless of etiology) do not behave well reproductively is an unresolved problem. Various mechanisms have been suggested, such as septal endometrial incompetence, or septal circulatory inadequacy.

Perhaps both of these play a role. However, clinical experience suggests that regardless of the details, asymmetrical uterine enlargement, in a septate uterus or in a T-shaped uterus, is undesirable, and predisposes to uterine irritability and expulsion of the uterine contents.

This arises from the observation that a uterus that repeatedly expulses a pregnancy from one horn will carry a pregnancy to term if there is a pregnancy in each of the horns.

If this evaluation is correct, the objective of therapy is to obtain a symmetrical cavity so that uterine enlargement is not hindered by the baggage of the opposite arm of the V or the T.

Treatment

In the event any correctable endocrine or metabolic causes of reproductive loss can be identified, it goes without saying that such disorders should be corrected before any surgical procedure is considered. However, in the event no endocrine or metabolic disorder can be identified, or if correction of such a defect does not produce a term pregnancy, surgical correction can be considered.

Selection of the most appropriate technique to remove or divide a septum requires the exercise of considerable judgment and experi-

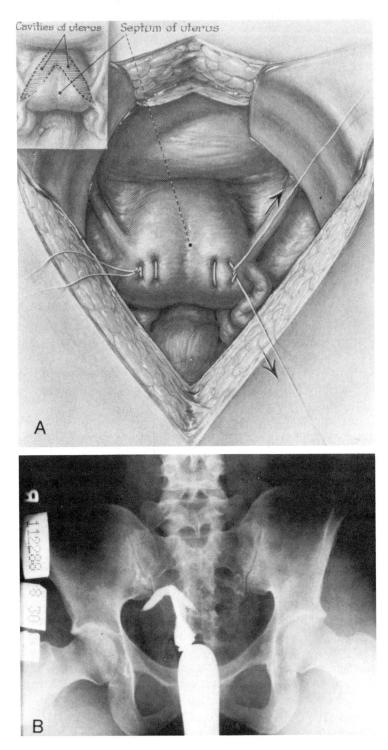

Figure 12.36.   *A,* A drawing of exterior of septate uterus. The inset shows the cavity. In this example, a median raphe can be noted, but this is not always visible. *B,* Hysterogram of the same patient.

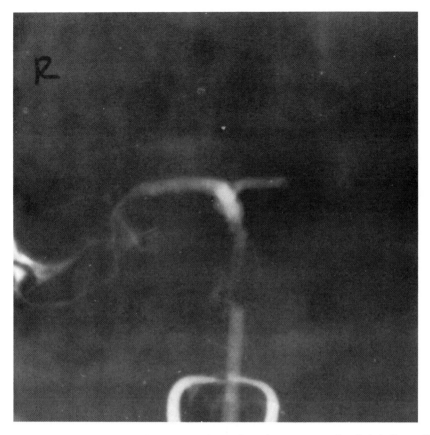

Figure 12.37.   A hysterogram of a T-shaped uterus in a patient who was exposed to diethylstilbestrol in utero.

ence. If the septum is "internal," i.e., occupies space that might be expected to belong to the endometrial cavity so that the hysterosalpingogram reveals a V-shaped image, transcervical resection by operative hysteroscopy seems to yield satisfactory results. However, if there is a hysterographic image approaching a T, operative hysteroscopy is inappropriate and dangerous, because there is often only a small intracavitary septum. These uteri are often, but by no means always, the result of exposure to diethylstilbestrol (DES), but occur spontaneously (Fig. 12.39). T-shapes resulting from DES exposure are special and are often quite small and generally easily distinguished from spontaneously occurring T's. The DES uteri have no resectable intracavity septum, and are clearly not suitable for hysteroscopic treatment.

Thus, the transcervical or abdominal approach must be selected according to the case. For example, DeCherney (4) found 72 of 103 patients suitable for hysteroscopic resection.

Abdominal surgical correction can be applied, not only to the V-shaped situation, but the T-shaped situation, including the special T's of DES exposure. In these cases, there is only a minimum or no septum to resect. The surgical goal, as stated above, is to obtain a cavity, which, when it enlarges, will be symmetrical.

THE TECHNIQUE OF TRANSCERVICAL CORRECTION

The technique for transcervical transection of a uterine septum is covered in a preceding chapter and will not be repeated here.

THE TECHNIQUE OF ABDOMINAL CORRECTION

The original Strassman procedure is unsuitable for correcting the defect in a septate uterus. Strassman operated only on a bicornuate uterus, as he worked in an era prior to hysterosalpingography, so that his only diagnoses

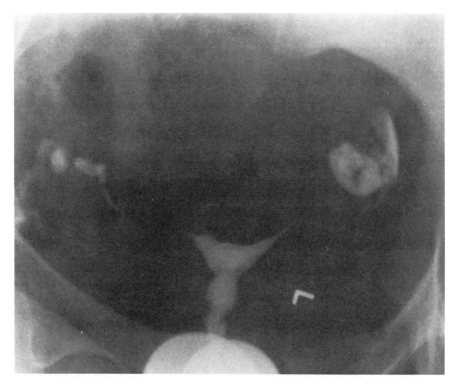

Figure 12.38. Hysterogram of a T-shaped uterus in a patient who was exposed to diethylstilbestrol. In this example, there is a deformity of the stem of the T.

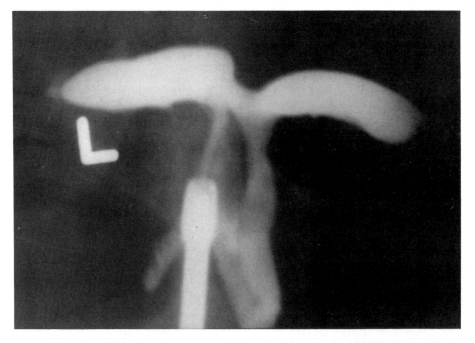

Figure 12.39. A hysterosalpingogram showing a "spontaneous" deformity. This patient had three midtrimester miscarriages. The external configuration of the uterus was quite normal. A symmetrical uterus was obtained by abdominal metroplasty. A term delivery ensued. It seemed unlikely that this deformity could have been satisfactorily corrected by hysteroscopic resection.

were made on the basis of bimanual examination and exploration of the endometrial cavity by curette or other means. Tompkins (18) and others have recommended a technique beginning by a sagittal midline incision in the uterus (Fig. 12.40). However, excision of the septum by wedge is an exceedingly satisfactory procedure and can be recommended. The technique is as follows:

The patient is positioned for the operation in the dorsal supine position. The abdomen may be opened either by a transverse or midline incision. The exterior configuration of the uterus, as has been previously mentioned, may

be quite normal. However, sometimes a median raphe may be noted. On palpation, the duplication of the uterus can often be confirmed.

It is convenient to outline the incision with brilliant green. This helps to be sure the incision is in the right place, because after the original incision is made, distortion often occurs. The position of the brilliant green and the lines of incision will depend upon the x-ray appearance of the configuration of the cavity. Prior to making the incision, three temporary sutures can be placed, one on each side at the insertion of the round ligaments, and one directly in the

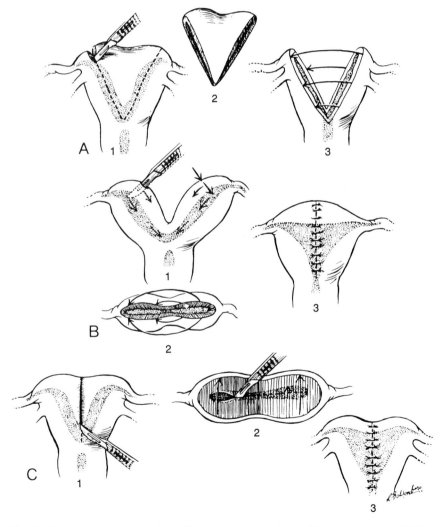

Figure 12.40.   *A,* Diagram of a method of repairing a small uterus by excision of a wedge. *B,* Diagram of the Strassman's technique of repair. This technique is applicable to a bicornuate uterus, but not so applicable to a septate uterus. *C,* The repair of a septate uterus by the Tompkin's technique.

midline in the area, which will be subsequently removed.

To control bleeding, up to 20 units of pitressin diluted in 20 ml of saline may be injected into the myometrium prior to making the uterine incision. This will produce blanching and diminish blood loss during the procedure. Sometimes pitressin may cause circulatory changes, so that the anesthesiologist must be alerted when this is being used. It is often entirely satisfactory to use only 10 units in all.

In this way, the possibility of circulatory changes is greatly diminished.

The uterine septum is surgically excised as a wedge, as indicated in the diagrams (Fig. 12.41). The incisions begin at the fundus of the uterus. In approaching the endometrial cavity, care must be taken that the cavity is not transected. The original incisions at the top of the fundus are usually within 1 cm and sometimes even less of the insertion of the fallopian tubes. However, if the incision is directed

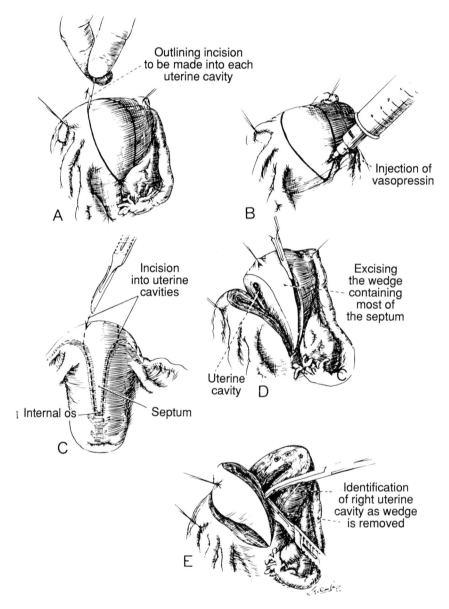

Figure 12.41. *A–E,* Various steps in the operative treatment of a septate uterus by excision of a wedge.

toward the apex of the wedge, there seems to be little danger of transecting the tube across its interstitial transit of the myometrium. After the wedge has been removed, sometimes major bleeding vessels can be noted. There seems to be a rather constant vessel near the top of the incision in the region of the tube. This is apparently the main branch of the uterine artery in this area. It is convenient to ligate this with very fine suture material, even though it may not be bleeding due to constriction by the pitressin. Generally, it is not necessary to ligate other vessels.

After the wedge has been removed, the uterus may be closed in three layers with interrupted stitches: chromic catgut (#00) on an atraumatic tapered needle in quite convenient, although synthetic absorbable materials are satisfactory. Two sizes of needles are used: a 1/2″ half-round needle for the inner and intermediate layers, and a large needle, 3/4″ half-round for the outer serosal layers. The inner layer of stitches must include about 1/3 of the thickness of the myometrium, as the endometrium itself is too delicate to hold a suture and will cut through. The suture is placed through the endometrium/myometrium in such a way that the knot is tied within the endometrial cavity. While the suture is being tied, an assistant presses together the two lateral halves of the uterus with his fingers and with the guy sutures, to relieve tension on the suture line and to reduce the possibility of cutting through. The stitches are placed alternately anteriorly and posteriorly. After the first few stitches are placed and before the first layer is completed, the second layer can be started to reduce tension. Indeed, as the operation proceeds, even the third layer can be inserted in the serosa, both anteriorly and posteriorly. While for a number of years #00 chromic catgut stitches have been used in the serosa, more recently, much finer synthetic suture material has been used to more precisely approximate the serosal edges of the uterus. Theoretically, this should cut down the opportunity for adhesions to the outside of the uterus, but whether this will make any practical difference in the ultimate end result is unclear. At the conclusion of the procedure, a single incision is visible beginning from the back of the uterus at

a position dictated by the depth of the septum and continuing anteriorly to a corresponding position in front. Most often, it has not been necessary to detach the peritoneal reflection of the bladder, but in the event there is a particularly deep septum, this may be necessary, and the final incision therefore will extend further down on the uterus, both posteriorly and anteriorly. If the bladder peritoneum was reflected, this will need to be replaced at this point. At the conclusion, the uterus appears rather normal in its configuration, but the striking feature will be the proximity of the intersections of the fallopian tubes. In placing the final sutures, it is exceedingly important that the interstitial portions of the fallopian tubes not be obstructed by the sutures.

The final size of the uterine cavity seems to be unimportant. Many times, the reconstructed cavity is quite small compared with a normal uterus. The symmetry is probably more important. A very small symmetrical cavity seems to function quite normally. Postoperative films often show small dog-ears, which are leftover tags from the original bifid condition of the uterus. Such dog-ears do not seem to interfere with function. Although a postoperative roentgenogram after such an operation cannot be considered normal, in the sense that it appears like a normal endometrial cavity, the uterus seems to function quite normally (Fig. 12.42).

Blood loss from the above procedure, if pitressin is used, is minimal. Diminished bleeding from pitressin lasts about 20 minutes, and the operation normally can be completed within this period of time.

If the duplication involves the cervix, which it does only rarely, it is important not to attempt to unify the cervix for fear of creating an incompetent cervix. Surgical reconstruction needs to be applied only to the corpus.

The above description relates to an intracavitary septum, many of which can be removed transcervically. The technique of abdominal metroplasty with very slight modification can be applied to T-shaped uteri, those due to diethylstilbestrol exposure, and those that occur spontaneously.

The goal is to unroof the center part of the crossbar of the T, and to restore the integrity of the uterus by uniting in the midline the residual

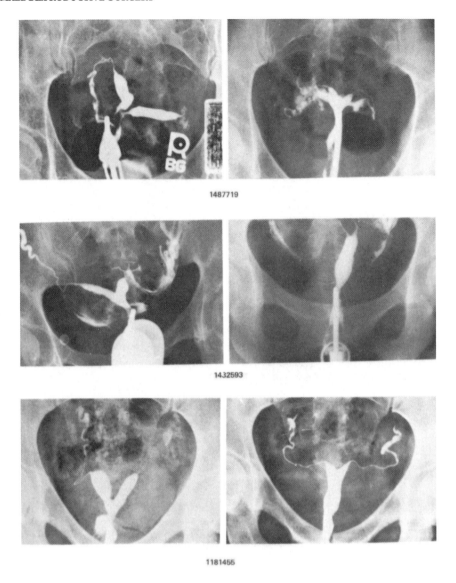

1487719

1432593

1181455

Figure 12.42. Hysterograms of three patients before (*left*) and after (*right*) wedge excision of the uterine septum. All three of these patients had repeated miscarriages prior to operation, and all three of the patients had term deliveries of normal children after the operation.

unroofed T, using a technique similar to that for unifying the two halves of the uterus after the removal of an intracavitary septum (Fig. 12.43).

Obstetrical Management

Healing in the nonpregnant uterus is probably not to be compared with healing after a cesarean section because myometrial healing after a term delivery takes place in a uterus that is undergoing involution. Thus, it might be expected that cesarean section wounds are less firmly healed than incisions in the nonpregnant uterus. Nevertheless, most patients who have had surgical reconstruction of a double uterus have been delivered by cesarean section. This can be recommended as a matter of precaution. Such patients have had a long, disappointing obstetrical experience. They are often in their late thirties, and in order to minimize the risk of an obstetrical catastrophe, an elective cesarean

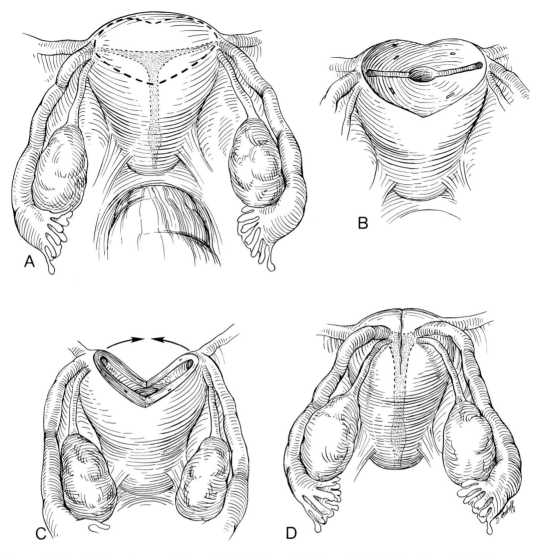

Figure 12.43. *A*, T-shaped uterus. Projected incision indicated by interrupted line. *B*, The T unroofed. *C*, The arms of the T are approximated. *D*, Final appearance.

section prior to the onset of labor seems the most conservative course to avoid the possibility of a uterine rupture.

To allow the uterine incision the best possible opportunity to heal, a delay in becoming pregnant after surgical reconstruction has generally been advised. The period of delay has been from 3–12 months, depending on the age of the patient. No difficulties have been encountered with this amount of time. Most patients have waited from 9–12 months before becoming pregnant. During this interval, it has been thought not advisable to recommend oral

contraceptives because of the progestational effect on the myometrium and the possibility that healing under this circumstance would be similar to postpartum healing. Therefore, mechanical contraception with diaphragm or condom has been recommended and has proven to be satisfactory as judged by the ultimate result.

Results

Hassiakos and Zourlas (9) reviewed comprehensively the results from transcervical division of uterine septa from 17 reports from 1974–1988.

Table 12.1. Reproductive Performance of Patients with a Double Uterus before and after Wedge Metroplasty (1936–1980)

Reproductive Performance	Pretherapy	Posttherapy
Number of patients with adequate follow-up	51	47
Number of patients pregnant	51 (100%)	45 (96%)
Number of patients with living children	3 (6%)	38 (81%)
Total pregnancies	165	66
Term	0 (0%)	50 (76%)
Premature	9 (5%)	4 (6%)
Abortion	156 (95%)	12 (16%)
Living children	4 (2%)	49 (74%)

There were 232 patients available, each of whom had had one or more miscarriages. These patients had a total of 585 pregnancies, of which 506 miscarried. There were 21 living children from these 585 pregnancies. Thus, this group qualified as being severely handicapped from a reproductive point of view. One hundred eight-three (78.9%) of the 232 patients became pregnant, and 155 (66.8%) carried to term. There were a total of 204 pregnancies, of which 24 (11.7%) miscarried. These results, although somewhat lower than those reported for abdominal metroplasty for similar types of patients (see Table 12.1), are reasonably satisfactory.

Of special interest in the Hassiakos review was the analysis of 36 patients from eight reports who had primary infertility. Eleven of these 36 (33.3%) became pregnant, but four of these miscarried, so that the term pregnancy rate was seven of 36, or only 19.4%. These data emphasize that extreme caution is required in attributing primary infertility to a uterine deformity.

PROBLEMS OF VERTICAL FUSION

Transverse Vaginal Septum: Obstructive

An obstructive transverse vaginal septum may be encountered in infancy. It may be a very serious problem because when it occurs, a large volume of mucus can collect above the obstruction, and such cases are often described in the literature as examples of hydromucocolpos. If such obstructions are not promptly relieved, there is the obvious potential for considerable impairment of subsequent reproduction. No systematic study, however, or even case reports of reproduction in individuals who in infancy had hydromucocolpos, have been noted.

As judged by a pedigree study of an inbred Amish community, there is impressive evidence that hydromucocolpos is the result of a rare autosomal recessive gene (Fig. 12.44).

The site of the obstruction may be anywhere along the vaginal canal, but most frequently is at the junction between the middle and upper third of the vagina (Fig. 12.45). The diagnosis of this condition in infancy is not easy, and many of these patients have been operated upon abdominally because of the palpation of a large mass in the lower abdomen. This mass has proven to be a tremendously distended vagina that has, in some instances, caused serious urinary tract obstruction because of its size. Fatalities have been reported. The diagnosis is difficult because there is no bulging at the outlet, since the obstruction is within the vagina (Fig. 12.46).

The most effective surgical therapy is an

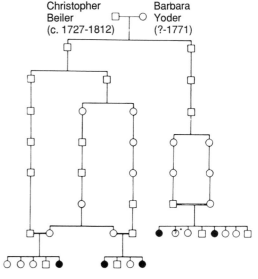

Figure 12.44. Pedigree pattern showing five patients affected with hydromucocolpos due to a transverse vaginal septum. The affected patients are shown in a solid black circle. The pedigree suggests that the lesion is due to a rare autosomal recessive disorder. (From McKusick et al: JAMA 1964;189:813.)

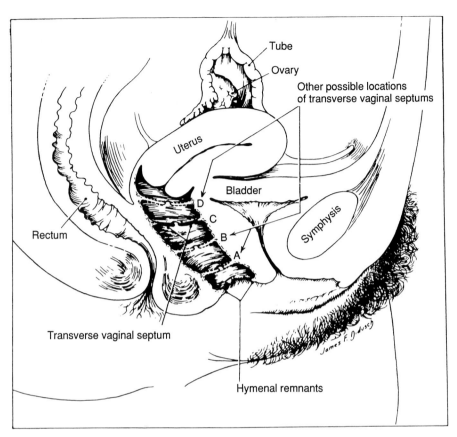

Figure 12.45. Diagram of various sites of occurrence for a transverse vaginal septum. The most common site is C at about the junction of the upper and middle third of the vagina. (From Bowman and Scott, Obstet Gynecol 1954;3:441.)

operation from below that removes the obstructive membrane. In most cases, this membrane is not very thick when encountered in infancy, but bilateral Schuchardt incisions may be required and should be carried out in order to be certain that the obstruction is relieved. Mandell et al. (12) have especially considered the operative approach to this problem.

It is possible to drain a large hydromucocolpos by needle aspiration under ultrasound guidance. However, permanent drainage must be provided coincident with the aspiration to prevent the consequence of the introduction of infection in an undrained space. This could cause the troublesome complication of a pyomucocolpos, which could destroy reproductive function.

Sometimes, an obstructive transverse vaginal septum does not give symptoms until after the onset of menstruation. The symptoms then are associated with obstruction to the outflow of

the menstrual blood. The character of the obstructing membrane may be quite different in the cases encountered in adults as compared with the situation in infancy. It is not clear why in infancy, in some cases, large amounts of mucus collect above the obstructing membrane, while in other cases, this does not seem to occur, and symptoms do not manifest themselves until after the onset of menstruation. Whether this is associated with the character of the obstructing membrane is uncertain, but, as mentioned, in the adult, many times the transverse vaginal septum may be quite thick-walled, making its removal more difficult. Indeed, a considerable segment of the vagina can be undeveloped, and if this segment is quite prolonged, so that it involves the whole lower portion of the vagina, congenital absence of the vagina with a uterus present arises. This situation may be considered to be an extreme form of transverse vaginal septum. This condition seems to be pathogenically quite different from the Rokitansky-Kuster-Hauser syndrome. This is because, with transverse vaginal septum, anomalies of the urinary tract are quite unusual, whereas they are quite common in the Rokitansky-Kuster-Hauser syndrome (Fig. 12.47).

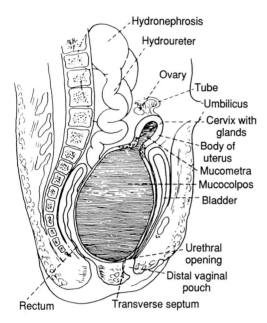

Figure 12.46 labels: Hydronephrosis, Hydroureter, Ovary, Tube, Umbilicus, Cervix with glands, Body of uterus, Mucometra, Mucocolpos, Bladder, Urethral opening, Distal vaginal pouch, Rectum, Transverse septum

Figure 12.46. Sagittal diagram of a patient with a transverse vaginal septum and the accumulation of a large amount of mucus, causing obstruction to the ureters.

A very puzzling situation exists when the vagina is undeveloped but the uterus is present, yet does not seem to function. This may occur when there is an associated amenorrhea of any cause, including that due to failure of development of the endometrium (Fig. 12.48).

When there is accumulation of menstrual blood, symptoms dominated by severe cyclic pain require therapy in the early teen years. If the obstructing membrane can be incised by multiple radial incisions with reanastomosis of the upper and lower vaginal segments, this is the preferred method (Fig. 12.49).

However, in some instances, the length of the obstructing transverse septum may be such that reanastomosis of the upper and lower segment is not possible. In that circumstance, the connection of the upper and lower segments may be accomplished by developing a space between the rectum and the bladder, as is done when there is complete absence of the vagina. The identification of the obstructed upper vagina may be troublesome, and it is important to distinguish it from the bladder anteriorly and the rectum posteriorly. The identification of the obstructed upper vagina is facilitated if there is a considerable amount of accumulated menstrual blood. For this reason, it is a disadvantage to have had the upper vagina drained abdominally, as has happened in

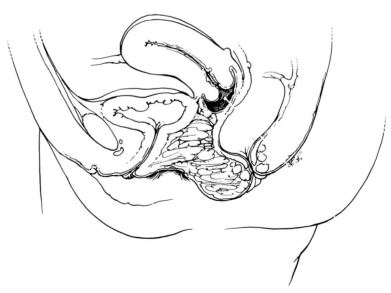

Figure 12.47. A sagittal diagram of a patient who might be considered to have congenital absence of the vagina with the uterus present. This may be considered to be an extreme example of a transverse vaginal septum.

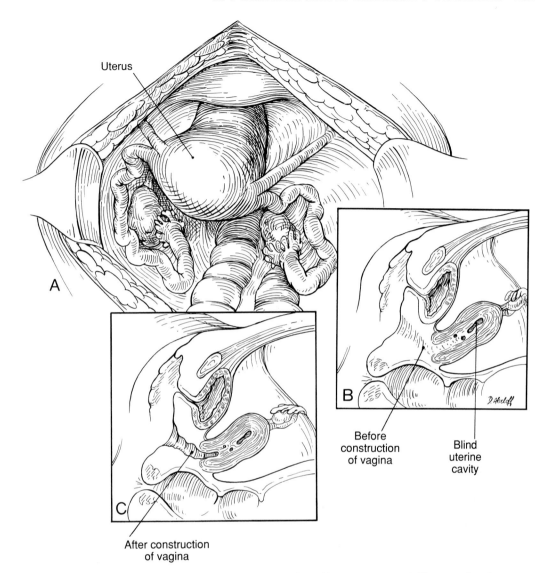

Figure 12.48. Patient with congenital absence of the vagina but with a uterus present. However, the uterus was nonfunctioning, as the endometrial cavity had not developed.

some instances when the accumulated blood in the upper vagina has created a mass of considerable size that was mistaken for some other intraabdominal structure and approached from above. When operating from below, it is often helpful to probe with an aspirating needle so that when menstrual blood is obtained, the identification of the vagina is certain.

After the upper vagina is opened and if the missing segment is such that the upper and lower portions cannot be reanastomosed, it is necessary to use an indwelling stent. A very satisfactory one can be made from Plexiglas or

other suitable plastic material. It is convenient to have it bulbous at one end and to have this end in the upper vagina so that as the dissected area contracts, the stent will be self-retaining (Fig. 12.50). This is particularly helpful in teenage patients, whose motivation to care for an indwelling stent is minimal. The Plexiglas stent will obviously require a channel through its center to provide for the egress of blood from cyclic menstruation. Such a stent may be left in place for 4–6 months. When it is removed—by making a lateral incision beside the stent, if necessary—it can be anticipated

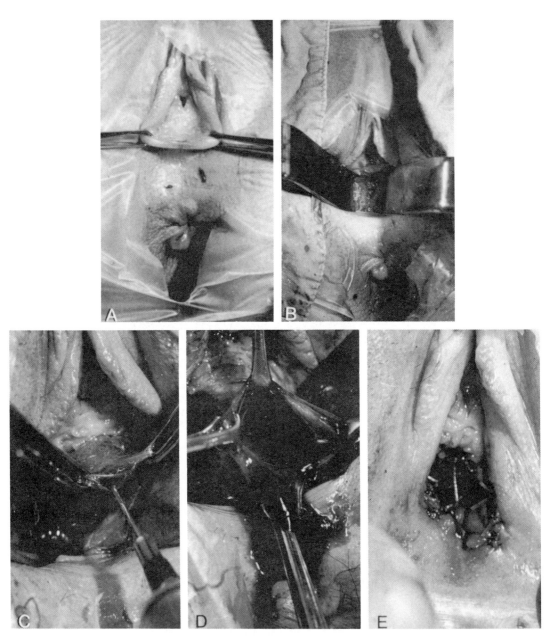

Figure 12.49. Patient with a transverse vaginal septum. *A,* Photograph of the external genitalia showing absence of the vaginal opening. *B,* Dissection between bladder and rectum. The blind vagina noticed in the depth of the incision. *C,* Aspiration of the blind vagina with thick blood in the aspirating syringe. *D,* Opening of the blind vagina. *E,* Suture of the upper and lower part of the vagina. In this case, the upper vaginal epithelium could be adequately mobilized to suture to the lower segment.

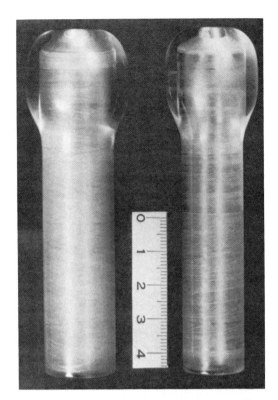

Figure 12.50. Two stents made of lucite for the treatment of a very long transverse vaginal septum, sometimes referred to as congenital absence of the vagina with the uterus present.

that the epithelium of the upper and lower vagina will have joined by the proliferation of the epithelium from above and below.

Following the removal of the original stent, vaginal dilation on a daily basis will be required for a period of 2–4 months to assure that undesirable contraction does not occur. However, if the size of the original Plexiglas stent was satisfactory, this should not be a major problem.

A very troublesome situation occurs when the defect in development includes the cervix. Thus, there is a functioning, but obstructed, uterine corpus and a defect in cervical and vaginal development. The vagina may be essentially absent, but in other cases, the vagina has been of adequate functional depth (Fig. 12.51).

Preservation of reproductive potential in this situation has been seldom achieved. In fact, there seems to be only one documentation of successful reproduction, that by Zarou et al. (19). Attempts to maintain a fistulous opening

between the endometrial cavity and the vagina are usually doomed to failure. After repeated dilatations over a number of years, both patient and surgeon are happy to solve the problem by the removal of the corpus of the uterus. For this reason, and because the fallopian tubes may also be malformed, it is realistic to recommend hysterectomy as initial primary therapy in these cases, with very few exceptions. Such was the conclusion of Geary and Weed (8) on the basis of experience with four cases of this unusual syndrome. Dillon et al. (5), after an experience with a single case, and a thorough review of the 17 previously reported cases up to that time, also recommended hysterectomy. On the other hand, Farber and Marchant (6) reported success in establishing a permanent fistulous opening between the uterine cavity and the cervix in four patients. However, at the time of the report, no pregnancies had occurred.

Incidentally, at the time of definitive surgery, very often the fallopian tubes are distorted, and endometriosis is widespread. At present, therefore, on the basis of the above considerations, hysterectomy seems the most suitable method of therapy, except in extenuating circumstances such as when there is only partial failure of the cervix to develop, or when there is a very short distance between the vagina and the endometrial cavity. In any case, successful subsequent reproduction seems to be very rare.

Transverse Vaginal Septum: Nonobstructed

Most often, a transverse vaginal septum is not complete and, therefore, the accumulation of mucus or menstrual blood is not a factor. However, such a partial transverse vaginal septum may cause dyspareunia or may develop a complication that compromises reproduction.

Occasionally, the opening in the transverse vaginal septum is so small that its identification is difficult. Such minimal lesions may give no dyspareunia, and pregnancies have occurred, making it clear that the sperm traversed the gap from the partial transverse septum to the cervix often a distance of 3–4 cm or longer (Fig. 12.52). On occasion, such small openings can be a problem, as in a patient delivered by

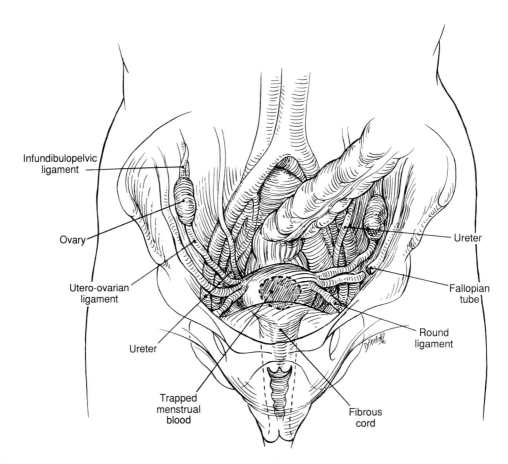

Figure 12.51. Drawing of a patient with congenital absence of the cervix, but with a functioning endometrial cavity. In this particular case, the fallopian tubes had no lumina, but the vagina was normally present. The right ovary was abnormally located. In this particular case there was no endometriosis because of the tubal obstruction, but in many instances endometriomas are present.

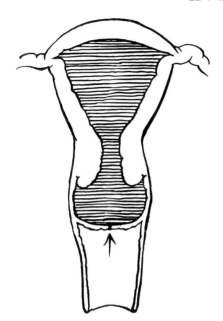

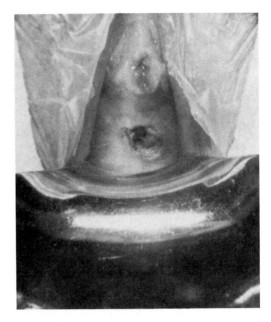

Figure 12.52. Diagram of a patient with a transverse vaginal septum containing a very thin opening. This patient became pregnant, was delivered by cesarean section, but postpartum had pyometra and polycopos above the point of obstruction.

Figure 12.53. Photograph of the transverse vaginal septum of the same patient shown in Fig. 12.52. This photograph was taken after the pinhole opening had been enlarged to allow draining of the pyocolpos.

cesarean section in whom the lochia was so profuse that it could not be accommodated through the pinpoint opening in the transverse vaginal septum with resulting obstruction, infection, and the necessity for emergency surgical drainage (Fig. 12.53).

References

1. Andrews MC, Jones HW Jr: Impaired reproductive performance of the unicornuate uterus and intrauterine growth retardation infertility and recurrent abortion in five cases. Am J Obstet Gynecol 1982; 144:173–176.

2. Azoury RS, Jones HW Jr: Cytogenic findings in patients with congenital absence of the vagina. Am J Obstet Gynecol 1966;94:178–80.

3. Barnes AB, Colton T, Gunderson J, et al: Fertility and outcome of pregnancy in women exposed in utero to diethystilbestrol. N Engl J Med 1980;302:609–613.

4. DeCherney AH, Russell JB, Graebe RA: Resectoscopic management of mullerian fusion defects. Fertil Steril 1986;45:726–728.

5. Dillon WP, Mudaliar NA, Wingate MD: Congenital atresia of the cervix. Obstet Gynecol 1979;54:126–129.

6. Farber M, Marchant DJ: Reconstructive surgery for congenital atresia of the uterine cervix. Fertil Steril 1976;27:1277–1282.

7. Garcia J, Jones HW Jr: The split-thickness graft technique for vaginal agenesis. Obstet Gynecol 1977; 49:328–332.

8. Geary WL, Weed JC: Congenital atresia of the uterine cervix. Obstet Gynecol 1973;42:213–217.

8a. Haney AF, Hammond CB, Soules MR, et al: Diethylstilbesterol-induced upper genital tract abnormalities. Fertil Steril 1979;31:142.

9. Hassiakos DK, Zourlas PA: Transcervical division of uterine septa. Obstet Gynecol Surv 1990;45:165–173.

10. Jones HW Jr, Mermut S: Familial occurrence of congenital absence of the vagina. Am J Obstet Gynecol 1972;114:1100–1101.

11. Kaufman RH, Binder GL, Gray PM Jr, et al: Upper genital tract changes associated with exposure in utero to diethylstilbestrol. Am J Obstet Gynecol 1977; 128:51–59.

12. Mandell J, Stevens PS, Lucey DT: Diagnosis and management of hydromucocolpos in infancy. J Urol 1978;120:262–265.

13. Muasher SJ, Jones HW Jr: Experience with diethylstilbestrol-exposed women in a program of in vitro fertilization. Fertil Steril 1984;42:20–24.

14. Park IJ, Jones HW Jr, Nager GT, et al: A new syndrome in two unrelated females: Klippel-Feil deformity, conductive deafness and absent vagina. Birth Defects: Original Articles VIII, New York: Alan R. Liss, Inc. 1971;311.

15. Strubbe EH, Thinjn CJP, Willemsen WNP, et al: Evaluation of radiographic abnormalities of the hand

in patients with Mayer-Rokitansky-Kuster-Hauser Syndrome. Genetics 1988;43:167–170.

16. Shokeir MHK: Aplasia of the mullerian system: Evidence for probable sex limited autosomal dominant inheritance. Birth Defects: Original Articles XIV(6C), New York: Alan R Liss, Inc., 1978:219.

17. Toaff R: A major genital malformation: Communicating uteri. Obstet Gynecol 1974;43:221–231.

18. Tompkins P: Comments on the bicornuate uterus and twinning. Surg Clin N Am 1962;42:1049–1062.

19. Zarou GS, Esposito JM, Zarou DM: Pregnancy following the surgical correction of congenital atresia of the cervix. Int J Gynecol Obstet 1973;11:143–146.

13

SURGICAL PROCEDURES FOR DISORDERS OF SEXUAL DEVELOPMENT

Howard W. Jones, Jr.

EXPERIMENTAL STUDIES OF SEXUAL DEVELOPMENT

A review of the classic studies of sexual development on the rabbit by Alfred Jost during the late 1940s and 1950s (48,49) is key to understanding human disorders of sexual development. The clinician can thereby recognize the pathogenesis of essentially all disorders of sexual development seen in the examining room.

In the rabbit, as in the human, during embryonic life, there is a phase of undifferentiated sex development, as far as the sex ducts are concerned. During this stage, there is a well-identified müllerian duct, a well-identified wolffian duct, a gonad that has not yet differentiated, and external genitalia that are ambiguous and undeveloped. The first critical experiment of Jost was the excision of the gonads of a fetal rabbit during the undifferentiated sexual stage. As a background, keep in mind that ductile differentiation and differentiation of the external genitalia are not due to a direct genetic message, but to products of the developing gonad. The genetic message behind sexual differentiation is directed entirely at gonadal differentiation. Thus, if in the indifferent stage, the gonad is destined to become a testis, the wolffian ducts will develop into the excretory ducts of the testis, the müllerian ducts will be inhibited and disappear, and the external genitalia will develop along masculine lines. On the other hand, if the gonad is destined to become an ovary, the reverse occurs, i.e., the wolffian ducts will wither, the müllerian ducts will develop, and the external genitalia do not masculinize, i.e., they develop along feminine lines. The critical experiments of Jost revealed that if he did a gonadectomy during the indifferent stage, regardless of whether that gonad was destined to become a testis or an ovary, the sex ducts developed along female lines. That is to say, the müllerian ducts persisted and developed, although not as actively as if an ovary had been present, the wolffian duct withered, and the external genitalia became feminine (Fig. 13.1).

The second critical experiment involved unilateral gonadectomy on a male rabbit. Thus, if one gonad was removed on day 19, i.e., during the indifferent sexual developmental stage, and the rabbit examined later, it was found that the wolffian duct developed into a vas deferens on the unoperated side, but on the operated side, the wolffian duct disappeared, and the müllerian duct developed on the way to being a uterus (Fig. 13.2).

In the third experiment, an embryonic testis was grafted into a female fetus onto the genital ridge on approximately day 20, i.e., during the indifferent duct stage. When the rabbits were

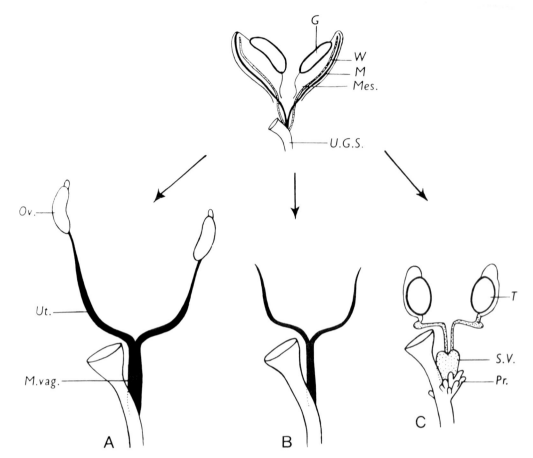

Fig. 13.1. Dissection of three rabbit fetuses. *A,* The undifferentiated stage (19 days old) identical in both sexes except for the histologic structure of the gonad. Notice the place of the gonad and of the sex ducts on the mesonephros; compare with Fig. 13.2. *B,* A male (28 days old); the testes are undergoing a still incomplete descent. *C,* A female (28 days old); the female rabbit has two uterine horns. *A* is 1.5 times as enlarged as *B* and *C.* Blad., bladder; Ext. Gen., external genitalia; gon., gonad; G. Tub., genital tubercle; K., kidney (metanephros); Mes., mesonephros; Ov., ovary; Ut., uterine horn; V. def., vas deferens.

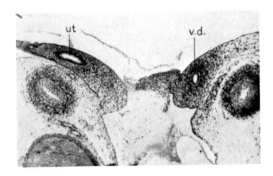

Figure 13.2. Section through the genital tract of a 28-day-old male rabbit fetus unilaterally castrated on day 19. Between the two ureters the genital ducts are seen. On the intact right side of the body, the vas deferens is seen (v.d.); on the gonadless left side a uterine horn (ut) developed, creating a lateral asymmetry.

examined on day 28, it was found that, where the grafts had been successfully placed, even though the graft was immediately adjacent to the ovary, the müllerian duct adjacent to the graft did not develop, but the wolffian ducts both on that side and the contralateral side were stimulated beyond the point they should have been at that stage of development. Furthermore, the external genitalia were somewhat masculinized. This experiment, as experiment number two, tended to confirm the fact that the inhibiting factor on the müllerian ducts was local in its action, but that the stimulus to maintain the wolffian ducts and to masculinize the external genitalia was rather general and probably exerted its effect by entry into the general circulation (Fig. 13.3).

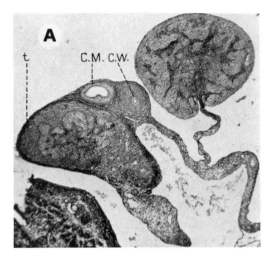

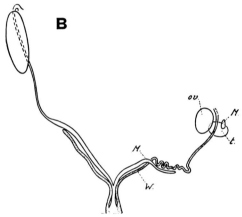

Figure 13.3. Testicular graft on a female rabbit fetus and masculinization of the genital tract. *A,* Histologic section showing the testicular graft (t) inserted on the mesosalpinx which contains the wolffian duct (C.W.) and a müllerian cyst (C.M.). *B,* Reconstruction of the genital ducts showing the grafted testis (t) near the ovary (ov); the müllerian duct (M, white) is locally inhibited; the wolffian duct (W, punctate) is unilaterally persistent. The fetal testis was grafted on the female fetus on day 20, and this fetus was sacrificed on day 28.

The fourth and final classical experiment was the substitution of various steroid crystals in the genital ridge of the female for the grafted testis. The most striking experiment was when a crystal of testosterone propionate was implanted on day 20 on an animal that was sacrificed on day 28. Contrary to the situation in experiment 3, the testosterone crystal did not duplicate exactly the situation when a male testis was grafted at that same time. The testosterone-implanted animal masculinized

the external genitalia and stimulated the wolffian duct, but there was no evidence of inhibition of the müllerian ducts (Fig. 13.4).

These experiments taken together indicate that during fetal development two positive influences emanate from the developing testis. The first of these inhibits the müllerian duct and does so by diffusion. It has variously been called the müllerian-inhibiting factor (MIF) or the antimüllerian hormone (AMH). The second influence from the testis seems to exert its influence by entering the general circulation and is responsible for the stimulation of the wolffian duct and its conversion into the excretory ducts of the testis. Furthermore, this general circulating product, probably testosterone itself, is responsible for the masculinizing of the external genitalia. Its role in masculinizing the external genitalia, however, may be that of acting as a substrate for dehydrotestosterone, which appears to be the active element in the masculinization process for those structures derived from the urogenital sinus.

Since the original experiments of Jost, the antimüllerian hormone has been purified. It is a product of the Sertoli cells and is a glycoprotein with a molecular weight of about 70,000 (46). Its purification is sufficient to have developed a radioimmunoassay, and with this new sensitive test, it has been found to be present in the serum of young males up until about the age of puberty. It cannot be found in girls or women, or in adult men (4,37). Its presence until puberty had led to the speculation that it may be a meiotic inhibitor in the absence of which spermatogenesis is initiated.

THE CRITERIA OF SEX: THE DEFINITION, NOMENCLATURE, AND CLASSIFICATION OF INTERSEXUALITY

The Criteria of Sex

Sex can be described in terms of at least seven characteristics, five of which are organic, four structural, one humeral, and the last two of which are psychogenic:

1. The sex chromosomes and the sex-determining genes;

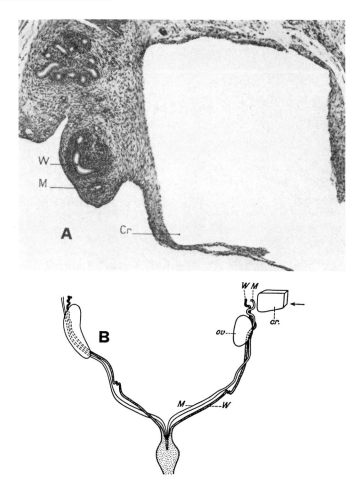

Figure 13.4. Masculinization of the genital tract of a female rabbit fetus by a crystal (Cr) of testosterone propionate implanted on day 20 (sacrificed on day 28). *A,* Histologic section showing the quadrate area, which are occupied by the crystal of androgen; müllerian (M) and wolffian (W) derivatives are present. *B,* Reconstruction of the genital tract showing the persistence of the complete wolffian duct (W, punctate); no inhibition of the müllerian duct (M, white) occurred. The arrow indicates the level of the section seen in *A.*

2. Gonadal structure;
3. Morphology of the external genitalia;
4. Morphology of the internal genitalia;
5. Hormonal status;
6. Sex of rearing;
7. Gender role of the individual.

The Sex Chromosomes and the Sex-Determining Genes

In 1949, Barr and Bertram (6) noted that it was possible to identify the sex of animals by the presence or absence of a specific chromatin body, the sex chromatin in the cells of the nerve nuclei in the brain. This quickly led to the discovery that when adequate preparations were available, nuclear morphology in almost all somatic cells could be used as an accurate indication of sex.

At one period in clinical medicine, a determination of the sex chromatin was a very useful clinical test; however, the technique is unreliable unless constantly used. For this reason, when confronted with a problem of intersexuality, contemporary practice requires a karyotypic examination by banding techniques. A proper karyotype will determine not only whether there are normal male or female chromosomes, 46XX or 46XY, but whether or not there is any structural abnormality of any of the chromosomes.

With the development of techniques for the identification of specific segments of DNA, several male specific sequences belonging to the Y chromosome have been identified. At this writing, the identification of these sequences is for the most part a research tool (63), but studies have been very helpful in elucidating the puzzling finding of certain problems. For example, in XX males, an examination of the DNA sequences has revealed a fairly constant finding of sequences normally found on the Y chromosome (23). This has led to the conclusion that the genetic message with the development of a testis has been the result of a meiotic error in the patient's father, whereby sequences on the Y chromosomes were abnormally translocated to the X.

Gonadal Sex

The identification of the sex of the gonad by microscopic examination is the basis for the well-known Klebs classification of hermaphrodites. It is obvious that various other criteria of sex identification are often in conflict with the gonadal sex. For example, in certain patients, there may be a contradiction between the gonadal sex and the sex of rearing. Adequate therapy often depends upon the proper identification of gonadal structure, and it certainly remains as perhaps the most important criteria of sexual identification. It must be emphasized, however, that gonadal identification is determined by microscopic and not gross examination. The gross appearance of gonads in cases of intersexuality may be deceptive.

The Morphology of External Genitalia

The morphology of the external genitalia is the criterion used by the obstetrician in assigning sex to the newborn. With a few exceptions, the sex of rearing is dependent upon the morphology of the external genitalia. If there is a contradiction between the predominant appearance of the genitalia and the sex of rearing, it was shown many years ago by Money et al. (57), that the patient often succeeds in coming to terms with a morphologic anomaly and assumes a role consistent with that of assigned sex and rearing. This is certainly not to say that such patients have no psychological difficulties—quite the contrary—the obstetrician's responsibility in assigning sex is indeed a grave

one when there is some ambiguity of the external genitalia.

The Morphology of the Internal Genitalia

In every normal embryo, as has already been mentioned, both the mesonephric (wolffian) and müllerian ducts are present and capable of development into perfect male or female internal genitalia, depending upon the hormonal signal from the testis. Whether this development occurs in a normal manner, or whether there is some development contradiction, as in the intersexual state, is of little importance with regard to assigned sex or gender role, both of which are largely dependent upon external morphology. Nevertheless, the development or atrophy of the sex ducts is of surpassing importance as far as function of the genital apparatus is concerned.

Hormonal Sex

The hormonal milieu is fundamental as a criterion of sex, but it is by no means identical with gonadal structure. The endocrine environment is an important determining factor for the morphology of the sex ducts and genitalia. It is also later responsible for such secondary sex characteristics as breast development, hair growth, bone growth, epiphysial fusion, fat distribution, general body habitus, and the like. Not only do the testes secrete estrogens that can feminize the body in the absence of androgenic action, but glands other than the gonads exert controlling hormonal influences of a contradictory type in some instances. The adrenals, for example, in the various forms of congenital adrenal hyperplasia, secrete large amounts of a virilizing hormone, probably testosterone, responsible for the hermaphroditic state in females. A proper recognition of the hormonal sex is therefore required for a proper understanding and therapy of many cases of intersexuality.

The Sex of Rearing

Of the various criteria of sex, the sex of rearing is the most obvious and can be recognized by the community as well as the physician. Assigned sex and rearing are critical factors in sex orientation. It follows that the sex of rearing is a most evident consideration in describing sex and should be a weighty factor in the therapeutic orientation of the physician.

Gender Role

The gender role can be defined as all those things a person says or does to disclose himself or herself as having the status of boy or man, girl or woman, respectively. It includes, but is not restricted to, sexuality in the sense of eroticism. Gender role is appraised in relation to such things as general mannerisms, deportment and demeanor, play, preferences and recreational interests, spontaneous talk and unprovoked conversation, casual comments, and finally, the individual's role to direct inquiry. A problem with gender role with no other aberration of sexual identification is a serious clinical complex of transsssexualism and will not be further considered in this text.

A Definition of the Hermaphroditic State

In a normal individual, all five organic and two psychologic criteria correspond to sex. The hermaphroditic state may be said to exist when there is a contradiction of one or more of the morphologic criteria of sex-chromosomal pattern, gonadal structure, morphology of external genitalia, and morphology of internal genitalia. Although the hormonal sex is often inconsistent in hermaphroditism, a sex contradiction of hormonal background may exist without hermaphroditism, as for example, with a virilizing tumor. Although the psychologic criteria of sex are of extreme importance, especially with regard to therapy of the hermaphroditic state, a conflict between them and other sex criteria is not necessary for a diagnosis of hermaphroditism. In fact, such a contradiction in the face of agreement of all of the organic criteria of sex is indicative of a psychiatric problem of transsexualism and transvestism and is quite distinct from hermaphroditism per se.

The Nomenclature and Classification of Hermaphroditism

Although any of the several criteria of sex might be the basis of a classification of ambisex-

ual individuals, the well-established classification of Klebs (51) is based upon the microscopic character of the gonad. According to this view, the state of true hermaphroditism can be considered to exist only if both male and female elements can be identified in the gonad. Klebs' original classification of true hermaphroditism is complex and attempts to give consideration to the various gonadal combinations that might exist. According to Klebs, 16 subdivisions were thought possible.

The Latin of the original classification is quite understandable when it is kept in mind that it refers only to the gonads with respect to the classification of true hermaphroditism. The adjectives *bilateralis, unilateralis,* or *lateralis* refer to ambisexual gonadal tissue on both sides, one side only or alternating (male one side; female other side), respectively. *Completus* is used to indicate gonadal tissue on both sides and *incompletus* is used to indicate that one side is devoid of all gonadal tissue. *Masculinus* or *feminus* followed by *dexter* (right) or *sinister* (left) is used to describe the character and side of the gonad opposite of a unilateral ovotestis.

Klebs further specified that ambisexual individuals with entirely male gonads should be identified as male *pseudo*hermaphrodites and ambisexual individuals with entirely female gonads should be identified as female *pseudo*hermaphrodites. Furthermore, according to Klebs, there are three forms of *pseudo*hermaphroditism: (1) *completus,* (2) *internus,* and (3) *externus.* As explained by Creevy (16), any *pseudo*hermaphrodite can be classified and described according to the Klebs concept by two adjectives. The first (male or female) indicates the nature of the sex gland. The second (external, internal, or complete) indicates whether it is the sex of the internal, external, or both groups of genitalia which differs from that of the gonad.

The female internal variety includes outwardly normal females with ovaries, but with such male vestigial remnants as a Gartner's duct, a rudimentary prostate, and vas deferens. The female external type has normal or rudimentary internal genitalia and ovaries but external genitalia resembling those of the male. In complete female *pseudo*hermaphroditism, both the external and internal genitalia would tend to be masculine in an individual with ovaries.

The male internal variety of *pseudo*hermaphrodite would possess testes and a well-developed uterus, tubes, and perhaps vagina. The male external variety would have testes but feminine external genitalia. In complete male *pseudo*hermaphroditism, the patient would have testes, but feminine internal and external genitalia.

Obviously, the Klebs classification is impractical because of its complexity. At the same time, it is incomplete in terms of current knowledge. Still, it has been described at some length because of its historic interest and because some hermaphrodites are described by its terms in current literature. Its widespread use and acceptance, in a simplified form, has made it desirable to continue to use gonadal sex as the basic criterion of any classification.

Before discussing the classification used in this book, a further word about nomenclature might prove clarifying. The terms *male* and *female* are preferably reserved to describe unequivocal biologic sex qualities, e.g., chromosomal arrangement or gonadal structure. They will generally not be used to describe a predominance of sex characteristics as applied, for example, to the external genitalia, nor will they be used to describe the sex of rearing. The terms *masculine, feminine, boy, girl, man,* or *woman* will be used to designate the predominance of sex characteristics without regard to whether the individuals described are *male* or *female.*

It is to be emphasized specifically that the use of the words *male* or *female* immediately before hermaphrodite implies nothing about that individual except that the individual has a testis or an ovary, respectively. It implies nothing with respect to the chromosomes, although they would generally but not always be in agreement; it indicates nothing about the anatomy of the external or internal genitalia, and it especially implies nothing with respect to the sex of rearing of that particular individual.

The terms intersexuality and hermaphroditism are used interchangeably and are considered synonymous.

Although we have retained the Klebs emphasis on gonadal structure, it has not been considered necessary to retain the prefix *pseudo*

in describing males or females with ambisexual development. *Male hermaphrodite* or *female hermaphrodite* is permissible in place of the obsolete male *pseudo*hermaphrodite or female *pseudo*hermaphrodite. This point of nomenclature stems from the thought that *pseudo* is redundant to describe an entirely male or entirely female gonad if *true* or *verus* be retained to describe the mixed gonad of *true hermaphrodite* or *hermaphroditismus verus.*

The classification of intersexuality used in this chapter is a simple one that recognizes: (*a*) male hermaphrodites; (*b*) female hermaphrodites; and (*c*) true hermaphrodites. Subclassifications within each group will be considered in the appropriate sections.

This book features only individuals who have ovarian or testicular development or both. Excluded are individuals with no gonadal tissue, i.e., those with only streak gonads. This is because the latter category of patients require essentially no reparative or constructive surgery and hence are beyond the scope of this treatise. In fact, the only surgery required for patients with streak gonads is excision of the streak if the individual has a Y chromosome.

MALE HERMAPHRODITISM

General Considerations

Genetic males with abnormal ectopic testes may have external genitalia so simulating the female at birth that the gonadal sex is not recognized (Figs. 13.5–13.7). At puberty, these individuals tend to masculinize or feminize, depending upon whether the abnormal testes secrete a biologic preponderance of androgenic or estrogenic hormones and on the receptivity of the end organs to these substances. Thus, the habitus of these individuals may develop to a typical android form without breast development or to a rather characteristic feminine form with excellent breast development. The external genitalia may be indistinguishable from those of a normal female. In other patients, the clitoris may be quite enlarged. In still other instances, there is fusion of the labia in the midline, resulting in what seems to be a hypospadic male urethra (Fig. 13.8). Under these circumstances, the individual is at

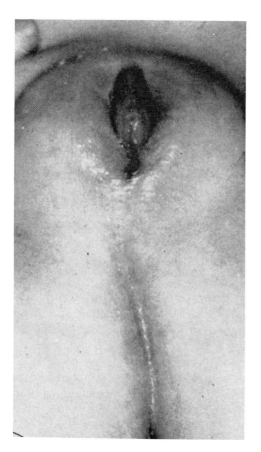

Figure 13.5. External genitalia of a 6-month-old girl whose true condition was recognized when a testis was discovered during an operation for inguinal hernia.

group, there are instances of a strong familial history. In spite of weak pedigree evidence in some forms of the disorder, it seems very likely that nearly all forms of male hermaphroditism have a genetic basis. Most male hermaphrodites have been reared as girls and women. Some have been quite successfully married and have been well adjusted with their sex partner. However, others as adults have been less than attractive women and have been the unfortunate victims of indecisive therapy. Psychiatric studies have indicated that if the aim of therapy is an emotionally well-adjusted person, best results are obtained by directing surgical, endocrinological, and psychiatric measures toward improving the feminine characteristics of the individual. Fortunately, this point of view coincides with the surgical and endocrine possibilities, for current surgical techniques can produce with relatively greater ease more satisfactory feminine than masculine external genitalia. Furthermore, in most patients, the testes of male hermaphrodites are nonfunctional as far as spermatogenesis is concerned, and no method now available shows promise of rendering them functional.

times reared as a man. A vagina of varying depth is usually present and often well developed. A cervix, uterus, and tubes may be developed to varying degrees, although müllerian structures are most often absent. Mesonephric (wolffian) structures may be grossly visible or identifiable by microscopic examination of appropriate tissue. Hair may be of typical feminine distribution or of masculine distribution and of sufficient quantity to require plucking or shaving.

In a special group, the axillary and pubic hair is congenitally absent. All cases so far reported have been amenorrheic in spite of the interesting theoretical possibility of uterine bleeding from endometrium stimulated by estrogen of testicular origin. There is no evidence of abnormal adrenal function. There may be no familial history of such disorders, but in the feminized group, and less frequently, in the nonfeminized

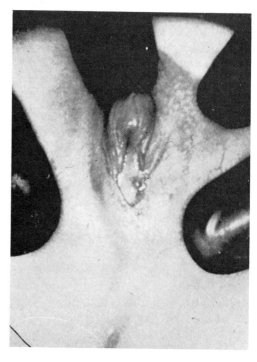

Figure 13.6. External genitalia of a 17-month-old male hermaphrodite reared as a girl.

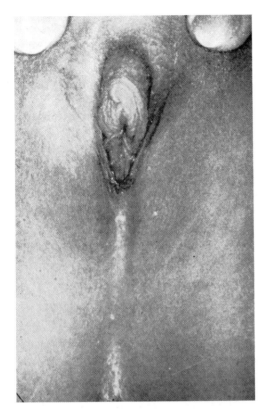

Figure 13.7. External genitalia of an 8½-year-old sister of the patient shown in Fig. 13.2. The condition of this girl was entirely unsuspected until she was examined as a result of the discovery of her sister's condition.

Not all male hermaphrodites are best reared as women, and when in a suitable patient there is a preponderance of masculine characteristics, the therapeutic efforts should, of course, be directed toward reinforcing these assets.

In the 1990s, all cases of male intersexuality with external ambiguity should be diagnosed in the nursery and therapy outlined in infancy. This has not always been the case, but experience with the consequences of late diagnosis should serve to emphasize the importance of careful study of any child with sexual ambiguity.

A DESCRIPTIVE CLASSIFICATION

All individuals classified as male hermaphrodites are genetic males in the sense that their chromosomes are 46,XY or a mosaic, one strain of which has a Y chromosome or a fragment of a Y. Their only gonadal tissue is testicular, albeit abnormal. The hermaphroditic states arises from the presence of a testis and external

genitalia that are feminine or are ambiguous as to sex, or from the presence of well-developed müllerian ducts.

For many years, a classification was used based on descriptive anatomical features. It follows:

A. Male hermaphrodites with ambiguous or predominantly masculine external genitalia and reared as men or women without potential for breast development.
   a. With rudimentary or no müllerian structures.
   b. With well-formed müllerian structures.
      1. Bilateral testes
      2. Unilateral testis, unilateral streak.
B. Male hermaphrodites with feminine or ambiguous external genitalia and best reared as women.
   a. Feminizing (androgen insensitivity syndrome)
   b. Masculinizing
   c. Mixed

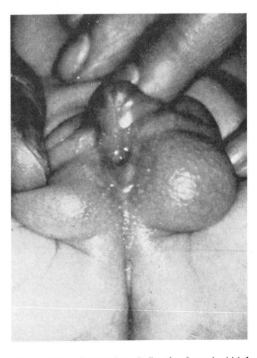

Figure 13.8. External genitalia of a 6-week-old infant whose sex was in doubt. Endoscopic examination revealed a 4-cm deep vagina but no cervix. The gonads were palpable in the inguinal canals. The phallus was of good size and was considered suitable for plastic correction toward the masculine side. He was classified as a male hermaphrodite because of the vagina, but the situation differed only in this detail from hypospadias.

Accumulated knowledge has made it possible to replace this descriptive classification with one based on pathogenesis and etiology (see below). While this is better with regard to understanding the development of the disorder, the older classification is useful to remember because it is therapeutically oriented. Thus, it may be helpful to place a given patient in each of the classifications: in the older, to help plan the surgical treatment, and in the newer, to understand the pathogenesis of the disorder.

AN ETIOLOGIC AND PATHOGENIC CLASSIFICATION

The classification follows:
I. Male hermaphroditism due to a central nervous system defect.
    A. Abnormal pituitary gonadotropin secretion
    B. No gonadotropin secretion
II. Male hermaphroditism due to a primary gonadal defect.
    A. Identifiable defect in biosynthesis of testosterone
       a. Pregnenolone synthesis defect (lipid adrenal hyperplasia)
       b. 3β-hydroxysteroid dehydrogenase deficiency
       c. 17α-hydroxylase deficiency
       d. 17–20-desmolase deficiency
       e. 17β-ketosteroid reductase deficiency
    B. Unidentified defect in androgen effect
    C. Defect in müllerian duct regression
    D. Familial gonad destruction
    E. Leydig cell agenesis
    F. Testicular dysgenesis
III. Male hermaphroditism due to peripheral end-organ defect
    A. Androgen-binding protein deficiency
    B. 5-reductase deficiency
IV. Male hermaphroditism due to Y chromosome defect

Even this detailed classification is by no means exhaustive. There are multiple subgroups within many and perhaps all of the above categories. As molecular studies are applied, it becomes evident that any of groups, especially those with an identifiable enzymatic problem can have that defect expressed as a result of a fault in any of the numerous steps from the gene itself to the enzyme or its modifiers.

Discussion of the nonanatomical aspects of each of the categories, while intrinsically interesting, is of only minimum significance to the surgical aspects of these cases. For this reason, the following discussions of each category will contain only the minimal information required for some insight into the pathogenesis of each of the categories. Emphasis will be on the anatomical defects of each of the categories. These, of course, are the focus of the surgeon's interest.

The Various Types of Male Hermaphroditism

MALE HERMAPHRODITISM DUE TO A CENTRAL NERVOUS SYSTEM DEFECT

Abnormal Pituitary Gonadotropic Secretion

Park et al. (69), reported a patient with slightly ambiguous external genitalia whose hermaphroditic state seemed to be the result of the secretion of a counterfeit gonadotropin.

This 27-year-old patient presented because of amenorrhea (Fig. 13.9). At birth, some abnormality of the genitalia was noted, but she was raised as a girl. Axillary and pubic hair developed at the normal age of 13 years. Breast development did not occur. At the age of 16, she received some cyclic Enovid with some breast development, but at the age of 22, an augmentation mammoplasty was carried out. No endocrine therapy was given except for the Enovid for a short period.

On physical examination, she was found to be 170 cm tall and weighed 58 kg. Her blood pressure was 110/80.

The general physical examination was essentially negative. The pattern of pubic hair was female. The external genitalia were characterized by some enlargement of the clitoris. The corpora measured 1×0.5 cm (Fig. 13.10). The urethra opened at the normal position for a female. The vaginal orifice was normal. The vagina was normally developed but was shallow, measuring only 4 cm deep. By bimanual examination and by rectal examination, no uterus was palpable. In the right inguinal canal,

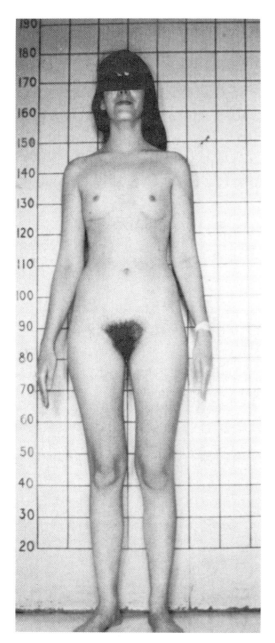

Figure 13.9. This 27-year-old patient complained of primary amenorrhea. The breast development was the result of an augmentation mammoplasty.

there was palpated what was thought to be a gonad, but nothing could be palpated on the left side.

The patient's karyotype was found to be 46,XY.

The patient was placed in the hospital on a laboratory metabolic protocol. Numerous data were collected. The essential and most impor-

tant finding was that she had a plasma testosterone of 53 ng/dl, a very low level for a male. Both FSH and LH were immunologically examined and found to be at menopausal levels. Total gonadotropins determined by a mouse assay also showed menopausal levels.

A key finding was that after the administration of exogenous human gonadotropin, the plasma testosterone rose immediately to 789 and 836 ng/dl at the end of the hCG stimulation. After discontinuing the hCG, but before gonadectomy, the testosterone value had returned to the prestimulation levels (Fig. 13.11).

Laparoscopy demonstrated that there was no müllerian duct development. A bilateral gonadectomy was performed by bilateral inguinal incisions.

Pathologic examination of the testes was of great interest (Fig. 13.12). A striking finding was that there was essentially no stimulation of the interstitial cells. The seminiferous tubules were lined with healthy-appearing Sertoli cells, but germ cells were absent.

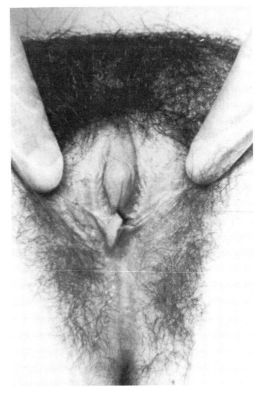

Figure 13.10. External genitalia of the patient shown in 13.9.

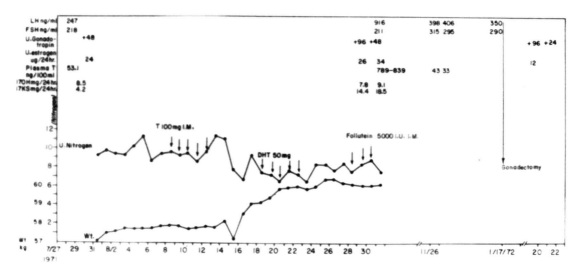

Figure 13.11. Chart of the metabolic studies of patient shown in Fig. 13.9.

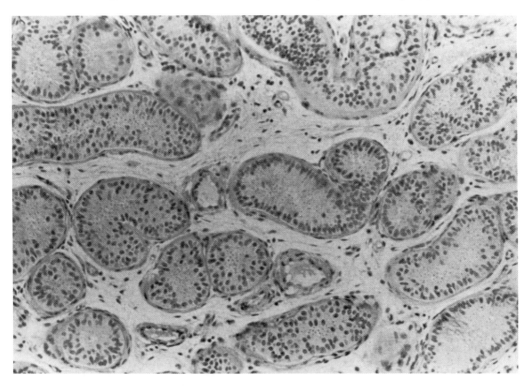

Figure 13.12. Histopathologic examination of the testis in patient shown in Fig. 13.9. Note healthy appearance of the Sertoli cells and the absence of unstimulated condition of the interstitial cells.

The most satisfactory explanation for the events that led to the male intersexuality in this case was a counterfeit gonadotropin, which was not recognized by the interstitial cells of the testes, but which assayed satisfactorily in the radioimmunoassay and indeed was recognized by the rat.

The surgical considerations were entirely with the removal of the testis to prevent tumor in this high-risk organ. The enlargement of the clitoris was not sufficient to warrant surgical consideration, and the vagina was of functional depth. It would be entirely possible that in other cases with less severe aberrations of the gonadotropin, the genitalia would be more ambiguous and that surgical reconstruction of the genitalia as discussed in the chapter on surgical treatment of hermaphroditism would be indicated.

No Gonadotropic Secretion

No liveborn fetuses have been reported with this particular category of disorders. Nevertheless, from a physiological point of view, this category is of great interest. Siler-Khodr et al. (87) reported a 36-week-old male fetus with an ambiguous external genitalia whose pituitary gland showed no detectable LH and FSH release in an in-vitro culture system.

By using a similar in-vitro culture system, they studied synthesis and release of pituitary gonadotropins from the adenohypophysis in 40 human fetuses. Among these 40 fetuses, one was the 36-week-old male fetus referred to above, with ambiguous external genitalia and undeveloped adrenals. There was no detectable LH and FSH release from the pituitary, although the pituitaries of the normal festuses released amounts considered to be normal. ACTH release was below normal, and growth hormone was at the low end of the normal range. It seems very likely that lack of pituitary gonadotropin secretion in this fetus was responsible for the incomplete masculinization of the external genitalia.

This finding is consistent with the observation of Jost (49), who found ambiguity of the external genitalia of the male rabbit following intrauterine decapitation. This experiment was interpreted to indicate the effect of the absence of pituitary gonadotropin.

It is interesting that in the anencephaly and in examples of congenital gonadotropin deficiency such as in Kallman syndrome, the genitalia are hypoplastic but not ambiguous. Bearn (7) has pointed out that in anencephaly, the pituitary gland is always present if carefully sought. This seems to explain why the male anencephalic fetus is not hermaphroditic.

The clinical evidence available from the patient with a counterfeit pituitary gonadotropin, discussed earlier, and the data from cases reported by Siler-Khodr indicate that pituitary gonadotropin is perhaps more critical in fetal gonadal stimulation than is chorionic gonadotropin.

Male Hermaphroditism Due to Primary Gonadal Defect

While various deficiencies in this category are listed under testicular defects, it is understood that nearly all of these heritable defects involve all body tissue. The chief organ of action and interest in connection with male hermaphroditism is the testis.

IDENTIFIABLE DEFECTS IN THE BIOSYNTHESIS OF TESTOSTERONE

To best understand these defects, the biosynthetic pathway of testosterone must be kept clearly in mind (Fig. 13.13). The diagnosis of a particular defect may be made by determining

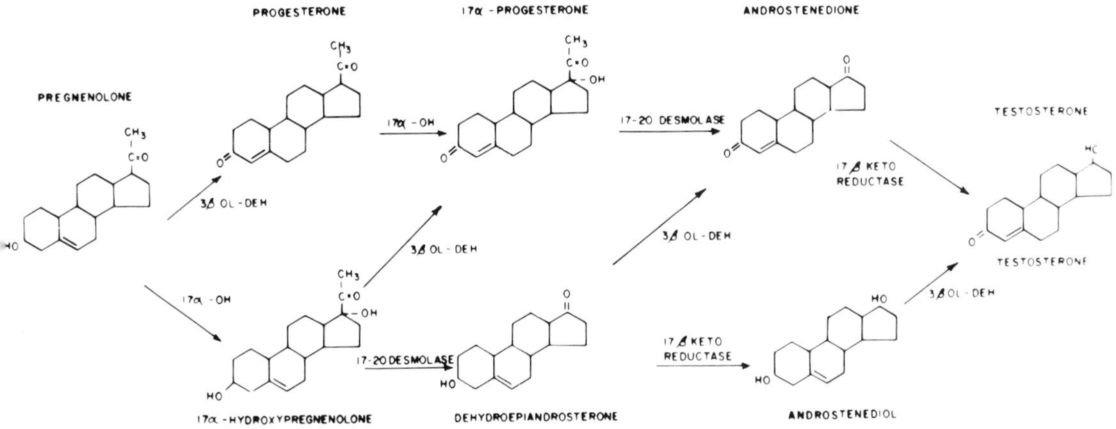

Figure 13.13. Diagrammatic representation of the intermediate steps in the biosynthesis of testosterone.

the various intermediate products. An enzymatic block, which, incidentally, is seldom complete, is indicated when there is an obvious accumulation of a substrate. In such cases, the serum concentration of testosterone is, as a rule, quite low. This, of course, is the proximate cause of the disorder.

After puberty, the determination of the intermediate metabolites presents no special problem. In infancy, however, when the gonadotropins are low normally, it is necessary to prime the patient with human chorionic gonadotropin to stimulate the interstitial cells to produce testosterone. When this is done, the levels of the intermediate metabolites become significant, so that the defect can be identified. In infancy during the first 2 months of life, the native LH is often sufficiently elevated so that the metabolites can be determined without prior priming, but if there is any uncertainty about this point, administration of hCG should resolve the difficulty.

Pregnenolone Synthesis Defect (Lipoid Adrenal Hyperplasia)

This category is included among male hermaphroditism largely for completeness. Severely affected patients do have ambiguity of the external genitalia and indeed are male hermaphrodites.

The first patient to be identified as having lipid adrenal hyperplasia was published by Prader and Gurtner (73), who reported the case of a female-appearing infant who died at the age of 6 weeks with symptoms of addisonian crisis. The autopsy revealed male gonads, a 46,XY chromosome complement, and very large adrenals filled with fat. They called the disease lipoid adrenal hyperplasia.

Degenhart (19) found evidence of unpaired 20-hydroxylation of cholesterol in these patients. Few survive infancy owing to the severe deficiency in the biosynthesis of cortisol, aldosterone, and other steroids.

3β-Hydroxysteroid Dehydrogenase Deficiency

Like patients with lipoid adrenal hyperplasia, individuals with a severe 3β-hydroxysteroid dehydrogenase deficiency are seriously ill because the 3β-hydroxysteroid dehydrogenase enzyme is required in the biosynthesis, not only of testosterone, but of cortisol, aldosterone, and the estrogens. As with many enzyme defects, there appears to be a spectrum of deficiency. Patients with severe difficulty are seriously ill and seldom survive through childhood.

Bongiovanni (10) first reported the 3β-hydroxysteroid defect. Parks et al. (70) published the cases of a most instructive family. In this family, an infant died in salt loss crisis from what seemed to be a congenital adrenal hyperplasia. There was a 13-year-old brother who had hypospadias, as well as severe salt loss. The children were genetic males. An autopsy on the 2-day-old patient showed large adrenal glands, perineal hypospadias, and a small phallus with chordee. The testes, scrotum, and vas deferens were grossly and microscopically considered to be normal.

The 13-year-old sibling had bilateral testes, hypospadias, and some breast development. He had been admitted to the hospital 13 times in the 13 years because of adrenal insufficiency.

As with the lipoid adrenal hyperplasia, individuals with 3β-ol-dehydrogenase difficulty are included in the rubric of male hermaphroditism largely for completeness. Their metabolic disturbances are so severe that they are often considered examples of salt-losing 21-hydroxylase deficiency in a female, and they must be distinguished from that. The sexual ambiguity of the male is inconsistent with a diagnosis of 21-hydroxylase deficiency in the female in that the latter have no testes in the scrotum.

During the 1980s, several cases of both males and females who have had very attenuated forms of this synthesis defect were reported. Such individuals have no abnormality of their external genitalia, but do have some metabolic disorders that can be treated by substitution therapy with cortisone or one of its analogs. These patients have no anatomical defect requiring surgical reconstruction. Cravioto et al. (14) have reviewed such cases.

17α-Hydroxylase Deficiency

Patients with a 17α-hydroxylase deficiency usually present with lack of pubertal development and hypertension (Fig. 13.14). The external genitalia of 46,XY patients appear entirely female or ambiguous (Fig. 13.15). Defective steroidogenesis results in inadequate conversion of progesterone to 17-hydroxyprogesterone and of pregnenolone to 17-hydroxy-pregnenolone. Consequently, inadequate androgen production among 46,XY patients with testes is responsible for inadequately virilized external genitalia. However, as with all enzyme defects, there seems to be a spectrum of incompetence. This is expressed by a wide spectrum in the appearance of the genitalia. Some may be quite feminine with relatively deep vaginas presumably of urogenital sinus origin, as seen in patients with the androgen insensitivity syndrome. On the other hand, there may also be complete fusion of the

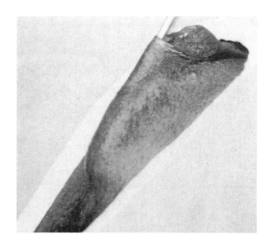

Figure 13.15. Photograph of external genitalia of patient shown in Fig. 13.14.

labioscrotal folds with total inhibition of vaginal development, as in the patient illustrated in the figures in this section. Phallic development is always limited, whereas the müllerian structures are uniformly totally inhibited.

Among 46,XX patients, pubertal development does not occur because of the inability of the ovary to produce estrogens. Hence, genetic females may not be diagnosed until secondary sexual characteristics fail to develop during pubertal years. However, among both XX and XY patients, spontaneous modest breast development may occur.

Because cortisol synthesis is also compromised by the 17α-hydroxylase defect, adrenocorticotropic hormone (ACTH) secretion is markedly increased. As the mineralocorticoid pathway does not require 17-hydroxylation, the excessive ACTH results in excessive production of 11-desoxycorticosterone, a potent mineralocorticoid. This increased production explains the hypertension that occurs regularly among patients with 17α-hydroxylase deficiency.

It is obviously important to make a precise diagnosis of this disorder as early as possible, as substitution therapy with cortisone or one of its analogues will reduce the ACTH elevation and thereby reduce the production of those intermediates that cause the hypertension. However, if the diagnosis is delayed, and the hypertension is longstanding, treatment may not be effective in reducing the hypertension.

Elevated luteinizing hormone level, and

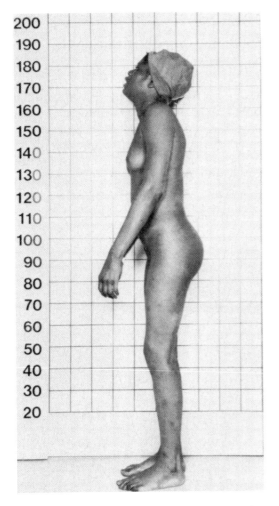

Figure 13.14. Lateral view of patient who proved to have 17α-hydroxylase deficiency.

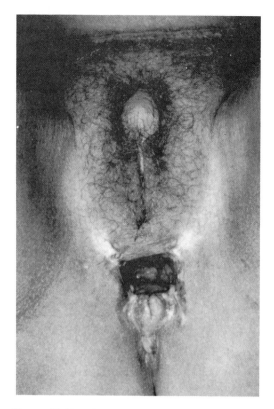

Figure 13.16. The postoperative appearance of the external genitalia of patient shown in Fig. 13.14.

inguinal hernias are not generally expected in males with this syndrome.

Reconstruction of the external genitalia according to the principles outlined in the section on reconstruction is required for patients with 17α-hydroxylase deficiency, if there is ambiguity. In some instances, (Fig. 13.16) where the vagina had been completely inhibited, the construction of the vagina through the perineum using the McIndoe split-thickness graft technique may be required.

Gonadectomy should be carried out (Fig. 13.17). Pathologic examination shows very active interstitial cells and seminiferous tubules with healthy-appearing Sertoli cells but no germinal cell elements (Fig. 13.18).

17-20-Demolase Deficiency

Zachmann et al. (98) were the first to recognize a specific 17-20 desmolase deficiency as a cause for male hermaphroditism. These workers reported two first cousins who had testes, a 46,XY chromosomal complement, and

ambiguous external genitalia. There was no salt-losing component. Another case was reported by Goebelsmann et al. (31), and an especially well-researched sibship was reported by Forest et al. (25).

As with other enzymatic defects, there seems to be a spectrum of abnormality even within a single sibship.

The diagnosis of this disorder is made by finding normal or elevated values for the C-21 compounds and the low values for the C-19 compounds under either basal or dynamic conditions. In the sibship studied by Forest et al. (25), the plasma concentrations of 10 C-21 progestagens or androgens measured by specific RIAs were found to be abnormally high under either basal or dynamic conditions, whereas basal levels of Δ4-androstenedione, dehydroepiandrosterone, and dehydroepiandrosterone sulfate were subnormal and failed to rise after ACTH stimulation both before and after castration. Meanwhile, levels of pregnenolone were extremely high under basal conditions and rose further after ACTH. All of the progestagens and cortisol were suppressed by dexamethasone. After hCG stimulation, either before treatment or during dexamethasone therapy, the rise in testosterone was less than 100 ng/dl, while the progestagens showed an abnormally high rise.

It was interesting that in a third member of the sibship studied by Forest et al. (25), there were only slight abnormalities of the genitalia,

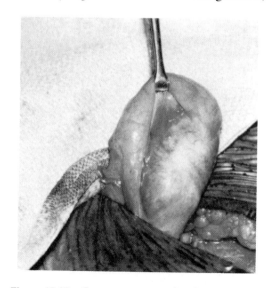

Figure 13.17. Gross appearance of testis at operation.

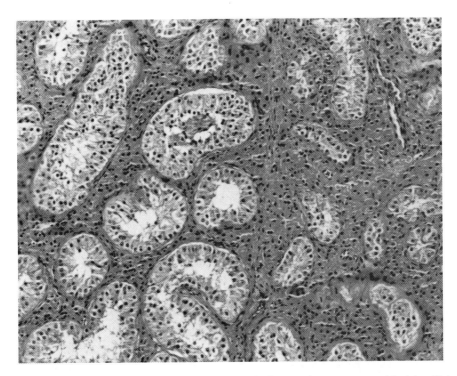

Figure 13.18. Histopathological examination of testis. Note the hyperactive appearance of the interstitial cells.

and it was suspected that he suffered from a very mild form of the same defect.

The familial occurrence of this disease suggests an autosomal recessive inheritance.

In the genitalia of the patients so far reported, there has been a spectrum of disorder varying from some fusion with a blind vaginal pouch to more complete fusion with little or no vaginal pouch.

It can be anticipated that with the report of more patients with this defect, a broader spectrum of abnormalities of the external genitalia will be found, as with the 17α-hydroxylase deficiency.

Surgical treatment will be required for the ambiguity of the external genitalia, as with the other enzyme defects, and the testes will obviously have to be removed in those patients reared as females, not only to remove any excess androgen production, but to eliminate this potential source of neoplastic transformation.

17β-Hydroxysteroid Dehydrogenase Deficiency

As judged by the number of case reports of this disorder, this deficiency seems to be some-what more frequent that the other enzyme deficiencies in the biosynthesis of testosterone. It is noteworthy that the study of Givens et al. (30) involved two sisters, and the study of Forest (25) involved the study not only of the proposita but of her niece. Rosler et al. (84) noted that this disorder was common among the Arab population in Israel.

The pedigree pattern provides strong evidence for an autosomal recessive mode of inheritance, and Tremblay et al. (92) has presented evidence that the involved gene is on the long arm of chromosome 17.

These patients, regardless of the age at which they present, do so with ambiguity of the external genitalia (Fig. 13.19). There are various degrees of fusion, although most cases have had rather feminine-appearing genitalia, and there has usually been no uncertainty about electing a female sex in rearing, although there are some exceptions. In the reported cases, a vagina of at least minimum depth has been found, and in some cases, the vagina has been deep enough for reasonable function. The clitoris has been moderately enlarged in some cases and enlarges if treatment is not undertaken prior to puberty.

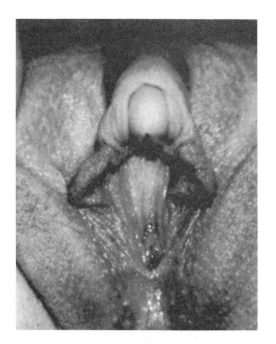

Figure 13.19. External genitalia of patient with 17β-hydroxysteroid dehydrogenase deficiency.

In individuals presenting in infancy, breast development is undeterminable, but after puberty, modest breast development has been noted for reasons that will be clear when the endocrine aspect of the disorder is discussed. But there have been some exceptions, and there has been failure of breast development in some patients well beyond the age of expected puberty (Fig. 13.20).

In no case has there been any müllerian structure so that the vagina ends blindly, and it is clear that the antimüllerian hormone has been normally active.

The plasma steroid analyses usually clearly make the diagnosis. If the individual is encountered in infancy, the abnormality can be accentuated by stimulation of the testes with hCG, as is true with all of the enzymatic defects in the biosynthesis of testosterone.

The essential difficulty is a problem in conversion of a double-bond oxygen at the 17 position to an OH. This is expressed in the conversion of Δ4-adrostenedione to testosterone so that the ratio of these substances is greatly elevated. It is also expressed in the conversion of estrone to estradiol, and this ratio is also elevated, although usually not to the extent of the androstenedione-testosterone ra-

tio. Typical values for androstenedione are in the range of 10 times the normal, and typical values for testosterone are half or less of the normal expected concentration for males. Estrone values are generally slightly elevated, and estradiol values markedly depressed, although an occasional case has been reported where the estradiol value has been normal for a male. Examination of these substances in the spermatic vein blood tends to exaggerate these abnormalities. In short, there is abundant evidence from studying the intermediate metabolites of a block in the conversion of the double-bond O at the 17 position to the hydroxyl group (Fig. 13.21).

It should be noted that for obvious reasons, there is no problem with the adrenal steroids, and thus, there is no systemic manifestation of mineralocorticoid difficulty.

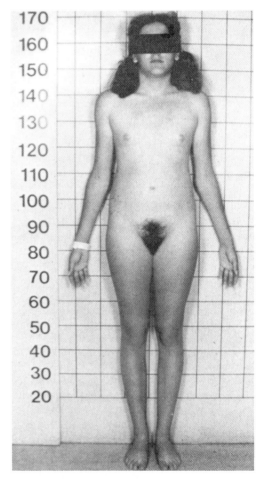

Figure 13.20. Photograph of patient shown in Fig. 13.19.

17β KETO-REDUCTASE

	NORMAL MALE	ng/dl PRE-OP	POST-OP
PROGESTERONE	.9 ± .2	22	<7
17 OH PROGESTERONE	110 ± 10	132	<10
ANDROSTENEDIONE	109 ± 20	1437	49
TESTOSTERONE	575 ± 150	303	12

Figure 13.21. Endocrine findings in patient shown in Fig. 13.19.

The treatment consists of reconstruction of the external genitalia where this is necessary (Fig. 13.22). In one case that came to our attention, an attempt had been made to convert the genitalia to male function, and this was a failure. It probably is safe to say that essentially all patients with this defect should be reared as females.

The testes need to be removed, and preferably prior to puberty, because they have some androgen production that will enlarge the clitoris unnecessarily and will cause masculine hair distribution, which is undesirable. They also need to be removed because of the predilection of such testes for neoplastic transformation (Fig. 13.23).

Unidentified Defect in Androgen Effect

Park et al. (63) called attention to a series of nine cases that seemed to have defective androgen action as judged by ambiguous external genitalia, but with inability to identify a specific enzymatic defect in the biosynthesis of testosterone.

The ambiguity of the external genitalia was similar to those patients who had identified enzymatic defects. The müllerian ducts were suppressed in all cases, and in several instances, there were affected sibs. Some, but not all of these patients were not adequately studied by contemporary techniques, and it is possible that the number of patients falling in this category will eventually be reduced or entirely eliminated when more complete studies are carried out in contemporary cases. Interestingly, the serum LH was uniformly elevated.

It may be that patients in this category suffer from some timing defect in the production of T by the developing gonad. It has been clear from the work of the experimental embryologist that sensitivity of the genital structures to testoster-

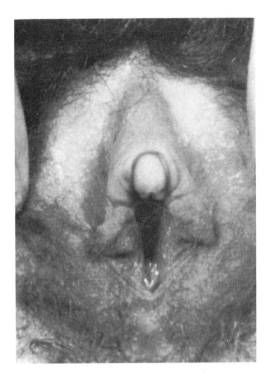

Figure 13.22. Postoperative appearance of external genitalia of patient shown in Fig. 13.19.

one during the period of their masculinization is confined to a very limited period in embryogenesis. If there is some failure of synchronization, it is quite possible that the abnormalities encountered would in fact be produced. But when the steroid values were determined many years later, no abnormalities could be found. On the other hand, the fact that these patients uniformly had elevated LH values suggests that there is some struggle in producing normal amounts of T.

At any rate, there is a category of cases where it has not been possible to identify a specific enzymatic defect and where the external genitalia are ambiguous, and the müllerian ducts suppressed. These patients clearly benefit by being reared as women. Cases with multiple congenital anomalies involving especially the heart, palate, jaw, and other organ systems, but having in common ambiguous external genitalia with only minor anomalies in the testes, could be included in this category. Greenberg et al. (32) have described several cases of this type. Ambiguity of the genitalia have also been reported with the VATER syndrome (88).

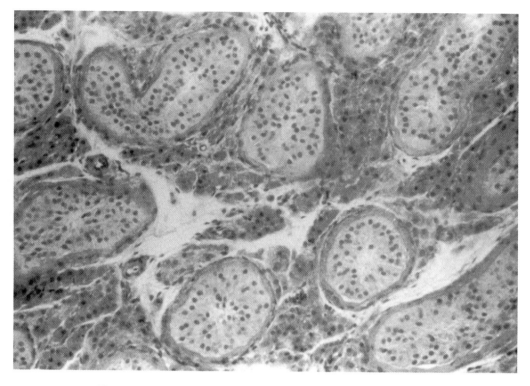

Figure 13.23. Histopathologic examination of testis shown in Fig. 13.19.

Treatments as with other patients in these general categories consist of such surgical reconstruction of the external genitalia, as appropriate, plus the removal of the gonads, and, of course, the use of exogenous estrogen at the appropriate time.

Defect in Müllerian Duct Regression

A number of patients have been reported in whom there has been failure of action of the antimüllerian hormone (AMH). This latter designation has been preferred by Natalie Josso rather than the previously used müllerian-inhibiting factor. It is the same substance.

Patients who have this difficulty generally have no ambiguity of the external genitalia that are normally developed for a male. There are some exceptions (Figs. 13.24–13.26). What is peculiar is that one or both testes are missing from the scrotum, and inguinal hernias, either unilaterally or bilaterally, are not at all uncommon. Such cases are sometimes referred to in the literature as *hernia uteri inguinalis*. Many times, it has come as a surprise to the operating surgeon

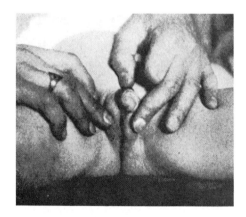

Figure 13.24. External genitalia of patient who proved to have hernia uteri inguinalis.

to discover that a uterus and fallopian tube were part of a hernia sac in what otherwise appeared to be a normal male (Figs. 13.27–13.29).

Naguib et al. (61) reported a family with this syndrome with two brothers and two affected maternal uncles. Such a pattern suggests X-linked inheritance, although an autosomal recessive determination with male limitation cannot be excluded.

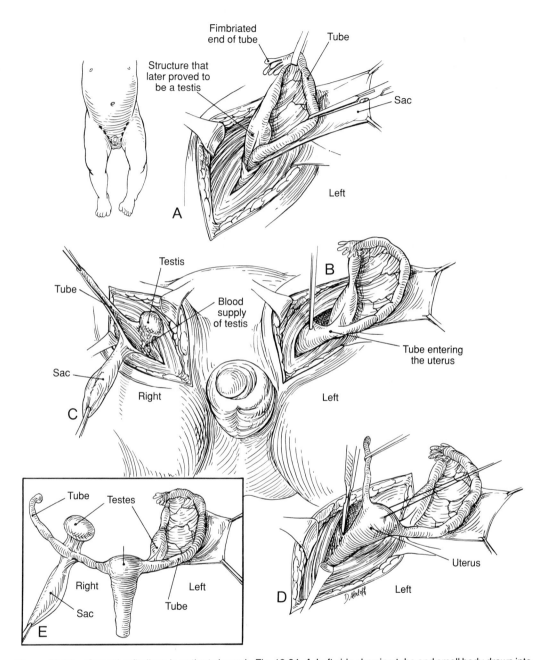

Figure 13.25. Operative findings in patient shown in Fig. 13.24. *A,* Left side showing tube and small body drawn into the incision. *B,* Further dissection showing the uterus. *C,* Right side showing a small testis near a fallopian tube connected with the uterus on the right side. No epididymis could be identified. *D,* Removal of fallopian and uterus. *E,* Reconstruction of condition as found at operation and confirmed by microscopic examination of tissue removed.

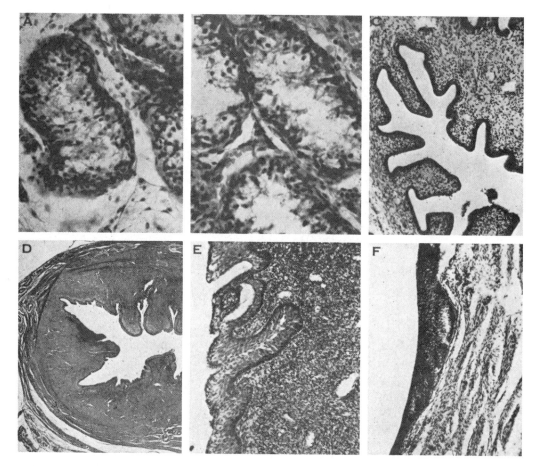

Figure 13.26. Pathologic examination of tissue removed in patient shown in Fig. 13.24. *A*, Section of right testis that was brought down into scrotum at operation (H & E × 250). *B*, Section of left testis which was practically identical to that of the opposite gonad ((H & E × 200). *C*, Section of fallopian tube (H & E × 75). *D*, Lower power view of uterus (H & E × 10). *E*, Higher power view of endometrium. *F*, Section of vagina. Epithelium rather atrophic (H & E × 75).

There is no concern or decision making in the sex rearing of these individuals when their external genitalia are entirely masculine (Figs. 13.30–13.33). The presence of the uterus is of relatively little importance, although the connection of the vagina to the urethra serves as a urethral diverticulum, and infection of the urine in this diverticulum sometimes indicates the removal of the uterus and the vagina down to the urethra to eliminate the problem of chronic urinary infection (Figs. 13.34–13.40).

As with retained testes, the question of neoplastic transformation arises, and they probably should be removed, bilaterally if within the abdominal cavity, and unilaterally if only one is descended (Figs. 13.41–13.43).

The abdominal testes do not have germ cells and have no spermatogenic potential, but patients who have had unilateral hernia uteri inguinalis have been found to have sperm counts in the oligospermic range. There are a few case reports of conception by individuals in this category, but the question of paternity always lends an element of uncertainty.

There is no clear evidence as to whether the difficulty in these cases is due to failure of the testis to produce the antimüllerian hormone or whether there may be some problem at the target area such as an absent receptor. It is entirely possible that both of these mechanisms operate in different circumstances.

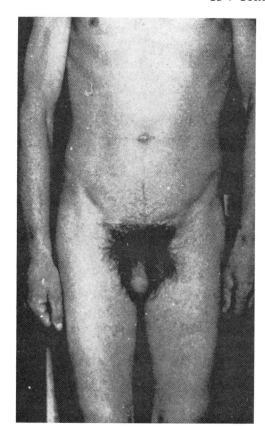

Figure 13.27. Photograph showing entirely normal external genitalia in patient who proved to have hernia uteri inguinalis.

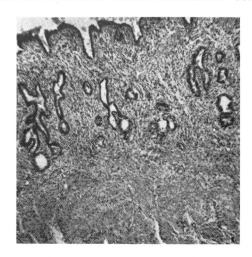

Figure 13.29. Histopathologic section of endometrial cavity of uterus removed from patient shown in Fig. 13.27.

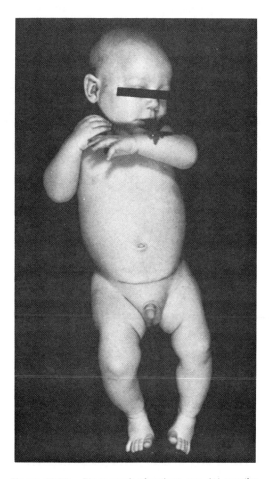

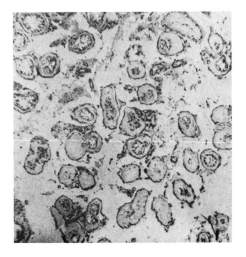

Figure 13.28. Pathologic section of atrophic testicular tissue removed from patient shown in Fig. 13.27.

Figure 13.30. Photograph of patient, age 4½ months. The only abnormality in this patient was absence of testes from the scrotum.

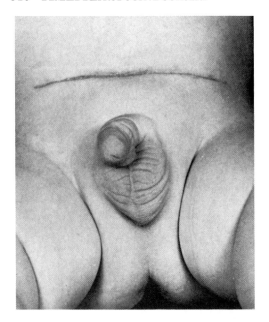

Figure 13.31. Photograph of external genitalia of patient shown in Fig. 13.30. The genitalia are perfectly formed, but there are no testes in the scrotum.

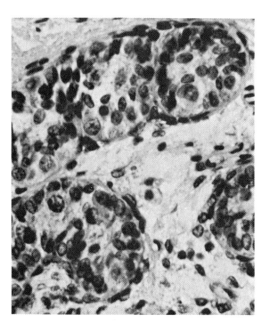

Figure 13.33. Histopathologic examination of testis in patient shown in Fig. 13.30. The seminiferous tubules contained mostly Sertoli cells, but there is an occasional germ cell in this 4½-month-old child. The interstitial cells are difficult to identify, but this is not unusual in an infant of this age (H & E × 600).

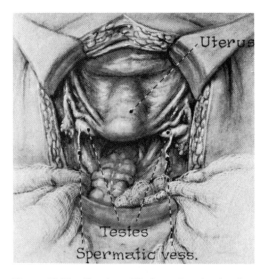

Figure 13.32. Drawing of findings at exploratory laparotomy in patient shown in Fig. 13.30.

Familial Gonadal Destruction

In this category of patients are individuals whose karyotype is 46,XY and who have surely had testicular function at one time. This is evidenced by various degrees of masculinization of the external genitalia or by various degrees of inhibition of müllerian ducts, but when seen later in life, these patients are found to have, on microscopic examination, no identifiable testis. There may be remnants, as in the case illustrated herein, but testicular tubules are completely absent. This syndrome has been referred to in the literature by variable names such as the "testicular regression syndrome" or "embryonic testicular syndrome," among others.

There seems to be a strong genetic tendency. For example, Park and Jones (42) reported two sibs illustrated in this section (Figs. 13.44–13.46), and Josso and Briard (47) reported two sibs and emphasized the variable phenotypic expression in these two individuals. Because of the familial occurrence of the disorder, the genetic background seems clear, although, as just mentioned, the phenotypic expression may have some variability.

Rios et al. (79) described such a patient and provided extensive hormonal studies. As might be expected, the plasma FSH and LH were elevated and responded in a normal fashion to LHRH. Plasma steroid levels in basic circumstances and after hCG stimulation and ACTH stimulation and dexamethasone suppression

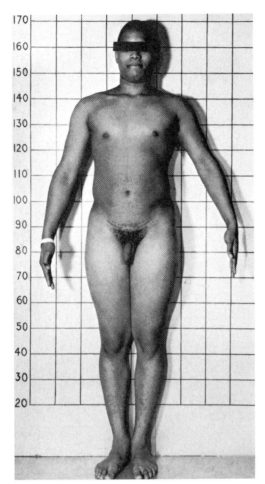

Figure 13.34. A healthy 17-year-old male whose only complaint was a right inguinal hernia and absence of testes from the scrotum.

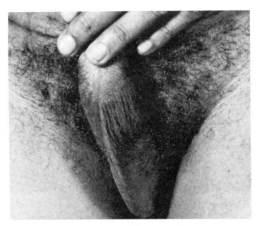

Figure 13.35. External genitalia of patient shown in Fig. 13.34.

showed normal adrenal function and essentially absent gonadal function.

The phenotypic expression, of course, depends entirely on the time sequence during embryonic life when testicular function was suppressed. In the cases illustrated herein, there were müllerian remnants and the ambiguity of the external genitalia without complete masculinization, but in other patients described with this syndrome, the müllerian ducts have been completely suppressed, and there have been variable degrees of masculinization of the external genitalia.

For the most part, these individuals have had sufficient ambiguity to have had the female gender elected as the sex of rearing, but in some instances, the masculinization of the external

genitalia has been such that a male sex of rearing was selected. Rosenberg (81) reviewed 20 cases.

Treatment consists of the removal of the gonadal tissue, which is quite small and usually can be identified only by removal of tissue at the terminal end of the spermatic vessels. In fact, the diagnosis cannot be made until such tissue is removed and examined microscopically.

Other therapy consists of reconstruction of the external genitalia according to the sex of rearing, which in most instances will be female, and the use of substitution endocrine therapy, as appropriate.

Leydig Cell Agenesis

A few cases have been described in which it was thought that the sexual ambiguity was due to agenesis of the Leydig cells.

The clinical manifestation is that of an individual who has had no androgen production by the testis. The external genitalia, therefore, are quite feminine. There may be some slight enlargement of the clitoris, but the müllerian ducts are completely inhibited (Fig. 13.47).

The findings in the Leydig cell agenesis syndrome are essentially identical to the findings in the patients who have counterfeit gonadotropin. Indeed, one cannot make a diagnosis of Leydig cell agenesis unless an effort has been made to stimulate the Leydig cells by the use of hCG. Therefore, the diagno-

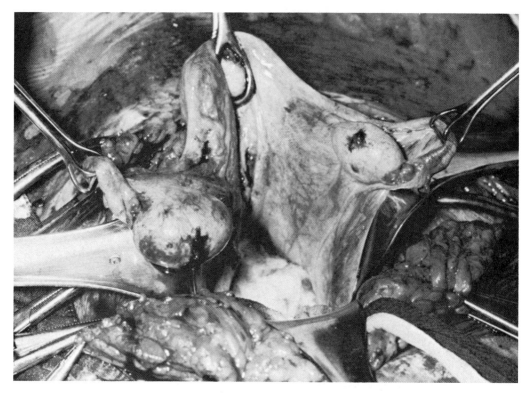

Figure 13.36. Photograph of operative situation in patient shown in Fig. 13.34. Note the rather normal-sized uterus and fallopian tubes with structures in the region of the ovaries that resemble testes.

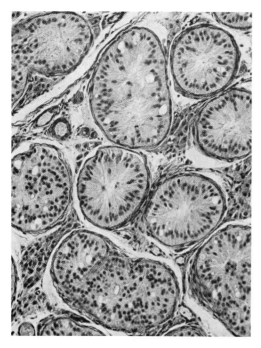

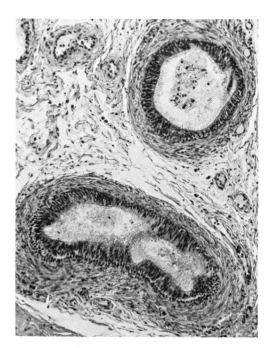

Figure 13.37. Histopathologic section of testis from patient shown in Fig. 13.34 (H & E × 150).

Figure 13.38. Section of epididymis in patient shown in Fig. 13.34 (H & E × 150).

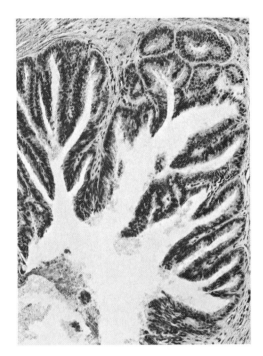

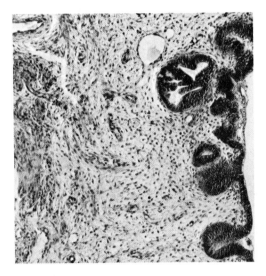

Figure 13.39. Section of tissue removed from deep in the pelvis. This is thought to represent seminiferous tubules from the patient shown in Fig. 13.34 (H & E × 150).

Figure 13.40. Photomicrograph of uterus showing rather attenuated endometrium in patient shown in Fig. 13.34 (H & E × 150).

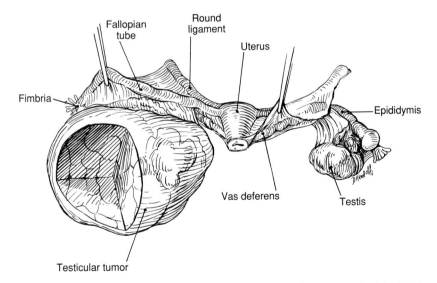

Figure 13.41. Specimen of a patient who had failure of the antimüllerian hormone and retained testes. Note the large tumor involving one of the testes.

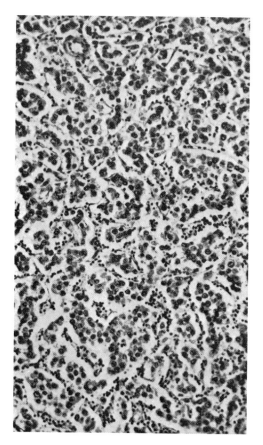

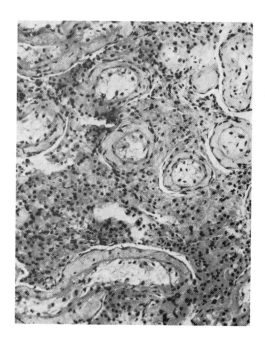

Figure 13.43. Microscopic appearance of the intraabdominal testis. The seminiferous tubules now contain few Sertoli cells and no spermatogenic cells. There is considerable thickening and hyalinization of the basement membrane of the tubular epithelium. This seems to occur in retained testes with time (H & E × 150).

Figure 13.42. Microscopic appearance of the testicular tumor. This is a typical seminoma or dysgerminoma (H & E × 150).

sis must be made with some reluctance unless it has been possible to make an effort to stimulate the Leydig cells.

As noted, the findings are essentially identical with those described for patients with abnormal gonadotropin secretion. This applies to the histologic examination of the testis, which is key. In those patients, as well as in the Leydig cell agenesis, no Leydig cells can be identified, although the Sertoli cells seem to be quite normal (Fig. 13.48).

Treatment consists of the removal of the testes, which presumably have a high risk for tumor formation, as they are located intraabdominally. Reconstruction of the external genitalia may be necessary, although this has not been necessary in the patients described to date, but might be if a spectrum of the disorder exists. The use of substitute therapy for breast development is required.

Dysgenetic Male Pseudohermaphroditism

Rajfer et al. (75) first emphasized a group of patients with severely dysgenetic testes, 46,XY karyotype, and various degrees of masculinization of the external genitalia. In the 10 instances described by these authors, the müllerian ducts were developed at least to a point that they were recognizable as such.

There is some uncertainty as to whether this really represents an entity distinct from the familial gonadal destruction syndrome. Indeed, it is very likely that this is a forme fruste of that same process. Nevertheless, in the syndrome under discussion, the testes are recognizable as such, and, as might be anticipated from the fact that all patients have müllerian ducts, the seminiferous tubules are quite dysgenetic. In addition, in the patients above the age of puberty, interstitial cells can be identified, as again might be anticipated from the fact that a good many individuals in this group have various degrees of masculinization of the exter-

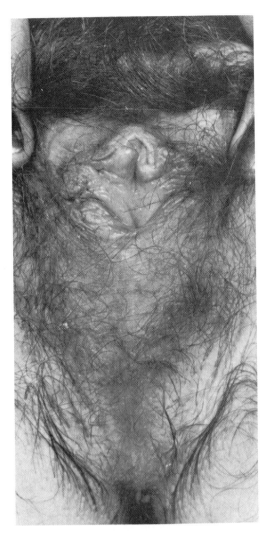

Figure 13.44. Photograph of external genitalia of patient with familial gonadal destruction.

nal genitalia. Rajfer et al. (75) emphasized the fact that this particular type of gonad had a high risk for neoplastic change, and indeed, in their 10 cases, three had gonadoblastomas or worse at an early age.

A subset of children with dysgenetic testes and ambiguous genitalia have diffuse glomerular disease and Wilms tumor. This triad was described by Drash (21), and has been referred to as the Drash syndrome. Several series of this generally fatal condition have been described (18).

As with several of the disorders in the male hermaphroditic group, precise diagnosis cannot be made until there has been an opportu-

nity to examine the gonads histologically. Treatment consists of the removal of the gonadal tissue, the reconstruction of the external genitalia to conform to the sex rearing of the individual, and the use of substitution endocrine therapy as appropriate.

MALE HERMAPHRODITISM DUE TO PERIPHERAL END-ORGAN DEFECT

Androgen Insensitivity (Testicular Feminization)

GENERAL CONSIDERATIONS

Although individual case histories had been reported before, it was in 1953 that Morris (58) collected 80 cases from the literature and added two of his own, and coined the term "testicular feminization." A vast literature has appeared about this disorder, and it has since been determined that the problem is due to an insensitivity to androgen, so that a more appropriate name might be androgen insensitivity. Nevertheless, the catchy phrase coined by Morris in 1953 has remained popular and is undoubtedly an acceptable clinical description for the condition.

CLINICAL FEATURES

An individual affected with this disorder has a female body type (Figs. 13.49–13.51). After puberty, there is normal and excellent breast development and female habitus. Such persons are normally identified as female at birth and reared as such. Breast development starts at puberty, often with a tendency to overdevelopment with poorly developed nipples. These patients become very attractive females, who are usually tall with long hands and feet and appear somewhat eunuchoid. The hair on the head is normal, and there is often scanty or no axillary and pubic hair, although there is some variation in the clinical expression of this particular finding.

There is no müllerian development. As mentioned, the external genitalia are quite feminine (Fig. 13.52). The clitoris is never enlarged. The labia, especially the labia minora, may be somewhat underdeveloped. The vaginal

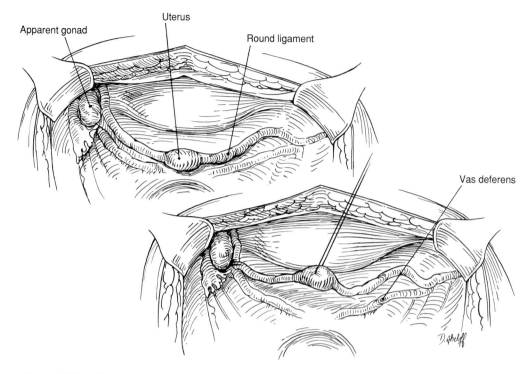

Figure 13.45.   Drawing of operative findings in two sisters, each of whom had familial gonadal destruction.

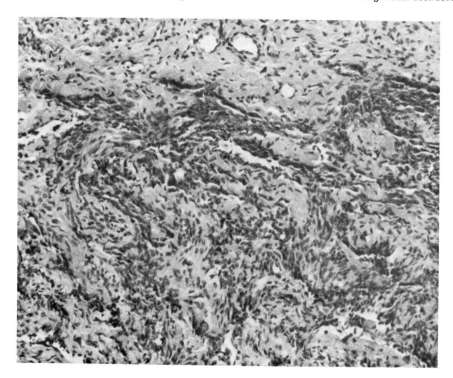

Figure 13.46.   Photomicrograph of only tissue that could be found that in any way resembled testis after making serial sections of what appeared to be a small gonad which was at the terminal end of the spermatic vessels.

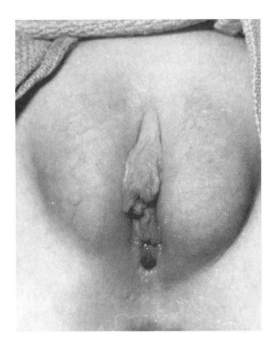

Figure 13.47. External genitalia of patient with Leydig cell hypoplasia.

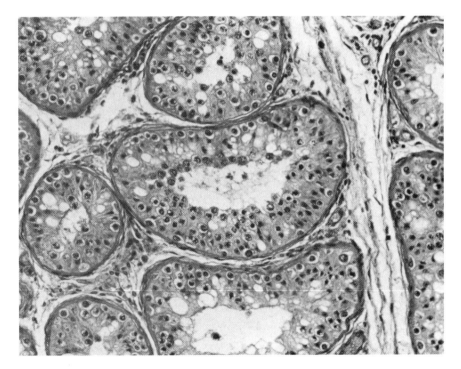

Figure 13.48. Photomicrograph of testis of patient shown in Fig. 13.47. In contrast to other types of male hermaphroditism, note the germ cells in these testes.

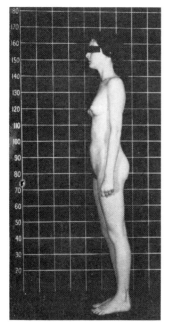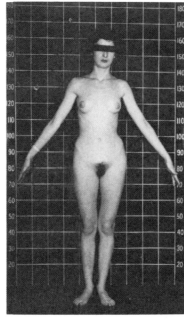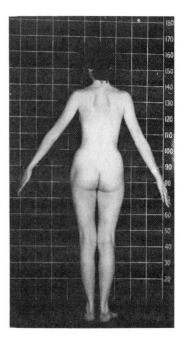

Figure 13.49. (*Left*), A lateral view of a patient with the androgen insensitivity syndrome.
Figure 13.50. (*Middle*), Anterior view of same patient shown in Fig. 13.49.
Figure 13.51. (*Right*), Posterior view of patient shown in Fig. 13.49.

cavity may be shallow and sometimes requires surgical lengthening. The vaginal mucosa is thoroughly estrogenized. Such patients consider themselves normal females and lead a normal female existence including a normal marital life. Such patients seek medical help because of amenorrhea, sterility, or inguinal masses. Dyspareunia from a short vagina may be a presenting symptom. A gonad in the inguinal canal in a hernia is a common feature. Atwell (3) reported than an inguinal hernia was associated in the testicular feminization syndrome in no less than 78% of the cases. This is in striking contrast to a very low anticipation of an inguinal hernia in a normal genetic female. Therefore, the presence of a hernia in a phenotypic female child must always raise the suspicion of this disorder.

The exact incidence of this disorder is difficult to state and apparently has not been recently estimated. Prader (74) designated an incidence of one of 20,000 males. Hauser (33) believed the incidence to be at least 10 times greater than that stated by Prader.

GENETIC CONSIDERATIONS

The pedigree pattern of these individuals is consistent with transmission as an X-linked recessive disorder. Thus, it is invariably transmitted through a phenotypically normal female (Fig. 13.53).

Except in a few cases of mosaicism and a very few cases of structural anomalies of the X chromosome, this disorder is associated with a normal 46,XY karyotype. The chromosomal anomalies described in association with this disorder are very likely entirely coincidental.

It was shown by Keenan et al. (50) that the basic defect was an inability of the cytosol receptor for testosterone (T) to bind T. Therefore, the target organs are unable to recognize T and translate it into a biological reality. While a defect in the cytosol receptor has been discovered in many cases of testicular feminization, it is interesting that some patients who are clinically indistinguishable from a typical example of this disorder seem to bind T in a normal fashion. It is now recognized that there are a

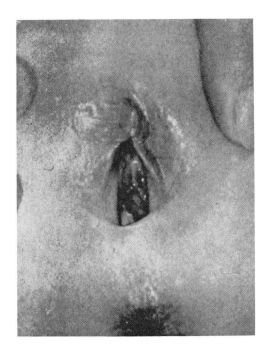

Figure 13.52. Photograph of the external genitalia of a 7-year-old girl who has relatively normal-appearing external genitalia. The vagina is of normal depth, but there is no cervix. The uterus is palpable by rectum, and it is very likely that the patient will feminize at puberty. She has a younger sister with identical findings.

number of different mutations that result in androgen insensitivity (11).

ENDOCRINE STUDIES

There is no impairment of the ability of the testis to produce testosterone and other steroids. There have been many studies on this point.

FSH values are often high, normal, or slightly elevated, but LH values are increased as much as 10-fold above the normal value for a male. Aono et al. (1) particularly studied the gonadotropin values in their response to GnRH. Following the injection of GnRH, there was a further increase in both LH and FSH. Both the testicular feminization patients and normal males showed no LH release following estrogen injection in contrast to normal females.

HISTOPATHOLOGY

The testes are usually normal in size and lie in the abdomen or sometimes in the inguinal canals

(Fig. 13.54). Seminiferous tubules are small and immature, dominated by Sertoli cells but with some spermatogonia and no spermatocytes. The Sertoli cells are often quite prominent and fill the tubules, obliterating the lumen. These cells are slender or oval with distinct cell borders and the cytoplasm is clear. Hyalinization of the basement membranes occurs at puberty in some but not in all cases. There is considerable Leydig cell hyperplasia and the Leydig cells occur in dense clusters or are scattered irregularly in small compact groups between the seminiferous tubules (Fig. 13.55).

Several authors have studied the ultrastructure of the gonads. Ultrastructurally, the tubules are lined by Sertoli cells that are considered to be immature but also to be lined by cells that are somewhat darker. The nature of these cells has been subject to some discussion. Ferenczy and Richart (22) consider these to be Sertoli cells in the process of atrophy. On the other hand, Damjanov and Drobnjak (18) seem to believe that they were identical with cells found in ovarian-like stroma in the interstitial tissue between the tubules. They seem to believe that these cells were responsible for the manifestation of the disorder, but this interpretation was made prior to the time when the cytosol receptor defect was elucidated, so that it is doubtful that it is necessary to make such an interpretation. The ultrastructure of the Leydig cells in the testis from testicular feminization is indistinguishable

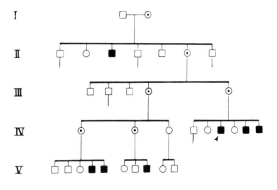

■ · Testicular feminization

Figure 13.53. Pedigree pattern typical for patients with testicular feminization.

from the ultrastructure of the Leydig cell in a normal testis.

The mesonephric (wolffian) duct derivatives were studied by Zourlas and Jones (99), who showed that they were extremely poorly developed in spite of a gross appearance to the contrary.

PSYCHOSEXUAL ORIENTATION

Individuals with this syndrome have completely female psychosexual orientation. This has been studied by many authors and is to be expected because the syndrome does not involve external malformations that might lead one to have some concerns about the sex of the individual.

Considering the inherent female psychosexual orientation of these individuals, the question naturally arises as to the desirability of complete disclosure to them of their genetic background. This is a troublesome problem, especially in the era of full disclosure. It is difficult to make a general rule, but it usually works well for the physicians to emphasize to these individuals their normalcy with regard to female characteristics. In the event that it is necessary to discuss the cytogenetics of the situation, it is important to point out that sexual orientation is not related to any one physical characteristic, but is related more to the social and psychological orientation imprinted by one's environment.

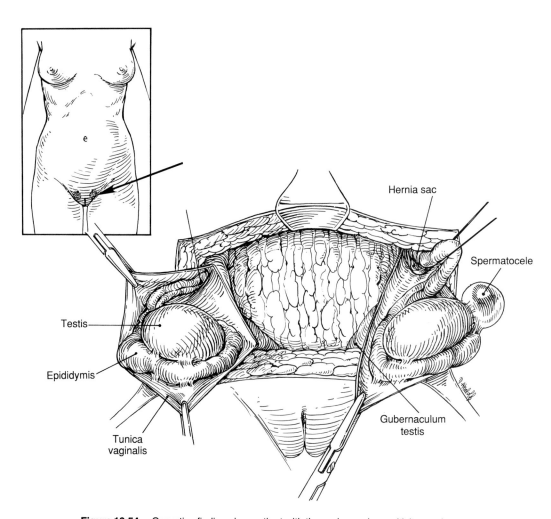

Figure 13.54. Operative findings in a patient with the androgen insensitivity syndrome.

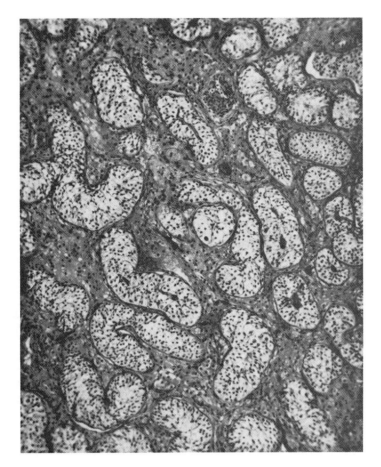

Figure 13.55.   Microscopic appearance of the testes of patient shown in Fig. 13.54.

TREATMENT

Essentially, no reconstructive surgery is required in these individuals because of the normal configuration of the external genitalia. Sometimes the vagina needs to be lengthened if it is particularly short.

The testes in these individuals are at high risk for neoplastic development. This was evident from the original study by Morris (58), who found that among 50 cases 30 years of age or older, there were malignant tumors, mostly seminomas. In addition to that, there were some tubular adenomas and cysts that were large enough to operate upon. It is therefore very important that the testes in these individuals be removed. Perhaps a case could be made for delaying such removal until after spontaneous puberty. Manuel et al. (56) showed that the

incidence of neoplastic change was no more than about 3% prior to the age of 10.

Following removal of the testes, exogenous estrogen therapy is necessary and desirable.

INCOMPLETE OR PARTIAL FORMS

A number of patients have been described who seem to have incomplete or partial manifestations of the testicular feminization syndrome. This is perhaps not surprising since many genetic disorders have a spectrum of phenotypic expression. Patients with the so-called incomplete form have ambiguity of the external genitalia, but they have breast development and moderate amounts of hair growth, and universally have had suppression of the müllerian duct derivatives (Figs. 13.56–13.58).

A number of sibships with the partial disorder have been described. Clearly, the pedigree

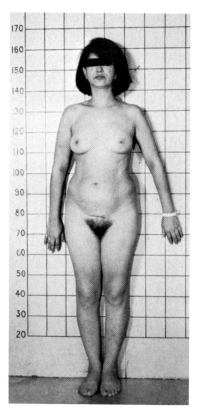

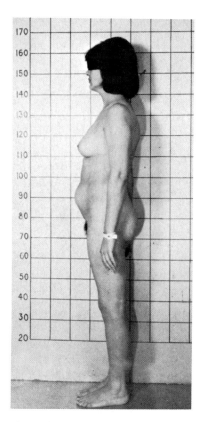

Figure 13.56. An example of the incomplete form testicular feminization. Note the rather normal pubic hair and the normal breast development.

Figure 13.57. Lateral view of same patient shown in Fig. 13.56.

patterns are essentially the same as with the complete form of testicular feminization (Fig. 13.59).

Therapy differs from the complete form only in that reconstructive surgery of the external genitalia is necessary, depending upon the degree of the malformation.

In addition to the incomplete form, several other syndromes have been described in the past that probably are really modest expressions of basically the same defect. These would include the Reifenstein syndrome (78), the Rosewater syndrome (83), the Gilbert-Dreyfus syndrome (29), and the Lubs syndrome (54). Each of these was originally assumed to be a distinct entity, but they all appear to be X-linked recessive disorders, and have been characterized by or suggestive of partial androgen insensitivity.

As some of the partial syndromes have considerable masculinization, a number of such individuals have been reared as males. In this circumstance, the undesirable breast development may need to be removed surgically.

Steroid 5α-Reductase Deficiency

An inherited form of male hermaphroditism has been found to be due to a 5α-reductase deficiency. This disorder has been studied in depth in an isolated community in the Dominican Republic by Peterson, Imperato-McGinley, and others (39), and updated later.

At birth, the affected males, who are karyotypically 46,XY, have a clitoral-like phallus, a bifid scrotum, and fused scrotolabial folds. The testes are often in the scrotolabial fold, but in some cases, have descended no further than the inguinal canals. However, in general, testicular descent is greater than in many other forms of male hermaphroditism. The wolffian structures are normally differentiated, but the müllerian

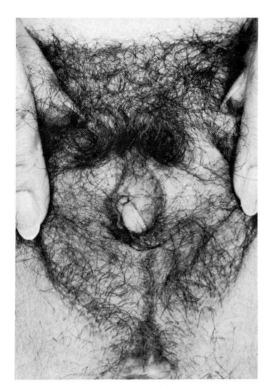

Figure 13.58. The external genitalia of patient shown in Fig. 13.56.

ducts are universally inhibited. At puberty, if they are untreated, a muscular male habitus develops with growth of the phallus and scrotum, the voice becomes deeper, but breasts never develop. The subjects have erections, ejaculations, and in the Santo Domingo environment, a libido directed toward females. Their body hair is somewhat decreased, and they have an absent beard and seem never to suffer from temporal hair regression. The prostate is quite small to palpation. A testicular biopsy reveals testes that are indistinguishable from normal.

The mean plasma levels of testosterone are at least normal and in many cases significantly higher than normal, but the mean plasma dihydrotestosterone (DHT) is significantly lower than in the normal subjects. Thus, the plasma T:DHT ratio ranges from 35–80, as compared with 8–16 normal subjects.

The mean plasma LH and FSH levels are significantly higher than normal. The metabolic clearance rate of testosterone and dihydrotestosterone are normal.

Inheritance is clearly autosomal-recessive with some sibling sisters showing the same biochemical defect, but of course no anatomical defect of the external genitalia. The obligate carrier parents seem to have an intermediate defect.

The serum endocrine studies suggest an inability to convert testosterone to dihydrotestosterone.

The study of patients with 5α-reductase deficiency gives insight into the requirements for masculinization of the male external genitalia. In patients with the 5α-reductase deficiency, male wolffian duct derivatives are normally formed and stimulated. This means that the epididymis, the vas deferens, and the seminal vesicles are normally formed and developed. On the other hand, male derivatives of the urogenital sinus are not at all well developed. This would, of course, include the urethra and the prostate, which are indifferently developed in patients with the 5α-reductase defect. The penis apparently is stimulated by both T and DHT, as such patients have a fairly well-developed organ, although the urethra is not formed, and the penis responds at puberty to increased amounts of testosterone production.

The effect of DHT and T on hair is interesting. It should be noted that these patients generally do not have facial hair, nor do they suffer from temporal baldness. This would imply that facial hair is a function of DHT, as contrasted to T.

The treatment of these patients has been related to their environment. In the isolated community in the Dominican Republic where the disorder is well-recognized by the villagers and where it is understood that masculinization will occur at puberty, many of these children seem to be successfully reared as males. On the other hand, in areas of the world where the appearance of this disorder seems to be sporadic and where the external genitalia are quite ambiguous, the preferred sex of rearing is probably female. In the latter case, it would be desirable to reconstruct the external genitalia to give a female cosmetic appearance. For female rearing, the testes should be removed to prevent the androgen surge at puberty, and because they are probably at potentially high risk for neoplastic development, although it would

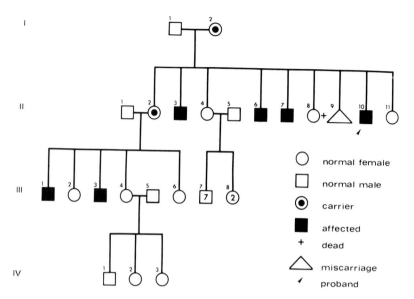

Figure 13.59.   Pedigree pattern of patient shown in Fig. 13.56. Note that the pedigree is identical to that of patients with the complete form of testicular feminization.

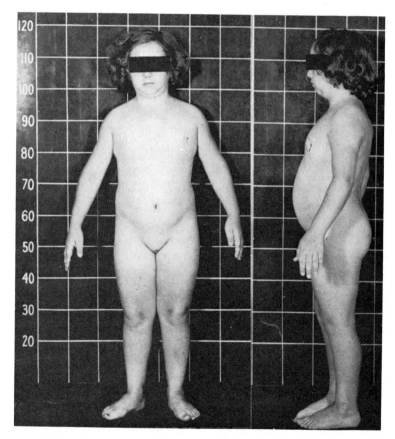

Figure 13.60.   Photographs anterior and lateral of a patient with a body type suggesting a Turner's syndrome, but who must be classified as a male hermaphrodite because of testicular tissue and a karyotype that showed a structural anomaly of the Y chromosome.

be difficult to document this particular point in this specific defect. In the case of castrated individuals who are reared as females, it would be necessary to use exogenous estrogen at the appropriate time.

Male Hermaphroditism Due to a Y Chromosome Defect

In male hermaphroditism, the majority of patients will have a normal male 46,XY karyotype. However, in a few patients who are technically male hermaphrodites—in that testicular tissue is present—a chromosomal abnormality will occur. The best known example of this is asymmetrical gonadal differentiation, which many times has a mosaic pattern 45,X/46,XY. However, there have been cases reported with structural anomalies of the Y chromosome (Figs. 13.60–13.65), and a few cases where a hermaphroditic condition existed with a testis where no Y chromosome was demonstrable in repeated examinations of the chromosomes of the peripheral blood.

As might be expected, a wide spectrum of body types occurs in this circumstance. Many times, shortness of stature is part of the syndrome. This is unusual in male hermaphroditism, but is explainable if the distal end of the Y chromosome is involved in the chromosomal abnormality.

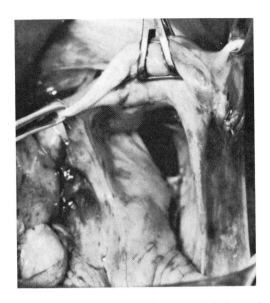

Figure 13.62. Photograph of operative findings of patient shown in Fig. 13.60. The fallopian tubes and ovaries are well developed. The numerous adhesions at operation were the result of a laparotomy done in infancy for purposes of identifying her sex. At that time, she was considered to be a normal female because of the presence of the uterus and structures that grossly were interpreted to be ovaries.

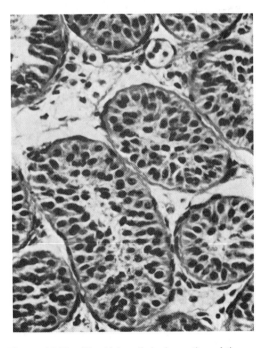

Figure 13.63. The histopathologic section of the gonads in patient shown in Fig. 13.60. It is a testis with healthy appearing seminiferous tubules.

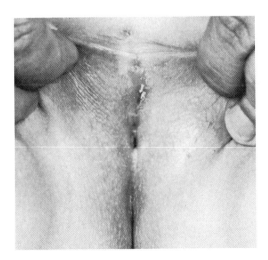

Figure 13.61. External genitalia of patient shown in Fig. 13.60.

As mentioned above, the clearest recognized syndrome with Y chromosomal defects is asymmetrical gonadal differentiation, where on one side a streak gonad is found; on the opposite side, a dysgenetic testis. In this circumstance, the testicular side often has inhibition of the müllerian ducts, whereas on the streak gonad side, the müllerian ducts are normally developed. The external genitalia are often quite ambiguous, but a vagina is present, and with proper reconstructive surgery, normal female genitalia result. The biggest difficulty from a somatic point of view in these patients is their stature, which, as mentioned above, tends to be short (Figs. 13.66–13.70).

Such patients require substitution therapy after removal of the gonads, but except for this difficulty, other somatic abnormalities have been quite unusual.

True Hermaphroditism

CRITERIA FOR DIAGNOSIS

It has been considered important to maintain the rigid criterion of a pathologic demonstration of both ovarian and testicular tissue before an individual can be accepted as a true hermaphrodite. A valid exception to this rule may be made if there has been positive microscopic identification of ovarian tissue plus viable sperm in the ejaculate. It is important to emphasize that the ovarian identification must include specific recognition of ovogenesis. Ovarian stroma is not sufficient to identify an ovary. Although viable sperm may be considered as positive identification of testicular tissue, uterine bleeding cannot be considered as positive identification of ovarian tissue. This is because estrogenic stimulation may be from

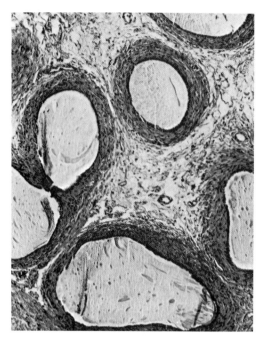

Figure 13.64. Photomicrograph of epididymis in patient shown in Fig. 13.60.

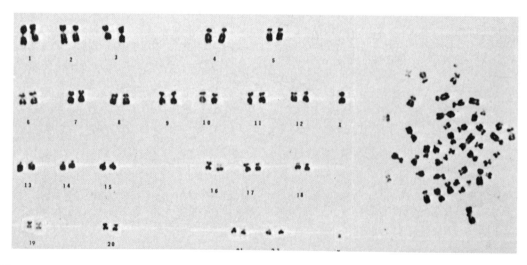

Figure 13.65. The conventionally stained karyotype of the patient shown in Fig. 13.60. Note that the Y chromosome is but a fragment and seems to have a deletion of portions of the long arm and portions of the short arm.

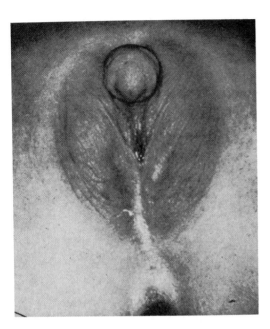

Figure 13.66.   Photograph of the external genitalia of a patient with asymmetrical gonadal differentiation.

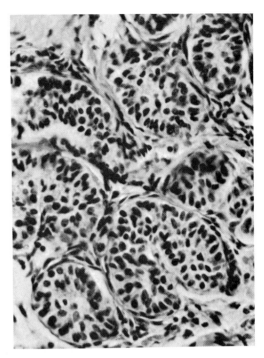

Figure 13.68.   Histopathological examination of the right testis (H & E × 400).

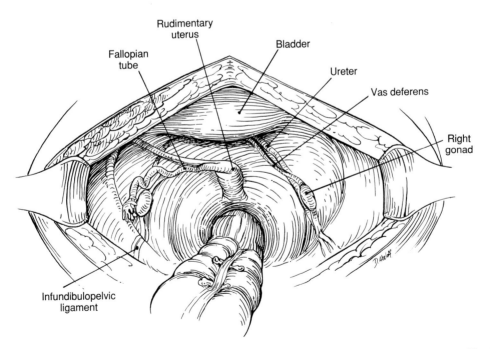

Figure 13.67.   The operative findings in the patient shown in Fig. 13.66. Note the unicornuate uterus with a left fallopian tube and round ligament. Examination of the gonad on this side showed no evidence of seminiferous tubules. Although the tissue seemed to be gathered in a structure that resembled a gonad, histopathologically it appeared to be a streak. The right side was a very poorly developed testis which seemed, however, to be adequate to suppress the development of the müllerian duct on its side.

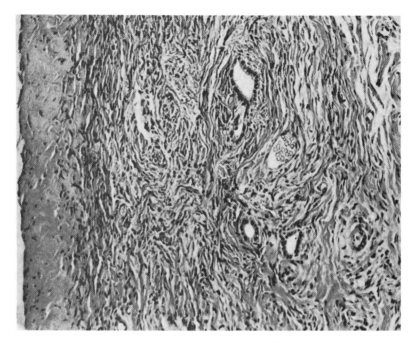

Figure 13.69. Histopathologic section of the left gonad. No evidence of testicular or ovarian structure could be found in many sections (H & E × 100).

extraovarian sources and indeed can arise from testicular tissue itself.

CLASSIFICATION OF HERMAPHRODITISMUS VERUS

The Klebs subdivision of hermaphroditismus verus recognized 16 possible groups. However, these groupings were made on theoretical conditions; many have not been recognized clinically, and further experience has shown that groups have appeared that were not provided for in the classification. For these reasons, it is best not to attempt to use the Klebs classification but to describe six groups, examples of which appear in the literature. This is an extension and enlargement of Young's classification (97), which itself was an attempted simplification of Klebs' groupings. It is as follows:

- Group I is the alternating variety. In this group there is an ovary on one side and a testis on the other. In many instances, the duct system on a given side corresponds in its development to the sex of the gonad on that side.
- Group IIa is the bilateral variety. In this group, there is an ovotestis on each side.
- Group IIb is the bilateral variety. There is a separate ovary and testis on each side.
- Group IIIa is the unilateral variety. In this group, there is an ovotestis on one side and ovary on the other.
- Group IIIb is the unilateral variety. A separate ovary and testis are on one side and an ovary is on the other.
- Group IIIc is the unilateral variety. In this group two ovotestes are on one side and an ovary is on the other.
- Group IV is the unilateral variety. An ovotestis on one side and testis on the other characterize this group.
- Group V is the unilateral variety. This group is characterized by an ovary and testis on the same side and no gonad on the other.
- Group VI is an incompletely studied group with an ovotestis on one side and the opposite gonad not examined.

Clinical Features

GENERAL

Aside from the difficult problem of assignment of a sex in a true hermaphrodite, the case

A review of the clinical and anatomical findings in true hermaphroditism is of interest. The following analysis is based on the study of 82 cases collected by Jones and Scott (42) and on 24 cases studied by van Niekerk (93). There has been no comprehensive review of the clinical anatomical correlative of true hermaphroditism since these studies. All patients in both series had a karyotypic study, at least on the peripheral blood. Patients were admitted to these collected series by virtue of having had a karyotypic analysis. The two series are treated separate by, as the van Niekerk study is based on the Bantu and provides some unique features not necessarily applicable to other groups.

MENSTRUATION

The presence or absence of menstruation is determined in some measure by the development of the uterus. A substantial number of true hermaphrodites have rudimentary or no development of the müllerian ducts. However, of those who have uteri that are developed well enough to menstruate, considerably fewer than one-half do so. Signs of cryptomenorrhea occur if there is a uterine anomaly and there is no communication to the outside. The Bantu group have development of the corpus without the cervix in about two-thirds of the examples. In the Jones and Scott collection, this deformity was noted in only about one in 10.

Among 32 patients with the XX genotype in the Jones and Scott group who were 14 or older and had uteri of various degrees of development, 12 had menstruated, 15 had not menstruated, and for five, there was no information. In the XY genotype, of three patients who were over 14, one had no period with a hypoplastic uterus, one had no uterus, and one had only a rudimentary uterus with no period. In the XX/XY genotype, among five patients who were over 14 and had a uterus, two patients in group III (OT:O) and one in group IV (OT:T) had menstruated and two had not. In the mosaic group other than the XX/XY genotype, among four patients who were over 14, two had no periods and for two, there was no information. Thus, about 38% of true hermaphrodites with XX genotype did menstruate by age 14, but no significant conclusion could

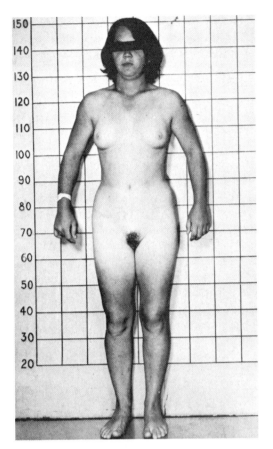

Figure 13.70. Photograph of the patient whose external genitalia are shown in Fig. 13.66 at 23 years of age. The secondary sex development is the result of exogenous estrogen.

of a person with bisexual gonads presents various unique clinical and pathologic pictures and also has the rewarding virtue of giving some insight into an understanding of normal human embryogenesis. The presence of bisexual gonads in the same person invariably seems to bring various degrees of ambisexual development. Often, there is an arresting discrepancy between the chromosomal sex and the structural development of the gonads. There are no characteristic features that clinically distinguish true hermaphroditism from other forms of intersexuality. Interestingly, the clinical picture of true hermaphroditism does not fit in with the clinical pictures associated with other examples of gross chromosomal anomalies. For example, there are very few patients with associated somatic anomalies, and mental retardation is almost unknown.

be drawn from other genotypes because of the limited number of cases. If we add the patients who have evidence of formation of corpus luteum cysts or chocolate cysts or signs of cryptomenorrhea, the actual percentage of those with uterine bleeding is higher. Those who menstruate do so at a little later age than normal.

In the van Niekerk series of 18 patients over 15, seven had amenorrhea, five menstruated, three had irregular periods, and five had cryptomenorrhea. Seven patients with a corpus but no cervix seemed to have had no sign of endometrial activity in the rudimentary corpus.

SEX OF REARING

The majority of reported true hermaphrodites have been reared as boys and men. This, of course, means that the greater number of such hermaphrodites have had rather masculine-appearing external genitalia. Of the 82 patients of Jones and Scott, 52 were reared as male and 18 were reared as female, and for 12, no information was given. If one eliminates group III (OT:O), the group with the most ovarian tissue (an ovotestis on one side and an ovary on the other), the preponderance of individuals who were reared as men becomes apparent. Among 52 patients who were raised as males, 21 belonged to group I (O:T), 11 belonged to group II (OT:OT), and 10 belonged to group III (OT:O). Among 18 patients who were raised as female, 12 belonged to group III (OT:O). Thus, except in group III (OT:O), the number of persons reared as male is greater in each group.

In the van Niekerk series, 19 were reared as males and five as females.

It must be emphasized that data on sex of rearing relates to the past. In view of the likelihood and desirability of diagnosis in infancy, a female sex of rearing should be selected much more often than it has been in the past. This is because at least half of such patients will have a 46,XX karyotype and there will be a predominance of ovarian tissue. Early removal of contradictory sex structures, including partial resection of gonads will enable reproduction as a female in some cases. Williams et al. (95) have reported such a case and cited four others. The testicular development in true hermaphroditism is usually less than normal, and it is extremely unlikely that reproduction as a male will occur.

BREAST DEVELOPMENT

Almost all true hermaphrodites who are old enough develop breasts (Fig. 13.71). In the XX genotype, of the 32 patients who were 14 or older, 29 developed breasts, and three had no breasts. Breasts may develop at the expected time of puberty, but often, development is delayed. We saw one patient in group III (OT:O) who started to have breast development at the age of 16 shortly after a contradictory ovotestis has been removed. The genotype of this patient was 46,XX/46,XY. Due to the limited number of persons who had reached puberty at the time of examination, no mean-

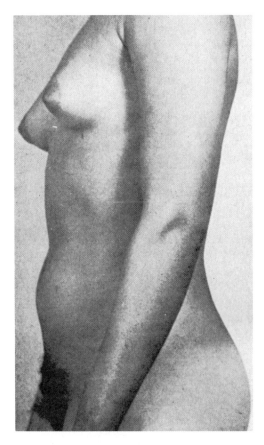

Figure 13.71. Feminine habitus with excellent breast development in a true hermaphrodite. (From Brewer, JI, Culver H: True hermaphroditism. JAMA 1952;148:431.)

ingful comparison could be made between different genotypes; however, breasts do develop in all genotypes.

Cytogenetic Findings

Because of the mixed gonads in this disease, the chromosomal complement has been very much studied in recent years. The first reported chromosomal findings (46,XX) in true hermaphroditism were given by Hungerford et al. (38). Since then, many authors have confirmed that the majority of true hermaphrodites have a chromosome complement of 46,XX, which is indistinguishable from the normal female karyotype.

Ferguson-Smith (23) reported the occurrence of XX/XXX true hermaphroditism, and since then, several other types of chromosomal complement have been reported. The obvious facts from the chromosomal study are that genotype-phenotype correlation is far from precise, and chromosomal analysis, while of great importance in the investigation of the disease, has a limited usefulness in the diagnosis and treatment of true hermaphroditism.

The following karyotypes have so far been reported.

46,XX

Repeated studies indicate that the majority of patients with true hermaphroditism have a karyotype indistinguishable from the normal female karyotype of 46,XX. This finding is of great interest, as it is one very rare proof that a testis can develop without an apparent Y chromosome.

46,XY

In these patients, the karyotypes are indistinguishable from those of the normal male. There is no characteristic feature associated with this genotype. Certainly, such patients are not masculinized more than the others, and they are an exception to the rule that ovarian tissue develops only when there are XX sex chromosomes.

46,XX/46,XY

Frequently, there is genetic evidence to prove that this type of chromosome comple-

ment is the result of chimerism by fertilization of two ova.

OTHER KARYOTYPES

In addition, many other types of chromosomal complement are reported: XX/XXYY, XX/XXY, XO/XY, XX/XXY/XXYYY, XX/XXX, XX/XY/XX, and XO/XX + fragment.

The majority of mosaic cases have a Y chromosome in at least one cell line. Those with the XO cell line in their genotype have a tendency to be short.

MOLECULAR GENETICS

In view of the finding of Y chromosome sequences on the X chromosome in XX males, it has been surprising that Y sequences have not been found in XX true hermaphrodites. This has lead to the possibility that sex determination may be a quantitative trait.

Thus, testicular development requires two doses, while ovarian development results with only one dose of the testicular determining gene or genes (23,28).

Gonadal Findings

LOCATION OF THE GONAD

The testicular tissue and the ovarian tissue can develop on the same side as a separate ovary or testis, or these two can be connected together as an ovotestis. The development of a testis on one side and ovary on the opposite side is also possible. The ovary usually occupies the position of the normal female ovary. The testis may also be located in the normal ovarian position, but it can be found at any level along the route of embryonic descent from abdomen to scrotum; very frequently, it is associated with an inguinal hernia. The ovarian tissue of the ovotestis is usually grossly distinguishable from the testicular tissue of the ovotestis by a raphe; very rarely, the testicular tissue can be completely intermixed or surrounded by ovarian tissue, thus making correct identification of the gonad extremely difficult (Figs. 13.72–13.74). Examination of the location of the contradictory gonadal development shows that there is no recognizable relationship between the location and karyotype. The contradictory testicu-

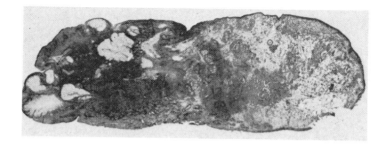

Figure 13.72. A longitudinal section through an ovotestis. Testis on the right, ovary on the left. Although there was a depression on the surface, there was minor comingling between the two portions (H & E × 3).

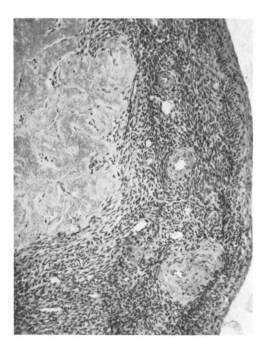

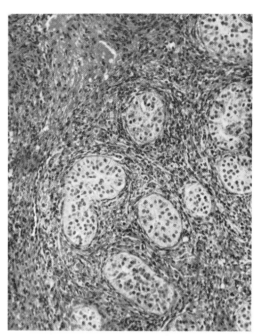

Figure 13.73. A section through the ovarian portion of the ovotestis shown in Fig. 13.72. The presence of numerous corpora albicantia was considered presumptive evidence of previous ovulation (H & E × 112).

Figure 13.74. A section through the testicular portion of the ovotestis shown in Fig. 13.72 (H & E × 112).

lar development occurs in all possible combinations (Table 13.1).

The interesting finding is that larger numbers of testes are located on the right side than on the left side in all types of true hermaphroditism (Table 13.2). In the XX genotype, 10 tests were located on the right side, while seven were located on the left side; four ovaries were located on the right side, and 24 were on the left side; 33 ovotestes were on the right side, and 15 were on the left. In the XY group, six testes were on the right side, and one was on the left side; four ovaries were on the right side, and

eight were on the left side; three ovotestes were on the right side, and three were on the left side. In the XX/XY genotype, five testes developed on the right side, and one developed on the left side; two ovaries developed on the right side, and eight developed on the left side; four ovotestes developed on the right side, and three developed on the left side. In the other groups with mosaicism, six testes were found on the right side, and two were found on the left side; four ovaries were on the right side, and four were on the left side; two ovotestes were on the right side, and three were on the left side.

As a whole, among 82 cases, 27 testes developed on the right side, while 11 developed

Table 13.1.   Hermaphroditic Groups by Karyotype

Karotype	Group						Total
	I (O:T)	II (OT:OT)	III (OT:O)	IV (OT:T)	V (OT: −)	VI (OT:?)	
XX	9	11	17	7	3	1	48
XY	6	1	4	1		1	13
XX/XY	6	2	3				11
XX/XXY	1	1			1		3
XY/XO	1				1		2
XX/XXX	1						1
XX/XXYY	1			1			1
XX/XXY/XXYYY							1
XO/XX + fragment	1						1
XX/XY/XXY	1						1
Total	27	15	24	9	5	2	82

Table 13.2.   Location of Gonad

	Right	Left
XX		
Testis	10	7
Ovary	4	24
Ovotestis	33	15
XY		
Testis	6	1
Ovary	4	8
Ovotestis	3	3
XX/XY		
Testis	5	1
Ovary	2	8
Ovotestis	4	3
Other mosaic group		
Testis	6	2
Ovary	4	4
Ovotestis	2	3
Total		
Testis	27	11
Ovary	14	44
Ovotestis	42	24

on the left side; 14 ovaries developed on the right side, while 44 ovaries developed on the left side; 42 ovotestes developed on the right side, and 24 developed on the left side.

Why more testicular tissue develops on the right side and more ovarian tissue develops on the left side is not known.

GONADAL PATHOLOGY

The testicular component of an ovotestis is usually separated by connective tissue from the ovarian component, but rarely, an intermixture of the two tissues is recognized. There is usually some indentation of the outer surface of the organ where the ovarian and testicular tissue unites (Fig. 13.72). The testicular part is composed of seminiferous tubules lined by Sertoli cells with very poor germ cell development (Fig. 13.74). After puberty, the germ cells are quite degenerate, and tubular degeneration with hyalinization is also seen. The interstitial cells seem to become hyperplastic. Estrogen secreted by adjacent or contralateral ovarian tissue is suggested very frequently as a cause for this change. Elevated gonadotropic hormone probably accounts for the interstitial cell hyperplasia. The presence of a testis apparently does not completely inhibit the function of the ovary, in view of the cyclic menstruation and breast development shown by many of these patients. Furthermore, the ovarian portion of an ovotestis often appears to be quite normal (Fig. 13.73).

Ductal System Development

THE DEVELOPMENT OF THE UTERUS

The development of the uterus from the müllerian ducts is of special interest, not only because of its clinical importance in making it possible for patients to menstruate, but also because there is suggestive evidence from the true hermaphrodite concerning the factors responsible for the normal development of the uterus.

There are more patients with uterine development in the group with genetic mosaicism or chimerism than in those with XY or XX genotype.

In the XX genotype, among 48 patients, 34 had uterine development of various extent; five had no uterus, six had but a rudimentary uterus, and for two, there was no information.

In the XY genotype, among 14 patients, eight had a uterus, three had no uterus, and one had a rudimentary uterus; for one, there was no information.

In the XX/XY genotype, among 11 patients, 10 had a uterus; for one there was no information. Among 10 patients who had various types of mosaicism other than XX/XY, seven had a uterus and two had no uterus; for one there was no information.

The most frequently encountered abnormality in the development of the uterus was that of hypoplastic uterus and absence of cervix. In 24 cases in the well-documented series by van Niekerk (93) it was shown that, among 19 patients who had a uterus, a total of 13 patients had a corpus uteri alone. In eight patients who had corpus uteri only, without cervix, and who had passed the age of 15 years, adenomyosis occurred in four cases, suggesting that obstruction was possibly the cause of adenomyosis. The more frequent development of a uterus was noted in group III (OT:O), and the more frequent suppression of uterine development was noted in group II (OT:OT), suggesting that complete or partial inhibition of the müllerian ducts was greatest when the inhibiting effects were of bilateral origin.

Table 13.3. Development of Tubes

	XX	XX/XY	XY	Other Mosaicism
Testicular side				
Testis with tube	0	3	3	(2) 1 XX/XXY/XXYYY
				1 XO/XY
Testis without tube		3	2	(2) 1 XO/XX + fragment
				1 XX/XXYY
Testis with vas deferens	5	?	?	?
No mention of duct or unknown	8	0	1	(3) 1 XX/XXYY
				1 XX/XXX
				1 XX/XY/XXY
No tube or vas deferens	2	0	0	0
Total	15	6	6	7
Ovarian side				
Ovary with tube	22	8	10	(5) 1 XX/XXY
				1 XO/XY
				1 XX/XXYY
				1 XX/XXX
				1 XO/XX + fragment
Ovary without tube	1	0	1	0
Ovary with rudimentary tube				(1) 1 XX/XXY
Ovaries with ductal system unknown	4	1		(1) 1 XX/XY/XXY
Total	27	9	11	7
Ovotesticular side (ovary and testis)				
With tubes	28	6	3	(1) XX/XXY/XXYYY
Without tubes	?	0	4	(2) 1 XX/XXY
				1 XX/XXY
With vas deferens	8	?	?	?
With rudimentary tube	1			
Both tube and vas deferens	5			
Proximal half vas deferens and distal half tube	1			
Ductal system unknown	5	1	1	(1) XX/XXY/XXYYY
Total	48	7	8	(4)

DEVELOPMENT OF FALLOPIAN TUBES OR VASA DEFERENTIA

The gonadal effect on the development of ductal systems, as expressed by the presence or absence of the tube or the vas deferens, is seen in Table 13.3. It is regrettable that the information on the fate of the wolffian duct is so sparse that no comparison can be made between each genotype.

In the XX genotype, the only one for which some information is available, there were a total of 15 testes with no adjacent tubes developed, while five vasa deferentia developed; two testes had no tube or vas deferens. There was no information in eight cases. There were a total of 48 ovotestes; in this situation, 28 tubes developed on the side of the ovotestis, while eight vasa deferentia developed. In five instances there was no information. There were five ovotestes that had both fallopian tubes and vasa deferentia; one case was interpreted as having development of the vas deferens at the proximal half and development of a tube at the distal half.

There were a total of 27 ovaries. Twenty-two tubes developed on the ovarian side; in five cases, tubes were not mentioned or were unknown. On the side where no gonad was found, one patient had no tube or vas deferens, and one patient was not mentioned.

As a whole, in the XX genotype, no tube developed on the side of a testis and, as far as the development of a tube is concerned, an ovotestis behaved more like an ovary than a testis (Fig. 13.75A). In other genotypes, on the basis of limited information, it seemed tubes did develop on the side of the testis. Thus, suppression of the müllerian ductal system is more complete in the XX genotype than in any others. The interesting observation was made by van Niekerk (93) in his limited series that on the side of an ovotestis the fimbriated end of a tube was almost always occluded. If this finding is reliable, the clinical situation is helpful in determining the nature of the gonad without a microscopic examination.

The reports made on vasa deferentia are few. The presence or absence of a vas deferens on the side where a tube has developed is not at all clear, since most often no microscopic examina-

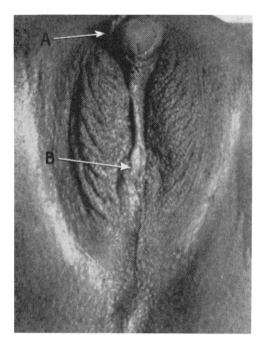

Figure 13.75. External genitalia. *A*, Phallus; *B*, The meatus of the urogenital sinus. Patient shown in Fig. 13.71 (From Brewer JI, Culver H: True hermaphroditism. JAMA 1952;148:431.)

tions have been carried out to detect the fate of the wolffian duct if a tube already has been identified by microscopic examination. In this respect, the number of vasa deferentia given in this series may not be correct.

DEVELOPMENT OF EPIDIDYMIS

The information regarding the epididymis is notoriously scanty if the gonad is other than a testis. Available information from the literature shows that among 53 ovotestes, 41 had an epididymis and 12 had no epididymis. Thus, on the side of an ovotestis, the epididymis develops. On the side of a testis, an epididymis is usually present, but on the side of an ovary, the presence or absence of the epididymis is totally unknown, although it is generally believed that it does not develop.

Among 24 ovotestes where clear information is available in regard to the development of both müllerian and wolffian ducts, 12 ovotestes had a tube and an epididymis on the same side, but the fate of the vas deferens is not known.

Six ovotestes had a vas deferens and an epididymis, but the fate of the tube is unknown; four ovotestes had a tube without an epididymis and the fate of the vas deferens is unknown. One ovotestis had a vas deferens without an epididymis and the fate of the tube is not known; one ovotestis had a tube, a vas deferens, and an epididymis. Thus, in the ovotestis, all or part of both ductal systems could develop simultaneously on the same side in the same person.

External Genitalia Development

One function of the embryonic testis is masculinization of the external genitalia. Examination of the external genitalia of true hermaphrodites showed that the true hermaphroditic testis and ovotestis were as competent in this function as was the testis of the patient with the virilizing type of male hermaphroditism. This influence is illustrated by the fact that the majority of reported true hermaphrodites have been reared as males. Even when the sex of rearing was female, the external genitalia were often described as ambiguous.

In this series of 82 patients, 52 were reared as male and 18 were reared as female, and for 12, the sex of rearing was not given. More persons were raised as male in the XX genotype

than in any other genotype. Also, 11 patients were described as having ambiguous external genitalia, except two of these had female type external genitalia with enlarged clitoris. Nevertheless, the masculinizing effect of the embryonic testis was not completely competent, as seen by the fact that of 82 patients, 67 had hypospadic urethras and variable phallic sizes not consistent with their somatic development. Among 72 patients with information available, three in the XX genotype (groups I, III, and IV), one in the XY genotype (group I), and one in the XX/XY genotype (group II) had a normal or nearly normal phallic urethra. Many persons who were listed as without a vagina on physical examination were found to have a vagina when they were examined by endoscopy. Frequently, the vagina shared the urogenital sinus with the urethra as their common external orifice (Fig. 13.76). With endoscopic examination or urography, more than two-thirds of these patients showed a vagina. The vagina was narrow in the majority of cases.

Among 48 patients with the XX genotype, 30 had a vagina, 11 had no vagina, and one had a rudimentary vagina; for six patients, there was no information. Among the 11 who had no vagina, it is not known how many had had an endoscopic examination. In 12 cases of XY

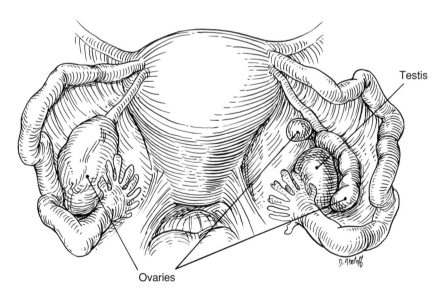

Figure 13.76. A patient with a 46,XX karyotype. Note that the right-sided testis has not inhibited the development of the tube in the presence of the ovary.

genotype, four patients had a vagina and four had no vagina; for four other patients there was no information. Among the four who had no vagina, only one was confirmed by endoscopy. In 11 cases of the XX/XY genotype, eight patients had a vagina and one had no vagina; in two cases there was no information. No endoscopy was done on the one patient who had no vagina. In 10 cases in the other mosaic groups, three patients had no vagina, but none of these was examined by endoscopy. For one case, there was no information.

Prostatic Development

Information on the prostate is very scanty and doubtless reflects the interest of the observer. Review of the literature indicates that among 67 cases where information was available, regardless of chromosomal study, 22 patients were described as having a prostate and 45 were described as not having a prostate. Even in the cases where an autopsy was performed, a prostate was not always identified. A case reported by De Moura (20), showed the lobe of the prostate on the side of the testis was bigger than the lobe on the ovarian side.

Principles of Treatment

The principles of treatment of patients who prove to be true hermaphrodites differ in no way from those for the treatment of hermaphroditism in general. These principles can be summarized here by stating that medical and surgical efforts should be directed toward removing contradictory organs and reconstructing the external genitalia in keeping with the sex of rearing. The special problem with this group is to establish with certainty the character of the gonad. This is particularly difficult where an ovotestis is concerned because its recognition by gross characteristics may be inaccurate. In rare instances, the gonadal tissue of one sex was completely imbedded within a gonadal structure primarily of the opposite sex. At the time of exploration, a biopsy, as well as a bisection of the gonad should be made and inspected in order to not miss the contradictory gonad.

FEMALE HERMAPHRODITISM DUE TO CONGENITAL ADRENAL HYPERPLASIA

Historical Introduction

Female hermaphroditism due to congenital adrenal hyperplasia is the most common disorder causing problems in sexual differentiation. It has been only since the discovery by Wilkins et al. (96) that cortisone successfully arrested the process of virilization associated with this disorder that the syndrome has been clearly understood. Female patients with this disorder, if untreated, not only have serious deformities of the external genitalia that sometimes lead to misidentification of sex, but they also have very serious metabolic disorders that cause accelerated bone growth as children, early fusion of the epiphyses with short stature as adults, and failure of female secondary sex characteristics to appear.

The first clear record of the abnormality is found in the writings of Crecchio (59), who in 1865, described in detail the history and autopsy findings of such a patient, although Crecchio himself did not recognize the association of the adrenal enlargement with the general clinical picture.

The history of Crecchio's patient is of interest. In June, 1820, a woman in Pales gave birth to a child whose sexual identity was the subject of considerable uncertainty. The child was raised as a female for 4 years, but at the age of 4, the name of Josephine was shortened to Joseph on the advice of a surgeon who declared that the patient was a male with cryptorchidism. Because of the sexual abnormality, and the less than normal body configuration, Joseph was somewhat ostracized from society. He smoked continually, turned against religion, and frequented cabarets, where he excelled in obscene stories. He died at the age of of 43.

The carefully described autopsy revealed an individual with a height of 156 cm with extremities much shorter than they should be in relation to the trunk. There was a small penis, but the urethral meatus opened at its base. There was no scrotum nor were testicles palpable. On opening the abdomen, a normal uterus and tubes were discovered. Furthermore, structures that appeared to be ovaries were in the normal position for these organs. The adrenal glands were almost as large as the kidneys, which were of normal size (Figs. 13.77–13.79).

Since this original description by Crecchio, numerous other cases have been observed. But since the recognition that the use of cortisone or its derivatives can arrest the process of

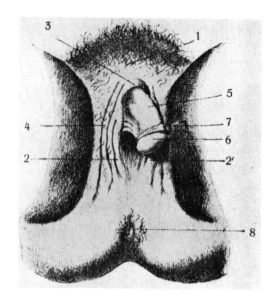

Figure 13.78. Joseph Martzo, a sketch of external genitalia.

virilization in these true females, it is, of course, exceedingly important to recognize the syndrome in infancy. If this is done, proper endocrinological treatment and suitable reconstructive surgery of the genitalia will yield a girl and woman who can enjoy a relatively normal life.

Pathologic Changes of the Adrenal Glands

Jones and Jones (40) had an opportunity to study 15 specimens from untreated patients with congenital virilizing adrenal hyperplasia. The adrenal alterations were described in detail. The adrenals in all cases were greatly enlarged over the normal for the age. The largest adrenals weighed 80 and 90 g, respectively, in a patient 27 years of age (Fig. 13.80).

Microscopic examination shows that the enlargement of the adrenal gland is due entirely to hyperplasia of the rreticular zone of the adrenal cortex. It is in the reticular zone that the sex steroids are formed. In general, the degree of hyperplasia seemed to increase with age in the study referred to above.

The zone fasciculata, which normally produces the glucocorticoids, i.e., cortisol, not only did not participate in the hyperplastic process, but was often unidentifiable, or if it

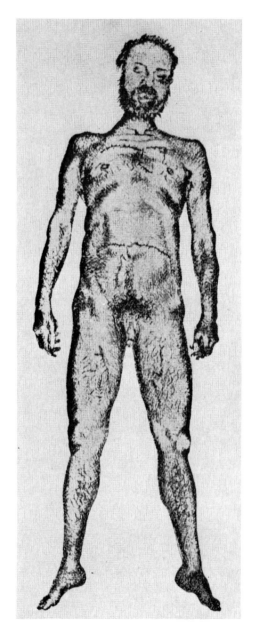

Figure 13.77. Joseph Martzo, a sketch made postmortem.

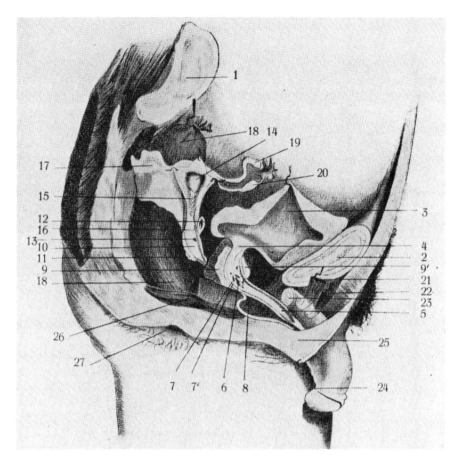

Figure 13.79. Joseph Martzo, sagittal view of internal genitalia as discovered at autopsy. The uterus (15) has been opened. The left tube (19) and ovary (20) are normal

was, was greatly attenuated and did not contain the large amount of lipid normally present in the fascicular zone of the normal adrenal.

The glomerular zone, which is associated with the production of the mineralocorticoids or aldosterone, was relatively unchanged from normal, although in some cases, it may have been even more prominent than normal.

The abnormality of the fasciculata is the fundamental pathologic change in this syndrome and all other changes pathologically and endocrinologically, and, therefore, clinically are the result of this fascicular abnormality (Figs. 13.81 and 13.82).

Endocrinological Abnormalities

The pathological changes referred to in the previous section are paralleled by disturbances in steroid metabolism that should normally occur in the zona fasciculata. It has been shown that the basic endocrinologic problem is a defect in the biosynthesis of cortisol (Fig. 13.83). There are four enzymatic steps required between Δ5-pregneninolone and cortisol, and patients have been described who have defects at each of these steps.

Chief interests in this chapter are in females with defects of 21-hydroxylation or of 17β-hydroxylation. These individuals have serious deformities of the external genitalia and are properly classified as patients with female intersexuality.

The 21-hydroxylase defect accounts for well over 95% of all female patients with congenital virilizing adrenal hyperplasia. The block causes an accumulation of the substrates immediately before it, principally 17-hydroxyprogesterone and to a lesser extent progesterone. Each of these products has a metabolite that is identifi-

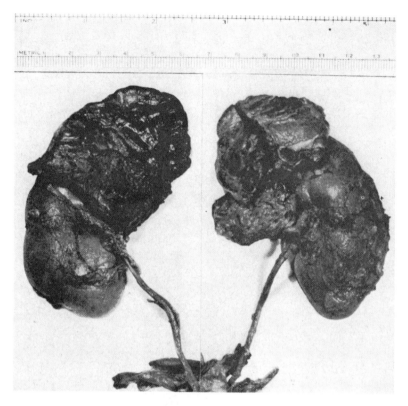

Figure 13.80. An autopsy specimen of a 9-month-old child with congenital virilizing adrenal hyperplasia. Note the huge size of the adrenals.

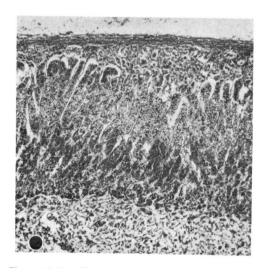

Figure 13.81. The normal adrenal of an adult. Autopsy specimen sudden death. The upper few cells are the zona glomerulosa. The middle zone occupies over half the space of the cortex and consists of the zona fasciculata showing characteristically foamy cytoplasm. The inner one-third of the cortex is occupied by the zona reticularis characterized by cells with darker staining eosinophilic cytoplasm (H & E × 50).

able in the urine; pregnanetriol in the case of 17-hydroxyprogesterone and pregnanediol in the case of progesterone. For many years, elevated pregnanetriol in the urine was a useful diagnostic procedure in determining the specificity of the enzyme block in patients with adrenal hyperplasia. However, much more reliable is the serum determination of 17-hydroxyprogesterone. In infants with this disorder, the 17-hydroxyprogesterone is very high indeed. Any confirmed value over 300 ng/dl is diagnostic. Progesterone may also be elevated, but proportionately nowhere near as great as the hydroxyprogesterone, and in some cases, may be entirely normal.

In the much rarer example of a problem of 11β-hydroxylase deficiency, the diagnosis depends on an elevation of 11-desoxycorticosterone in the blood serum. This defect accounts for no more than 2 or 3% of all patients affected by enzymatic defects of the adrenal.

In the normal situation, homeostasis between the adrenal and the pituitary and hypothalamus is maintained by a seesaw effect between the adrenocorticotropic hormone (ACTH) and cortisol. ACTH stimulation is essential for the normal production of the glucocorticoids, i.e., cortisone, and for the adrenal production of androgens and estrogens by the zona reticularis.

If there is a problem with the biosynthesis of cortisol at any of the required enzymatic steps, the feedback or cortisol on the central mechanism will be decreased, with the result that the ACTH output of the pituitary gland will be greatly above normal. The adrenal gland reacts in the only way possible, namely by excess output of the products of the zona reticularis. This results in great hyperplasia of this zone with a great increase in the estrogens and androgens normally produced from this zone. During embryonic life and in infancy, and during adulthood in the event no treatment is given, there will be a biologic preponderance of androgens. These androgens in intrauterine life abnormally affect the development of the external genitalia. However, the excess output of estrogens and androgens has undesirable metabolic side effects. Bone growth is greatly stimulated during infancy and childhood, and fusion of the epiphyses occurs prior to the attainment of adult height. In addition to that, the excess sex steroid production feeds back on the gonadotropic function of the central mechanisms, with the result that puberty is not initiated in a cyclic manner, breast development never occurs, menstruation does not begin, and the patient is troubled by great excess of hair on the body and face.

Clinical Aspects

21-HYDROXYLASE DEFICIENCY

If the diagnosis is not made in infancy, an unfortunate series of events occurs (Figs. 13.84–13.86). Because the adrenals secrete an abnormally large amount of virilizing steroid, even during embryonic life, such infants are born with abnormal genitalia. In the fully developed

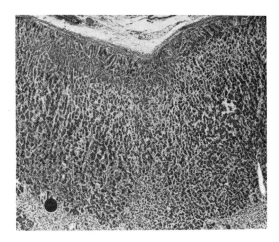

Figure 13.82. A section of the adrenal of a patient 29 years of age with congenital virilizing adrenal hyperplasia. Note the remarkable hyperplasia of the zona reticularis (H & E × 27).

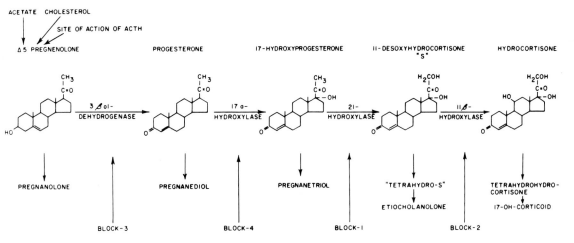

Figure 13.83. Enzymatic steps in the biosynthesis of cortisol.

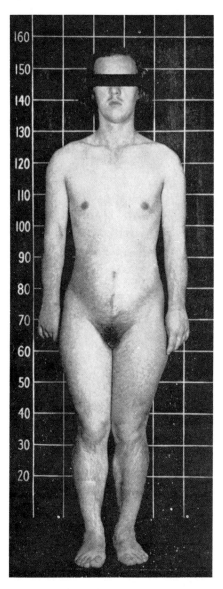

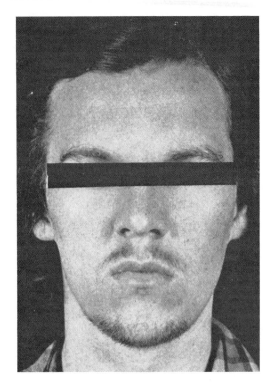

Figure 13.85. Same patient as shown in Fig. 13.84. The mustache and chin whiskers are the result of 3 days without shaving.

Figure 13.84. A 16-year-old-female with congenital virilizing hyperplasia. It was untreated. Note the short extremities that give a stocky build. The hirsutism and lack of breast development are also noted.

case, there is fusion of the scrotolabial folds, and in rare instances, there is the formation of a penile urethra. The clitoris is greatly enlarged so that it may be mistaken for a penis. There are, of course, no gonads palpable within the fused scrotolabial folds, and their absence has sometimes given rise to the mistaken impression of male cryptorchidism, especially if there is a penile urethra. There is usually a single meatus at the base of the phallus, and the vagina

enters the persistent urogenital sinus in a rather consistent fashion. An occasional case is encountered where no communication does in fact occur between the vagina and urogenital sinus. However, in most cases, vaginal communication is in relation to the caudal urogenital sinus derivatives, i.e., beyond the portion of the urogenital sinus, which gives rise to the female urethra. In no case of virilization in the female due to congenital adrenal hyperplasia has the androgenic influence been sufficient to completely suppress the development of the vagina. There is some variation in the point of communication between the vagina and the urogenital sinus. In cases of severe masculinization, the point of juncture tends to approach the region of the bladder, but from a practical point of view, there is usually no problem with the internal vesicle sphincter. In sum, there are various degrees of masculinization apparently depending on the time and severity of the androgenic exposure during intrauterine life (Figs. 13.87–13.92).

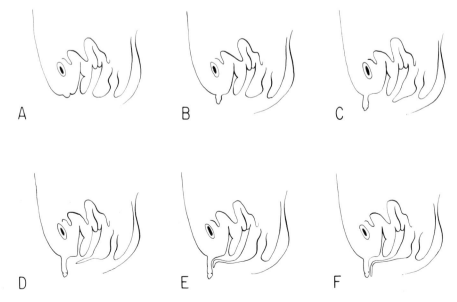

Figure 13.86.   The external genitalia of the same patient shown in Fig. 13.84.

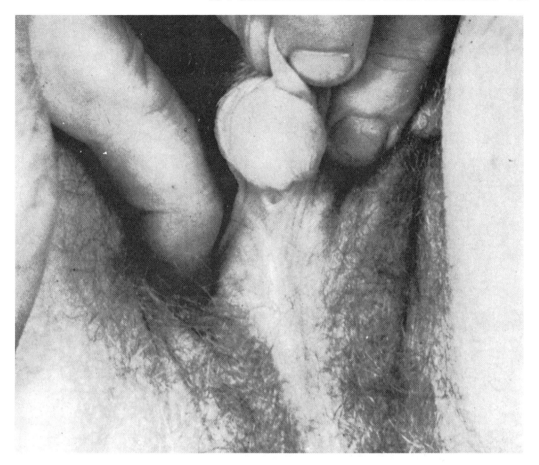

A   B   C

D   E   F

Figure 13.87.   A diagrammatic representation of the various degrees of abnormality of the external genitalia in patients with congenital virilizing adrenal hyperplasia.

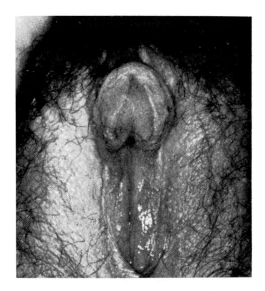

Figure 13.88. External genitalia of a 10-year-old patient with 21-hydroxylase deficiency. The genitalia are of a type B deformity as shown in Fig. 13.87.

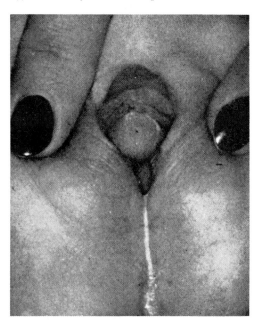

Figure 13.89. External genitalia of a 4-year-old child with 21-hydroxylase deficiency. The external genitalia correspond to type D, as shown in Fig. 13.87.

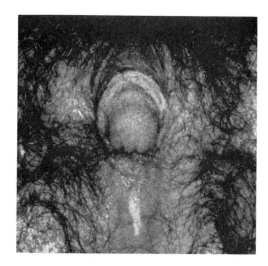

Figure 13.90. External genitalia of an 8-year-old child with 21-hydroxylase deficiency. The external genitalia correspond to type D, as shown in Fig. 13.87.

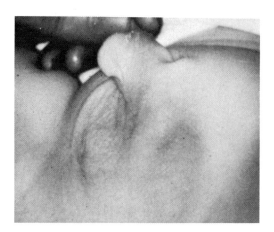

Figure 13.91. External genitalia of a patient with 21-hydroxylase deficiency. The genitalia correspond to type E, as shown in Fig. 13.87.

reach 1½–3 years of age before the growth of the genitalia is sufficient to attract attention.

The unfortunate somatic difficulties with bone growth and short adult stature, of course, affect the male as well as the female in untreated circumstance.

Both males and females with virilizing hyperplasia may have the complicating syndrome of electrolyte imbalance. In infancy, it is manifested by vomiting, progressive loss of weight, dehydration, and unless recognized promptly, may lead to death. Such episodes are really a form of addisonian crisis. The condition is sometimes misdiagnosed as congenital pyloric

Although our principal concern in this chapter is with females afflicted with this abnormality, it should be mentioned that adrenal hyperplasia occurs in the male. Under these circumstances, the clinical picture has been designated as macrogenitosomia precox. In this situation, the penis is often large at birth, but patients may

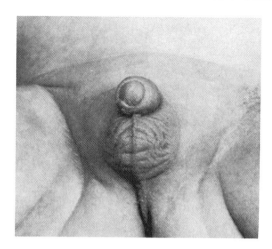

Figure 13.92. External genitalia of a female child with complete scrotolabial fusion. The genitalia are quite indistinguishable from those of a normal male except for the absence of testes in the scrotum. The deformity corresponds to type F, as shown in Fig. 13.87.

stenosis. The characteristic finding is an exceedingly low serum sodium and a high potassium value. Any serum sodium below normal must be regarded with suspicion, and any value below 120 Eq/ml requires energetic therapy.

THE ATTENUATED FORM OF 21-HYDROXYLASE DEFICIENCY

Jones and Jones (40) suggested that some patients with oligomenorrhea, hirsutism, and infertility might represent an attenuated form of the 21-hydroxylase deficiency. This was confirmed by the studies of Rosenwaks et al. (82). Such patients have the symptoms referred to above, and have an elevated value for 17-hydroxyprogesterone in the blood serum. In addition, they respond in a characteristic manner to an ACTH stimulation test. The ovulatory malfunction, and therefore the infertility, can be overcome by the use of cortisone. Anatomical defects of the genitalia are slight and practically never require surgical attention.

11β-HYDROXYLASE DEFICIENCY

Individuals with this disorder are quite unusual. Such individuals may not have as severe deformity of the external genitalia as those with the 21-hydroxylase deficiency. However, they may have the complicating factor of hypertension. This is probably due to

the excess concentration of 11-desoxycorticosterone (Compound S). There may be considerable variability in the clinical and biochemical aspects of this disorder (98).

Genetic Aspects of Virilizing Adrenal Hyperplasia Therapy

It seems clear that the gene or genes for 21 hydroxylation are closely linked to HLA loci on the short arm of chromosome 6. Different forms of 21-OH deficiency seem to be associated with characteristic HLA types. The simple virilizing disease is typically associated with HLA-13W51/5. The severe salt wasting form is associated with HLA-(A3); BW 47; DR7, and HLA-BW 60/40. Thus, there is reason to believe that the gene controlling aldosterone biosynthesis may not be the same gene controlling 21-hydroxylation in the adrenal zona fasciculata (90).

The aim of therapy is to replace the deficiency of cortisol so that the excessive level of ACTH is suppressed. Administration of glucocorticoids not only supplies the deficient hormone, but inhibits the overproduction of the estrogens and androgens. Thus, it is hoped that virilization will be controlled and normal growth and development will occur. This includes normal pubertal development menstruation, and reproduction.

Klingensmith et al. (52) studied the effects of therapy. They found relatively normal growth and development if therapy began soon after birth, although there were some exceptions. In those patients who had reached reproductive age, fertility seemed to be somewhat compromised, and cesarean section was required for delivery because of cephalopelvic disproportion.

The suggested replacement dose is 20–25 mg of cortisol per square meter of body surface per day. The endocrinological therapy can best be managed by a pediatric endocrinologist. Lifetime replacement therapy is required.

In the salt-wasting form of the disease, in addition to cortisol replacement, desoxycorticosterone, and later 9α-fluohydrocortisone, are necessary, as well as additional salt in the diet.

Surgical correction of the masculinized external genitalia in the female is required in almost all cases. This should be carried out as early as feasible, and is best performed by the gynecological surgeons experienced in this area. Details of the surgical reconstruction of the external genitalia are laid out below.

Female Hermaphroditism not due to Adrenal Hyperplasia

Virilizing congenital adrenal hyperplasia is by all odds the most common cause of female intersexuality among genetic females. Nevertheless, fetal masculinization of the external genitalia does occur in otherwise normal females who have been subject to some virilizing influence during intrauterine life. Such patients, contrary to those with the adrenogenital syndrome, do not have postnatal elevations of androgenic substances, and as they grow older, they do not show precocious development, nor are they subject to the metabolic difficulties associated with the adrenal disorder. On the contrary, at the expected time of puberty, the nonadrenal patients will feminize normally and ovulate and have menstruation, except perhaps among the subgroup where there are associated anomalies of the müllerian ducts, where menstruation is precluded because of a uterine anomaly.

The diagnosis of female hermaphroditism not due to adrenal hyperplasia depends upon ambiguity of the external genitalia, the demonstration of a normal female karyotype, and the absence of an adrenal disorder. The relationship of the vaginal orifice and the female urethral meatus to the persistent urogenital sinus is essentially the same in the nonadrenal type of disorder as in the difficulty caused by adrenal hyperplasia. The differential diagnosis among the various conditions causing female-hermaphroditism is usually self-evident, but the differentiation of such patients from those with true hermaphroditism may be exceedingly difficult, and in some circumstances, actually require gonadal biopsy to make the diagnosis with certainty (42).

CLASSIFICATION

Patients with nonadrenal female pseudohermaphroditism may be seen under a variety of pathogenetic and etiological circumstances, and may be classified in three main groups: one related to maternal androgen, exogenous or due to maternal tumor; a special or "nonspe-cific" group, associated with congenital malformations and an idiopathic group.

MATERNAL ANDROGEN

Exogenous

In 1938 masculinization of the female external genitalia was first noted in patients whose mothers had been treated because of habitual or threatened abortion with certain steroid compounds that were used because of their progestational activity. However, as it turned out, such compounds also were androgenic and caused the birth of several genetic females with masculinization of the external genitalia, but with no abnormalities of the internal genitalia. In the early 1960s, several hundred patients with this disorder were observed, but after the realization that the synthetic progestational agents were also virilizing, their use was discontinued. Patients with this disorder are rarely seen today, except for those unrecognized at birth and identified only later (Fig. 13.93) and for patients whose mothers have inadvertently taken androgenic substances without realizing that they were pregnant.

Ovarian Androgenic Tumor

Several patients have been observed with masculinization of the external genitalia at birth whose mothers were found to have an ovarian tumor. In several instances, this was a specific virilizing tumor, but several cases have been observed where the tumor was nonspecific, i.e., of an epithelial type, but nevertheless, the tumor seemed to have induced androgen production from the stroma of the ovary.

A great variety of neoplasms have been found causing this disorder (Table 13.4). While the source of the androgen is clear in some of the tumors, such as the Leydig cell tumor, in others, the role of the tumor at the cellular level in producing the androgen is speculative. However, it is assumed that in the case of the epithelial tumors, the mere presence of the tumor stimulates the surrounding cells to androgenic activity by an unknown mechanism. While androgenic or other steroidal activity can be stimulated in the ovarian stroma in the nonpregnant state by the presence of an epithelial tumor, this reaction seems to be greatly

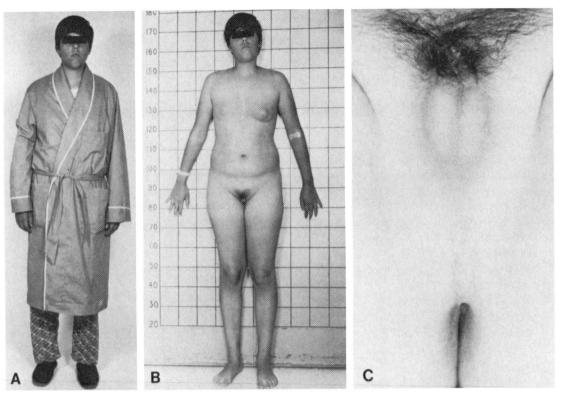

Figure 13.93. Female hermaphroditism caused by the maternal ingestion of an androgenic substance. Although the penis was small at birth and testes were not identified in the scrotum, the child was reared as a male. *A,* Appearance of the patient at age 15. *B,* The same patient showing spontaneous breast development which began at age 11. *C,* Photograph of external genitalia showing complete fusion of the scrotolabial folds and a small penile urethra. At the age of 15, a hysterectomy and bilateral salpingo-oophorectomy were carried out. Testicular prostheses were inserted and exogenous androgen administered.

enhanced by the action of the pregnancy protein hormones, particularly human chorionic gonadotropin (hCG). This was clearly illustrated by the patient with a Krukenberg tumor reported by Connor et al. (13), where the extremely high serum levels of testosterone observed during pregnancy were found to return to normal after delivery of the child, but were later found to be stimulated to the high pregnancy levels by the exogenous administration of hCG during the nonpregnant state.

All degrees of masculinization of the scrotolabial folds and enlargement of the clitoris have been observed in the ovarian tumor group. The degree of fusion and the enlargement of the clitoris is presumably related to the time during pregnancy of the androgenic exposure. For fusion, early exposure is obviously required, presumably by tumors that were present prior

Table 13.4. Histological Appearance of Virilizing Ovarian Tumors in Pregnancy[a]

Histology	Number of Patients
Arrhenoblastoma	8
Leydig cell tumor	5
Brenner tumor	2
Lipoid cell tumor	2
Adrenal-rest-cell tumor	
Granulosa-theca-cell tumor-thecoma	5
Krukenberg tumor	6
Dermoid cyst	2
Hyperthecosis + cystoma simplex	1
Mucinous cystadenoma	3
Papillary mucinous cystadenoma (possibly malignant)	1
Mucinous-cystadenocarcinoma	1

[a]From ref. 94.

to pregnancy, but not producing androgen in sufficient quantities to inhibit ovulation. As the clitoris will respond by growth to androgen at any time during pregnancy, this organ will grow from androgenic ovarian tumors that are active in the latter half of pregnancy and give rise to undesirable clitoral size when there is little or no fusion of the scrotolabial folds.

As with the exogenous maternal androgen group, the internal generative organs are quite normal. This is in keeping with the data from the experimental embryologists, who have demonstrated no effect on the development of the müllerian ducts or on the ovary by maternally administered androgenic steroid compounds.

Furthermore, no permanent reproductive functional impairment of these affected individuals has been observed, and normal reproduction can be expected. However, surgical reconstruction of the masculinized external genitalia is, of course, necessary.

Luteoma of Pregnancy

Special attention is required when the luteoma of pregnancy is a source of virilization. These lesions are important because it is very likely that most cases of masculinized female genitalia classified in the past as idiopathic were in fact cases with masculinization associated with luteomas of pregnancy.

The luteoma was first described by Sternberg and Barclay (89), who provided classical information about its gross and microscopic characteristics.

The luteoma of pregnancy is not a neoplasm; rather, it is a solid tumor that is probably hCG-dependent, and characteristically disappears after pregnancy. These tumors may reach 10 or even 12 cm in size at times, although are usually smaller. They are mostly unilateral, but in some cases, a biopsy of the apparently normal ovary has revealed a microscopic luteoma. The tumor has a fleshy appearance and usually is yellow to brown in color, and may be characterized by darker areas of hemorrhage. Microscopically, the tumor is composed of cells with uniform nuclei and abundant cytoplasm. The cells appear similar to those of normal lutein cells, hence the name. Mitoses can be seen but are infrequent. The lesion is entirely benign. These lesions can produce numerous androgens, under circumstances that are not at all understood.

As with other virilizing influences in pregnancy, not all luteomas result in the birth of a masculinized fetus, in spite of causing considerable maternal virilization. Thus, in the review of Verhoeven et al., (94) from the eight cited maternally virilizing luteomas, there were born four female children, of whom two showed partially masculinized external genitalia. Hensleigh and Woodruff (36) in their review cite additional cases.

The luteoma of pregnancy must be distinguished from multiple lutein cysts of pregnancy, sometimes referred to as hyperreactio luteinalis (Table 13.5). This ovarian reaction is the same as that seen in many instances with hydatidiform mole or chorioepithelioma. At times, hyperreactio luteinalis is associated with a normal pregnancy, and may be virilizing to

Table 13.5. Hyperreactio Luteinalis and Luteoma of Pregnancy[a]

Hyperreactio Luteinalis	Luteoma of Pregnancy
Multiple cystic tumors, generally bilateral	Solid tumors, generally large, often bilateral
Increased incidence with excessive hCG, i.e. mole	No relation to excessive hCG—some arise postpartum
More common in primigravida white patients	More common in multigravid black patients
Also associated with twins, erythroblastosis, toxemia and patients with ovulation disorders	Not associated with any of these conditions
About 25% of non-molar cases reported to have virilization; increased measurable androgens in molar pregnancies but no clinical virilization.	Between 10 and 50% in reported series have clinical virilization
No reported fetal masculinization even when mother is virilized	Female fetus masculinized in half of cases with maternal virilization

[a]From ref. 36.

the mother. However, to date, among 24 cases reviewed by Hensleigh and Woodruff (36), hyperreactio luteinalis does not seem to have been associated with fetal masculinization. It is mentioned at this point, however, not only to distinguish it from the luteoma, but especially because there are data relating to the placental androgenic barrier. Hensleigh et al. (36) reported a patient with secondary amenorrhea and hirsutism and her ovaries enlarged so that each had a diameter of approximately 25 cm. The cardinal clinical finding was marked maternal virilization but no fetal masculinization. At the time of delivery, the maternal arm vein testosterone was 15,000 ng/dl, while the cord blood level in the unaffected female child was only 465 ng/dl. Interestingly, at the same time, there was an increase in fetal cord blood estradiol to 33 ng/ml, a sevenfold increase, as compared with normal cord levels. Thus, the placenta seemed to have been aromatizing testosterone at a sufficient rate to prevent the masculinization of the female child. Another facet of the protective mechanism may be the increased fetal exposure to potent estrogens, which may buffer the influence of any androgens that reach the fetus.

It is likely that sooner or later a female child masculinized by hyperreactio luteinalis will be observed. Presumably, masculinization in this circumstance, as with other virilizing circumstances, would eventuate if the protective mechanism of the placenta were overwhelmed or were deficient.

ADRENAL ANDROGENIC TUMORS

Curiously, some patients who have adrenal tumors that produce large amounts of androgenic steroids nevertheless continue to menstruate regularly and become pregnant. These individuals seem to be relatively insensitive to amounts of androgen that could masculinize the normal woman and cause her to be amenorrheic. Such an interpretation is quite speculative in the absence of any specific study. Nevertheless, pregnancies in women with virilizing adrenal adenomas do occur, and Murset et al. (59) reported such a patient who gave birth to a genetic female with complete fusion of the scrotolabial folds and a large penile urethra.

When this child was 7 years of age, the mother was found to have an adrenal tumor, which at that time produced 83.8 mg/24 hr or urinary 17-ketosteroids (normal, 3–10 mg/24 hr) and 27.9 μg/24 hr of urinary testosterone (normal 2–10 μg/24 hr). The defect in the child had been so severe at birth that the sex was considered to be male, and the child was so reared. The diagnosis was not made until the child was 7 years of age when uterus, tubes, and ovaries were discovered during an operation which carried out under the misdiagnosis of cryptorchidism.

Thus, virilizing adrenal adenomas must be considered as an androgenic source when confronted with a genetic female with masculinized genitalia.

SPECIAL OR NONSPECIFIC

Masculinization of the external genitalia can occur associated with a variety of other somatic anomalies. With the publication of the first edition of Jones and Scott (41), five such patients were identified and designated as special. That designation has been retained. Since that time, a number of additional cases have been described. For example, Park et al. (66) were able to collect 15 examples, and Park et al. (67) reported two sisters with masculinization of the external genitalia and numerous other somatic abnormalities. Carpentier and Potter (12) also contributed patients with masculinization of the external genitalia in a review of fetuses and stillborns with renal agenesis. Among 30 males studied, 22 had normal-appearing external genitalia, while seven had no or a poorly developed phallus with cryptorchidism, seven had normal external genitalia, and four had a hypertrophied clitoris that resembled a male phallus. Thus, it seemed that if anomalies of the external genitalia were present, the phallus in the male tended to be larger than normal.

In this section of special female hermaphrodites are included only individuals with masculinization of the external genitalia and abnormal female karyotype, but, in addition, these individuals have somatic anomalies involving a variety of systems. The uterus generally is present, but in some has not been present, and when present, a double uterus is a frequent finding. Anomalies of the upper urinary tract range from bilateral renal agenesis in the series studied by Carpentier and Potter (12), but in the surviving group may include a variety of upper urinary tract anomalies including bilateral hydronephrosis of a considerable degree. Imperforate anus or anorectal atresia are common lower gastrointestinal tract anomalies. A fistula between the lower urinary tract and the rectum or the vagina is a frequent observation. In the case described by Park et al. (66), there was abnormal function of the thyroid gland, the pituitary gland, and the patient had ectodermal dysplasia with deafness, dwarfism, and pancreatic hypoplasia with mental retardation. This was a unique finding.

Park et al. (67) described two sisters with masculinization of the external genitalia with normal development of the müllerian ducts, but with amenorrhea apparently due to a hypothalamic disorder. Their gonadotropins were low at the time they were reported in their late teens. These patients have been followed through their late twenties and have remained amenorrheic and hypogonadotropic. Their unique features were widespread disturbances of the bones resulting in hypoplasia of the mandibula, hypoplasia of the maxilla, disturbances of the long bones with fusion of the humerus and ulna, and other disturbances of the small bones of the feet (Fig. 13.94). There was consanguinity of the parents, strongly suggesting that the difficulty described was due to an autosomal recessive disorder. The etiology of the other patients in the special group is entirely unknown, as most of the other described patients are sporadic with no familial history.

The cause of the masculinization of the external genitalia is entirely unknown. There does not seem to be any undue masculinization of the mother in such cases, nor is there any progressive masculinization of the patient, so that the disturbance of the external genitalia is unexplained. Many of these individuals die from serious complications of their somatic difficulties, but in the event that they seem to be in generally good health, revision of the external genitalia for the provision of vaginal function is, of course, desirable.

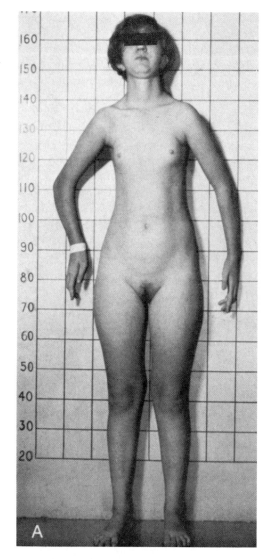

Figure 13.94. *A,* Female hermaphrodite of the special variety. Anterior view. Note the anomaly of the elbow. *B,* External genitalia of the same patient shown in *A. C,* Internal genitalia of the same patient shown in *A.*

IDIOPATHIC

Traditionally, in discussing nonadrenal female pseudohermaphroditism, provision has been made for an idiopathic group of patients. There are individuals who have masculinization of the external genitalia, no other somatic abnormality, and no continuing virilization. Generally, the source of the masculinization was not identified. However, in reviewing cases

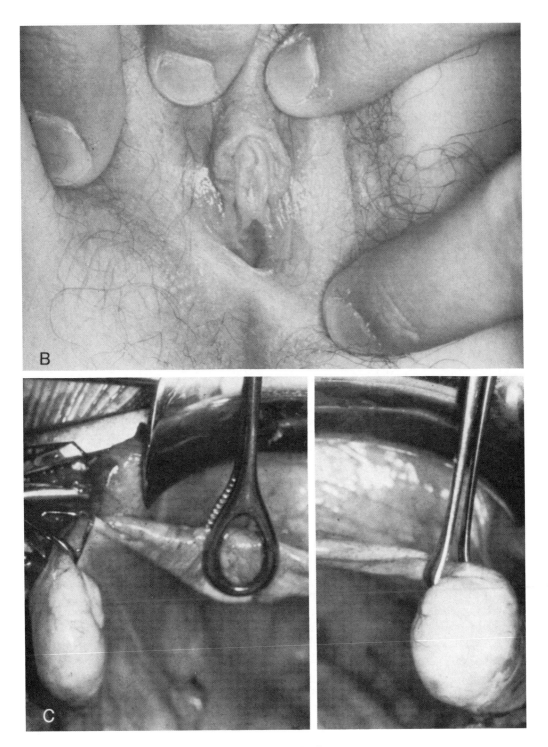

Figure 13.94.   *B–C.*

reported as idiopathic, it is interesting that on several occasions, it was noted that the mother complained during pregnancy of increased virilization, such as troublesome acne, or the abnormal growth of hair. The virilization characteristically disappeared after pregnancy. Thus, it is entirely possible that the cases previously described are not idiopathic and, indeed, are examples of masculinization of the external genitalia due to luteomas of pregnancy.

From a practical point of view, therefore, when one is confronted with a newborn with masculinization of the external genitalia and no evident cause of masculinization, it is important to secure as promptly as possible a serum testosterone level on the mother. The involution of the luteoma of pregnancy requires several days, and even with modest or no maternal masculinization, elevated testosterone levels have been observed under such circumstances. Luteomas of pregnancy can thus be a cause for masculinization in individuals who otherwise would be considered to have unexplained ambiguity of the external genitalia.

DIAGNOSIS AND TREATMENT

All individuals in this category have a normal female karyotype of 46,XX. Attention is called to their hermaphroditic state by virtue of ambiguity of the external genitalia. As a group, these individuals must be distinguished on the one hand from genetic females who have virilizing adrenal hyperplasia, and on the other hand, from true hermaphroditism. In the case of the former, elevated urinary 17-ketosteroids or elevated 17-hydroxyprogesterone is diagnostic. With the latter, a positive assay for H-Y antigen is very suggestive that true hermaphroditism exists. However, as reported by Jones et al. (43), this test may be less than completely reliable in true hermaphroditism. Therefore, at present, the only sure way that true hermaphroditism can be eliminated is by exploratory laparotomy.

With the diagnosis of adrenal hyperplasia and true hermaphroditism eliminated, the diagnosis within the nonadrenal female pseudohermaphrodites is usually fairly simple. A maternal history of the ingestion of androgen should be sufficient to make the diagnosis in this group,

which nowadays is not very frequently. A pelvic examination of the mother should reveal any enlarged ovary with the possibility of a virilizing tumor. With the very rare circumstance of maternal virilizing adrenal tumor, an examination of maternal urinary 17-ketosteroid excretion and/or serum values of androgens should lead to a suspicion. In the subgroup of individuals with somatic abnormalities, the diagnosis is quite evident, and a history of consanguinity of the parents would strengthen this impression.

Fortunately, the anatomical difficulty with the external genitalia is essentially the same, regardless of the virilizing source and regardless of the particular category in which these individuals are found. As indicated above, the anatomical defect is basically the same as with virilizing adrenal hyperplasia.

The treatment of the individual is fortunately much simpler than with virilizing adrenal hyperplasia, as no indication exists for systemic treatment of any kind. The only necessary procedure is surgical reconstruction of the external genitalia at a very early age, i.e., as soon as the diagnosis is made. Details of this operative procedure are considered in a separate chapter, and are also described in Jones and Scott (42).

CONSTRUCTION OF FEMININE EXTERNAL GENITALIA
Gynecologic Operative Procedures

Sexually ambiguous external genitalia exhibit defects in the urogenital sinus derivatives that are remarkably constant regardless of the etiology of the anomaly. These genitalia differ only in their degree of malformation and occupy an intermediate position between the genitalia of a normal female on one hand and a normal male on the other. As already noted, the anomaly may be anatomically the same whether the etiologic factor is congenital adrenal hyperplasia, male hermaphroditism, true hermaphroditism, or another syndrome. This is understandable when the embryology of the genitalia is recalled. Also, it is important to understand that without a virilizing factor, either from the normal embryonic testis or from the abnormal virilizing source, as the adrenal in congenital adrenal hyperplasia, the urogenital sinus will invariably develop along female lines. However, if there is a virilizing influence, there will be more or less fusion of the scrotolabial folds in such a manner that the vagina is suppressed altogether or is concealed from the outside. A urethra will be formed for varying distances along the entire length of the penis. Therefore, the operative procedure to reconstruct ambiguous genitalia into feminine genitalia is essentially the same, regardless of the type of intersexuality.

In reconstruction of the external genitalia on feminine lines, the surgical anatomy is of considerable importance. This is especially true with respect to the site of communication of the vagina with the urogenital sinus. This point is discussed in the section on adrenal hyperplasia. Again, the vaginal communication is almost always in relation to the caudal urogenital sinus derivatives. This means that the vagina communicates with that portion of the urogenital sinus which in a male gives rise to the membranous portion of the male urethra and which in the female becomes the vaginal vestibule. It is almost never in communication with the portion of the urogenital sinus that becomes the prostatic urethra in the male or the entire urethra in the female. Bargy et al. (5) restudied those relationships and confirmed the arrangements just described. This is of considerable surgical importance, for it means that the anomalously persistent urogenital sinus may be boldly incised to the vaginal communication without fear of disturbing the urinary sphincter. Such an anatomic finding tallies with the clinical observation that hermaphrodites with anomalies of the external genitalia as a rule do not have problems of urinary continence.

Hendren and Crawford (34) identified a few patients in whom the vagina entered the urogenital sinus in that portion from which the posterior urethra is derived. While we recognize this variation in the point of junction, it remains our opinion that the communication is seldom sufficiently posterior to be concerned about urinary continence.

It is our belief that the reconstruction operation is best carried out before 18 months of age. The key to the operation is the identification of the vagina, and if by sounding this can be identified soon after birth, the operation may be conveniently done at any time. In any case, the operation cannot be satisfactorily completed until the vagina can be identified. The objective is to complete the procedure at a time when the structures are of a size to permit ease of handling and yet prior to the age when the anomalies may prove embarrassing. If the patient is first seen at an older age, the operation may be carried out at any time. There is no reason to delay operation until puberty, and there are many psychological advantages to proceed as early as possible.

Most hermaphrodites reared as girls will have a vagina or vaginal pouch, although in some instances it will be quite rudimentary. However, in a minority of circumstances, there will be no vagina whatsoever, in spite of ambiguity of the external genitalia, which requires rearing as a female. The operative procedure must conform to the anatomy and will therefore be considered under several categories.

THE BASIC OPERATION FOR PATIENTS WITH A VAGINA

The operation is, in essence, a modification of one described at length by Young (97), which had been carried out previously by various surgeons, notably in Europe. Neugebauer, for instance, describes incision of the urogenital sinus in cases of hermaphroditism (97).

In patients with adrenal hyperplasia, reconstruction of the external genitalia will be the only operation performed in the average case. However, when exploratory laparotomy is necessary to remove contradictory sex structures in other types of intersexuality or to establish the diagnosis, reconstruction of the genitalia may be accomplished at the same operation.

When the operation is carried out at the ideal age, the structures are so small that it is impossible to introduce a finger into the urogenital sinus, so that all tissues must be handled throughout the operation by means of small and delicate tissue forceps. It is also necessary to have available small hemostatic forceps and tiny scissors. Fine suture material, like #00000 synthetic suture on an atraumatic needle, is used throughout.

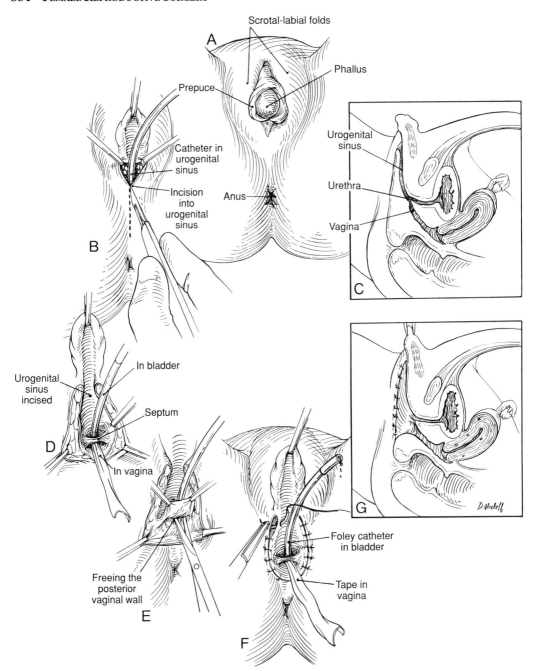

Figure 13.95. *A,* The external genitalia of an 18-month-old patient with female hermaphroditism due to congenital adrenal hyperplasia. The operation is the same, regardless of the etiology of the deformity. *B,* Beginning of the operation. Incision into the urogenital sinus. If the external meatus is large enough and the urogenital sinus will accommodate it, it is sometimes possible to introduce a catheter into the bladder through the urethra and introduce a sound into the vagina beside this. When the structures are large enough, this maneuver greatly facilitates the operative procedure by assuring their identification. *C,* Lateral view, which better shows the relations of the various structures. In this patient, where the anomaly was due to congenital virilizing adrenal hyperplasia, the development of the müllerian ducts was entirely normal for a female. *D,* Situation after incision of the urogenital sinus. *E,* With the glass catheter in the bladder, the posterior vaginal wall is freed as far as necessary to make it possible to bring it to the skin edge without undue tension. *F,* The operative situation after the edges of the vagina are sutured to the skin and after the edges of the mucous membrane of the urogenital sinus are also sutured to the skin along the line of incision. *G,* Lateral view at the completion of the operation.

As a preliminary to the operation, the urogenital sinus may be thoroughly investigated with a small McCarthy panendoscope to determine accurately the position and size of the vaginal communication. If sound or catheter can be easily introduced into the meatus of the urogenital sinus and into the vagina, the endoscopy may be omitted. Special care is needed not to introduce the sound into the urethra, for the urogenital sinus is incised on

the instrument to within 2 or 3 cm of the anus; if the sound is in the urethra by mistake, there is danger of incising the latter structure (Fig. 13.95). After the urogenital sinus has been incised, the urethral orifice may be discovered in the normal position for the female urinary meatus. A small Foley catheter may then be introduced through the urinary meatus for purposes of identification throughout the remainder of the operation. To attach the edges

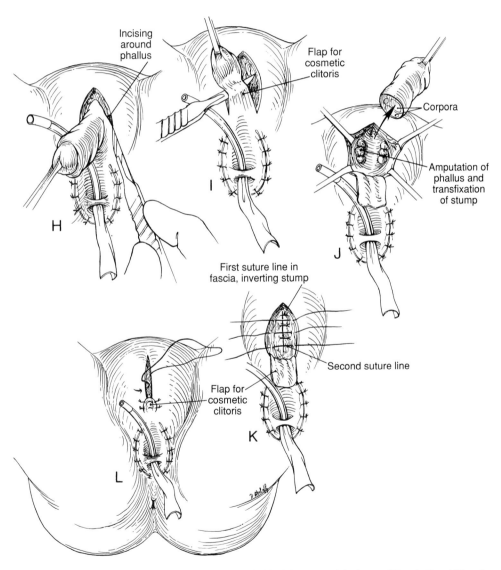

Figure 13.95. *Continued. H*, The beginning of the elliptical incision around the base of the phallus. *I*, The shape of the incision to preserve the flap of mucous membrane along the ventral surface of the phallus. This mucous membrane is used to fashion a small cosmetic clitoris. *J*, The amputation of the phallus with transfixion of the stump. *K*, The stump is buried, drawing the fascia together in the midline. *L*, Final stages of the operation showing a tiny cosmetic clitoris. The size of this clitoris will vary from case to case and gives a remarkably normal appearance to the external genitalia, especially after some pubic hair appears.

of the vagina to the skin, it is usually necessary to free the vagina posteriorly and laterally to secure sufficient mobilization to have these structures meet without tension. It is unnecessary to free the vagina anteriorly, as this would require its separation from the urethra, and sufficient mobilization can ordinarily be obtained by lateral and posterior dissection. When sufficient freedom has been secured, the edges of the vagina may be secured to the skin with interrupted of #00000 suture on an atraumatic reserve cutting needle. In an infant, four or five such stitches around the edge of the vagina are usually sufficient. The edges of the incised sinus membrane may then be sutured to the skin anteriorly, as shown in the illustration. An umbilical tape or a small sponge impregnated with Vaseline may be introduced in the vagina to assure its patency.

Attention is directed to the enlarged clitoris. This may be simply amputated with the fashioning of a nonfunctioning cosmetic clitoris. This technique was used for years. Several children so treated now have normal adult sexual function, so that the technique can still be useful.

However, a newer technique gives a somewhat better cosmetic result. This procedure attempts to preserve a shell of the glans on a pedicle flap. The shaft of the clitoris is subtotally resected and the stumps reanastomosed (Fig. 13.96). The nerve supply to the glans is severed during this procedure so that sensation in the glans is diminished. However, sexual function seems to be satisfactory.

Rajfer et al. (76) have suggested a dorsal approach to the subtotal resection of the corpora (Figs. 13.97–13.101). This has the advantage of preserving the ventral nerve supply and should preserve sensation in the glans. While this is theoretically desirable and can be recommended for suitable cases, as mentioned above, lack of clitoral sensation does not seem to be an important point in the later erotic behavior of patients treated by procedures which sever the dorsal nerves to the glans.

Several other authors have suggested minor variations to the basic procedure described above (6,33,37,39,61).

The indwelling catheter may be left in place for a few days until the edema of the surrounding structures has subsided. This is particularly useful in children with metabolic disorders where accurate urine collection is desirable. A pressure dressing for 24 hr is useful.

Special Operations

OPERATIONS FOR MINOR DEFORMITIES

In some patients, especially among those with enlargement of the clitoris due to maternal androgen, the clitoral enlargement is primarily the result of growth of the prepuce with little or no enlargement of the corpora or glans. This may be true regardless of the degree of fusion of the scrotolabial folds. In such a circumstance, the fleshy clitoris may be removed without disturbing the corpora or glans by a butterfly incision, drawing together the defect from side to side by interrupted stitches (Fig. 13.102).

OPERATION WHEN THE VAGINAL ORIFICE IS DIFFICULT TO LOCATE

As previously mentioned, identification and catheterization or sounding of the vaginal orifice preoperatively is the key to a successful one-stage procedure. It is very seldom that it can be found at operation if it has not been previously identified. However, if it cannot be located by sounding, it can sometimes be seen by endoscopy; often, the reverse is the case, and it can be sounded but not seen. When sounding and vision both fail, immediately prior to surgery it is well worth attempting to introduce a small (No. 4 or 5) ureteral catheter into the vagina by blindly probing through the endoscope along the posterior wall of the urogenital sinus. Sometimes, when worked successfully, this finds the orifice. If so, the catheter can be left within the vagina as a guide to the surgical exposure of the area (Fig. 13.103). In the event that the vaginal orifice cannot be located by any of these maneuvers, a planned two-stage operation may be indicated. At the first stage, the objective would be to obtain cosmetically female genitalia by removing the clitoris and partially excising the urogenital sinus without exteriorizing the vagina. The exteriorization of the vagina may conveniently be postponed until

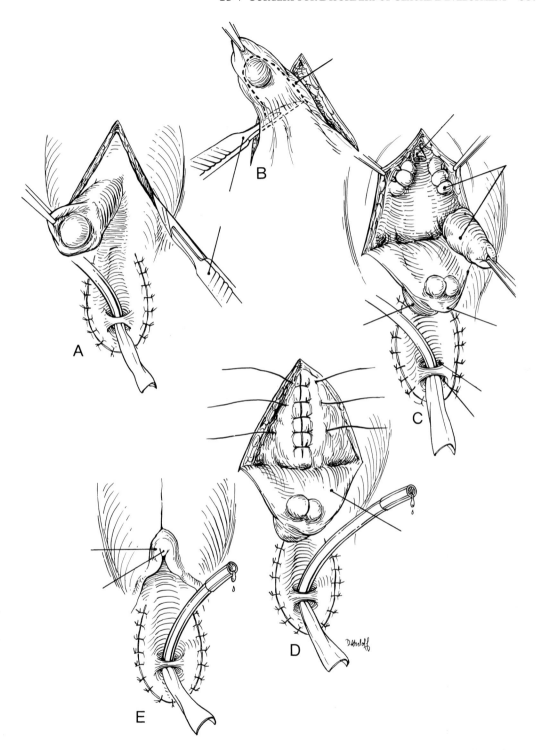

Figure 13.96.   The clitoral flap technique. *A,* The initial incision. *B,* The flap must be as wide as possible at the base to preserve the circulation for the glans. The glans cannot be totally preserved, as the blood supply will be insufficient to maintain it. It must be as thin a shell of the glans as possible. *C,* The shaft of the phallus has been removed. *D,* There has been some closure of the space from which the corpora were removed. *E,* The flap has been sutured into place.

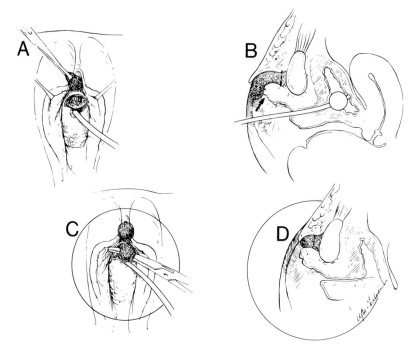

Figure 13.97. Operation of Rajfer et al. *A,* Corpora are approached and removed through a posterior incision in the phallus. *B,* Diagram of the excised portion of the corpora. *C,* The corpora are removed and stumps approximated. *D,* Diagram of the operative procedure.

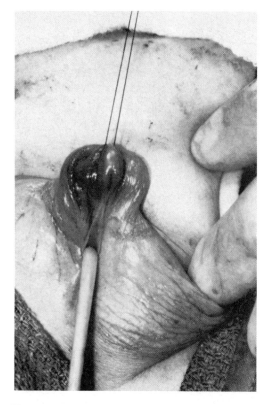

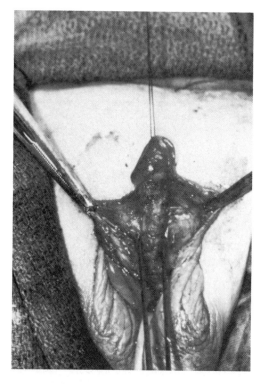

Figure 13.98. Operation of Rajfer et al. Photograph of patient at the beginning of the operative procedure.

Figure 13.99. Operation of Rajfer et al. Photograph of patient with the corpora exposed through dorsal incision.

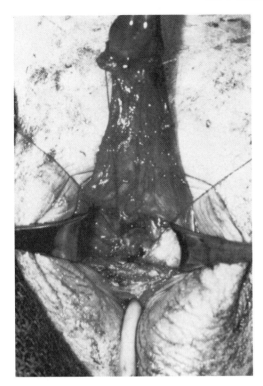

Figure 13.100. Operation of Rajfer et al. The corpora have been removed.

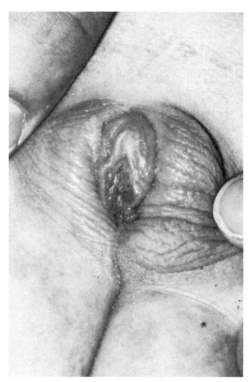

Figure 13.101. Operation of Rajfer et al. (1978). A postoperative photograph of patient several days after the operation.

a later date, when identification of the vaginal orifice by sounding becomes possible.

OPERATION WHEN THE VAGINA IS IMPERFORATE

Very rarely (only three times in about 350 operations, in personal experience) the vagina does not communicate with the urogenital sinus (Fig. 13.103). This is, perhaps, not astonishing, as the point of communication of the vagina with the urogenital sinus is homologous with the hymenal area, and very rarely in an otherwise normal female is the hymen imperforate. For such a circumstance, we have found it helpful to pass a sound downward from above to identify the vagina in the perineum. With such a guide, the edges of the vaginal epithelium can be located and sutured to the skin (Fig. 13.104). Until the uterus enlarges somewhat from its infantile state, the cavity is not large enough to accommodate even a uterine sound. Therefore, if such an operation is contemplated, it should not be done until

there is palpable enlargement of the uterus at the onset of puberty.

OPERATION WITH A POSTERIOR FLAP

Sometimes it is difficult, especially in patients with copious and subcutaneous fat, to approximate the vagina with the skin, particularly posteriorly. When such a situation is anticipated, the flap technique advocated by Fortunoff et al. (26) has been used successfully (Fig. 13.105).

OPERATIONS FOR DEEP VAGINO-SINUS COMMUNICATION

Hendren (35) has been especially interested in patients whose vagino-sinus communication involves the proximal urethra. He has advocated an operation that disconnects the vagina from the urethra and repositions the vaginal orifice in the perineum. In his hands, this seems to have been satisfactory for some patients. The procedure requires positioning the new vaginal

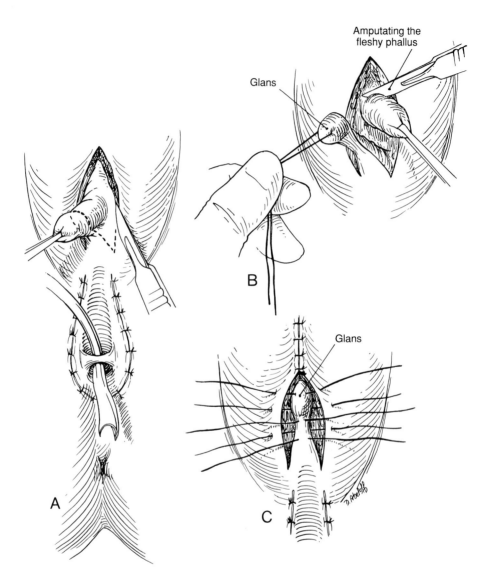

Figure 13.102.   Operative procedure when it is not necessary to remove the corpora or glans. In the drawing above, the clitoral portion of the operation was associated with incision of the urogenital sinus, but in other instances, the latter aspect of the procedure is unnecessary.

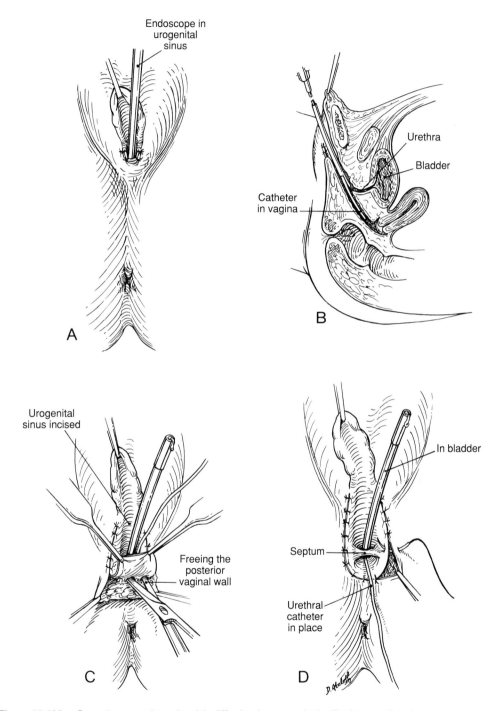

Figure 13.103.   Operative procedure when it is difficult to locate vaginal orifice by sounding. An operative endoscope can be used to probe with a small ureteral catheter. *A,* The orifice is enlarged to accommodate the endoscope. *B,* The tip of the catheter has found the vaginal opening and entered the vagina. *C,* Freeing the posterior vaginal wall with the ureteral catheter in the vagina and a stiff catheter in the urethra. *D,* The vaginal portion of the operation is complete.

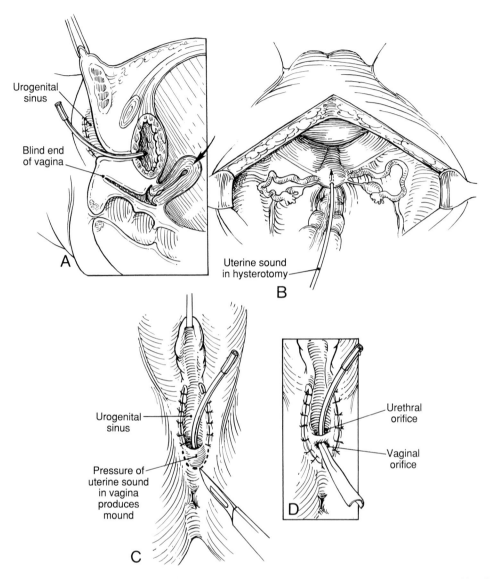

Figure 13.104. *A,* The situation in a patient where the vaginal orifice was imperforate. *B,* A uterine sound has been passed through the fundus into the vagina. *C,* The tip of the sound can be palpated in the perineum. *D,* The completed procedure.

orifice in the perineum. This is sometimes cosmetically not entirely satisfactory. (Fig. 13.106). The vast majority of patients with ambiguous external genitalia and a vagina have a vagino-sinus communication well distal to the proximal urethra so that the procedure advocated by Hendren does not often need to be considered.

RESULTS OF OPERATIONS

The various operations described above can be applied to ambiguous genitalia of various etiologic origins. The results of the application of these procedures in patients with virilizing adrenal hyperplasia were reviewed by Jones and Verkauf (44), and results for this particular etiological situation can perhaps be used as an index of results of the operation applied to other disease entities.

The complete operation (cosmetic correction and exteriorization of the vagina) cannot always be carried out. In addition, it may be important to construct cosmetically female genitalia, even though the vagina cannot be exteri-

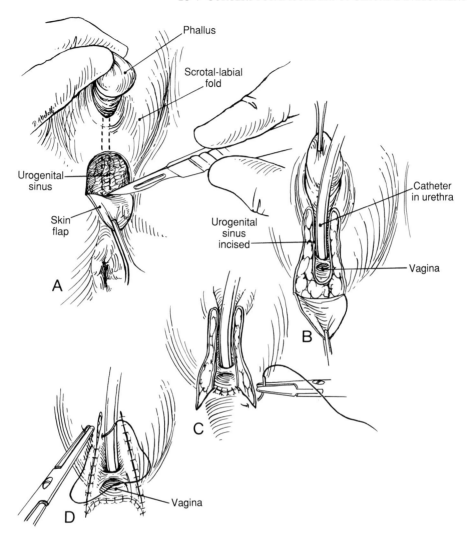

Figure 13.105. A posterior flap technique for use when it is anticipated that there will be difficulty bringing the vaginal orifice to the outside.

orized in the initial operation. However, among patients under 18 months of age, it has been possible to do the operation in by far the majority of cases (Table 13.6).

In 84 patients with congenital adrenal hyperplasia, the success of the operative procedure was evaluated by determining the number of patients requiring reoperation in relation to the age at which surgery was done. This review showed that as long as the vagina could be identified, the complete operation could be carried out successfully, regardless of age (Tables 13.7 and 13.8). It should also be noted that the severity of the deformity had no relation to

the end results. Similar follow-up results were reported by Randolph et al. (77).

Secondary Operations

Secondary operations upon the vaginal outlet may be required. This is the case if the basic operation is deliberately done in two stages for whatever reason. This may be indicated if the vaginal orifice is not readily identifiable, and it seems desirable to construct cosmetically acceptable female genitalia at a very early age. Under this circumstance, the clitoroplasty can be done in the newborn era and the vagina

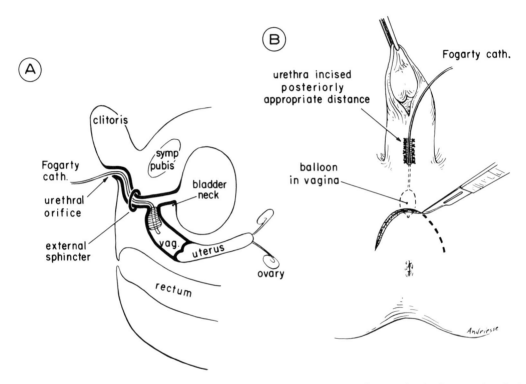

Figure 13.106. A perineal pull through vaginoplasty according to Hendren. *A,* Sagittal view in diagram of vaginal communication very high in the urogenital sinus. A small Fogarty catheter is placed in the vagina to aid in its manipulation and localization. *B,* The location of the initial incision in relation to the balloon in the vagina. (From Hendren WH: Clin Plastic Surg 1980;7:207.) A perineal pull through vaginoplasty according to Hendren. *C,* Flap retracted posteriorly and dissection carried along anterior wall of the rectum until the vagina as identified by the balloon is approached. *D,* Vagina identified by the Fogarty balloon catheter. The vagina is open. Care should be taken to allow flap of vagina distal so that there will be no problem in closing the urethra. *E,* The urethra is closed. Clips are placed on the vagina to bring it down to the perineum. *F,* Vagina is further mobilized. (From Hendren WH: Clin Plastic Surg 1980;7:207.) A perineal pull-through vaginoplasty according to Hendren. *G,* The edge of the vagina is attached to the original flap of perineal skin. *H,* Anterior and lateral flaps are attached. Note the use of drain in the perivaginal space (From Hendren, WH: Clin Plastic Surg 1980;7:207.)

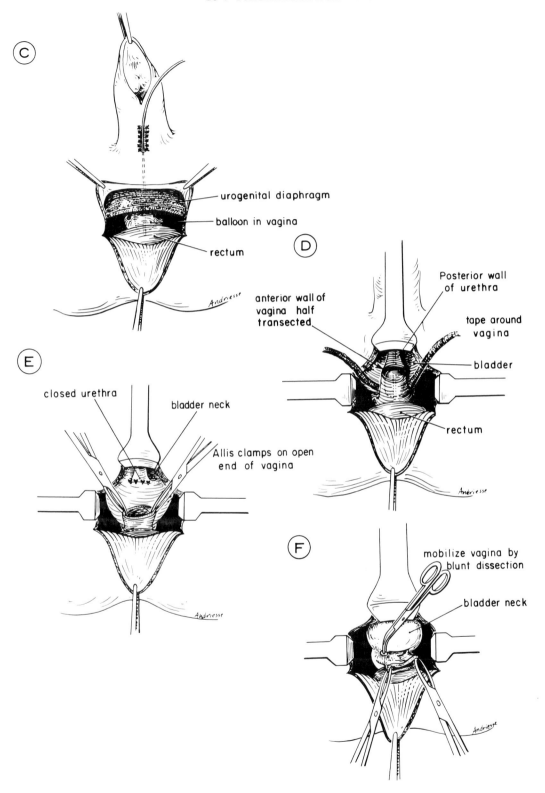

Figure 13.106. *C–F.*

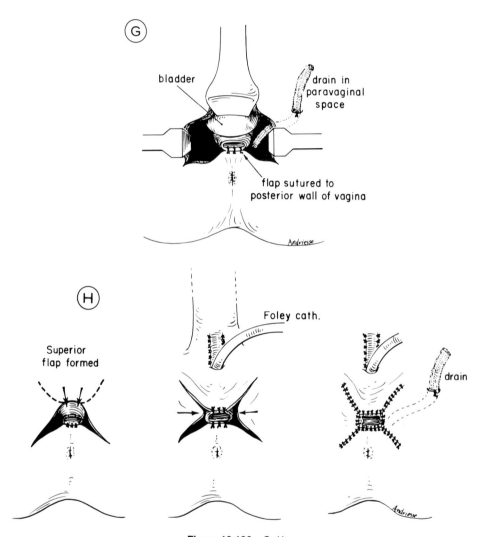

Figure 13.106   *G–H.*

exteriorized at a much later date. In this circumstance, the operation for exteriorization is really part of the basic operation described above.

However, even when the complete operation is attempted at an early age, the vagina is sometimes not satisfactorily exteriorized. The principal difficulty here is failure to carry the midline incision far enough posteriorly. This circumstance requires a second procedure, which in essence completes the first one by continuing the midline incision far enough posteriorly (Fig. 13.107).

At other times, there may be contraction at the vaginal outlet even if the operation is adequately done in the first instance. In this circumstance, a minor revision of the vaginal orifice is required. The vaginal orifice may be enlarged by making an incision in the midline and closing it at 90° to the original axis of the incision (Fig. 13.108). These procedures are

relatively minor and can often be done on an outpatient basis.

OPERATIONS FOR PATIENTS WITHOUT A VAGINA

It is sometimes appropriate to construct female genitalia for genetic male individuals who are reared as females, but whose deformity does not include any vaginal development. In such patients, endoscopic or radiographic visualization by injection of radiopaque medium through the external meatus reveals only a urethra with no vaginal diverticulum. These patients are of two types: (*a*) hypospadic and sometimes cryptorchid males with a penis so small that female rearing is thought desirable; and (*b*) those with micropenis.

Patients in the first category, that is, those listed as hypospadic males with a very small penis are often categorized as individuals with intersexuality of hermaphroditism, especially if they are reared as females, as indeed some patients may best be. According to the concept and classification expressed in Jones and Scott (45), such patients should be characterized as having intersexuality only if a vaginal out-pouching, however small, can be demonstrated arising from the urogenital sinus.

Table 13.6. Initial Operation on Genitalia at Johns Hopkins Hospital in 84 Females with Congenital Adrenal Hyperplasia Reared as Females

Operation[a]	Number of Patients
Clitorectomy	7
Circumcision	1
Clitorectomy + exteriorization of urogenital sinus	9
Clitorectomy + exteriorization of vagina	52
Excision of clitoral stump + exteriorization of vagina	1
Partial clitorectomy, transplantation of glans clitoris + exteriorization of vagina	1
Circumcision + exteriorization of vagina	4
Exteriorization of vagina[b]	9
Total	84

[a]Cosmetic reduction in size of labia also done in four cases.
[b]Six of these had previous clitorectomy at another hospital.

Table 13.8. Relationship of Age at Surgery to Success of Surgery

Age	Number of Cases	Number of Patients Requiring No Further Surgery	Success Rate (%)
0–2 mo	5	2	40
3–18 mo	16	14	87.5
19 mo–5 yr	43	34	79.1
6 yr–12 yr	9	9	100
12 yr and over	11	10	91.9
Total	84	69	82.1

Table 13.7. Relationship of Success of Operation to Preoperative Identification of Vagina

Vagina Identified	Successful Completion of Initial Operation	Reoperation Necessary	Unsuccessful Completion of Initial Operation	Reoperation Necessary
Yes (65)	64	4	1	1
No (11)	3	0	8	8
No information (2)	2	0	0	0

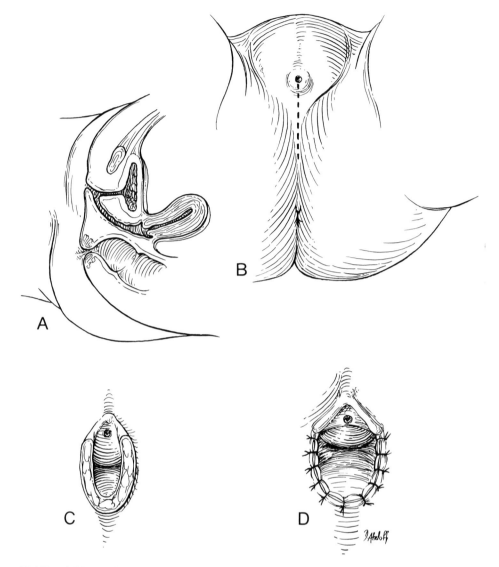

Figure 13.107. *A,* Situation for reoperation on the vaginal outlet when the operation has really not been completed at the first procedure. *B,* The posterior incision. *C,* The vagina is exposed. *D,* The closure.

As defined by Amrhein et al. (2), micropenis may be considered to exist if the stretched penile length is below two standard deviations from the mean in an individual without hypospadias and with a normal 46,XY karyotype.

Individuals in either of these categories are not anatomically or pathogenitically homogeneous. For example, the majority of patients with micropenis have been noted to have rudimentary testes on pathological examination (45) but the etiology of all testicular deficiency usually is not known. However, Najar and Taklarj (61a) described a sibship of five individuals with this condition, thus providing important evidence that in some patients, a genetic etiology is very likely.

In spite of what seems to be testicular immaturity by microscopic examination, when the testes are examined in infancy, it can be noted that the testes of such patients must have been competent enough to masculinize the external genitalia to some degree in the hypospadic patients and completely in the micropenis patients. Thus, when testicular incompetence can be demonstrated, it does not seem to have existed in early embryonic life, espe-

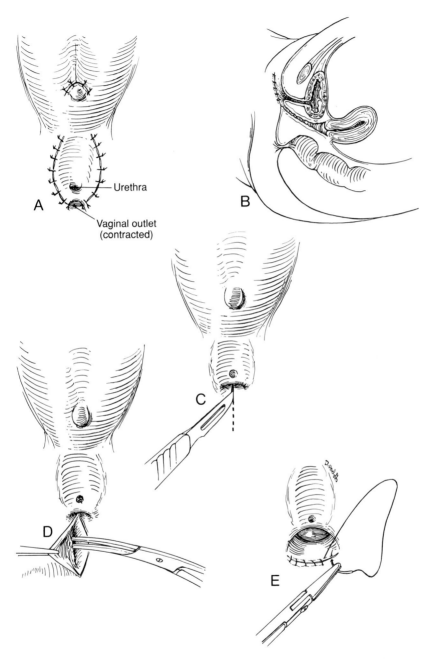

Figure 13.108. Reoperation for contraction of the vaginal outlet. *A,* The lines of the original incision are shown, but the vaginal orifice is shown as contracted in this situation. *B,* The lateral view of the same situation. *C,* The incision through the posterior edge of the contracted vaginal outlet. *D,* Dissecting the vagina from the skin flap. *E,* The closure of the incision at 90° to the direction of the original incision.

cially with respect to the antimüllerian hormone. Failure of the testes seems to have occurred sometime close to but after about the 12th embryonic week, for at that time fusion is complete, but penile growth occurs subsequently to this period.

It has been shown that in most of these patients, androgen binding seems quite normal (2).

In our opinion, sex reassignment should be seriously considered in those patients with a newborn penile length of 2 cm or less with or without hypospadias, especially if the penis shows other malformations as, for example, no identifiable glans or corpora. Sex reassignment can also be considered if the length is longer than 2 cm, if the organ shows serious anatomical deficiencies of the type just noted.

In the type of patients under consideration, the glans is most often not identifiable. The corpora cavernosa and the corpus spongiosum seem undeveloped, so that the urethra is little more than a tube with a wall thickness of a maximum of 2 or 3 mm with or without hypospadias, the covering skin is often redundant, and can be stretched beyond the urethral tube. In ascertaining penile length, the length of the urethral tube is the most important measurement, not the length of the stretched skin.

In some instances, the scrotum is fairly well developed, especially if the testes have descended into the scrotum (Fig. 13.109). In other cases, even if the scrotolabial folds are completely fused, the scrotum is essentially undeveloped. Thus, the perineum appears quite flat so that with the attenuated urethra, the patient appears to have no genitalia at all (Fig. 13.110).

SURGICAL TECHNIQUE

White the technique about to be described is most useful in patients with hypospadias with a penis of micropenis dimensions, or with micropenis, it can also be applied to male individuals who have had a slough of the penis following circumcision (Fig. 13.111). In such unfortunate patients, the scrotum is normally developed and provides adequate material for the fashioning of labia.

The objectives of surgical construction in infancy are:

1. The removal of testes;
2. The provision of the labia lateral to the vaginal orifice, which will be created at a much later date;

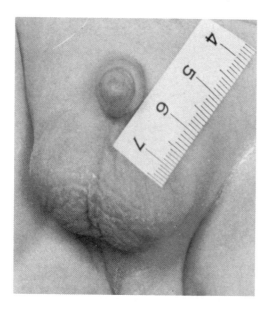

Figure 13.109. A patient with micropenis but with testes descended into the scrotum.

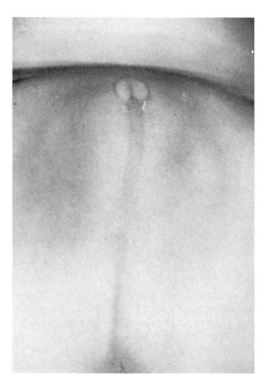

Figure 13.110. A patient with micropenis with little scrotal development with testes that are undescended.

3. Repositioning of the urethral orifice to a location more normal for a female;
4. The provision of a cosmetic clitoris.

These objectives can be accomplished in greater or lesser degree, depending on the situation of the particular case.

The operation begins by bilateral Y-incisions to convert the scrotum into labia. Normally, the scrotum is positioned too far anteriorly to be lateral to the normal position of a vaginal orifice; hence, the necessity for the bilateral Y-V-plasty. There is a limit to the distance that the lower tip of the stem of the Y can be carried for fear that tension will cause the separation of the edges. Ideally, the bilateral incisions should reach at least to the level of and lateral to the anterior edge of the anus. The testes can usually be removed through the Y-plasty incisions (Fig. 13.112). However, occasionally, a separate inguinal incision is useful. If the testes are located interabdominally, a laparotomy will be necessary. To this point, the operation is the same whether or not there is hypospadias.

The urethral orifice is now repositioned by incising in the midline for a suitable distance and suturing the urethral epithelium to the edges of the skin. The length of the incision will depend on whether or not there is complete urethral fusion. There is a limit to which this incision can be carried posteriorly for fear of compromising the circulation to the scrotal flaps. However, the objective is to lower the orifice to a position that will direct the urinary stream into the toilet bowl from a normal female sitting position (Fig. 13.112C).

A second-stage Y-V-plasty is sometimes necessary to complete the posterior translocation of the divided scrotum (Fig. 13.112D).

Where there is a hypospadias or, indeed, where there is a complete penile urethra, the glans is seldom well developed, so that this structure is not available for cosmetic purposes. However, as mentioned, there may sometimes be redundant skin that can be trimmed in order to give a better cosmetic result. The immediate cosmetic result has usually been quite satisfactory from this procedure, but if there was initially no scrotum, a flat perineum may remain.

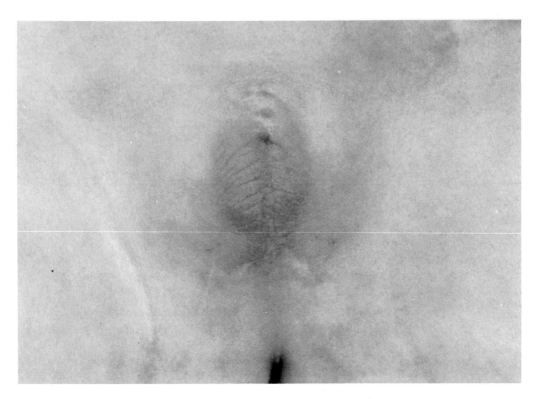

Figure 13.111.   Photograph of child with total slough of the penis following circumcision.

Rock and Jones (80) reviewed 34 patients with microphallus of whom 15 were above the age of 17 and therefore required a functional vagina. The technique of the vaginal procedure as applied to this special group of patients is shown in the figures (Figs. 13.113–13.117).

There are three subgroups easily identified in the figures.

Pyschosexually, patients with disorders just described develop and differentiate a satisfactory feminine gender identity.

As noted earlier, it is always necessary to

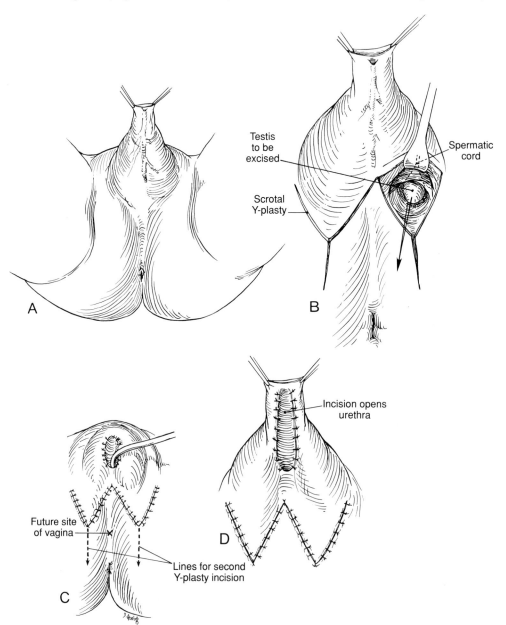

Figure 13.112. *A*, Patient with micropenis. *B*, The beginning of the operative procedure showing the bilateral Y-plasty and excision of the testis, although in this case, the urethra came to the end of the small fleshy phallus. The operative procedure is basically the same in patients with hypospadias where there would be ambiguity of the external genitalia and a phallus insufficient for normal male function. *C*, Completed first stage of the operative procedure converting the external genitalia to a cosmetically female appearance. *D*, Shown in this diagram are the lines for the second stage Y-plasty to bring the posterior flaps far enough posterior to be lateral to the future site of the vaginal orifice.

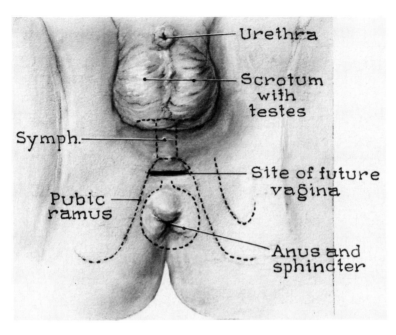

Figure 13.113. *Group A,* Anatomic findings include well-developed scrotum with, in most instances, descent of both testes. The angle between the pubic rami is quite acute, as seen with an android pelvis. These patients should receive gonadectomy with revision of the external genitalia. A bilateral Y-plasty bringing the scrotal folds down to the site of the future vagina is usually performed prior to 2 years of age.

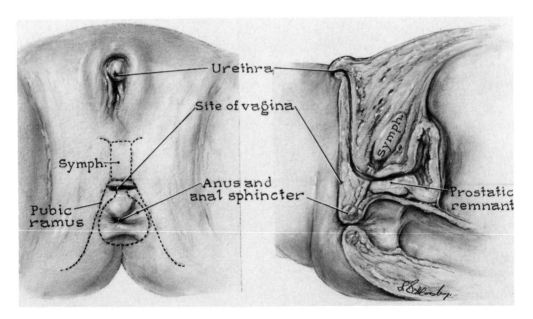

Figure 13.114. *Group B,* There is an acute angle between the pubic rami. The space between the lower portion of the pubic symphysis and the anal sphincter may be limited. The scrotal folds are less well-developed. It is necessary to incise the urethra to a point where the patient may void into the toilet. The gonads are usually removed prior to 2 years of age.

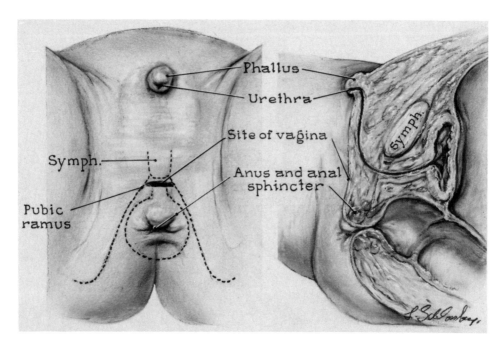

Figure 13.115.   *Group C,* The space between the two pubic rami is limited. The perineum is flat. Revision of the external genitalia includes an incision of the urethra to a point where the patient may void into the toilet when sitting. Further cosmetic surgery is, in most instances, not possible.

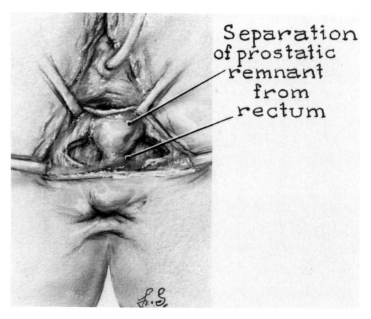

Figure 13.116.   A transverse incision is made just above the rectal sphincter. The space is developed laterally. The levators have been incised. The prostatic remnant must be sharply dissected from the rectum to allow the space to be fully developed to the peritoneum.

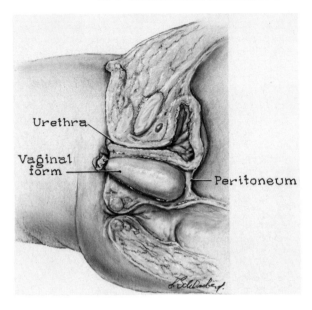

Figure 13.117.   The form with attached skin graft has been placed into the neovagina.

remove the testes in any male intersex because of the high risk of neoplasia in such cases. This has been discussed in detail by Manuel (56), Rutgers (85), Besheti (8), and Savage (86).

References

1. Aono T, Miyake A, Kinugasa T, et al: Absence of positive feedback effect of oestrogen on LH release in patients with testicular feminization syndrome. Acta Endocrinol 1978;87:259.

2. Amrhein JA: Studies of androgen production and binding in 13 male pseudohermaphrodites and 13 males with micropenis. J Clin Endocrinol Metab 1977;45:32.

3. Atwell JD: Inguinal hernia and the testicular feminization syndrome in infancy and childhood. Case report and review of the literature. Br J Surg 1962;49:365–371.

4. Baker ML, Metcalfe SA, Hutson JM: Serum levels of müllerian inhibiting substance in boys from birth to 18 years, as determined by enzyme immunoassay. J Clin Endoc Metab 1990;70:11–15.

5. Bargy F, Laude F, Barbet JP, Houette A: The anatomy of intersexuality. Surg Radiol Anat 1989;11:103–107.

6. Barr ML, Bertram EG: A morphological distinction between neurones of the male and female, and the behaviour of the nucleolar satellite during accelerated nucleoprotein synthesis. Nature 1949;163:676–677.

7. Bearn JG: Anencephaly and the development of the male genital tract. Acta Paediatr Hung 1968;9:159.

8. Besheti M, Hardy BE, Manser K, et al: Neoplastic potential in patients with disorders of sexual differentiation. Ped Urol 1987;24:404–407.

9. Bissada NK, Sakati N, Woodhouse NJY, et al: One-stage complete genital reconstruction for patients with congenital adrenal hyperplasia. J Urol 1987; 137:703–705.

10. Bongiovanni AM: Unusual steroid pattern in congenital adrenal hyperplasia: deficiency of 3-hydroxydehydrogenase. J Clin Endocrinol Metab 1961;21:860–862.

11. Brown TR, Migeon CJ: Androgen receptors and abnormal male sexual differentiation. Adv Exp Med Biol 1986;196:227–255.

12. Carpentier PJ, Potter EL: Nuclear sex and genital malformation in 48 cases of renal agenesis with special reference to nonspecific female pseudohermaphroditism. Am J Obstet Gynecol 1959;78:235.

13. Connor TB, Ganis FM, Levin HS: Gonadotropin-dependent Krukenberg tumor causing virilization during pregnancy. J Clin Endocrinol Metab 1968; 28:198.

14. Cravioto MD, Ulloa-Aguirre A, Bermudez JA, et al: A new inherited variant of the 3-hydroxysteroid dehydrogenase-isomerase deficiency syndrome evidence for existence of two isoenzymes. J Clin Endoc Metab 1986;63:360–367.

15. Crecchio L: Ann Hyg 1865;25:178.

16. Creevy CD: Pseudohermaphroditism: report of five cases. Int Surg Digest 1933;16:195–212.

17. Curry CJR, Carey JC, Holland JS, et al: Smith-Lemli-Opits Syndrome - Type II: Multiple congenital anomalies with male pseudohermaphroditism and frequent early lethality. Am J Med Gen 1987;26:45–57.

18. Damjanov I, Drobnjak P: Ultrastructure of the gonad in the testicular feminization syndrome. Pathol Europ 1974;9:249–257.

19. Degenhart HJ, Visser HKA, Boon H, et al; Evidence for deficient 20-cholesterol-hydroxylase activity in

adrenal tissue of patients with lipoid adrenal hyperplasia. Acta Endocrinol 1972;71:512–518.

20. De Moura AC, Pinto Basto L: True hermaphroditism. J Urol 1946;56:725.

21. Drash A, Sherman F, Hartmann LH, Blizzard RM: A syndrome of pseudohermaphroditism, Wilms tumor, hypertension, and degenerative renal disease. J Ped 1970;76:585.

22. Ferenczy A, Richart RM: The fine structure of the gonads in the complete form of testicular feminization syndrome. Am J Obstet Gynecol 1972;113:399–409.

23. Ferguson-Smith MA, Affara NA: Accidental X-Y recombination and the aetiology of XX males and true hermaphrodites. Phil Trans R Soc Lond, 1988; 322:133–144.

24. Forest MG, de Peretti E, Campo-Paysaa EA: Cas familial de pseudohermaphrodisme masculin par deficit en 17-retoreductase. Ann Endocrinol (Paris) 1979;40:545–546.

25. Forest MG, Lecornu M, de Peretti E: Familial male pseudohermaphroditism due to 17-20-desmonlase deficiency. I. In vivo endocrine studies. J Clin Endocrinol Metab 1980;50:826–833.

26. Fortunoff FS, Latimer JK, Edson M: Vaginoplasty technique for female pseudohermaphrodites. Surg Gynecol Obstet 1964;118:545.

27. Gallo GE, Chemes HE: The association of Wilms tumor, male pseudohermaphroditism and diffuse glomerular disease (Drash syndrome): report of eight cases with clinical and morphological findings and review of the literature. Ped Path 1987;7:175–189.

28. German J: Gonadal dimorphism explained as a dosage effect of a locus of the sex chromosomes, the gonad differentiation locus (GDL). Am J Hum Genet 1988;42:414–421.

29. Gilbert-Dreyfus M, Sebaoun M, Alexandre C, et al: Etude d'un cas familial d'androgyioism avec hypospadias grave, gynecomastie et hyperoestrogenie. Ann Endocrinol (Paris) 1957;18:93–101.

30. Givens JR, Wiser WL, Summitt RL, et al: Familial male pseudohermaphroditism without gynecomastia due to deficient testicular 17-ketosteroid reductase activity. N Engl J Med 1974;291:938.

31. Goebelsmann U, Zachmann M, Davajan V, et al. Male pseudohermaphroditism consistent with 17-20-desmolase deficiency. Gynecol Invest 1976;7:138–156.

32. Greenberg F, Gresik MV, Carpenter RJ, et al: The Gardner-Silengo-Wachtel or Genito-Palato-Cardiac syndrome: male pseudohermaphroditism with micrognathia cleft palate, and conotruncal cardiac defect. Am J Med Gen 1987;26:59–64.

33. Hauser GA: Testicular feminization. In: Overzier C, ed. Intersex. New York: Academic Press, 1963;261–282.

34. Hendren WH, Crawford JD: Adrenogenital syndrome: The anatomy of the anomaly and its repair. J Pediatr Surg 1969;4:49.

35. Hendren WH: Surgical management of urogenital sinus abnormalities. J Pediatr Surg 1977;12:339.

36. Hensleigh PA, Woodruff JD: Differential maternal fetal response to androgenizing luteoma or hyperreactio luteinalis. Obstet Gynecol Surv 1978;33:262.

37. Hudson PL, Dougas I, Donahoe PK, et al: An immunoassay to detect human müllerian inhibiting substance in males and females during normal development. Clin Endoc Metab 1990;70:16–22.

38. Hungerford DA, Donelley AJ, Nowell PC, et al: The chromosome constitution of a human phenotypic intersex. Am J Hum Genet 1959;2:215.

39. Imperato-McGinley J, Gautier T, Peterson RE, et al: The prevalence of 5α-reductase deficiency in children with ambiguous genitalia in the Dominican Republic. J Urol 1986;136:867–873.

40. Jones HW Jr, Jones GS: The gynecological aspects of adrenal hyperplasia and allied disorders. Am J Obstet Gynecol 1954;68:1330.

41. Jones HW Jr, Scott WW: Hermaphroditism, Genital Anomalies and Related Endocrine Disorders, 1st ed. Baltimore: Williams & Wilkins, 1958.

42. Jones HW Jr, Scott WW: Hermaphroditism, congenital anomalies and related endocrine disorders, 2nd ed. Baltimore: Williams & Wilkins, 1971.

43. Jones HW Jr, Rary JM, Rock JA, et al: The role of the H-Y antigen in human sexual development. Johns Hopkins Med J 1979;145:33.

44. Jones HW Jr, Verkauf BS: Surgical treatment in congenital adrenal hyperplasia: age at operation and other prognostic factors. Obstet Gynecol 1970;36:1.

45. Jones HW Jr, Park IJ, Rock JA: Technique of surgical sex reassignment for micropenis and allied conditions. Am J Obstet Gynecol 1978;132:870.

46. Josso N: Anti-müllerian hormone: new perspectives for a sexist molecule. Endocrine Reviews 1986; 7:421–433.

47. Josso N, Briard M: Embryonic testicular regression syndrome: Variable pheotypic expression in siblings. J Pediatr 1980;97:200–204.

48. Jost A: Recherches sur la differenciation sexuelle de l'embryon de lapin. I. Introduction et embryologie genitale normale. Arch Anata Micros Morphol, Expt 1947a;36:151.

49. Jost A: Biologie des Androgenes chez l'embryon, vol 3, Masson & Cie, Paris 1955;160.

50. Keenan BS, Meyer WJ III, Hadjian AJ, et al: Syndrome of androgen insensitivity in man: Absence of 5α-dihydrotestosterone binding protein in skin fibroblasts. J Clin Endocrinol Metab 1974;38:1143–1146.

51. Klebs E: Handbuch der pathologischen Anatomie. A Herschwald, Berlin, 1876.

52. Klingensmith GJ, Garcia SC, Jones HW Jr, et al: Glucocorticoid treatment of girls with congenital adrenal hyperplasia: Effects on height, sexual maturation, and fertility. J Pediatr 1977;90:996.

53. Kogan SJ, Smey P, Levitt SB: Subtunical total reduction clitoroplasty: a safe modification of existing techniques. J Urol 1983;130:746–748.

54. Lubs HA, Ruddle FM: Applications of quantitative karyotype to chromosome variation in 4400 consecutive newborns. Pfizer Symposium on Human Population Cytogenetics, 1969.

55. Mandell J, Haskins JM, Hammond MG: Surgical correction of external genitalia and lower genitourinary tract of markedly virilized child. Ped Urol 1988;31:234–236.

56. Manuel M, Katayama KP, Jones HW Jr: The age of occurrence of gonadal tumors in intersex with a Y chromosome. Am J Obset Gynecol 1976;124:293–300.

57. Money J, Hampson JC, Hampson JL: Hermaphroditism: recommendations concerning assignment of sex, change of sex, and psychologic management. Bull Johns Hopkins Hosp 1955;97:284–300.

58. Morris JM: Syndrome of testicular feminization in male pseudohermaphrodites. Am J Obstet Gynecol 1953;65:1192–1211.

59. Murset G, Zachmann M, Prader A, et al: Male external genitalia of a girl caused by a virilizing adrenal tumor in the mother. Acta Endocrinol Copenh 1970; 65:627.

60. Mussinelli F, Armando C, Cipollini TL: Trends in conservative clitoroplasty. Scand J Plast Reconstr Surg 1986;20:147–152.

61. Naguib KK, Teebi AS, Farag TI, et al: Familial uterine hernia syndrome: report of an Arab family with four affected males. Am J Med Gen 1989;33:180–181.

61a. Najar S, Taklarj N: The syndrome of rudimentary testes: occurrence in five siblings. J Pediatr 1974;84:199.

62. Oesterling JE, Gearhart JP, Jeffs RD: A unified approach to early reconstructive surgery of the child with ambiguous genitalia. J Urol 1987;138:1079–1082.

63. Page DC, Mosher R, Simpson EM, et al: The sex-determining region of the human Y chromosome encodes a finger protein. Cell 1987;51:1091–1104.

64. Park IJ, Jones HW Jr: Familial male hermaphrodite with ambiguous external genitalia. Am J Obstet Gynecol 1970;108:1197–1205.

65. Park IJ, Jones HW Jr, Bias W: A true hermaphroditism with 46,XX/46,XY chromosome complement. Obstet Gynecol 1970;36:377–387.

66. Park IJ, Johanson A, Jones HW Jr, Blizzard RM: Special female hermaphroditism associated with multiple disorders. Obstet Gynecol 1972a;39:100.

67. Park IJ, Jones HW Jr, Melhem RE: Nonadrenal familial female hermaphroditism. Am J Obstet Gynecol 1972b;112:930.

68. Park IJ, Aimakhu VE, Jones HW Jr: An etiologic and pathogenetic classification of male hermaphroditism. Am J Obstet Gynecol 1975;123:505–518.

69. Park IJ, Burnett LS, Jones HW Jr, Migeon CJ, Blizzard RM: A case of male pseudohermaphroditism associated with elevated LH, normal FSH, and low testosterone possibly due to the secretion of an abnormal LH molecule. Acta Endocrinol 1976;83:173.

70. Parks GA, Bermudez JA, Anast CS, et al: Pubertal boy with the 3-hydroxysteroid dehydrogenase defect. J Clin Endocrinol Metab 1971;33:269–278.

71. Peterson EP, Musich JR, Behrman SJ: Uterotubal implantation and obstetrics outcome after previous sterilization. Am J Obstet Gynecol 1977;128:662–667.

72. Peterson RE, Imperato-McGinley J, Gautier T, et al: Male pseudohermaphroditism due to steroid 5α-reductase deficiency. Am J Med 1977;62:170–191.

73. Prader A, Gurtner HP: Das syndrom des pseudohermaphroditismus masculinus bei kongenitaler nebennierensinden-hyperplasie ohne androgenuber-produktion (adrenaler pseudohermaphroditismus masculinis). Helv Paediatr Acta 1955;10:397–412.

74. Prader A: Gonadendysgenesie und testiculare feminisierung. Schweiz Med Wochenschr 1957;87:278–285.

75. Rajfer J, Mendelsohn G, Arnheim J, Jeffs RD, et al: Dysgenetic male pseudohermaphroditism. J Urol 1978;119:525.

76. Rajfer J, Ehrlich RM, Goodwin WE: Reduction clitoroplaty via ventral approach. J Urol 1982; 128:341.

77. Randolph J, Hung W, Rathlev MC: Clitoroplasty for females born with ambiguous genitalia: a long-term study of 37 patients. J Ped Surg 1981;16:882–887.

78. Reifenstein EC Jr: Hereditary familial hypogonadism. Proc Am Fed Clin Res 1947(abstr);3:86.

79. Rios EP, Herrera J, Bermudez JA: Endocrine and metabolic studies in an XY patient with gonadal agenesis. J Clin Endocrinol Metab 1974;39:540–547.

80. Rock JA, Jones HW Jr: The construction of the neovagina in women with a flat perineum. Am J Obstet Gynecol 1989;160:845–853.

81. Rosenberg C, Mustacchi Z, Braz A, et al: Testicular regression in a patient with virilized female phenotype. Am J Med Gen 1984;19:183–188.

82. Rosenwaks Z, Lee PA, Jones GS, et al: An attenuated form of congenital virilizing adrenal hyperplasia. J Clin Endocrinol Metab 1979;49:335.

83. Rosewater S, Gwinup G, Hamwi GH: Familial gynecomastia. Ann Intern Med 1965;63:377–385.

84. Rosler A, Kohn G: Male pseudohermaphroditism due to 17α-hydroxysteroid dehydrogenase deficiency: studies on the natural history of the defect and effect of androgens on gender role. J Steroid Biochem 1983;19:663–674.

85. Rutgers JL, Scully RE: Pathology of the testis in intersex syndrome. Seminars in Diagnostic Pathology 1987;4:275–291.

86. Savage MO, Lowe DG: Gonadal neoplasia and abnormal sexual differentiation. Clin Endoc 1990;32:519–533.

87. Siler-Khodr TM, Morgenstern LL, Greenwood FC: Hormone synthesis and release from human fetal adenohypophysis in vitro. J Endocrin Metab 1974;39:891–905.

88. Sofatzis JA, Alexacos L, Skouteli HN, et al: Malformed female genitalia in newborns with the VATER association. Acta Pediatr Scand 1983;72:923–924.

89. Sternberg WH, Barclay DL: Luteoma of pregnancy. Am J Obstet Gynecol 1966;95:165.

90. Stoner E, Dimartino-Hardi J, Kuhnle U, Levine LS, Oberfield E, New MI: Is salt-wasting in congenital adrenal hyperplasia due to the same gene as the fasciculata defect? Clin Endocrinol 1986;24:9.

91. Sun G-C, Zhong A-G, He W, et al: Reconstruction of the external genitals and repair of skin defects of the perineal region using three types of lateral groin flap. Ann Plast Surg 1990;24:328–334.

92. Tremblay Y, Ringler GE, Morel Y, et al: Regulation of the gene for estrogenic 17-ketosteroid reductase lying on chromosome 17 cen→q25. J Biol Chem 1989;264:20458–20462.

93. van Niekerk WA: True Hermaphroditism: Clinical, Morphologic, and Cytogenetic Aspects. Hagerstown, Maryland: Harper & Row, 1974.

94. Verhoeven ATM, Mastboom JL, Van Leusden HAIM, et al: Virilization in pregnancy co-existing with an (ovarian) mucinous cystadenoma. A case report and review of virilizing ovarian tumors in pregnancy. Obstet Gynecol Surv 1973;28:597.

95. Williamson HO, Phansey SA, Mathur RS: True hermaphroditism with term vaginal delivery and a review. Am J Obstet Gynecol 1981;141:262.

96. Wilkins L, Lewis RA, Klein R, Rosemberg E: The suppression of androgen secretion by cortisone in a case of congenital adrenal hyperplasia. Bull Johns Hopkins Hosp 1950;86:249.

97. Young HH: Genital abnormalities, hermaphroditism and related adrenal diseases. Baltimore: Williams & Wilkins, 1937.

98. Zachmann M, Hamilton W, Vollmin JA, et al: Testicular 17,20-desmolase deficiency causing male pseudohermaphroditism. Acta Endocrinol Suppl (Copenh) 1971;155:65.

99. Zourlas PA, Jones HW Jr: Clinical histologic and cytogenetic findings in male hermaphroditism. II. Male hermaphrodites with feminine external genitalia (testicular feminization). Obstet Gynecol 1965;25:768–778.

IN-VITRO AND OTHER ASSISTED REPRODUCTIVE TECHNOLOGIES

Howard W. Jones, Jr.

INTRODUCTION

The purpose of a chapter on assisted reproduction (AR) in a book on reparative surgery involves more than providing procedural details. It also can inform the surgeon of the current role of assisted reproduction as a supplement, occasionally as an alternate, and sometimes, even as the only method of overcoming a barrier to reproduction. To accomplish this purpose, it seems necessary to describe, at least in broad outline, the various steps required to complete a cycle of assisted reproduction.

OPTIONS FOR ASSISTED REPRODUCTION

In-vitro fertilization (IVF) followed by embryo transfer (ET) was the method originally developed to overcome problems of infertility not amenable to therapy then available. More recently, variations on the theme of IVF have been described. These include gamete intrafallopian transfer (GIFT), zygote intrafallopian transfer (ZIFT), transcervical intrafallopian transfer (TIFT), and many other alternatives. This chapter will describe the basic steps and requirements for IVF, followed by comments pointing out the variations from this standard imposed by the alternatives.

IN-VITRO FERTILIZATION

Indications

In-vitro fertilization was originally designed to overcome infertility caused by absence of or nonfunctional fallopian tubes. With the passage of time, this original indication has been supplemented by many others. The procedure has been found useful for a certain percentage of cases attributable to inadequate spermatogenesis on the part of the male. It has been found useful for certain cases of endometriosis. It has been used successfully where there have been antisperm antibodies in the female, as well as in the male. It has been used in the rare cases where there seemed to be a particularly hostile cervix besides the immunological reasons. It has been found useful in refractory cases of anovulation, and has been used successfully to overcome the combination of difficulties caused by intrauterine exposure to diethylstilbestrol (DES). Finally, it has been applied when the exact cause of the infertility has been unidentifiable, i.e., to the so-called "normal" infertile couple.

With the use of donor eggs, the indications for in-vitro fertilization can be extended to include individuals suffering from premature menopause, or who have had the ovaries surgically removed or who were born without ovaries. It can be used where there are serious genetic defects and danger of transmission from the mother to the child, and in those cases being identified with more frequency where there seems to be an intrinsic egg problem demonstrated by repeated failure of IVF, which is probably also genetic in origin.

The indications can be extended even further if the use of a surrogate uterus is considered acceptable. It could then include the treatment of patients who, for whatever reason, do not have a uterus, such as those born with the Rokitansky-Kuster-Hauser syndrome, that is, with congenital absence of the uterus and vagina, and could include patients who have required a hysterectomy but whose ovaries produce oocytes. This type of surrogacy needs to be distinguished from surrogacy where the surrogate supplies the genetic component to the surrogacy procedure. In this latter circumstance, IVF is not required. It is a completely different biological concept and a somewhat different social and ethical situation.

Required Investigations

Before undertaking a cycle of IVF, it is necessary to confirm the status of the uterus. As a minimum, a routine hysterosalpingogram of contemporary vintage is necessary, not only to rule out any possible congenital defects, but to determine the configuration of the cavity and to ensure the absence of suspected synechiae or filling defects. Hysteroscopy is extremely useful if the hysterosalpingogram reveals an abnormality.

Evaluation of the internal genitalia is required. Most patients who are candidates for IVF will have had laparoscopy at some point in their workup or treatment. The records of this examination can usually be all that is required. However, if there is any doubt about the status of the internal genitalia, and if there is doubt that some other form of therapy might be applicable, contemporary laparoscopy is an essential part of the investigation.

The endocrine profile of a patient is most useful in predicting the patient's response to stimulation for maximizing the number of eggs available for an IVF cycle, and indeed for counseling the patient on the expectation of success in in-vitro fertilization. Currently, in the Norfolk program, this profile is carried out on the third day of a regular menstrual cycle by determining what might be referred to as basal values for follicle stimulating hormone (FSH), luteinizing hormone (LH), and for estradiol. For other patients, depending on the history, additional endocrine assays might be extremely useful; for example: prolactin, testosterone, 17-hydroxyprogesterone, and so forth.

In addition, an accurate evaluation of the semen is a sine quo non known for a cycle of in-vitro fertilization. A "standard" semen examination may be inadequate. An adequate estimation using the "new" morphology has been found to be exceedingly helpful in the Norfolk experience (8). Included in the semen examination should be a bacteriological investigation. Positive cultures for ureaplasma urealyticum are very common. This organism's relationship to infertility remains to be established, but the condition should be treated. Positive cultures for pathogenic organisms are a very poor prognostic sign, and every effort should be made to eliminate infection in the male prior to undertaking a cycle of in-vitro fertilization.

Patient Selection

As implied in the previous section, the candidate for IVF must have a uterus that is suitable for reproduction and one in which the ovaries are available for follicular aspiration. The latter is almost always the case with the use of transvaginal aspiration. It is necessary that the endocrine status and the semen examination be suitable. Further details of the pros and cons of the latter two situations will be described in the following sections. Over and above these requirements in suitable patients, there are other considerations:

A major factor in successful IVF is the age of the female partner. Generally, in patients with a chronological age of 40 and above, the effectiveness of IVF falls off rapidly. Furthermore, pregnancies are more apt to spontaneously miscarry at these ages. There are, of course, exceptions to this general rule that make it difficult to set an age cutoff. In considering patients who are 40 and above, certain other factors come into play, such as the endocrine profile of the patient, particularly the level of FSH under basic conditions. Generally, if the FSH is above 15 MIU on day 3 of a spontaneous menstrual cycle, the expectation of success in in-vitro fertilization diminishes, as will be described in the section on stimulation. In the Norfolk program, the oldest patient who delivered a normal child at term was 43 years of age, although it must be said that there have been very few patients who have been tried at or above this age.

A program of IVF is emotionally draining. It is therefore important to evaluate the emotional stability of the couple, and during the IVF program to offer emotional support.

As of this writing, the reimbursement from insurance sources for IVF has been very small. The financial aspect of the program, therefore, needs to be thoroughly understood by the patient prior to initiating a program. However, the patient should know that the cost for IVF is somewhat less than the cost for a tubal surgery, and the results with even one cycle of IVF are comparable to the expectation of tubal surgery in the average situation (20).

Harvest Cycle

Assuming that the patient is acceptable from all points of view for the program, there are several options with respect to harvesting the oocyte. This may be done: (*a*) in the natural cycle; (*b*) in the modified natural cycle; and (*c*) in the cycle stimulated by various combinations of gonadotropins or clomiphene and including GnRH agonists in various combinations.

The Natural Cycle

Historically, Steptoe et al. (16) worked initially with stimulated cycles, but were unsuccessful and found success obtainable only by the use of the natural cycle. The natural cycle proved to be quite inconvenient, had a low pregnancy rate, and for this reason has been generally discontinued.

Modified Natural Cycle

To overcome the inconvenience in a natural cycle, and yet benefit from its inexpensiveness in that costly drugs and monitoring are not required, a technique has been developed using HCG injection as a substitute for the spontaneous LH surge. In this way, the timing of aspiration can be controlled, with its attendant conveniences to the patient and to the staff. Such programs can be useful in patients where cost is a factor, or in patients where one cannot anticipate much more than a single egg by stimulation. The results have not been spectacular, but it is possible to achieve a very modest pregnancy rate and a modest term pregnancy rate. Current technology indicates that these rates are about 5% (11).

Stimulated Cycle

To obtain multiple eggs, various types of stimulation have been tried in the normal menstrual cycle. These include clomiphene, clomiphene plus human menopausal gonadotropin (hMG), follicle stimulating hormone (FSH), and various combinations of these agents. In addition, there has been widespread use of various GnRH agonists prior to stimulation. As this is written, the best results seem to be obtained by using a GnRH agonist selectively, depending upon the endocrine profile of the patient, or depending upon observation of the patient in a previous cycle of stimulation. In general, patients seem to fall into two groups:

1. If the basal E_2 value on day 3 of the menstrual cycle is below 30 pg/mL, and if the basal FSH value is not elevated, i.e., is not above 15 MIU, and if the LH value is equal to or greater than 15 MIU/mL, patients should do extremely well beginning the GnRH agonist therapy at midluteal phase in the cycle preceding the one of expected harvest. When this is done, the menstrual period generally appears at the expected time and stimulation with gonadotropins, either hMG alone or a combination of FSH and hMG can be begun on the third day of the menstrual cycle, as has been traditionally done, without GnRH agonist suppression. With an average patient mix, roughly half of all patients will fall into this category.

2. On the other hand, if there is a tendency for the FSH to be elevated above 15 MIU, almost regardless of the LH level, luteal phase suppression of the pituitary with a GnRH agonist is apt to result in the necessity to use very large amounts of menopausal gonadotropin or FSH, or a combination, in order to acquire sufficient response to harvest a reasonable number of eggs. In this circumstance, the use of GnRH agonist seems to work better if it is started on the second, or at the latest, the third day of the menstrual cycle, according to the "flare-up" technique, to be followed by gonadotropin stimulation on day 3 or 4 of the cycle.

There is a fundamental difference in the physiological concept in using the GnRH agonist in these two circumstances. With the use of luteal agonist therapy, an attempt is being made to allow eggs to accumulate without gonadotropin exposure as they come into the gonadotropin-sensitive phase, so that when gonadotropins are used, there will be a small pool of eggs that will be relatively synchronized in their response to the gonadotropin. In patients who have a basal elevation of FSH, even though they are normally menstruating, the probability of accumulating a reasonable pool of eggs by luteal gonadotropins suppression is very low. In this circumstance, the flare-up technique is used, not so much for its gonadotropin enhancement, but to prevent the inadvertent LH surge. This surge is apt to occur in patients where the number of harvested eggs is limited. Using the flare-up technique as described, the number of eggs harvested will be limited, but will be greater than can be expected without the use of the agonist, as stimulation may be continued sufficiently long to maximize oocyte recruitment without having it hampered by an inadvertent LH surge.

In patients who have third day FSH values above 15 MIU or are demonstrated low responders as determined by previous attempts at stimulation regardless of age, the patient needs to be aware of the fact that large numbers of eggs will never be obtained from her, no matter what stimulation is used with current knowledge (17). In some instances, the use of the natural cycle may yield results comparable to those following the flare-up technique.

Monitoring

No matter what method of stimulation is selected, the patient must be monitored to determine optimum time for oocyte aspiration. Monitoring is generally done by determination of serum estradiol on a daily basis, and the observation by ultrasonography, either abdominally or preferably transvaginally, of follicular development. Each method of stimulation has its unique values, and it cannot be stated arbitrarily that follicular size is accompanied by oocyte maturation of a certain stage, except in terms of the method of stimulation being used.

The details involved in this determination are beyond the scope of this chapter. In general, however, egg harvest will occur somewhere around day 10 or 12 of the menstrual cycle, when the leading follicles are from 18–20 mm in diameter after they have received exogenous hCG as a surrogate for the spontaneous LH surge, which in many instances is suppressed by gonadotropin stimulation, and is always suppressed when a GnRH agonist is used.

Oocyte Aspiration

Oocyte aspiration and preembryo transfer are the only two quasisurgical procedures involved in IVF.

Until about 1989, many programs utilized laparoscopic technique for oocyte harvest. However, most programs now use some form of ultrasound-guided needle aspiration, and, for the most part, this is transvaginal (Figs. 14.1, 14.2). There are many commercial manufacturers of equipment for this procedure. The essential requirement is that the vaginal transducer be of suitable length and of a diameter that is comfortable for the patient. From a technical point of view, it needs to be at least 5 MHz, or better yet, probably 7–7.5 MHz.

A number of studies, including one from Norfolk, have demonstrated that there is no difference in the number of eggs harvested transvaginally vs. laparoscopically. Furthermore, these eggs fertilize and cleave, as do eggs harvested in other ways, so that the pregnancy rates by the two methods of aspiration are essentially comparable (4). Patients who have experienced both laparoscopic pickup and transvaginal pickup uniformly prefer the transvaginal route, as it requires a very short outpatient hospital stay, general anesthesia is generally not required, and there is less general discomfort with the transvaginal procedure.

On some occasions, it is desirable to inspect the pelvic viscerae to be sure that IVF is the proper therapy for a particular case. In that circumstance, laparoscopic oocyte pickup can be used, along with the diagnostic procedure.

In-Vitro Fertilization and Culture

The handling of the aspirated follicular fluid and the identification of any egg therein is a

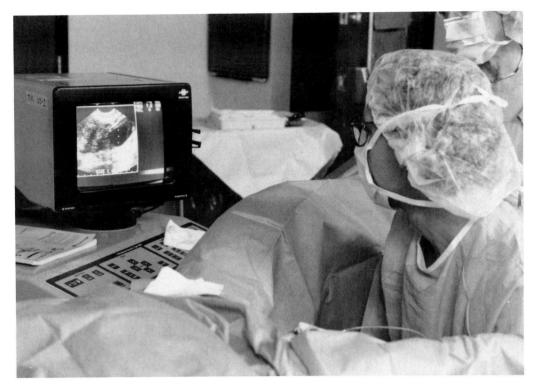

Figure 14.1. Oocyte aspiration by means of vaginal ultrasound guidance. Note the image on the screen, with the dotted line indicating the path of the aspirating needle, which cannot be seen in this view. The operator watches the screen as the needle is advanced to penetrate the follicle.

highly specialized field. For best results, it is necessary not only to identify the egg, but to determine its meiotic maturational state. This is vital, because the time of insemination needs to be determined by the maturational state. Thus, eggs that are harvested in meiosis-II, i.e., by the identification of a polar body at the time of aspiration, may be inseminated as soon as the sperm can be prepared, i.e., within about 2 hr of aspiration. On the other hand, if eggs are aspirated in meiosis-I, results are best if the egg is allowed to proceed in vitro to meiosis-II, and insemination takes place about 3 hr after the identification of the polar body. This requires repeated observation of the egg, indeed through the night, if necessary. Eggs that eject the polar body within 15 hr may be considered as preovulatory eggs, and their biological behavior is essentially equivalent to eggs that are harvested in meiosis-II. Eggs in meiosis-I that take longer than 15 hr to eject the polar body, and eggs that are harvested in prophase will

often mature to meiosis-II, can be inseminated, will fertilize, and will cleave. However, on transfer, the probability of pregnancy in this group is far less than that achieved with mature eggs (19).

Based on these experiences, standard handling of eggs and an estimation of their maturational stage by a determination of the corona do not yield the best results.

Preembryo Transfer

There are two main issues in embryo transfer. The first is the question of when it should be done, and the second is how it should be done. Evidence from Diaz et al. (2) suggests that under normal circumstances, the embryo reaches the uterus somewhere between 3–5 days after ovulation. If the goal is to simulate nature, this would mean that the preembryo should be cultured in vitro until this time. However, culture in vitro probably results in

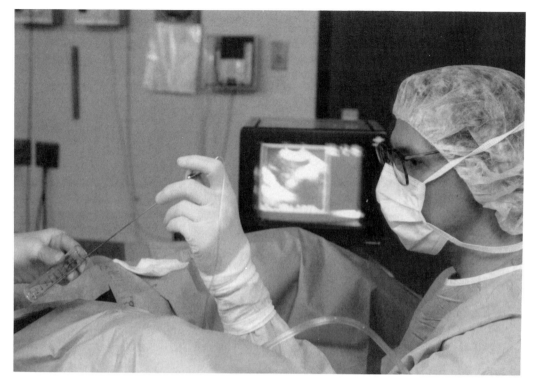

Figure 14.2. The needle has now been removed from the follicle, and the operator is washing the needle by additional suction. The follicular aspirant and the washing solution are collected in the trap, which is not visible in this photograph.

some delay in cell division, and for that reason, it has been the practice to transfer the embryo into the uterus at an earlier time on the theory that the uterine environment is probably better for cell division than the in-vitro environment. Various times have been used, but about 48 hr after insemination, i.e., when the preembryo has reached the 4–6 cell stage, seems to give the best results. In the Norfolk program, a trial at 72 hr was made, but this did not make any difference in the results, and resulted in some incubator clutter.

The current practice in almost all programs is to use some type of transcervical transfer. There are many commercial catheters available for this purpose. In the Norfolk program, a small Teflon catheter is passed through the cervix with the patient in the knee/chest position to allow the transfer to take place with the fundus of the uterus in the lowest possible position. The transfer is a quasisurgical procedure, but no anesthesia or other preparation is required. The catheter is passed for a predetermined distance through the cervix so that the eye of

the catheter comes to rest within 1 cm from the top of the fundus (Fig. 14.3). The preembryo is transferred into the fundus with a small amount of culture fluid (30 μl), followed by a very small amount of air to assure that the preembryo has been ejected from the catheter. Subsequent to the procedure, the catheter is withdrawn and irrigated, and the flushings carefully observed under the microscope to insure that the preembryo has been ejected from the catheter (Fig. 14.4).

It is customary to have the patient remain in a prone position for 3–4 hr following the transfer.

The Inefficiency of Human Reproduction

To understand the odds of achieving pregnancy in any single cycle by IVF, it is necessary to understand that human reproduction is remarkably inefficient. There have been a number of studies in this field with striking similarity of results (10). These studies indicate that

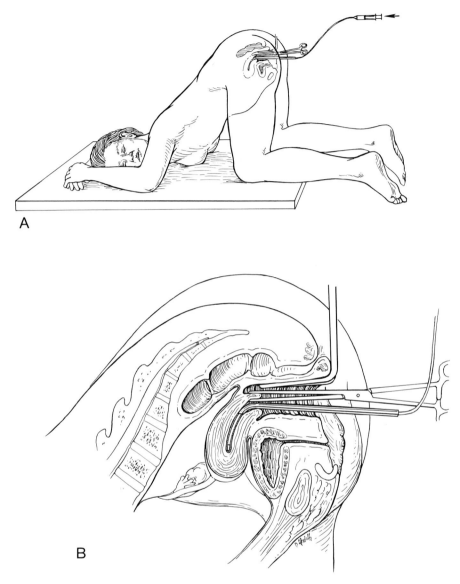

Figure 14.3. *A*, Knee-chest position assures that the fundus is below the cervix at the transfer. *B*, With a simple retractor blade in the vagina, a tenaculum can be applied to the posterior lip of the cervix.

the probability of becoming pregnant and carrying a pregnancy to term among patients who eventually become pregnant is somewhere between 20–25%, and many studies have calculations less than this. The nonfertile cycles seem to be the result of failure of an oocyte to fertilize, or more commonly, the fertilized egg does not develop normally and either does not implant or results in an extremely early miscarriage. A number of studies have found that, at the chromosomal level, the incidence of chromosomal abnormalities in ovulated eggs may

be in the neighborhood of 30%. Similar studies with the sperm show a much lower incidence of abnormality, but it must be remembered that in order to examine the chromosomes of the sperm, a sperm must be able to penetrate a surrogate egg, such as that of the hamster, in order to decondense and have the chromosomes available for analysis. Thus, 8–10% abnormality figures found by this technique probably represent an understatement of the problem (9). Furthermore, the chromosomal examinations of early concepti that have been

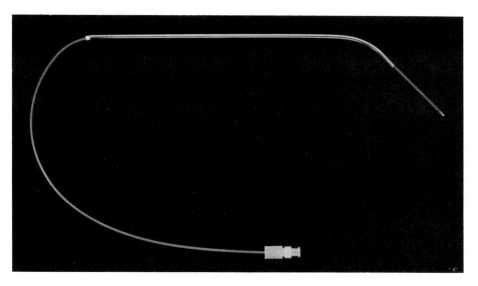

Figure 14.4. Transfer catheter and carrying tube. (Courtesy of Cook Urological, Inc.)

aborted have shown that in early miscarriages, two-thirds of the cases examined show chromosomal difficulties (14). There is, therefore, every reason to believe that the inefficiency of human reproduction is a sorting-out of the abnormal gametes and concepti. One aspect of natural selection is being observed.

Results

In estimating the results from IVF, it is very helpful for the patient to know that the results achieved are not dissimilar from the results in any one cycle of natural reproduction. This is not to say that IVF is as efficient as natural reproduction per cycle. In-vitro fertilization attains its efficiency by the use of multiple eggs, which does not happen in natural reproduction, and the results are enhanced by cryopreservation and other procedures that are unnatural processes.

The quotation of a single figure for the expectation of pregnancy by IVF can only be an average figure and, therefore, is only a very rough approximation to the true expectation for a particular couple. In this sense, it can be misleading.

Keep in mind that in calculating a pregnancy rate, there is no uniformity in the factors used for the numerator or the denominator.

For the numerator, there is the option of using: (*a*) an early transient rise in the β-hCG—

a "chemical pregnancy"; (*b*) a higher and persistent rise in the β-hCG and the identification of pregnancy by ultrasound, i.e., a clinical pregnancy; (*c*) the presence of a pregnancy identified by ultrasound at 20 weeks or greater, sometimes referred to as a continuing pregnancy; or (*d*) a term delivery. The factors entering into the denominator can also be variable. They could be (*a*) those patients who entered treatment, i.e., attempts; (*b*) those patients who come to egg harvest, i.e., an aspiration cycle or, in short, a cycle; or (*c*) those who come to transfer.

Thus, in evaluating pregnancy rates, it is extremely important to ascertain what figure is being used in the numerator and what figure is being used in the denominator.

It is becoming more common to express rates as clinical pregnancies per transfer, although attempts or cycles may sometimes be used in the denominator.

Pregnancy rates, if based on a numerator other than term pregnancy, necessarily include ectopic pregnancies and pregnancies destined to terminate in a spontaneous abortion.

In addition to these statistical matters, the pregnancy rate is significantly influenced by the medical status of the couple. These factors include such things as the age of the couple, particularly of the female partner, the endocrine profile of the female partner, the cause of the infertility in the female partner, and the semen quality and method of estimating sperm quality of the male.

There is an additional confounding factor in estimating the pregnancy rate as stated by an individual program. IVF results are very much influenced by the patient mix. They can also be influenced by temporary, and often unidentifiable vagaries in program results, sometimes attributed to variations in laboratory quality, and sometimes in spite of impeccable laboratory quality control. Thus, figures, to be at all meaningful, must be of a substantial number of consecutive cases and over a sufficient period of time to truly represent the ups and downs of in-vitro fertilization. Consecutive experience of at least 1 year with a minimum of 300 patients should be a minimal requirement.

Having pointed to the vagaries of IVF data, it nevertheless may be of some use to the patient and surgeon to have an average value for an average couple. The results for IVF as reported by the IVF-ET Registry for calendar year 1988 (6) show that from 135 clinics for 13,647 retrieval cycles, there were 11,821 transfers, 2,243 clinical pregnancies, and 1,657 deliveries. This gives a term delivery rate of 12.1% based on retrieval cycles, a 14.0% based on transfers, and a 26.2% miscarriage rate (Table 14.1).

Individual program rates will vary. For example, for the 1990 academic year (July 1, 1989–June 30, 1990), Norfolk treated 483 consecutive patients by some form of gonadotropin stimulation. There was a term delivery rate of 21% based on cycles, 24% based on transfers, and a 28% miscarriage rate. Complete rates may be seen in Table 14.2.

GIFT-ZIFT-TIFT

Gamete intrafallopian tube transfer (GIFT), zygote intrafallopian tube transfer (ZIFT), and

Table 14.1. Pregnancy Results—U.S. Registry 1988[a]

		Number	Percent		
			A	B	C
A	Cycles	12647			
B	Transfers	11821	87		
C	Pregnancies	2243	16	19	
D	Term	1657	12	14	74

[a]Fertil Steril 1990; 53:13–20.

Table 14.2. Pregnancy Rates—Norfolk, July 1, 1989–June 30, 1990

		Number	Percent		
			A	B	C
A	Cycles	483			
B	Transfers	438	91		
C	Pregnancies	144	30	33	
D	Term	103	21	24	72

transcervical intrafallopian transfer (TIFT), and several other alternative methods to standard IVF have been proposed.

GIFT requires laparoscopy. In this procedure, the patient is stimulated and monitored, as for IVF. Egg harvest is carried out by laparoscopy. Usually, four mature eggs are mixed with sperm, which are prepared as for IVF, and two eggs with sperm introduced into each fallopian tube through the fimbriated ostium. Generally, GIFT is used only on patients who were stimulated in such a way that it could be anticipated that four, or at least three eggs with sperm could be introduced into the tubes.

For GIFT, patients must have normal functioning fallopian tubes. The method has the disadvantage that fertilization is not observed, and if the procedure fails, fertilization remains an untested phenomenon. Thus, its use in patients with male problems has become quite problematic.

The results for GIFT, as reported by the IVF-ET Registry for 1988, show that in 3080 retrieval cycles, there were 846 pregnancies (27%), and 654 (21%) deliveries. Results for individual programs will, of course, vary above and below these average figures. It is important to note that it can be misleading to compare results for GIFT with results for IVF or other alternate methods for several reasons. First, GIFT patients must have at least one functional tube. For a comparison, patients in other study groups must have the same tubal competence as tubal status is an index of pelvic pathology that can greatly influence results of any method of assisted reproduction. Second, the number of eggs transferred in any comparative group must be the same. Third, the number of patients stimulated and not retrieved, i.e., the cancellation rate, needs to be known in each group.

Thus, to evaluate the results between groups, there can be no shifting of patients from one treatment group to another, depending on the results of stimulation.

A knowledge of the implantation rate, i.e., the number of sacs identifiable by ultrasound, as a percentage of the eggs transferred, is a very useful index that is becoming more widely used, and overcomes some, but not all, of the difficulties mentioned in the preceding paragraph.

Asch et al. (1) reported an implantation rate of 19.1% for 596 eggs transferred by the GIFT technique.

ZIFT differs from GIFT in that fertilization is observed prior to transfer in the tube in the ZIFT process. Thus, two procedures are required. Egg harvest can be accomplished by the standard transvaginal ultrasound-guided route, and 24 hr later, after fertilization is established, the pronuclear oocytes, i.e., the prezygotes, are transferred by laparoscopy into the tubes with the same technique used for the GIFT procedure. Results from the ZIFT technique are limited. For 1988, 385 stimulation cycles for ZIFT were reported to the IVF-ET Registry. Of these, 355 (92%) resulted in egg retrieval, and 275 (91% and 77%) in a transfer, but the number of zygotes transferred were not included in the data. There were 97 pregnancies (25%, 27%, and 35%) and 71 deliveries (18%, 20%, and 26%). Asch et al. (1), reported an implantation rate of 18.8% for 154 transfers. Thus, according to Asch, the implantation rates for ZIFT and GIFT were essentially the same.

TIFT has been developed to overcome the disadvantages of the laparoscopy, and yet take advantage, of transferring any eggs and sperm or prezygotes into the fallopian tubes. Current techniques for TIFT, i.e., transcervical intrafallopian transfer into the tubes involve special instruments for blind catheterization. Some groups have reported that ultrasound monitoring during catheterization has been helpful. Developmental studies are underway with catheterization of the tubal ostia by hysteroscopic visualization. Only limited data are available for this technique. Scholtes et al. (15) reported a pilot study among 38 patients with unexplained infertility. They reported a 23% pregnancy rate per retrieval cycle for TIFT, as compared with a 20% rate for IVF in their

clinic for the same type of patient during the same time interval. There was thus no demonstrated advantage of using the TIFT procedure in this series.

A larger question concerns the necessity to use assisted reproduction for patients with patent tubes, especially for the "normal" infertile group. There is some evidence that the multiple eggs resulting from the stimulation used for follicular recruitment is the key to the pregnancy enhancement in this group. For example, Hovatta et al. (5) reported a 10.4% pregnancy rate per cycle from stimulation alone. Dodson et al., (3) had earlier reported pregnancy rates of 17% for patients with endometriosis and open tubes, 29% for patients with cervical factor difficulty, and 19% for idiopathic infertility. These rates are very comparable to the rates for normal reproduction, as indicated in an earlier discussion.

CRYOPRESERVATION

Cryopreservation has provided a significant supplement to the pregnancy rate for assisted reproduction. This supplement may add up to 5% to the fresh rate quoted in the section on "Results," depending upon the number of fertilizing eggs that are cryopreserved.

Cryopreservation may be carried out during fertilization, i.e., in the pronuclear stage, or later, at the four-cell stage up to blastocyst. The most consistent and satisfactory results occur if cryopreservation takes place during the pronuclear stage, although some programs prefer to use later stages. In addition to medical factors, there is an ethical point to consider. Those who are persuaded that a human personality, with all its implications, begins at the completion of fertilization, might regard cryopreservation as morally acceptable if carried out during fertilization, i.e., during the pronuclear stage, but might have moral concerns if carried out after fertilization is complete.

The technique of cryopreservation has been facilitated by the development of automatic equipment by many manufacturers. Such equipment lowers the temperature in programmable stages. The concepti can be stored for many years (Fig. 14.5).

With contemporary methods of stimulation

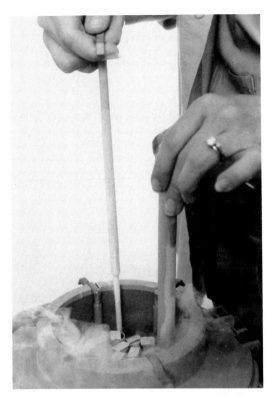

Figure 14.5. The cane holding the frozen prezygote is being lowered into the storage tank cooled by liquid nitrogen. The cryopreserved prezygote can easily be maintained through the reproductive life of the prospective parents.

and an average patient mix, about one-half of all couples will have sufficient numbers of eggs fertilized to transfer up to four developing preembryos and have one or more eggs available for cryopreservation. The results from cryopreservation and the augmentation of results by cryopreservation, as might be expected, depends upon the number of eggs cryopreserved (18) (Tables 14.3 and 14.4).

The decision to utilize cryopreservation initiates a future obligation to prospective parents to use them for childbearing, or to agree to one of several options for their alternate utilization. These obligations may be burdensome and need to be thoroughly understood prior to utilizing the technique (7).

MICROFERTILIZATION

Infertility due to the male is far more prevalent than is generally appreciated. This becomes even truer as more refined techniques are developed to identify males with impaired sperm. IVF can overcome a segment of this handicapped population; however, below certain limits, IVF is inadequate. For example, in Norfolk, a live birth has not resulted if the sperm population was below 1.5 million (13). However, pregnancy resulting in miscarriage has occurred with counts below 1.5 million,

Table 14.3.   Outcome of Cryo-thaw Transfers[a]

Outcome	Number of Preovulatory Oocytes		
	1–5	6–10	>10
% Cycles with cryopreservation	10%[b]	62%[c]	88%[d]
# Preovs frozen/cryo cycles[e]	1.2[b]	2.7[c]	7.8[d]
Cryo embryos thawed to date/	60%	70%	62%
total cryo embryos	(9/15)	(152/217)	(279/447)
Cryo survival	44%	70%	75%
Embryos surviving/embryos	(4/9)	(106/152)	(208/279)
thawed			
# Preembryos[f] transferred/thaw	0.6	2.1	4.7
Implantation rate	0% (0/9)	8.6% (13/152)	9.3% (26/279)
—sacs/embryo thawed			
—sacs/embryo transferred	0% (0/4)	12.3% (13/106)	12.5% (26/208)
Pregnancy rate/thaw cycle	0% (0/7)	24% (12/49)	41% (18/44)
Ongoing pregnancy rate/thaw cycle	0% (0/7)	16% (8/49)	27% (12/44)

[a]From Toner et al., Human Reproduction 1991; 6:284–289.
[b]< [c]< [d]$P < 0.05$
[e]: Mean number.
[f]Includes preembryos from immature oocytes.
Preovs = preovulatory oocytes; cryo = cryopreserved

Table 14.4. Pregnancy Augmentation by Cryopreservation[a]

Outcome	Number of Preovulatory Oocytes		
	1–5	6–10	>10
Known Performance			
(fresh + cryo[f] to date)			
—pregnancy rate	31.1%[b]	45.7%[c]	61.5%[d]
—ongoing pregnancy rate	22.2%[b]	28.3%[b]	41.5%[c]
Total Expected Performance			
(fresh + cryo to date = projected cryo)			
—pregnancy rate	31.1%[b]	50.0%[c]	85.5%[d]
# pregnancies/[s]stimulation cycles	22.2%	31.4%[c]	58.3%[d]
—ongoing pregnancy rate			
# ongoing pregnancies/[s]stimulation cycles			

[a]From Toner et al., Combined impact of the number of preovulatory oocytes and cryopreservation Human Reproduction 1990; 6:284–289.
[b] < [c] < [d]P < 0.05
[e]Of preembryos yet to be thawed.
[f]Cryo = cryopreserved; stim cycles = original cycle of ovarian stimulation.

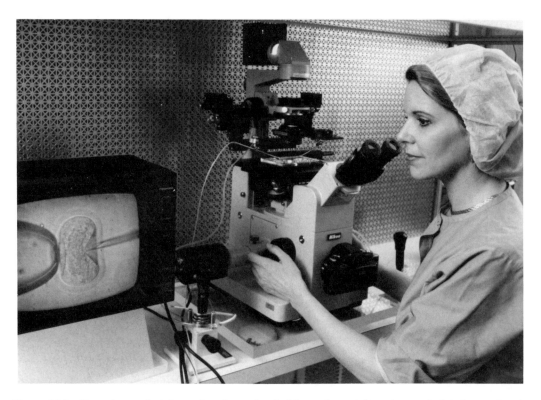

Figure 14.6. The micromanipulative setup, the embryologist carrying out the micromanipulated procedure by viewing the image on the monitor.

raising the possibility that inadequacy in total sperm count is accompanied by individual sperm inadequacy, either at the chromosomal or possibly the gene level in such individuals.

Nevertheless, for patients with a count below 1.5 million, microfertilization is an experi-mental possibility. There are several alternate techniques available, all requiring micromanip-ulative capability (Fig. 14.6). Thus, an individ-ual sperm may be injected into the cytoplasm of the egg (Fig. 14.7). As an alternative, the single sperm may be placed in the perivitelline space

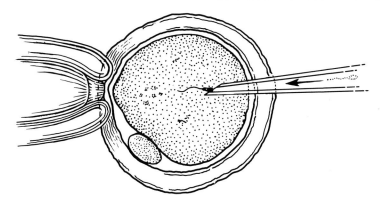

Figure 14.7. Diagram of the cytoplasmic injection of a spermatozoa.

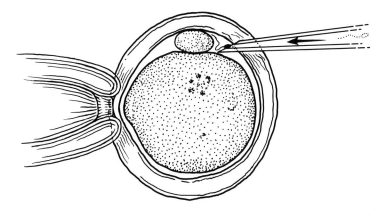

Figure 14.8. Diagram of the perivitilline placement of spermatozoa.

(Fig. 14.8). Another technique that has been utilized has been to partially dissect the zona (PZD) or to drill the zona to provide a passageway through the zona for sperm that are incapable of transiting this barrier normally (Fig. 14.9).

A very limited number of pregnancies have been reported using one or another of these techniques (12). However, the data concerning the severity of the male defect are inadequately described in contemporary terms to be completely sure that fertilization in those cases would not have occurred without the use of micromanipulative procedures.

DONOR GAMETES

Donor sperm have been used for many years as a substitute for gametes from a male who was incapable of producing fertilization. This has been true in programs of artificial insemination

donor (AID), and to a much more limited extent, in IVF when adequate numbers of sperm could not be produced for the use of fertilization in vitro.

It has only been since the development of in-vitro techniques that donor eggs have been available and useful. They can be used for women who have had a premature menopause, who have congenital absence of the ovaries, or surgical absence, or who have known genetic defects of a Mendelian type that they do not wish to transmit to their offspring. Donor eggs can also be used for egg defects that have become apparent through IVF programs where repeated failure to fertilize has probably resulted from abnormal eggs. This latter category of defects is somewhat nebulous, probably genetic in nature, but it is clearly established by repeated IVF failure under optimum conditions.

Donor eggs may become available from

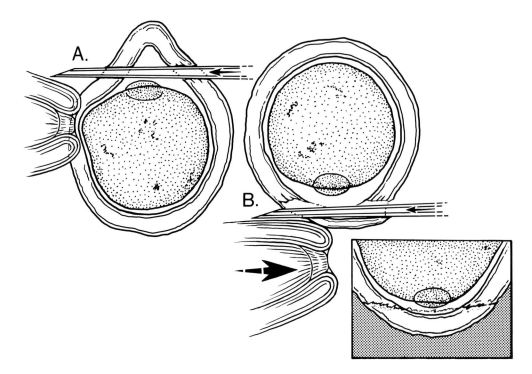

Figure 14.9.   Diagram of the zona pellucida dissection.

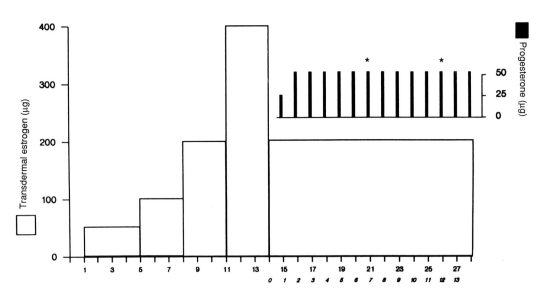

Figure 14.10.   A diagram of the supplementation used in the donor egg program when the patient has essentially no ovarian function. Transdermal estrogen is given from day 1–5 at the rate of 50 μg, from 5–8 at the rate of 100, from 8–11 at the rate of 200, and from 11–14 at the rate of 400. During the luteal phase, the transdermal estrogen is kept constant at 200 μg. Progesterone supplementation is essentially 50 mg per day beginning on day 16, although 25 mg per day are given on day 15. In a mock cycle, endometrial biopsies are obtained on day 21 and again on day 26 to be sure that the supplementary dosages are satisfactory. *Endometrial biopsy.

Table 14.5. Donor Egg Pregnancies (Norfolk Data)

		#	%A	%B
A	Transfers	133		
B	Pregnancies	37	28	
C	Ongoing/Term	32	24	86

patients who have adequate eggs for their own reproductive purposes, especially if, for whatever reason, they choose not to use cryopreservation. On the other hand, eggs may also be available from specific family donors or anonymous donors who receive an operative procedure, such as tubal sterilization in exchange for eggs.

It is possible in patients who do not have functioning ovaries to prepare the endometrium by the use of exogenous estrogen/progesterone so that pregnancies occur and develop, and normal children are delivered (Fig. 14.10). The results of donor egg programs indicate that the expectancy of pregnancy per egg is approximately the same as in a normal IVF situation (Table 14.5).

References

1. Asch RH: Implantation rates with assisted reproduction: intrauterine versus tubal transfers. Abstract 497, VII World Congress on Human Reproduction, June 26–July 1, 1990, Helsinki, Finland.
2. Diaz S, Ortiz ME, Croxatto HB: Studies on the duration of ovum transport by the human oviduct. Am J Obstet Gynecol 1980;137:116–121.
3. Dodson WC, Whitesides DB, Hughes CL Jr, et al: Superovulation with intrauterine insemination in the treatment of infertility: a possible alternative to gamete intrafallopian transfer and in vitro fertilization. Fertil Steril 1987;48:441–445.
4. Flood JT, Muasher SJ, Simonetti S, et al: Comparison between laparoscopically and ultrasonographically guided transvaginal follicular aspiration methods in an in vitro fertilization program in the same patients using the same stimulation protocol. J in Vitro Fertil Embryo Trans 1989;6:180–185.
5. Hovatta O, Kurunmaki H, Tiitinen A, et al: Direct intraperitoneal or intrauterine insemination and superovulation in infertility treatment: a randomized study. Fertil Steril 1990;54:339–341.
6. In vitro fertilization-embryo transfer in the United States. 1988 results from the IVF-ET Registry. Medical Research International and the Society for Assisted Reproductive Technology. Fertil Steril January, 1990; 53:13–20.
7. Jones HW Jr: Cryopreservation and its problems. Fertil Steril 1990;53:780–784.
8. Kruger TT, Acosta AA, Simmons KF, et al: Predictive value of abnormal sperm morphology in in vitro fertilization. Fertil Steril 1988;49:112–117.
9. Martin RH: A comparison of chromosomal abnormalities in hamster egg and human sperm pronuclei. Biol Reprod 1984;31:819–825.
10. Mills JL, Simpson JL, Driscoll SG, et al: Incidence of spontaneous abortion among normal women and insulin-dependent diabetic women whose pregnancies were identified within 21 days of conception. N Engl J Med 1988;319:1617–1623.
11. Muasher SJ, Kruithoff C, Webster S, et al: Natural Cycle In Vitro Fertilization. Submitted for publication, 1990.
12. Ng S-C, Bongso A, Sathananthan H, et al: Micromanipulation: its relevance to human in vitro fertilization. Fertil Steril 1990;53:203–219.
13. Oehninger S, Acosta AA, Morshedi M, et al: Corrective measures and pregnancy outcome in in vitro fertilization in patients with severe sperm morphology abnormalities. Fertil Steril 1988;50:283–287.
14. Plachot M, Mandelbaum J, Junca AM, et al: Cytogenic analysis and developmental capacity of normal and abnormal embryos after IVF. Human Reprod 1989; 4(Suppl):99–103.
15. Scholtes MCW, Roozenburg BJ, Alberda A Th, et al: Transcervical intrafallopian transfer of zygotes. Fertil Steril 1990;54:283–286.
16. Steptoe PC, Edwards RG, Purdy JM: Clinical aspects of pregnancies established with cleaving embryos grown in vitro. Brit J Obstet Gynaecol 1980;87:757–768.
17. Toner JP, Brzyski RG, Oehninger S, et al: Combined impact of the number of preovulatory oocytes in cryopreservation IVF outcome. Human Reprod 1990;5:1004–1008.
18. Toner JP, Philput C, Jones GS, et al: Basal follicle stimulating hormone (FSH) level is a better predictor of in vitro fertilization (IVF) performance than age. Fertil Steril, in press.
19. Veeck L: Extracorporeal maturation. Annals of the New York Academy of Sciences, N.Y. Volume 442, 1985. In Vitro Fertilization and Embryo Transfer, (eds) Seppala N, Edwards RG, pp 357–367.
20. Watson AJS, Gupta JF, O'Donovan P, et al: The results of tubal surgery in the treatment of infertility in two non-specialist hospitals. Brit J Obstet Gynaecol July, 1990;97:561–568.

INDEX

Note that page numbers in *italic* denote figures; and italic "*t*" denote tables.

Abdominal metroplasty
  for septate uterus, *274–276*
  for T-shaped uterus, *275–277*
Abdominal myomectomy, 119–*122*
Abdominal pain, of ectopic pregnancy, 171
Abdominal retractor, 38, *39*
ACTH. (*see* Adrenocorticotropic hormone)
Ad Hoc Committee of International Federation of Fertility
    and Sterility, classification of tubal procedures, 147*t*
Adenyomyosis, 114
Adhesiolysis
  in endometriosis, 229
  hysteroscopic, 133–134*t*
  laser techniques for, 68
  results of, *13–14t*
Adhesions
  clinical significance of, 6–7, 14
  foreign materials and, 190
  formation, suture methods and, 190
  incidence of, 5–6*t*
  infertility and, 7
  intestinal obstruction and, 6–7
  intrauterine (*see* Interuterine synechiae)
    classification of, 135*t*, *136*
    hysteroscopic lysis of, 133–134*t*
  from ovarian surgery, 202
  pelvic pain and, 7
  periovarian, 190
  peritubular, 190
  prevention of formation, 7–*13*
    in abdominal myomectomy, 122
    anti-inflammatory drugs for, 11–12*t*
    barrier solutions for, 10–11
    fibrin deposition and, 7
    limitations in, 11
    mechanical barriers and, 8–9*t*
    peritoneal lavage and, 7–8
    procoagulants and, 8
    by removal of fibrin deposits, 13
  second-look laparoscopy and, 165–166
  tuboovarian, 206
Adhesolysis. (*see* Adhesiolysis)
Adnexal torsion, management of, 195
Adrenal androgenic tumors, female hermaphroditism and,
    349
Adrenal glands, pathologic changes in female hermaphro-
    ditism, of congenital adrenal hyperplasia, 338–*341*
Adrenal hyperplasia
  congenital, female hermaphroditism of, 337–352

lipoid, male hermaphroditism of, 300
  virilizing therapy for, genetic aspects of, 345–346
Adrenocorticotropic hormone (ACTH)
  cortisol biosynthesis and, 341
  in 17α-hydroxylase deficiency, 301
AFS. (*see* American Fertility Society)
Allis-Adair clamps, 121, 122
Ambisexual individuals, nomenclature and classification of,
    292–293
Amenorrhea, danazol-induced, 215–216
American Fertility Society (AFS)
  classification
    of endometriosis, *212*–213
    of intrauterine adhesions, *136*
    of tubal procedures, 148
  report form, standardized, 28
American National Standards Institute (ANSI), 67
AMH. (*see* Antimüllerian hormone)
Androgen insensitivity
  clinical features of, 315, *318–319*
  differential diagnosis of, 247
  endocrine studies for, 319
  general considerations, 315
  genetic considerations for, 318–*319*
  histopathology of, 319–*321*
  incomplete or partial forms of, 321–*323*
  psychosexual orientation in, 320
  treatment of, 321
Androgens
  for endometriosis, 213–214
  exogenous maternal, female hermaphroditism and, 346,
    347
Androstenedione, postoperative levels, in laparoscopic
    techniques for ovulation induction in PCO, 200
Anovulation, from polycystic ovary disease, 198
ANSI (American National Standards Institute), 67
Antimüllerian hormone
  activity failure of, male hermaphroditism of, 306–*313*
  identification of, 289
Antinuclear antibody (ANA), in endometriosis, 209
Antiprogestational agents, for ectopic pregnancy manage-
    ment, 187–188
Appendiceal endometriosis, 221
Argon laser
  clinical applications of, 64
  emissions of, 64
Aspirators, for laparoscopy, 52–*53*
Assisted reproduction
  cryopreservation and, 388–*389*

by gamete intrafallopian tube transfer, 237–238, 387–388

in-vitro fertilization. (*see* In-vitro fertilization)

microfertilization techniques for, 389–391

options for, 379

by transcervical intrafallopian tube transfer, 388

using donor gametes, 391–393

by zygote intrafallopian tube transfer, 388

Atom, basic structure of, 61, *62*

B cells, in endometriosis, 209

Backstop, for lasers, 65–66

Barrier solutions, for prevention of adhesion formation, 10–11

Bayonet microsurgical forceps, 42

Benson-Durfee transabdominal isthmic cerclage, 101–103

Biochemical markers, of ectopic pregnancy, 172–174

Biopsy forceps, 51, *52*

Bohr's law, 60

Bone anomalies, in Rokitansky-Kuster-Hauser syndrome, 249, *252*

Brain dressing forceps, *41*

Breast development, in true hermaphrodites, *330*–331

Buxton stitch, 190

Buxton uterine clamp, 39, *40*

CA-125, in endometriosis, 211

Carbon dioxide, for uterine distention in hysteroscopy, 23, 55–56

Carbon dioxide laser
  for adhesolysis, 68
  emissions of, 62–*63*
  for endometriosis, 227–229
    peritoneal vaporization method, 218, *219*
    surgical outcome of, 235*t*
  impact site of, 63–64
  power densities of, 66
  for uterine nerve ablation, 234

Carboxymethyl cellulose (CMC), 10

Castroviejo forceps, 42

Castroviejo needle holder, for laparotomy, 42, *44*

CD4/CD8, in endometriosis, 209

Cefazolin, in irrigation solutions, adhesion formation and, 8

Cerclage
  indications for, 103*t*
  during pregnancy, 97
    Benson-Durfee transabdominal isthmic procedure, 101–103
    for incompetent cervical os, 97–*103*
    McDonald technique for, 97–*99*
    results of, 100–101
    Shirodkar-Barter procedure for, 99–*102*
    Wurm procedure for, 101, *103*

Cervical dilation, hysteroscopy and, 24

Cervical stenosis, 107, *109–110*

Cervix
  congenital absence of, 283–*285*
  conization of, 107
  incompetence. (*see* Incompetent cervical os)

Chemotherapy, for ectopic pregnancy, 185, 187

Chi-square test, 86–87*t*

Chondroitin sulfate, 10

Clinical trial, randomized, 79–80

Coherent light, 61

Computer software, for multivariate analysis, 90

Confounding variables, 88*t*

Congenital anomalies
  of fallopian tube, 157–158
  uterovaginal. (*see* Uterovaginal anomalies)

Continuous variables, 81

Cornual polyps, 159

Cornual resection, for ectopic pregnancy, 185

Corticosteroids, postoperative adhesion formation and, 11

Cortisol biosynthesis
  adrenocorticotropic hormone and, 341
  in female hermaphroditism of congenital adrenal hyperplasia, 339–*341*

CPR (cumulative pregnancy rate), *83*–85

Crile-Wood needle holder, for laparotomy, 42, *44*

Cryo-thaw transfers, outcome of, 389*t*

Cryopreservation, 388–*389*, 389*t*, 390*t*

Culdocentesis, for diagnosis of ectopic pregnancy, 172

Cullen uterine elevator, 39, *40*

Cumulative pregnancy rate (CPR), *83*–85

Cystectomy, laparoscopic, 195–*199*

Danazol
  adverse effects of, 215
  to decrease endometrial lining, 127
  for endometriosis, 206, 215–216
  with surgery, for endometriosis, 235

D&C, postoperative intrauterine synechiae and, 129–130

Deafness, in Rokitansky-Kuster-Hauser syndrome, 248, *250*

17–20Demolase deficiency, 302–303

Dependent variables, 80–81

Dermoids, 194–195

Dextran
  prevention of adhesion formation and, 10–11
  side effects of, 10–11

Dichotomous variables, 81

Diethylstilbestrol exposure (DES exposure)
  in-vitro fertilization for, 379
  T-shaped uterus and, 265, *271–272*
  uterine anomalies of, 271, *272*

Dihydrotestosterone, in steroid 5α-reductase deficiency, 323

Directors, for laparotomy, 43–44, *45*

Donor gametes, 391–*393*

Doppler flow studies, of ovarian artery, for diagnosis of ectopic pregnancy, 174

Dysgenetic male pseudohermaphroditism, 314–315

Dysmenorrhea, in endometriosis, uterine nerve ablation and, 234

Ectopic pregnancy
  diagnosis of, 170–171
    by biochemical markers, 173–174
    by culdocentesis, 172
    by hCG levels, 172–*173*
    by progesterone levels, 173

Ectopic pregnancy
  diagnosis of—*continued*
    by ultrasound, 174–*175*
  expectant management of, 188
  future reproductive success and, 170, *171*
  laparoscopic treatment of, 69–*70*
  location of, *170*
  medical management of
    by antiprogestational agents, 187–188
    by chemotherapy, 185, 187
    by prostaglandins, 187
  pathology of, 174–175, *176*
  signs and symptoms of, 171*t*
  surgical management of, 188
    by cornual resection, 185
    by laparoscopic salpingectomy, 181, 185, *186*
    by linear salpingostomy, 175–*181*
    by salpingectomy, 181, *184*–185
    by second-look laparoscopy, 185
    by segmental resection, 180–*183*
    by tubal abortion, 185
Electrocautery
  instrumentation, for laparotomy, 44–*46*
  in salpingectomy, 185
  in segmental resection, 180–*183*
ELISA (enzyme-linked immunosorbent assay), 172
Embryology of ovary
  deviations from normal, 192–*194*
  normal, 192
Embryonic testicular syndrome. (*see* Familial gonadal
    destruction)
Endocoagulation, of endometriosis, 228–*229*
Endocrine profile, for in-vitro fertilization, 380
Endoloop, 558–*559*
Endometriosis
  adhesiolysis for, 229
  androgens for, 213–214
  appendiceal, 221
  assisted reproductive technologies for, 237–238
  classification of, 211–*213*, 214*t*
  conservative surgery for, 217
    surgical outcome of, 235–236*t*
  diagnosis of, 210–211*t*
  expectant therapy for, 213
  fertilization and, 207–208
  gonadotropin-releasing hormone agonist for, 216–217
  histogenesis of, 205–206
  hormonal-surgical combined therapy for, 234–235
  intestinal, 221
  laparoscopic therapy for, 227–*230*
  laser technique for, 70, *72*–73
  natural history of, 206
  ovarian
    resective surgery for, 229, 231–*233*
    surgical management of, 218, *220*–222
  pathophysiology of, 206–209*t*
  peritoneal, 218, *219*, 228–*231*
  preimplantation development and, 207–208
  presacral neurectomy for, 223, *226*–227
  prevalence of, 206
  progestogens for, 214–215

  pseudocapsule formation by endometriomas, 72–73
  surgical outcome for, 235–236*t*
  surgical reconstruction procedures for, general consider-
    ations of, 217–218
  surgical therapy for, 238
  symptoms of, 209–210
  of urinary tract, 221
  uterine nerve ablation for, 234
  uterine suspension techniques for, 221–223, *224*–225
Endometrium
  anatomy of, 113
  appearance of, in proliferative phase, 24
Endosalpingitis, 146
Endoscopes
  description of, 47–*48*
  magnification for, 37–38*t*
Endoscopy
  for ablation of endometriosis, 228
  instrumentation for, 46–*48*
  preparation of operative field, 36
Enzyme-linked immunosorbent assay (ELISA), 172
Epididymis, development in true hermaphrodites, 335–
    336
α Error, 79
β Error, 79
Estradiol, in endometriosis, 207
Estrogen receptors, in uterine myomas, 115
Estrogen therapy
  for cervical mucus improvement, 107
  for endometrial proliferation, 133
Excision
  of ovarian endometriosis, 218, *220*
  of peritoneal endometriosis, 218, *219*
Expectant therapy, for endometriosis, 213
Explanatory variables, 80
External genitalia
  development, in true hermaphrodites, *336*–337
  female
    construction of in female hermaphroditism, 352–
      375
    masculinization of, 349–*350*
  morphology of, 291
  reconstruction of, in 17α-hydroxylase deficiency, *302*

Fallopian tube forceps, *41*
Fallopian tubes
  ampullary mucosa of, 26
  congenital anomalies of, 157–158
  development, in true hermaphrodites, 334*t*, *335*
  diagnostic examination of, 24, *26*–29, 147
  infertility and, 146–148*t*
  proximal obstruction, on hysterosalpingography, 19
  reconstructive surgeries of
    classification of, 147*t*
    neosalpingostomy, 151–*157*
    salpingolysis, 148–*150*
    salpingoplasty, *150*–151
  second-look laparoscopy, 165–166
  segmental resection of, for ectopic pregnancy, 180–*183*
  transcervical catheterization of, 162
  tubal anastomosis, 158–*165*. (*see* Tubal anastomosis)

Familial gonadal destruction, male hermaphroditism of, 310–311, *315–316*

Fecundability. (*see* Pregnancy rate)

Female, use of term, 293

Female hermaphroditism

  construction of female genitalia

    basic operation for patients with vagina, 353–*359*

    general considerations, 352–353

    in hypospadias patient with micropenis, surgical technique for, *370–375*

    operation for deep vagino-sinus communication, 359, 362, *364–366*

    operation for minor defects, 356, *360*

    operation when vagina is imperforate, 359, *361–362*

    operation when vaginal orifice is difficult to locate, 356, 359, *361*

    operation with posterior flap, 359, *363*

    operations for patients without vagina, 367–375

    results of operations, 362–363, 367t

    secondary operations for, 363, 367–369

  due to congenital adrenal hyperplasia

    attenuated form of 21-hydroxylase deficiency, 345

    endocrinological abnormalities in, 339–341

    genetic aspects of virilizing adrenal hyperplasia therapy, 345–346

    historical introduction of, 337–339

    11β-hydroxylase deficiency, 345

    21-hydroxylase deficiency and, 341–*345*

    pathologic changes of adrenal glands and, 338–*341*

  external genitalia construction in, 352–375

  not due to congenital adrenal hyperplasia, 346–352

    adrenal androgenic tumors and, 349

    classification of, 346

    diagnosis and treatment of, 352

    exogenous maternal androgen and, 346–*347*

    idiopathic, 350, 352

    luteoma of pregnancy and, 348–349t

    ovarian androgenic tumor of mother and, 346–348t

    special or nonspecific cases of, 349–350

Fertilization, endometriosis and, 207–208

Fibrin deposits

  prevention of, 7

  removal of, postoperative adhesion formation and, 13

Fibrinolysis, in peritoneum, 4–5

Fibroids, uterine, infertility and, 115

Fimbrica ovarica, elongated, 158

Fimbrioplasty

  for distal tubal obstruction, 148

  laser techniques for, 67–68

Flapper valve, of trocar, 49–50

Flare-up technique, 381–382

Follicle stimulating hormone

  postoperative levels, in laparoscopic techniques for ovulation induction in PCO, 200

  in steroid 5α-reductase deficiency, 323

Folliculogenesis, in endometriosis, 207

Forceps

  atraumatic grasping types, *50*

  biopsy types, 51, *52*

  for laparoscopy, *50–52*

  for laparotomy, 39, *41–42*

  traumatic grasping types, *51*

Frank technique, for Rokitansky-Kuster-Hauser syndrome, *252–258*

Gamete intrafallopian tube transfer (GIFT), 238, 387–388

Gender role, 292

Genital tract, of female rabbit fetus, maculinization of, 289, *290*

Gestrinone, for leiomyomata uteri reduction, 117

GIFT (gamete intrafallopian tube transfer), 387–388

Gilbert-Dreyfus syndrome, 322

Gilliam procedure, modified, 221–223, *224–225*

Glycine, for uterine distention in hysteroscopy, 24

GnRH agonists. (*see* Gonadotropin-releasing hormone agonists)

Gonadal sex, 291

Gonadectomy

  for 17α-hydroxylase deficiency, *302*

  sexual development effects of, *287–288*

Gonadotropin-releasing hormone agonists

  for endometriosis, 206, 216–217

  leiomyoma and, 115

  for leiomyomata uteri reduction, 117, 119

  side effects of, 217

  with surgery, for endometriosis, 234–235

  use of, prior to myomectomy, 119

Gore-Tex surgical membrane, 8

Hazard rate, *83*

β-hCG. (*see* Human chorionic gonadotropin)

hCS (human chorionic somatomammotrophin), in ectopic pregnancy, 188

Healing, of smooth muscle, in nonpregnant uterus, 113–114

Helium-neon laser, 64

Hemostatic instruments, for laparoscopy, 51, 53, *54–55*

Heparin, in irrigation solutions, adhesion formation and, 8

Hermaphroditism

  definition of, 292

  female. (*see* Female hermaphroditism)

  male. (*see* Male hermaphroditism)

  nomenclature and classification of, 292–293

  sex of rearing for, 330

Hermaphroditismus verus. (*see* True hermaphrodites)

Hernia uteri inguinalis, *306–313*

hMG/IUI, for endometriosis-associated infertility, 238

Hormonal sex, 291

Hormonal-surgical combined therapy, for endometriosis, 234–235

HSG. (*see* Hysterosalpingography)

Human chorionic gonadotropin (hCG)

  for diagnosis of ectopic pregnancy, 172–173

  disappearance of, after linear salpingostomy vs. salpingectomy, 175–176, *177*

  discriminatory zone for ectopic pregnancy diagnosis and, 174

  patterns of production, in ectopic pregnancy, 172–*173*

Human chorionic somatomammotrophin (hCS), in ectopic pregnancy, 188

HUMI/HUI device, 39

Hydromucolpos, *278–279*
11β-Hydroxylase deficiency
    in female hermaphroditism of congenital adrenal hyper-
        plasia, 339–340
    virilizing adrenal hyperplasia therapy, genetic aspects of,
        345–346
17α-Hydroxylase deficiency, 300–*302*
21-Hydroxylase deficiency
    attenuated form of, 345
    clinical aspects of, 341–*345*
    in female hermaphroditism of congenital adrenal hyper-
        plasia, 339
    virilizing adrenal hyperplasia therapy for, genetic aspects
        of, 345–346
17-Hydroxyprogesterone
    in female hermaphroditism diagnosis, 352
    in female hermaphroditism of congenital adrenal hyper-
        plasia, 339–340
3β-Hydroxysteroid dehydrogenase deficiency, 300
17β-Hydroxysteroid dehydrogenase deficiency, 303–*305*
Hyperreactio lulteinalis, 348*t*
Hypospadias
    with micropenis, surgical technique for, 370–*375*
    operations for, 367–*370*
Hypothesis testing, 77, 78–79*t*
Hyskon (Pharmacia), 11, 23, 127
Hyskon reaction, 23
Hysterosalpingography
    of cervical stenosis, 107
    contraindications for, 20
    diagnostic accuracy of, 19–20*t*
    evaluation of fallopian tube, 147
    for evaluation of uterine cavity, 19–20*t*
    of leiomyomata uteri, *116*
    technical errors in, 21–22*t*
    techniques for, 20–22
    of uterine disorders, 114
    vs. laparoscopy, 19
Hysteroscope, panoramic operating, development of, 127
Hysteroscopy
    complications of, 22*t*
    for grading of intrauterine adhesions, 134–135*t*
    indications for, 19–20
    instrumentation for, 55–58
    laser techniques for, 73–*74*
    for lysis of intrauterine adhesions/synechiae, 132–*133*
    of myomas, 116
    report form, standardized, 24, *25*
    for resection of submucous myomas, 127–*128*
        contraindications for, 127
        results of, 128, 129*t*
        surgical technique for, 127–*128*
    technique for, 22–*24*
    for uterine cavity examination, 19–20
    of uterine disorders, 114

Ibuprofen, postoperative adhesion formation and, 12*t*
Idiopathic female hermaphroditism, 350, 352
Immune response, in endometriosis, 209
Immunofluorometric assay (IFMA), for hCG, 172
Imperforate hymen, differential diagnosis of, *247–248*

In-vitro fertilization
    culture techniques, 382–383
    for endometriosis-associated infertility, 237
    fertilization and conception rates, with endometriosis,
        207–208
    harvest cycle for, 381
    indications for, 379–380
    inefficiency of human reproduction and, 384–385
    modified natural cycle and, 381
    monitoring of, 382
    natural cycle and, 381
    oocyte aspiration for, 382–*383*
    patient selection for, 380–381
    preembryo transfer, 383–*386*
    required investigations for, 380
    results of, 386–387*t*
    stimulated cycle and, 381–382
Incision, for abdominal myomectomy, *120*, *121–122*
Incompetent cervical os
    diagnosis of, 95–96*t*, 110
    etiology of, 94–95
    incidence of, 94
    surgical techniques for, 103–*109*
    therapy for, 110
        cerclage during pregnancy, 97–*103*
        conservative method of, 96–97
        historical aspects of, 94
Independent variables, 80–81
Infertility
    data, special features of, 80–81
    follow-up therapy, nonuniform, impact of, 81
    investigations, measurements of outcome, 80
    peritoneal adhesions and, 7
    tubal factors in, 146–148*t*
Instrumentation. (*see also specific instruments*)
    for laparoscopy, 48–*55*
    for lasers, 64–*66*
Insufflators
    for hysteroscopy, 55–56
    for laparoscopy, *49*
Interceed, 9*t*
Interleukin-1, in endometriosis, 208
Internal genitalia, morphology of, 291
Intersexuality. (*see Hermaphroditism*)
Intestinal obstruction, by intraperitoneal adhesions, 6–7
Intrauterine synechiae
    adjunctive therapy for, 133*t*
        results of, 133–135*t*
    classification of, by hysterogram, *32*
    definition of, 128–129
    diagnosis of, 131–*132*
    etiology of, 129–130
    historical aspects of, 128
    incidence of, 129
    pathophysiology of, 130
    symptoms of, 130–131*t*
    therapy for, 132, 133*t*
IRP, 172
Irrigating solutions, for peritoneal lavage, prevention of
        adhesion formation and, 7–8
Irrigators, for laparoscopy, 52–*53*

IS, 172
IVF-ET, 166

Jury trials, vs. surgical trials, 77–78t

Kallman syndrome, 299
Karyotype
    examination, by banding technique, 290–291
    of true hermaphrodites, 331, 333t
Kelly clamp, 122
17-Ketosteroids, in female hermaphroditism diagnosis,
    352
Kirschner abdominal retractor, 38, 39
Kleppinger bipolar electrocautery forceps, 180, 185
Knot tying, microsurgical procedure for
    in laparoscopy, 34–35
    in laparotomy, 32–33
KTP/532 laser, 64

Laparoscopes
    magnification powers of, 210–211t
    types of, 48–49
Laparoscopy
    for adhesolysis, laser applications in, 68
    contraindications for, 27
    for cystectomy, 195–199
    for dermoid cyst removal, 195
    for diagnosis of ovarian or pelvic mass, 195
    for electrical thermal coagulation, in endometriosis, 236t
    for endometriosis therapy, 227–228, 230–231
    evaluation of fallopian tube, 147
    indications for, 27
    instrumentation for, 48–55
    for linear salpingostomy, patient positioning for, 176–
        177
    microsurgical technique for, 32–35
    peritoneal adhesions and, 5–6t
    for peritoneal endometriosis, 228–231
    report form, standardized, 28, 29
    for resection of leiomyomata uteri, 124
    resection, surgical technique for, 124–126
    for salpingectomy, 181, 185, 186
    second-look, 165–166
        postoperative pregnancy rates for, 13–14t
    suture materials for, 58–59
    technique of, 27–28
    vs. hysterosalpingography, 19
Laparotomy
    for endometriosis, 217
    instrumentation, scissors, 42, 43
    instrumentation for, 38–46
    microsurgical technique for, 32–33
    for resection of ovarian cyst, 196–197
    of Rokitansky-Kuster-Hauser syndrome, 248
    vs. laparoscopy, 6
Lasers
    instrumentation for, 64–66
    in laparoscopic technique for ovulation induction in
        PCO, 202
    physics of, 61–62
    power density of, 66

quartz fibers for, 65
    safety considerations for, 66–67
    surgical applications of, 68–74. (see also specific surgeries)
    surgically useful types of, 61–64. (see also specific types of
        lasers)
    for tuboplasty, 147
    for vaporization of peritoneal endometriosis, 228, 231
Leiomyomata uteri
    clinical management of, 114
    diagnosis of, 116–117t
    etiology of, 115
    incidence of, 114–115
    laparoscopic resection of, 124
    medical management of, 117–118
    pathophysiology of, 117, 118t
    recurrence, after myomectomy, 123–124t
    surgical management of
        by abdominal myomectomy, 119–122
        development of cleavage plane, 120, 122
        by hysteroscopic resection, 127–128
        by laparoscopic resection, 124–126
        prevention of adhesions, 120
        repairing myometrial defect, 121, 122
        results from, 122–124t
        by transcervical myomectomy, 125
        by vaginal myomectomy, 125
    symptoms of, 115–116
Leydig cell agenesis, male hermaphroditism of, 311, 314,
    317
Life-table analysis, 80, 81–82, 85
Life-table method, 81–82
Lighting
    for endoscopy, 46
    for microsurgery, 36
Linear salpingostomy, for ectopic pregnancy, 175–181
Lipoid adrenal hyperplasia, 300
Logistic model, 90
Logistic regression, 88–90
Logistic regression coefficients, 89–90
Logit model, 90
Loop ligature, 58–59
Loupes, 36, 37
Lubs syndrome, 322
Luteinized unruptured follicle syndrome (LUF), 207
Luteinizing hormone
    postoperative levels, in laparoscopic techniques for ovu-
        lation induction in PCO, 200
    in steroid 5α-reductase deficiency, 323
Luteinizing hormone (LH), homology with hCG, 172
Luteoma of pregnancy, female hermaphroditism and,
    348–349t

Magnetic resonance imaging, of uterine myomata, 116,
    118
Magnification system, for microsurgical technique, 36–38
Male, use of term, 293
Male hermaphroditism
    of central nervous system defect
        from abnormal pituitary gonadotropic secretion, 296–
            299
        with no gonadotropic secretion, 299

Male hermaphroditism—*continued*
  classification, etiologic and pathogenic, 296
  from 17–20demolase deficiency, 302–303
  descriptive classification for, 295–296
  due to defect in Müllerian duct regression, 306–313
  due to peripheral end-organ defect, 315, 318–337
  due to primary gonadal defect, *299–315*
  due to unidentified defect in androgen effect, 305–306
  due to Y chromosome defect, *324–329*
  etiologic and pathogenic classification for, 296
  of familial gonadal destruction, 310–311, *315–316*
  general considerations of, 293–295
  from 17β-hydroxysteroid dehydrogenase deficiency,
    303–*305*
  in Leydig cell agenesis, 311, 314, *317*
  true, criteria for diagnosis, 326, 328
Mattress sutures, 190
McDonald cerclage technique, 97–*99*
McIndoe procedure, for Rokitansky-Kuster-Hauser syn-
    drome, 253–*258*
Mechanical barriers, for prevention of adhesion formation,
    8–9t
Medrogestone, for leiomyomata uteri reduction, 117
Menorrhagia, reduction or resolution, after abdominal
    myomectomy, 123t
Menstrual flow, endometriosis and, 205
Menstruation, in hermaphroditismus verus, 329–330
Methotrexate, for ectopic pregnancy management, 185,
    187
Methyltestosterone, for endometriosis, 213–214
Metroplasty, wedge, for double uterus, surgical results of,
    277–278t
Metzenbaum scissors, 42, *43*
Microfertilization, 389–*391*
Microinfertility bipolar forceps, 44, *45*
Microinfertility forceps, *41*
Microscope, operating, advantages of, 36–*37*
Microsurgery
  data adjustment for confounding variables, 88t
  definition of, 31
  historical aspects of, 31
  instrumentation for, 38–*59*
  for laparoscopy, 32–*35*
  for laparotomy, 32–*33*
  magnification system for, 36–*38*
  needles for, 57–58
  operating room staff for, training of, 35–36
  operative field for, preparation of, 36
  pregnancy success and, 166
  principles of, 31
  surgeon for, training of, 35
  for tubal anastomosis, pregnancy success after, 162–165t
MIF (Müllerian-inhibiting factor), 289
Miscarriage, due to double uterus, 266
Morcellator, 53–*54*
Mosquito hemostatic forceps, *41*
Müllerian anomalies, classification of, 246
Müllerian ducts
  aplasia or dysplasia of. (*see* Rokitansky-Kuster-Hauser
    syndrome)
  embryonic development of, 252–253

lateral fusion problems of, 258–*269*
  paraovarian cysts and, 194
  regression defect in, male hermaphroditism of, 306–*313*
Müllerian-inhibiting factor (MIF), 289
Müllerian tract anomalies, endometriosis and, 205
Multiple linear regression, 89
Multiple logistic regression, 89
Multivariate analysis, 88–*90*
Myomas
  malignancy in, 115
  recurrence of, after myomectomy, 123–124t
  submucous, hysteroscopic resection of, 127–128
Myomectomy
  abdominal
    incision for, *120*, 121–122
    open abdomen, 119–*121*
  laparoscopic, 124–*126*
  for leiomyomata uteri, 114
  surgical principles of, 123t
  transcervical, 125
  vaginal, 125
Myometrium, 113

Nd:YAG laser. (*see* Neodymium:YAG laser)
Needle holders, for laparotomy, 42, *44*
Needles, for microsurgical techniques, 57–58
Neodymium:YAG laser
  emissions of, 64
  impact site of, 64
Neosalpingostomy
  for distal tubal obstruction, 148
  laparoscopy for, 152–154
  operative technique for, 151–*154*
  results of, 154–157t
Nonsteroidal anti-inflammatory drugs (NSAIDs), postop-
    erative adhesion formation and, 11–12t
Null hypothesis, 78

Occupational Safety and Health Administration (OSHA),
    67
Odds ratio, 90
Omentum, adhesion formation and, 5–6
Oocyte aspiration, for in-vitro fertilization, 382–*383*
Oophorectomy, paradoxical, value of, 191
Operating room staff, for microsurgery, training of, 35–36
Operative sheaths, for hysteroscopy, *56–57*
Oral contraceptive pills, fibroid risk and, 115
Outcome. (*see also* Pregnancy rate)
  of infertility investigation, measurements of, 80
Ovarian androgenic tumor, maternal, female hermaphro-
    ditism and, 346–348t
Ovarian artery
  anatomy of, 191–192
  Doppler flow studies of, for diagnosis of ectopic preg-
    nancy, 174
Ovarian cysts
  benign, resection of, 194–196
  laser techniques for, 70–*71*
  resection of, by laparotomy, 196–*197*
Ovarian endometriosis, surgical management of, 218,
    220

Ovarian reconstructive surgery
    anatomic relationships and, 191–*194*
    for endometriosis, 229, 231–*233*
    indications for, 190
    laser techniques for, 70–*72*
    techniques for, 196–*198*
Ovarian tumors, benign, resection of, 194–196
Ovarian wedge resection, by laparotomy, 200, *201*
Ovary(ies)
    anatomy of, 191–*194*
    malposition of, 193
    prepubertal, 191
    stimulation with exogenous gonadotropins and intra-
        uterine insemination, 238
    supernumerary, *193*
Ovary forceps, *41*
Oviduct, physiologic functions of, 146
Ovulation
    in endometriosis, 207
    induction surgery
        laparoscopic surgery for, 200–202
        for polycystic ovarian disease, 198, 200–202
Oxidized regenerated cellulose (ORC), 8–9

Paraovarian cyst, 194–195
Paraovarian tumor, 195
Pelvic cavity, diagnostic examination of, 24, *26–29*
Pelvic pain, peritoneal adhesions and, 7
Perimetrium, 113
Peritoneal adhesions. (*see* Adhesions)
Peritoneal endometriosis, 228–231
Peritoneal fluid
    composition of, 2–3
    in endometriosis, 208–209
Peritoneal lavage, prevention of adhesion formation and,
    7–8
Peritoneum
    adhesions. (*see* Adhesions)
    fibrinolytic activity of, *4–5*
    fluid absorption and, 2–3
    repair of, *3–4*
    surface of, 2
Pharmacia (hyskon), 11, 23, 127
Phocomelia, Rokitansky-Kuster-Hauser syndrome and,
    252
Pitressin (vasopressin), 119, 121, 124–125
Plasminogen activator activity (PAA), *4–5*
Pneumoperitoneal needle, for laparoscopy, 49
Polycystic ovary disease
    histologic findings in, 198
    laser technique for, 70, *72*
    ovulation induction, laparoscopic surgery for, 200–
        202
    ovulation induction surgery for, 198, 200
Polyps, uterine, hysteroscopic laser procedure for, 73
Population parameter, 78
Postabortion infection, uterine synechiae and, 129
Postpelvic inflammatory disease (PID)
    endogenous, 146
    exogenous, 146

Power density, of lasers, 66
Pregnancy
    ectopic. (*see* Ectopic pregnancy)
    effect on endometriosis and, 206
    in obstructed rudimentary horn, 260, *262*
    prognosis for, following surgery for distal tubal obstruc-
        tion, 69
    repeated loss, preconception evaluation of, 117*t*
    uterine myoma and, 115
Pregnancy rates
    adjusting for incomplete and variable follow-up, 81
    after adjunctive therapy for intrauterine synechiae, 133–
        135*t*
    after linear salpingostomy, 176
    after myomectomy, 122–123
    after neosalpingostomy, 154–157*t*
    after radical vs. conservative surgery for ectopic preg-
        nancy, 187*t*
    after second-look laparoscopy, 166
    constant hazard rate calculation, *83*
    from cryo-thaw transfers, 389*t*
    cumulative, *83–85*
    from donor gametes, 393*t*
    following tubal anastomosis, 162–165*t*
    following conservative surgery for endometriosis, *237*
    following danazol therapy and, 216
    following surgical adhesion lysis, *13–14t*
    from in-vitro fertilization, 386–387*t*
    in infertility research, 81
    by life-table analysis, 81–82
    by life-table method, 81–82
    statistical analysis
        when follow-up is not uniform, 81–*86*
        when follow-up is uniform, 86–90*t*
Pregnenolone synthesis defect, 300
Preimplantation development, endometriosis and, 207–
    208
Presacral neurectomy, for endometriosis, 223, *226–227*
Probability distribution, 78
Probability value (p value), 78
Probes
    for laparoscopy, 50
    for laparotomy, 43–44, *45*
Procoagulants, for prevention of adhesion formation, 8
Progesterone
    in ectopic pregnancy, 173
    in endometriosis, 207
    with gonadotropin-releasing hormone agonist, for endo-
        metriosis, 217
    for uterine myoma reduction, 117
Progestin, 127
Progestogens
    for endometriosis, 214–215
    for leiomyomata uteri reduction, 117
Prostaglandins
    for ectopic pregnancy management, 187
    in endometriosis, 208–209
Prostate, development, in true hermaphrodites, 337
Proteolytic enzymes, 13
Proximal tubal obstruction, tubal-cornual anastomosis for,
    206–207

Pseudohermaphroditism
 definition of, 292–293
 male dysgenetic, 314–315

Quantum, 60
Quartz fibers, for lasers, 65

Radioimmune assay (RIA), 172
Radioreceptor assay (RRA), 172
Random variable, 78
Randomization, 79–80
Reamers, for laparotomy, 43–44, *45*
Rearing, sex of, 291–292
Reifenstein syndrome, 322
Reperitonealization, 6
Reproduction, human, inefficiency of, 384–385
Resectoscope, for hysteroscopy, 56–57
Retroperitoneal endometriosis, 228–229
Reversal of sterilization
 results of, 162–165*t*
 by tubal anastomosis, 158–*163*
Rokitansky-Kuster-Hauser syndrome
 bone anomalies of, 249, *252*
 diagnosis of, 246–*248*
 etiology of, 252–*253*
 internal anomalies in, 248–*250*
 surgical correction of, 252–258
 transverse vaginal septum anomalies of, *280*
Rosewater syndrome, 322
RU-486, for ectopic pregnancy management, 187–188
Rubin's cannula, *21, 27, 28*
Rudimentary horn
 noncommunicating, 260, *262*
 obstructed, pregnancy in, 260, *262*
Rugal folds, presence of, on hysterosalpingography, 147

Saline, for uterine distention in hysteroscopy, 23–24
Salpingectomy
 for ectopic pregnancy, 181, *184*–185
 laparoscopic, for ectopic pregnancy, 181, 185, *186*
 postoperative pregnancy success rates for, 185, 187*t*
Salpingitis isthmic nodosa, 159
Salpingolysis, technique for, 148–*150*
Salpingoovariolysis, probability of conception and, *13*
Salpingoplasty, *150–151*. (*see also* Neosalpingostomy)
Salpingoscopy
 for diagnostic evaluation of fallopian tubes, 24, *26–27*
 evaluation of fallopian tube, 147
 technique for, *26–27*
Salpingostomy, laser techniques for, 67–68
Sample statistic, 78
Scalpels, laparoscopic, 51–*53*
Scissors
 for laparoscopy, 51–*53*
 for laparotomy, 42, *43*
Second-look laparoscopy
 after oviduct reconstruction, 165–166
 for ectopic pregnancy, 185
Segmental resection, for ectopic pregnancy, 180–*183*
Semen examination, for in-vitro fertilization, 380

Septate uterus
 correction of
  Tompkin's technique for, *273–274*
  by wedge excision, *274–277*
 metroplasty for, 73, *74*
 surgical results for, 277–278*t*
Sex
 criteria of, 289–290
 gender role and, 292
 of gonads, 291
 hermaphroditic state and, 292
 hormonal, 291
 karyotypic evaluation of, 290–291
 morphology
  of external genitalia, 291
  of internal genitalia, 291
  of rearing, 291–292, 330
Sex chromosomes, 290–291
Sex-determining genes, 290–291
Sexual development, experimental studies of, *287–290*
Sexually transmitted diseases, postpelvic inflammatory disease and, 146
Sheaths, for hysteroscopy, 56–*57*
Shirodkar-Barter cerclage procedure, 99–*102*
Shirodkar clamp, 39, *40*
Siegler Hellman clamp, 39, *40*
Silicone-plastic cuff, for incompetent cervical os, 97
Smith-Hodge pessary, 97
Software, for multivariate analysis, 90
Sonography, of uterine synechiae, 131
Sounding of uterine cavity, in diagnosis of intrauterine synechiae, 131
Sperm, donor, 391–*393*
Split-thickness graft, for Rokitansky-Kuster-Hauser syndrome, *254–255*
Spontaneous abortion, with leiomyomata, 118*t*
Spontaneous emission, 60, *61*
Spot size of laser, power density and, 66
Statistical analysis
 when follow-up is not uniform, 81–*86*
 when follow-up is uniform, 86–*91*
Statistical testing
 bias and, 91
 of hypothesis, 78–79
 sample size determination and, 79
 surgical trials vs. jury trials, 77–78*t*
Steroid 5α-reductase deficiency, 322–323, 325
Steroid hormones, endometriosis maintenance and, 205–206
Stevens scissors, 42, *43*
Stimulated emission of radiation, theory of, 60
Strassman procedure, 271, 273
Stress urinary incontinence, leiomyoma and, 115–116
Student's t test, 87–88
Suction/irrigation equipment, for laparotomy, 38–39
Surgeon, training of, for microsurgical technique, 35
Surgical trials, vs. jury trials, 77–78*t*
Surgicel, 9
Suture materials, for microsurgical techniques, 58–*59*
Suture methods, adhesion formation and, 190

T cells, in endometriosis, 209
T-clamps, 121, 122
T-shaped uterus
  abdominal metroplasty for, 275–277
  diethylstilbestrol exposure and, 265, 271–272
Telescopes, for endoscopy, 47–48
Teratoma, cystic
  benign, 194–195
  malignant, 194–195
Testicular feminization. (*see* Androgen insensitivity)
Testicular grafting, in female rabbit fetus, 288–289
Testicular regression syndrome. (*see* Familial gonadal destruction)
Testosterone
  biosynthesis of, *299*
    identifiable defects in, 299–305
  postoperative levels, in laparoscopic techniques for ovulation induction in PCO, 200
Tetracycline, in irrigation solutions, adhesion formation and, 8
Thalidomide, Rokitansky-Kuster-Hauser syndrome and, 252
Thermocoagulation, 54–55
  of endometriosis, 228–229
TIFT (transcervical intrafallopian tube transfer), 388
Tissue plasminogen activator, 13
Tompkin's technique, for septate uterus correction, 273–274
Touhy needle, 49
Traction test of Bergman and Svenerund, 95
Transcervical fallopian tube catheterization, 162
Transcervical intrafallopian tube transfer (TIFT), 388
Transcervical myomectomy, 125
Trocar, 49–50
True hermaphrodites
  breast development in, *330*–331
  classification of, 328
  cytogenic findings in, 331, 333*t*
  epididymis development in, 335–336
  external genitalia development in, *336–337*
  fallopian tube development in, 334*t*, *335*
  general clinical features, 328–329
  gonadal location in, 331–333*t*
  gonadal pathology in, *332*–333
  menstruation and, 329–330
  molecular genetics of, 331
  prostate development in, 337
  treatment principles for, 337
  uterus development in, 333–334
  vasa deferentia development, 334*t*, *335*
Trumpet valve, of trocar, 49
Tubal abortion, for ectopic pregnancy, 185
Tubal anastomosis
  laser techniques for, 70–*71*
  macrosurgical vs. microsurgical technique, 158–159
  results of, 162–165*t*
  technique of
    for ampullary-ampullary anastomosis, 160, *162*
    for interstitial/ampullary anastomosis, 160–161, *163*
    for isthmic-ampullary anastomosis, 159–160, *161*

  for isthmic-isthmic anastomosis, 159, *160*
Tuberculous endometritis, 130
Tubolysis, 148
Tuboplasty, by second-look laparoscopy, 165
Type I error, 79
Type II error, 79

Ultrasound
  in diagnosis of ectopic pregnancy, 174–*175*
  transvaginal probe, ectopic pregnancy diagnosis and, 174
Unicornuate uterus, 263, *267*
Urinary tract anomalies, in Rokitansky-Kuster-Hauser syndrome, 249
Urinary tract endometriosis, 221–222
Urogenital system, mesodermal components of, 194
Uteri avovalus, 136, *137*
Uterine cavity, diagnostic examination of, 19–20*t*
Uterine cervix, incompetent. (*see* Incompetent cervical os)
Uterine clamps, for laparotomy, 39, *40*
Uterine fibroids, treatment of, with GnRH agonists, 119*t*
Uterine incision, for abdominal myomectomy, *120*, 121–122
Uterine lesions, benign, hysteroscopic laser procedure for, 73–74
Uterine nerve ablation, for endometriosis management, 234
Uterine reconstructive surgery, 113
Uterine surgery, laser techniques for, *73–74*
Uterine suspension techniques, for endometriosis, 221–223, *224–225*
Uterotubal implantation, 162
Uterovaginal anomalies
  abdominal correction of, 271, *273–277*
  classification of, 246
  failure of lateral fusion of vertical septa
    nonobstructed, 263, 265–*271*
    obstructed, 258–265
  of lateral fusion, 258–269
  obstetrical management for, 276–277
  reproductive failure in
    pathogenesis of, 269
    treatment of, 269, 271
  surgical results, 277–278*t*
  transcervical correction of, 271
  vertical fusion problems, 278–285
Uterus
  acquired defects of, 114–*119*
  agenesis of. (*see* Rokitansky-Kuster-Hauser syndrome)
  anatomy of, 113
  anomalies of, in diethylstilbestrol exposure, 271, *272*
  bicornuate, classification of, 265, *266*
  blood supply of, 113
  congenital anomalies of, 136, *137*. (*see also* Uterovaginal anomalies)
  development, in true hermaphrodites, 333–334
  diagnostic techniques for, 114
  differentiation of septate vs. bicornuate, 19
  double, 258–*261*
    classification of, 265, *266*

Uterus
  double—*continued*
    diagnosis of, 265–266, 269
  intrauterine synechiae. (*see* Intrauterine synechiae)
  lateral fusion, nonobstructive failure of, 136–*141*
  nonpregnant, smooth muscle, healing of, 113–114
  septate, classification of, 265, *266*
  T-shaped, 271, *272*
    diethylstilbestrol exposure and, 265, *271–272*
  unicornuate, 263, *267*
Uterus didelphys, with double vagina, 258–*259*

Vagina
  agenesis of. (*see* Rokitansky-Kuster-Hauser syndrome)
  congenital absence of, with uterus present, 280–*283*
  congenital anomalies of. (*see* Uterovaginal anomalies)
  double, with double uterus, 258–*259*
  transverse septum, obstructive, 278–*283*
  transverse septum anomalies, nonobstructed, 283–*285*

Vaginal myomectomy, 125
Vaginal septum, failure of lateral fusion
  nonobstructed, 263, 265–*272*
  obstructed, 258–*265*
Vaporization or coagulation, of endometriosis, 70, *72–73*
Vasa deferentia, development, in true hermaphrodites,
    334*t, 335*
Vasopressin (Pitressin), 119, 121, 124–125
VATER syndrome, 305
Verres needle, 49
Video/photography equipment, for endoscopy, 46–*47*

Wolffian duct, 194
Wurm cerclage, 101, *103*

Y chromosome defect, male hermaphroditism of, *324–329*

ZIFT (zygote intrafallopian tube transfer), 388
Zygote intrafallopian tube transfer (ZIFT), 388